Biochemistry

for the Pharmaceutical Sciences

Charles P. Woodbury, Jr., PhD
Associate Professor
Department of Medicinal Chemistry and Pharmacognosy
University of Illinois at Chicago
College of Pharmacy
Chicago, Illinois

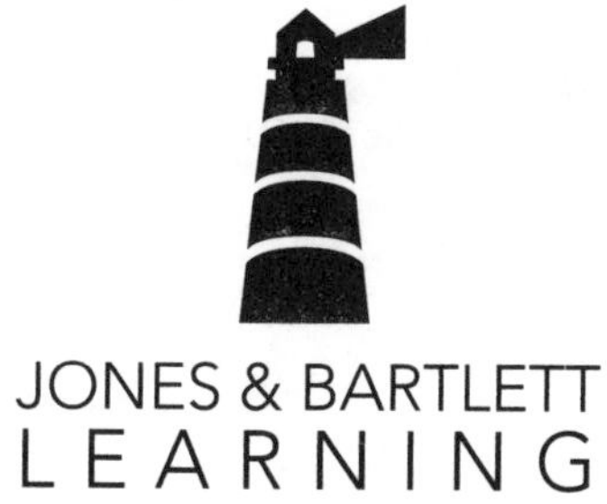

JONES & BARTLETT
LEARNING

World Headquarters
Jones & Bartlett Learning
40 Tall Pine Drive
Sudbury, MA 01776
978-443-5000
info@jblearning.com
www.jblearning.com

Jones & Bartlett Learning Canada
6339 Ormindale Way
Mississauga, Ontario L5V 1J2
Canada

Jones & Bartlett Learning International
Barb House, Barb Mews
London W6 7PA
United Kingdom

Jones & Bartlett Learning books and products are available through most bookstores and online booksellers. To contact Jones & Bartlett Learning directly, call 800-832-0034, fax 978-443-8000, or visit our website, www.jblearning.com.

Substantial discounts on bulk quantities of Jones & Bartlett Learning publications are available to corporations, professional associations, and other qualified organizations. For details and specific discount information, contact the special sales department at Jones & Bartlett Learning via the above contact information or send an email to specialsales@jblearning.com.

The author, editor, and publisher have made every effort to provide accurate information. However, they are not responsible for errors, omissions, or for any outcomes related to the use of the contents of this book and take no responsibility for the use of the products and procedures described. Treatments and side effects described in this book may not be applicable to all people; likewise, some people may require a dose or experience a side effect that is not described herein. Drugs and medical devices are discussed that may have limited availability controlled by the Food and Drug Administration (FDA) for use only in a research study or clinical trial. Research, clinical practice, and government regulations often change the accepted standard in this field. When consideration is being given to use of any drug in the clinical setting, the health care provider or reader is responsible for determining FDA status of the drug, reading the package insert, and reviewing prescribing information for the most up-to-date recommendations on dose, precautions, and contraindications, and determining the appropriate usage for the product. This is especially important in the case of drugs that are new or seldom used.

Production Credits
Publisher: David Cella
Acquisitions Editor: Katey Birtcher
Associate Editor: Maro Gartside
Production Director: Amy Rose
Senior Production Editor: Renée Sekerak
Production Assistant: Sean Coombs
Marketing Manager: Grace Richards
Manufacturing and Inventory Control Supervisor: Amy Bacus
Composition: Laserwords Private Limited, Chennai, India
Cover Design: Kate Ternullo
Cover Image: © Sebastian Duda/ShutterStock, Inc.
Printing and Binding: Courier Kendallville
Cover Printing: Courier Kendallville

Library of Congress Cataloging-in-Publication Data
Woodbury, Charles P.
Biochemistry for the pharmaceutical sciences / Charles P. Woodbury Jr.
p. ; cm.
Includes bibliographical references and index.
ISBN-13: 978-0-7637-6384-8
ISBN-10: 0-7637-6384-5
1. Biochemistry. 2. Metabolism. 3. Pharmacy. I. Title.
[DNLM: 1. Biochemical Phenomena. 2. Pharmacology—methods. QU 34]
QP514.2.W66 2012
612'.015—dc22
2010047696

6048

Printed in the United States of America
15 14 13 12 11 10 9 8 7 6 5 4 3 2 1

Contents

Chapter 7 Models for Enzyme Kinetics 171

Chapter 8 Basic Concepts in Metabolism 195

Chapter 10 Mitochondria and the Citric Acid Cycle 257

Chapter 11 Respiratory Complexes and ATP Synthesis 283

Preface

This text is based on my course for first-year students in our PharmD curriculum. These students have taken organic chemistry and are taking physiology concurrently, and they need to gain a background in enzymology and in primary metabolism for their upcoming courses in drug therapy. At the University of Illinois at Chicago, we only spend about one semester on classical biochemical topics. Keeping in mind that we are not preparing students for a career in biochemical research, we therefore need a shorter, less detailed, and less expensive alternative to the available large biochemistry textbooks.

This text follows a traditional organization for a course in biochemistry. There are four main divisions in the text. The first five chapters are largely reviews of topics from organic and basic physical chemistry; then two chapters on enzymes; then eight chapters on primary metabolism; and lastly a chapter on topics at the level of molecular biology: DNA replication and repair, and transcription and translation of genetic messages.

Chapter 1 starts with basic thermodynamic concepts, just enough to help in later explanations of metabolic strategies. Then comes a series of chapters that introduce (or review) the chemistry of the fundamental building blocks of biochemistry: carbohydrates, amino acids, nucleic acids, and lipids. These chapters go from the level of the monomer up to the level of the polymer (or in the case of the lipids, to the level of the biomembrane). Material at the beginning of these chapters may be skipped by students who are well-prepared from their organic chemistry course, though I do recommend that some time be taken with the latter half of each of these chapters, as the topics here are generally not covered in organic chemistry courses.

Next there are two chapters on enzymology. Chapter 6 is on enzyme mechanisms, while Chapter 7 deals with mathematical aspects of enzyme kinetics and inhibition. I believe this approach keeps students interested by making their first contact with enzymology close to their previous study of reaction mechanisms in organic chemistry. The discussion of enzyme mechanisms starts with those we can regard as "classical": ribonuclease A and chymotrypsin. Then carbonic anhydrase introduces the use of metal ion cofactors; cofactor use is elaborated upon in later chapters, for example in discussions of the transaminases, of pyruvate dehydrogenase, and of phenylalanine hydroxylase. Cooperativity and allosterism are introduced via hemoglobin and aspartate transcarbamoylase.

In the second of these chapters on enzymology, the presentation of the mathematics of enzyme kinetics is deliberately kept simple, with little derivation of equations (not a useful exercise for future pharmacists, in my opinion). The Michaelis-Menten model is emphasized, as is competitive inhibition. There is a very brief introduction to drug design of enzyme inhibitors as well.

The main meat of the text comes after we finish with enzymology. Chapter 8 discusses the conventions and basic concepts in metabolic biochemistry: pathways, feedback, and other unifying ideas. Then we move into sugar metabolism and energy generation for the cell (Chapter 9). Glycolysis is first, then gluconeogenesis and glycogen metabolism. After working through the tricarboxylic acid cycle and the notion of anaplerosis, we get to respiratory complexes and the coupling of ATP synthesis in the mitochondrion to proton pumping. This is followed by a short chapter on the pentose phosphate pathway and the generation of reducing power for biosynthesis and protection against oxidative agents.

After this, it is time to deal with energy production from lipids; we also need to treat lipid biosynthesis (Chapter 13). Next comes the metabolism of amino acids (Chapter 14). I have deliberately emphasized their use as a fuel for the cell over their biosynthesis, to maintain an emphasis on energy generation for the cell. I wrap up the presentation of primary metabolism with the synthesis and breakdown of the building blocks of DNA and RNA.

The last chapter is an altogether too brief treatment of cellular transactions with DNA and RNA. This material is typically the subject of multiple chapters in the large encyclopedic textbooks of biochemistry, and I have compressed all of this into one chapter. Necessarily I have left out much; my excuse is that I wished to keep the book to a reasonable length, and my hope is that most, if not all, of the students using this book will have taken a course in modern cell biology, where these topics have received their due attention.

The Questions for Discussion at the end of each chapter are intended to spur in-class review and elaboration of the topics in that chapter. Acquiring the proper specialized vocabulary is necessary in the study of any scientific subject. Toward this end, I have included a short glossary of terms used in this text.

Through this organization and approach, and these helpful features, *Biochemistry for the Pharmaceutical Sciences* makes this important topic accessible to students.

Acknowledgments

First, I must acknowledge the support of the Department of Medicinal Chemistry and Pharmacognosy, University of Illinois at Chicago. I especially appreciate the encouragement of Dr. Judy Bolton, Head of the Department. I must also thank my colleagues, Dr. Douglas Thomas and Dr. Joanna Burdette, for their critique of portions of the manuscript.

I also wish to thank the reviewers whose detailed criticisms greatly improved the text.

In preparing several of the figures of proteins and nucleic acids, I have used the Swiss-PdbViewer (also known as DeepView) to visualize structures from the Protein Data Bank. Those wishing to learn more about this highly useful program should visit the web site at http://www.expasy.org/spdbv. The authors of the program have requested that I cite their publication as well: N. Guex and M.C. Peitsch (1997) *Electrophoresis* 18:2714–2723.

Finally, I must thank the many students who have patiently pored over my lecture notes (the precursor to this text), and just as patiently inquired why I had misspelled this, contradicted myself there, and mis-drew that structure or diagram. Their critiques contributed very substantially to this book.

Acknowledgments

Reviewers

Cassandra S. Arendt, PhD
Assistant Professor
Pacific University School of Pharmacy

John H. Block, PhD, RPh
Professor Emeritus of Medicinal Chemistry
College of Pharmacy, Oregon State University

Tracey Boncher, PhD
Associate Professor of Medicinal Chemistry/Biochemistry
Ferris State College of Pharmacy

Michael R. Borenstein, RPh, PhD
Associate Dean
Temple University School of Pharmacy

William Chan, PhD
Professor
Thomas J. Long School of Pharmacy and Health Sciences
University of the Pacific

Ganesh Cherala, PhD
Assistant Professor
College of Pharmacy, Oregon State University
Oregon Health & Science University

Gemma P. Geslani, MS, PhD, MPH
Associate Professor of Biochemistry
St. Louis College of Pharmacy

Reza Karimi, RPh, PhD
Assistant Dean for Academic Affairs and Assessment, Associate Professor
Pacific University School of Pharmacy

Evgeny Krynetskiy, PhD, DSc
Associate Professor
Temple University School of Pharmacy

John C. Matthews, PhD
Professor of Pharmacology
University of Mississippi School of Pharmacy

Sigrid C. Roberts, PhD
Assistant Professor
Pacific University School of Pharmacy

CHAPTER 1

Biochemical Thermodynamics

Learning Objectives

1. Define and use correctly the terms *system, closed, open, surroundings, state, energy, temperature, thermal energy, irreversible process, entropy, free energy, electromotive force (emf), Faraday constant, equilibrium constant, acid dissociation constant, standard state,* and *biochemical standard state.*
2. State and appropriately use equations relating the free energy change of reactions, the standard-state free energy change, the equilibrium constant, and the concentrations of reactants and products.
3. Explain qualitatively and quantitatively how unfavorable reactions may occur at the expense of a favorable reaction.
4. Apply the concept of coupled reactions and the thermodynamic additivity of free energy changes to calculate overall free energy changes and shifts in the concentrations of reactants and products.
5. Construct balanced reduction–oxidation reactions, using half-reactions, and calculate the resulting changes in free energy and emf.
6. Explain differences between the standard-state convention used by chemists and that used by biochemists, and give reasons for the differences.
7. Recognize and apply correctly common biochemical conventions in writing biochemical reactions.

Basic Quantities and Concepts

Thermodynamics is a system of thinking about interconnections of heat, work, and matter in natural processes like heating and cooling materials, mixing and separation of materials, and—of particular interest here—chemical reactions. Thermodynamic concepts are freely used throughout biochemistry to explain or rationalize chains of chemical transformations, as well as their connections to physical and biological processes such as locomotion or reproduction, the generation of fever, the effects of starvation or malnutrition, and more. Thermodynamics uses a set of technical terms that may seem somewhat artificial, but that are necessary for clarity and conciseness in thinking about thermodynamic problems. Thermodynamics also relies on three general statements about the behavior of matter—the "laws" of thermodynamics—that reflect long experience in dealing with energy, equilibria, and natural processes and their tendencies.

Terminology

Thermodynamics uses a specialized and precise vocabulary in its explanations of natural processes, to give more rigor to its deductions about these phenomena.

- A *system* is whatever part of the universe we are interested in, in terms of thermodynamics. *Closed* systems cannot exchange matter across their boundaries; *open* systems, however, can pass matter back and forth across their boundaries.
- The *surroundings* are everything else in the universe that lie outside the boundaries of the system. It can include reservoirs of heat energy or of matter, mechanical devices to perform or absorb work, and so on. The system could be, for example, a collection of biochemicals in aqueous solution in a beaker or flask, while the surroundings would be the water bath, lab bench, and other apparati around the beaker of dissolved biochemicals. **Figure 1-1** contains examples of some simple systems and their surroundings.
- The overall *state* of a system refers to its temperature, pressure, composition (e.g., how many moles of each constituent; their presence as gas, liquid, or solid), and perhaps other properties such as electrical charge or electrical potential. When matter, heat, or some other form of energy crosses from the surroundings into the system (or if it leaves the system and passes into the surroundings), the system reaches a new state. For example, chemical reactions might take place in the beaker, changing its composition, and perhaps liberating some heat that would cause the volume of solution to expand slightly. This heat might pass over to the water bath, outside the system, and warm the surroundings.
- *Pressure* (P) is defined as the force exerted per unit area. The SI unit of pressure is the Pascal (Pa). For reference, atmospheric pressure is 101,325 Pa.
- Pressure multiplied by volume (V) has the dimensions of *energy* (E), so that volume or pressure changes are often related to work done on or extracted from a system. The SI unit for energy is the joule (J).
- The common scale of *temperature* used in thermodynamics is the absolute or Kelvin scale; the unit is the Kelvin (K). 0°C equals 273.15 K. The absolute zero of temperature on the Kelvin scale is the point where all thermal motion would cease; it corresponds to −273.15°C.
- The *thermal energy* of a system is related to motions on the atomic or molecular level. For each gas particle in an ideal monatomic gas at temperature T, the energy is

$$E = \frac{3}{2} k_B T \qquad (1\text{-}1)$$

Here k_B is Boltzmann's constant, equal to 1.38066×10^{-23} J/K. Per mole of ideal monatomic gas, the energy is $\frac{3}{2} RT$, where R is the gas constant, equal to 8.3144 J/mol-K.

In thermodynamics, the concepts of systems and surroundings are quite general. For example, the concept of system could be extended to include living cells or even whole organisms, along with a suitable enlargement of the notion of "boundaries" and "surroundings."

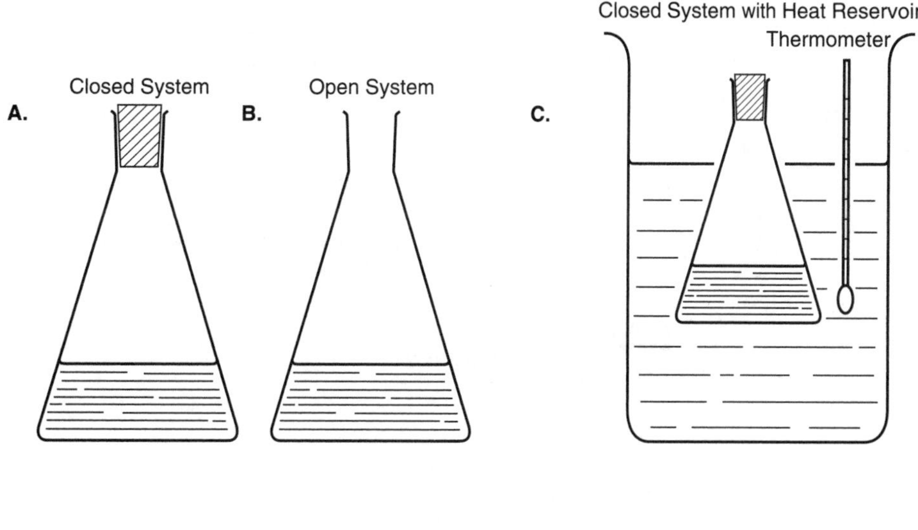

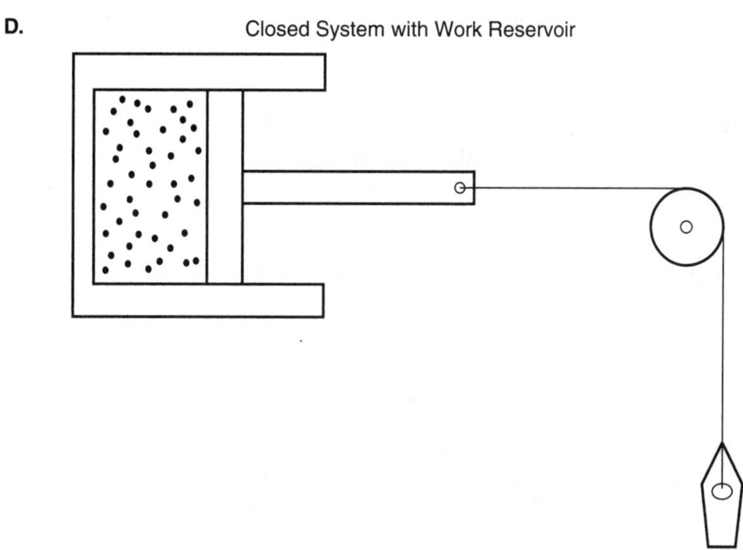

Figure 1-1 Simple thermodynamic systems. **A, B.** Open and closed systems: The stoppered flask cannot exchange matter with the surroundings. **C.** A closed system (stoppered flask) in contact with a heat reservoir (water bath). **D.** A closed system (gas in piston-cylinder) in contact with a work reservoir (weight-pulley).

First Law: Energy Conservation

The *first law of thermodynamics* states that energy is conserved. The forms of energy can be interconverted, but the sum of the energies must remain constant. This includes mechanical work and heat, as well as less apparent chemical or electrical changes.

- If the energy of a closed system in state A is E_A, and if the system passes to a different state B, with a different energy E_B, then the energy change for this process is

$$\Delta E = E_B - E_A \tag{1-2}$$

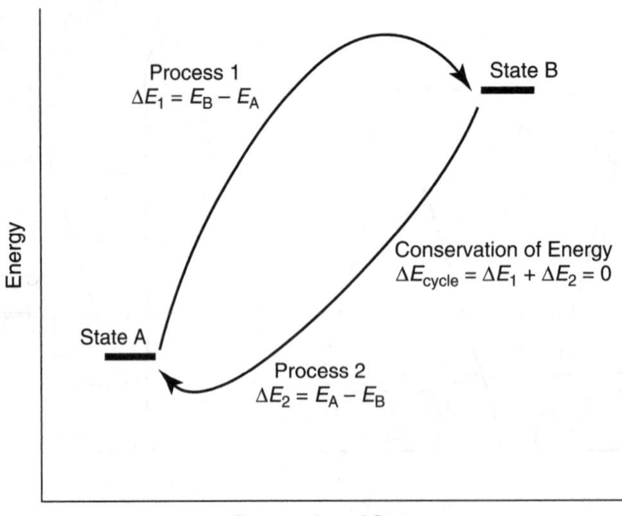

Figure 1-2 The first law of thermodynamics: energy conservation in a cyclic process.

- A negative sign for ΔE implies that the system has a lower energy in state B than in state A; informally, B is energetically "downhill" from A.
- For a *cyclic process,* taking a closed system from state A to B and back to A, ΔE is zero (**Figure 1-2**).
- In terms of exchanges of heat (ΔQ) and work (ΔW), the change in energy for a closed system is

$$\Delta E = \Delta Q + \Delta W \tag{1-3}$$

- More generally, ΔE for a particular system is equal in magnitude, but opposite in sign, to the total energy change for all other systems (including the surroundings) involved in the change of the first system.

For energy exchange processes at constant pressure, thermodynamics introduces a new quantity, called *enthalpy* (H). The enthalpy function is defined by

$$H = E + PV \tag{1-4}$$

At constant pressure (the conditions under which most biochemical experiments are performed), the change in enthalpy accounts for both work and heat exchanges. The change in enthalpy is then

$$\Delta H = \Delta E + P\Delta V \tag{1-5}$$

As with ΔE, in a cyclic process that takes a closed system to another state and then back to precisely the original state, ΔH for the system is zero. For many biochemical systems and processes at constant pressure, the change in volume is small. Under these conditions the term $P\Delta V$ is often negligible compared to ΔE in Equation 1-5; then the change in enthalpy is very nearly the same as the change in energy.

Second Law: Entropy and the Direction of Spontaneous Change

Many natural processes are observed to proceed spontaneously in one direction, but never in the opposite direction; that is, they are *irreversible* (**Figure 1-3**). For example, two inert gases spontaneously mix throughout their container uniformly, but the mixture is not observed to

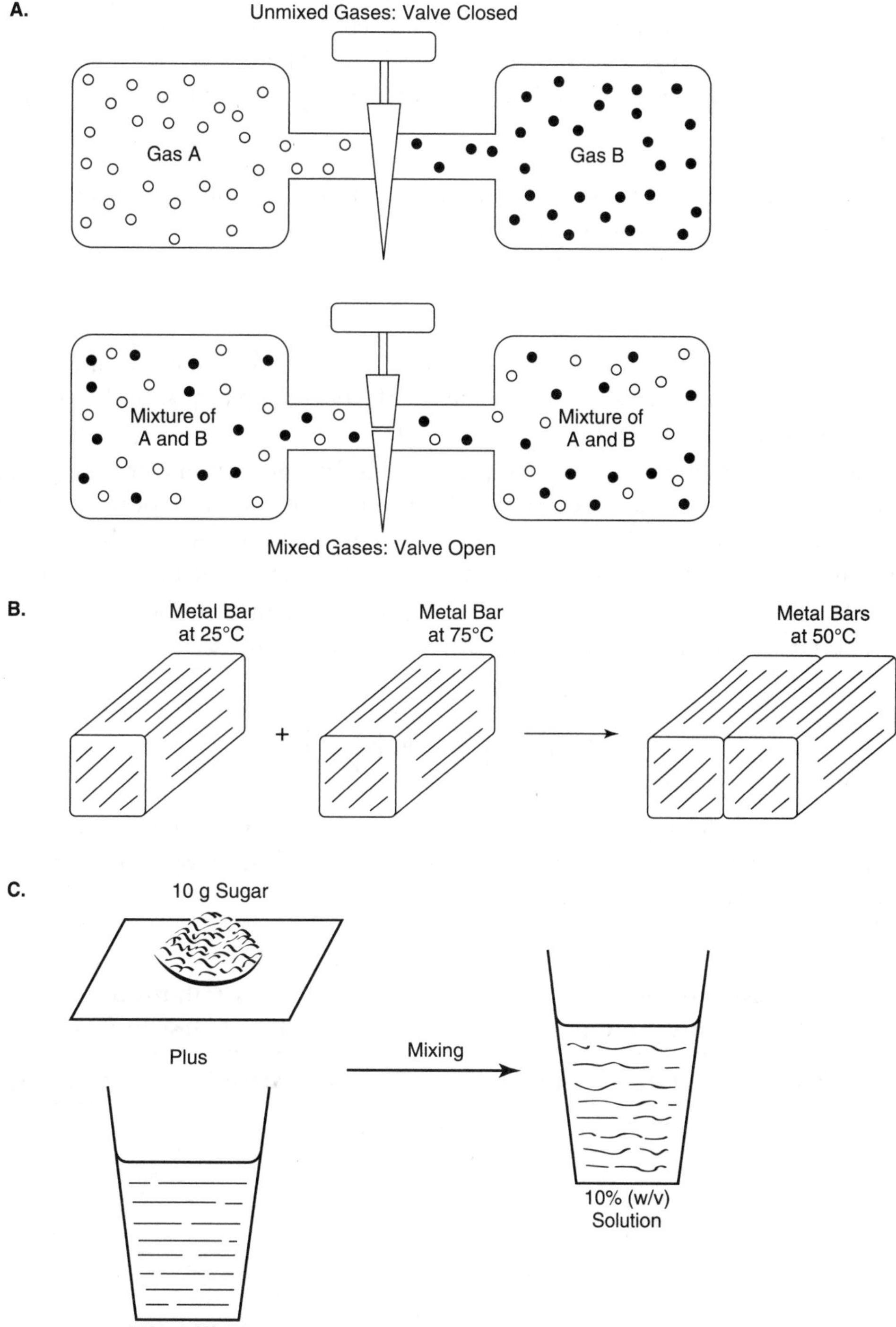

Figure 1-3 Spontaneous irreversible processes. **A.** Mixing of inert gases. **B.** Temperature equilibration of two metal bars. **C.** Dissolution of sugar (sucrose) in water.

spontaneously segregate into dense clumps of one gas and the other. Hotter objects in contact with cooler ones spontaneously transfer heat to the cooler object, but the cooler object does not become cooler and the hotter object even warmer. Common sugar (sucrose) dissolves in water to form a solution, but that solution does not spontaneously separate back into pure water and solid sucrose. The direction of change in these processes is not predicted by the first law. Instead, the second law of thermodynamics introduces a new thermodynamic quantity, called *entropy* (S), to help explain such spontaneous changes, including their direction and magnitude. The units of entropy are joules per mole-Kelvin (J/mol-K).

Entropy is closely connected to notions of order and disorder, sometimes in a very general and abstract way.

- The entropy of a system is proportional to the logarithm of the number of ways of arranging the system, down to the quantum level:

$$S = k_B \ln W \qquad (1\text{-}6)$$

  where W is the number of arrangements of the system with the same overall energy. **Table 1-1** compares arrangements and the value of W for a simple quantum system of two molecules and four available states.
- The meaning of "arrangements," "order," or "mixing," in connection with entropy, can refer to positions or orientations in space, but also includes freedom of motion (i.e., rotations, translations, and vibrations) and distributions over quantum energy levels. Such motions and quantum distributions must be considered, for example, in chemical reactions.
- For a change from a state A where there are W_A arrangements available to the system, to a different state B with W_B arrangements, the change in entropy is

$$\Delta S = S_B - S_A = k_B \ln\left(\frac{W_B}{W_A}\right) \qquad (1\text{-}7)$$

- The overall entropy change ΔS for the system depends only on the initial and final states of the system. This is similar to the energy change, ΔE, which likewise depends only on the initial and final states of the system.

Distribution 1 (W = 4; more ordered)				**Distribution 2 (W = 6; less ordered)**			
State 1	**State 2**	**State 3**	**State 4**	**State 1**	**State 2**	**State 3**	**State 4**
ab				*a*	*b*		
	ab			*a*		*b*	
		ab		*a*			*b*
			ab		*a*	*b*	
					a		*b*
						a	*b*

Table 1-1 Two Molecules, *a* and *b*, with Four Available States

- A simple version of the second law is that the entropy S of the system plus that of the surroundings must increase in an irreversible process, and it remains constant in a reversible process. In terms of changes in entropy for the system and surroundings, this relationship is expressed as follows:

$$\Delta S_{\text{system}} + \Delta S_{\text{surr}} \geq 0 \qquad (1\text{-}8)$$

The equality holds for reversible changes, the inequality for irreversible (and spontaneous) changes.

Spontaneous changes are associated with a positive entropy change; spontaneous processes also result in a greater overall state of "mixing" or disorder. Very disordered systems have a high entropy, whereas highly ordered systems have a low entropy. A crystal, which has long-range ordering of its atoms, is a good example of a low-entropy system, while a hot gas of the same atoms would have a much greater disorder and a much higher entropy. The mixing process in Figure 1-3, for example, clearly leads to greater disorder and a positive entropy change. The entropy change involved in the temperature equilibration process is more subtle, but can be thought of as the net result of matching the cooling and ordering of atoms in the hot metal bar against the greater thermal disorder gained by the atoms in the bar that is warmed up.

Illustrating the entropy change for a chemical reaction is more difficult yet. If we view the reaction as distributing the particles (atoms, molecules) of a system over a broader range of energy levels, then this process increases the disorder of the system. Hence, the entropy increases; ΔS is positive for such a chemical reaction (**Figure 1-4**). Conversely, a process that collects otherwise dispersed particles into a narrow set of positions, or a limited set of energy levels, would have a negative value for ΔS. Indeed, it is quite possible to have chemical reactions with negative entropy changes, when the products are more "organized" or "ordered" than the reactants, in terms of distributing them over energy levels.

If a system can exchange heat or matter with its surroundings, then the system can have a decrease in entropy (an increase in its ordering). The surroundings, however, undergo an

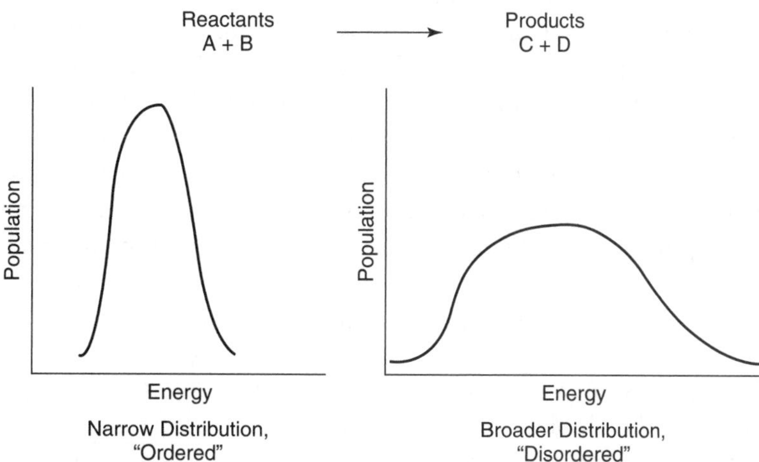

Figure 1-4 Chemical reactions that spread the system over more states will have positive entropy changes.

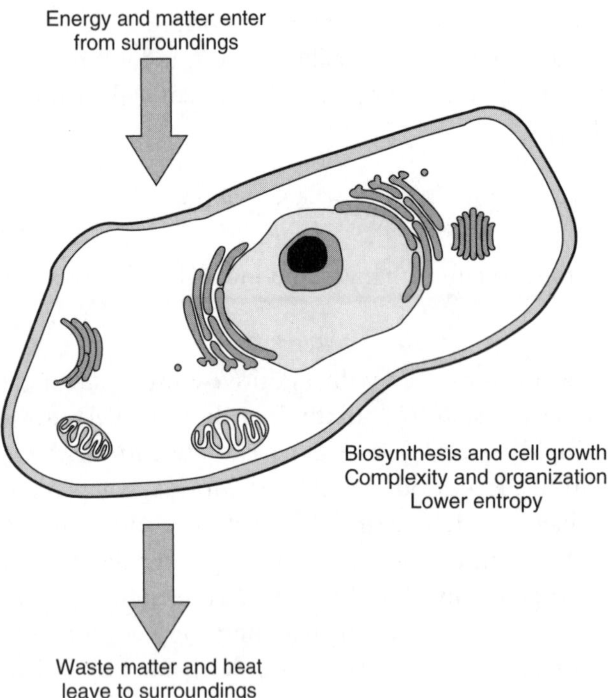

Figure 1-5 Living systems are open systems and order themselves by using energy and matter from the surroundings.

increase in their entropy. In this way, an influx of energy to a system can produce more order in that system. Living systems exploit such energy fluxes to order or organize themselves; however, their surroundings must become ever more disordered or disorganized as a result of this activity (**Figure 1-5**).

Third Law: An Absolute Scale for Entropies

There are several ways to state the third law of thermodynamics. One version says that it is not possible to reach absolute zero in temperature through any finite series of processes. Another states that as the temperature approaches absolute zero, the magnitude of the entropy change in a reversible process also approaches zero. While these formulations may be helpful to physicists and material scientists, a more chemically relevant version of the third law is that the entropy of a pure substance is zero when that substance is in a physical state such that there is no contribution to the entropy from translation, rotation, vibration, configuration, or electronic terms. The substance must be perfectly ordered, with no disorder from any motions or spatial disarrangements. As a mathematical equation, this version of the third law can be written as

$$\lim_{T \to 0} S = 0 \text{ (perfectly ordered substance)} \tag{1-9}$$

A (hypothetical) physical state that matches these criteria is that of a perfectly ordered crystalline chemical, at the absolute zero of temperature. Note that a gas or liquid would still have some disorder as the temperature approached absolute zero (in making this statement, we set aside quantum physics anomalies such as liquid helium).

With a perfect crystal, there is of course, no contribution from alternative configurations of the molecules (there is only one "arrangement" in a perfectly ordered material); also, there are no rotational or translational contributions to the entropy. As the temperature drops, lattice vibrations and electron distributions in the crystal drops to the lowest permitted quantum level, so that vibrational and electronic contributions to the entropy also approach zero. Thus chemists use the convention that S is zero for pure compounds in the most stable crystalline form, at the absolute zero of temperature. This sets the scale for entropies of chemical compounds, so-called absolute entropies, with zero entropy attained at the zero of temperature, and more positive entropy values occurring as the temperature rises.

The entropy of a substance does depend on the temperature. For a reversible change in temperature from T_1 to T_2, the change in entropy is given by

$$S_2 - S_1 = \int_{T_1}^{T_2} \frac{C\,dT}{T} \tag{1-10}$$

where C is the heat capacity of the substance. With the convention that S for a pure substance is zero at absolute zero temperature, this last equation allows calculation of the entropy at any higher temperature, provided that the heat capacity function C is known. Because C is always a positive quantity, any increase in temperature increases the entropy; rising temperature leads to more disorder in the system.

The third law of thermodynamics sets a zero point for entropy values and allows the calculation of values of the entropy for chemical compounds. With these entropy values, along with measurements of other thermal properties of those compounds, one can predict the equilibrium constant for a chemical processes using a quantity called the free energy.

Free Energy Changes

The ΔS criterion given in the second law of thermodynamics is insufficient to determine the spontaneity of a process for a system that is connected to its surroundings. What complicates things here is the exchange of heat, work, and matter with the surroundings. Supplying energy or matter to the system can overcome unfavorable changes in ordering the system, thereby making the overall process (for system and surroundings) spontaneous even though, from the system's point of view, the entropy change is not at all favorable. To determine the spontaneity of such processes, a broader, more inclusive quantity that takes such changes into account is needed. For processes taking place at constant pressure, the Gibbs free energy G is just the quantity needed.

- G is defined as a composite of enthalpy and the entropy:

$$G = H - TS \tag{1-11}$$

- Changes in G depend only on the initial and final states of the system; for a process going from state A to state B,

$$\Delta G = G_B - G_A \tag{1-12}$$

- Spontaneous changes have a negative value for ΔG, while nonspontaneous processes have a positive ΔG. If ΔG is zero, then the system is at equilibrium.

- In terms of changes in enthalpy and entropy, for processes at constant temperature:

$$\Delta G = \Delta H - T\Delta S \tag{1-13}$$

Formally, ΔG measures the available work in a spontaneous process—that is, how much work can be extracted by doing the process. This includes chemical "work," or the conversion of reactants to products, which is our main interest. In particular, the use of ΔG enables quantitative predictions for biochemical reactions, the energetic bases for life processes. Evaluation of ΔG allows prediction of whether a process will tend to occur naturally (spontaneously) or whether it is at equilibrium. The connection of ΔG to conditions for equilibrium allows prediction of the way an equilibrium will shift, and how far.

The free energy criterion for a spontaneous process, $\Delta G < 0$, says nothing about the *rate* at which the process occurs. Although many spontaneous processes occur at a moderate to rapid rate, this is not universally true. Many thermodynamic processes occur at extremely slow rates, even though the free energy change is quite negative. A familiar example is the kinetic stability of diamond relative to graphite. Here ΔG at room temperature is -2.9 kJ/mol for the diamond-to-graphite conversion, so diamonds are thermodynamically unstable with respect to graphite. The rate of conversion, however, is so slow that, for all practical purposes, it does not occur; thus diamond can be described as kinetically stable but thermodynamically unstable. This distinction will turn out to be an important one when we discuss biochemical reaction pathways later in this book.

A constant passage of matter and energy through living systems occurs such that living systems are not at thermodynamic equilibrium; in fact, they are generally very far from equilibrium. Living organisms exploit the flux of matter and energy to promote their internal organization, a higher state of order, or a state of lower entropy in the thermodynamic sense. Clearly, certain nonspontaneous processes (usually involving chemistry) takes place in achieving such organization. It is also obvious that counterbalancing spontaneous processes must occur for the living system to maintain its life processes overall. Thermodynamics, especially the use of ΔG, can help us make sense of the combination of favorable and unfavorable processes that permit life to continue.

Chemical Equilibria

There is a very close connection between the free energy change for a chemical process and the equilibrium constant for that process. To predict which way a reaction might spontaneously proceed, or the amounts of chemicals formed or depleted by setting up a chemical reaction, one needs to study the free energy change and the associated equilibrium constant for that process. This can be particularly important in biochemistry, where many reactions share products and reactants. The products of one reaction may be the reactants for another, and careful dissection of the various free energy changes is needed to understand the direction and magnitude of the overall change in the biochemical system. This line of study will be very useful in later chapters in understanding how metabolic pathways such as glycolysis or the citric acid cycle function.

Basic Equations

For the reaction

$$a\mathrm{A} + b\mathrm{B} \rightleftharpoons c\mathrm{C} + d\mathrm{D} \tag{1-14}$$

the *equilibrium constant* K_{eq} is given by

$$K_{eq} = \frac{[C]^c[D]^d}{[A]^a[B]^b} \tag{1-15}$$

where [A], [B], and so on are the equilibrium concentrations of the reactants and products.

The Gibbs free energy change ΔG for a chemical reaction is given by

$$\Delta G = G(\text{products}) - G(\text{reactants}) \tag{1-16}$$

The free energy of j moles of a species I can be written as

$$G_I = j \times \overline{G_I^\circ} + j \times RT \ln [I] \tag{1-17}$$

where $\overline{G_I^\circ}$ is the free energy per mole of that substance under standard conditions of temperature, pressure, and concentration.

Setting up conditions that define a "standard state" gives a reference point for free energy changes relative to this state. Recall that the third law of thermodynamics sets a "zero point" for entropy changes, but that there is no corresponding zero point for energy (or enthalpy) changes; thus we need a way to set a scale for free energy changes. Using standard states for substances (e.g., gases, liquids, or solutions) is the chemist's way of setting that scale. In biochemistry, the standard concentration for a solution is typically one molar, unit concentration. Other standard state conditions are one atmosphere of pressure and a temperature of 298 K.

For the reaction shown in Equation 1-14, the free energy change is

$$\Delta G = c\overline{G_C} + d\overline{G_D} - a\overline{G_A} - b\overline{G_B} \tag{1-18}$$

Notice the inclusion in this relation of the stoichiometric coefficients a, b, c, and d. This equation can be expanded to

$$\begin{aligned}\Delta G = c \times G_C^\circ + c \times RT \ln[C] + d \times G_D^\circ + d \times RT \ln[D] \\ -a \times G_A^\circ + a \times RT \ln[A] - b \times G_B^\circ + b \times RT \ln[B]\end{aligned} \tag{1-19}$$

Grouping terms then leads to

$$\Delta G = \Delta G^\circ + RT \ln\left(\frac{[C]^c[D]^d}{[A]^a[B]^b}\right) \tag{1-20}$$

The quantity ΔG° is the *standard state free energy change,* the free energy change for the reaction if all components are in their *standard state* (a temperature of 298 K, atmospheric pressure, and unit concentration). This is different from the free energy change ΔG when the components are at arbitrary and non-unit concentrations [A], [B], [C], and [D]. The quantity ΔG but not ΔG° determines whether the system is at equilibrium.

At equilibrium ΔG is zero, by definition. This gives the connection to the equilibrium constant for "standard chemical conditions":

$$\Delta G^\circ = -RT \ln K_{eq} \quad \text{or} \quad K_{eq} = e^{-\Delta G^\circ/RT} \tag{1-21}$$

The second (exponential) relation shows that even small changes in the (standard) free energy can lead to large values of the equilibrium constant.

Biochemical Standard States

For reactions involving the release or uptake of protons, the species H^+ appears as a reactant or product. It is clear that the concentration of protons influences the equilibrium. But biological systems are typically buffered at around pH 7, where the hydrogen ion concentration is smaller by a factor of 10^7 than for the standard state of one molar $(\text{pH} = 0)$. Many hydrolysis reactions also exist in which water appears as a reactant or product. Reactions of biochemical interest almost always are studied in dilute aqueous solution, where the concentration of water remains essentially constant at 55.6 molar.

As an example, consider the following hydrolysis reaction:

$$\text{1,3-}bis\text{-phosphoglycerate} + H_2O \rightleftharpoons \text{3-phosphoglycerate} + HPO_4^{2-} + H^+ \quad (1\text{-}22)$$

Strictly speaking, the free energy change for this reaction should be written as

$$\Delta G = \Delta G^\circ + RT\ln\left(\frac{[\text{3-phosphoglycerate}][HPO_4^{2-}][H^+]}{[\text{1,3-}bis\text{-phosphoglycerate}][H_2O]}\right) \quad (1\text{-}23)$$

Because we expect neither $[H^+]$ nor $[H_2O]$ to change much, we can separate out the logarithmic terms in $[H^+]$ and $[H_2O]$ from the other concentrations:

$$\Delta G = \Delta G^\circ + RT\ln\left(\frac{[\text{3-phosphoglycerate}][HPO_4^{2-}]}{[\text{1,3-}bis\text{-phosphoglycerate}]}\right) + RT\ln\left(\frac{[H^+]}{[H_2O]}\right) \quad (1\text{-}24)$$

Because the last logarithmic term is essentially constant, we can combine it with the ΔG° term and write this as a combined $\Delta G'^\circ$. In essence we have defined a new standard state for the 1,3-*bis*-phosphoglycerate, the phosphate, and the 3-phosphoglycerate. This *biochemical standard state* is defined as pH 7, 298 K, 1 atmosphere pressure, and unit concentrations for chemicals other than water or protons.

Notice that we have a new symbol for the standard free energy change: $\Delta G'^\circ$. However, just as ΔG° is not the criterion for spontaneity for regular chemical reactions (under nonstandard conditions, we should use ΔG), neither is $\Delta G'^\circ$ the appropriate criterion for biochemical reactions. Instead, we should (for biochemical reactions, at pH 7) use $\Delta G'$.

Acid–Base Equilibria

Many biochemicals contain acidic or basic functional groups, and the state of titration of these groups plays an important role in their biological function (e.g., stability of conformation, enzymatic catalysis, binding of other molecules). Examples of such groups include the following:

- Acidic carboxyl groups of amino acids and acidic metabolites such as citric and lactic acids
- Basic amino groups of amino acids, amino sugars, and biological amines such as spermidine
- Side chains of several amino acids containing groups that can act as weak acids or bases, such as the phenolic hydroxyl group in tyrosine, the thiol group of cysteine, and the imidazole ring of histidine

The Henderson-Hasselbach equation connects the *acid dissociation constant* with the solution pH. For an acid dissociation reaction of a simple acid HA to its conjugate base A^-,

$$HA \rightleftharpoons H^+ + A^- \tag{1-25}$$

the acid dissociation constant K_a is given by

$$K_a = \frac{[H^+][A^-]}{[HA]} \tag{1-26}$$

This rearranges to

$$[H^+] = K_a \cdot \left(\frac{[HA]}{[A^-]}\right) \tag{1-27}$$

Taking negative logarithms gives

$$-\log[H^+] = -\log K_a - \log\left(\frac{[HA]}{[A^-]}\right) \tag{1-28}$$

With the usual definitions of pH and pK_a, this gives

$$pH = pK_a + \log\left(\frac{[A^-]}{[HA]}\right) \tag{1-29}$$

If the concentrations of the undissociated acid HA and the conjugate base A^- are equal, as when the acid is half-dissociated, then the logarithmic term on the right is cancelled, and the pH then equals the pK_a. Such a situation occurs at the midpoint of the acid's titration curve (**Figure 1-6**). At this pH, the solution has its maximum buffering capacity (buffers are solutions that minimize changes in pH upon addition of either acid or base).

Coupling of Reactions

Many individual biochemical processes are nonspontaneous by themselves and have positive ΔG values. However, by adding a second, spontaneous reaction with a (sufficiently) negative

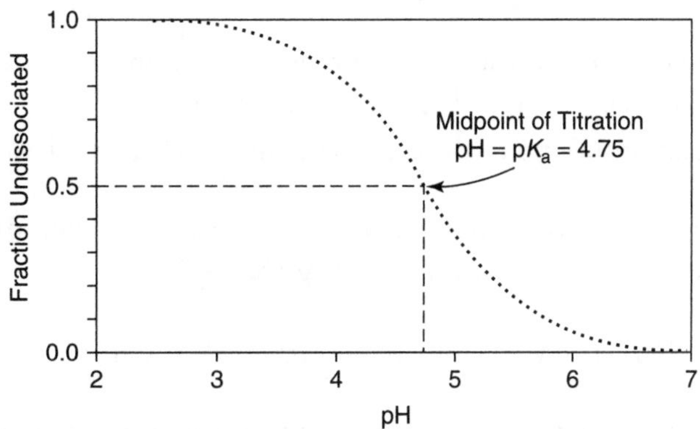

Figure 1-6 Monoprotic acid titration curve. The midpoint pH corresponds to the acid's pK_a.

ΔG, the sum of the two reactions may result in an overall negative ΔG and, therefore, become overall spontaneous. This practice is referred to as *coupling* the reactions.

For example, consider two reactions with their associated free energy changes under standard conditions:

$$\text{A} \rightleftharpoons \text{B} + \text{C}, \quad \Delta G'^{\circ} = +5 \text{ kJ/mol} \qquad \text{C} + \text{D} \rightleftharpoons \text{P}, \quad \Delta G'^{\circ} = -15 \text{ kJ/mol} \quad (1\text{-}30)$$

The first reaction is not spontaneous under standard conditions, but the second is; B (and C) will *not* form spontaneously from A under standard conditions.

Now suppose that, for biological reasons, it would be desirable to drive the conversion of A over to B. This can be done by combining or coupling the unfavorable first reaction with the favorable second reaction, thereby taking advantage of the tendency of C to react with D. The net result is

$$\text{A} + \text{D} \rightleftharpoons \text{B} + \text{P}, \quad \Delta G'^{\circ} = +5 + (-15) \text{ kJ/mol} \quad \text{or} \quad \Delta G'^{\circ} = -10 \text{ kJ/mol} \quad (1\text{-}31)$$

The coupled reaction is now spontaneous under standard conditions. Thus feeding in A and D leads spontaneously to the formation of B and P, at standard concentrations all around. The coupling of unfavorable reactions with favorable ones appears widely throughout biochemistry, and we will see several examples of this phenomenon in later chapters.

Reduction–Oxidation Reactions (Redox)

Reduction–oxidation (*redox*) reactions occur when one chemical species loses electrons and another gains electrons. The species losing electrons is *oxidized,* and the species gaining electrons is *reduced*. Redox reactions involve free energy changes just like any other chemical reaction, and the tendency for a redox reaction to proceed depends on whether there is a favorable free energy change for that reaction.

Organisms exploit the free energy released by the oxidation of fuel molecules to do biological "work," including biosynthesis, transport, and mechanical work. The passage of electrons from the fuel molecules down to the ultimate electron acceptor, molecular oxygen, is overall a spontaneous process. Coupling to unfavorable (but desirable) reactions occurs at several steps in this process. The reactions are often complex, and many different intermediates carry electrons in these pathways. Redox reactions will appear throughout later chapters of this book as we discuss the breakdown of foodstuffs and the biosynthesis of complex biological molecules.

Redox reactions can be analyzed using *redox couples.*

- Redox couples are the pair of reactions that together add up to the overall reaction but that individually show which species is losing or gaining electrons.
- The individual reaction in one of these redox couples is called a *half-reaction.*

A simple, familiar example is the transfer of a pair of electrons from metallic zinc to copper ions, as might occur in an electrochemical cell (**Figure 1-7**):

$$\text{Zn}(s) + \text{Cu}^{2+}(aq) \rightleftharpoons \text{Zn}^{2+}(aq) + \text{Cu}(s) \quad (1\text{-}32)$$

For clarity we have by the notation (s) that the native metals are in the solid state; the notation (aq) indicates that the metal ions are dissolved in aqueous solution. The metallic zinc Zn(s)

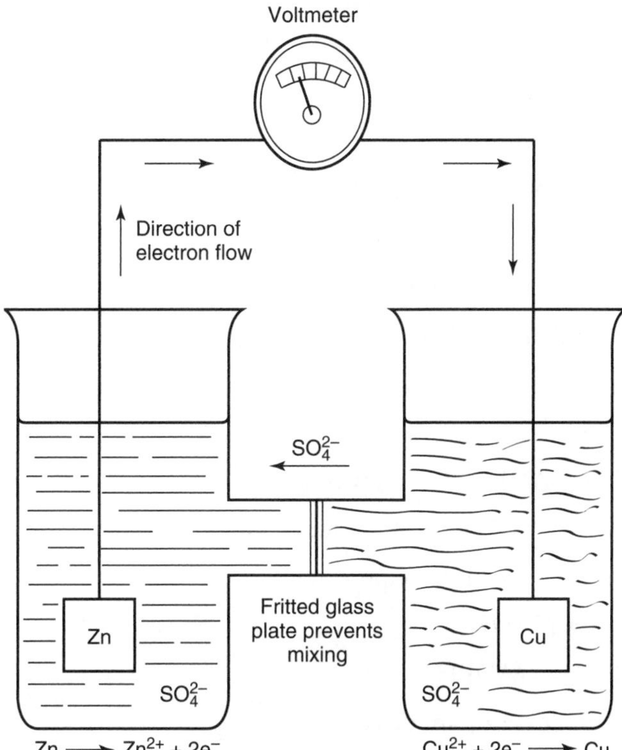

Figure 1-7 Electrochemical cell showing the oxidation of zinc and the reduction of copper.

is oxidized to $Zn^{2+}(aq)$, while the copper ions, written as $Cu^{2+}(aq)$ in Equation 1-32, are reduced to metallic copper or Cu(*s*). The individual half-reactions for the zinc and copper are

$$\mathrm{Zn}(s) \rightleftharpoons \mathrm{Zn}^{2+}(aq) + 2\mathrm{e}^-$$
$$\mathrm{Cu}^{2+}(aq) + 2\mathrm{e}^- \rightleftharpoons \mathrm{Cu}(s) \quad (1\text{-}33)$$

Each of these half-reactions has a certain tendency to occur—that is, a certain standard-state free-energy change can be associated with it. Historically, the energy changes for these electron transfer reactions were determined by using electrical circuits and electrochemical cells and by measuring the voltage generated by the cell with standard concentrations of reactants. The electrical current that flowed was attributed to an *electromotive force* (*emf*), which was measured in volts.

By convention, these voltages are now tabulated for reactions written as reductions, and the result for a given half-reaction is expressed as a standard half-cell reduction potential, or E°. Another convention has set the emf for the reduction of the hydrogen ion to H_2 at precisely zero volts (under certain highly specific conditions, including a pH equal to zero; this is the so-called standard hydrogen electrode).

For biochemical reactions, a pH of 7.0 makes more sense, so biochemists use a set of standard biochemical emf values E'° for biochemical half-reactions at pH 7 but are coupled to the standard hydrogen electrode at pH 0. **Table 1-2** collects a number of such half-reactions and their reduction potentials. Because the solvent is assumed to be water, the notation (*aq*) can be dropped.

Half-reaction	E'°(volts)
$\frac{1}{2}O_2 + 2H^+ + 2e^- \rightarrow H_2O$	0.816
$Fe^{3+} + e^- \rightarrow Fe^{2+}$	0.771
$O_2 + 2H^+ + 2e^- \rightarrow H_2O_2$	0.295
Ubiquinone + $2H^+ + 2e^- \rightarrow$ ubiquinol	0.045
Fumarate + $2H^+ + 2e^- \rightarrow$ succinate	0.031
$2H^+ + 2e^- \rightarrow H_2$ (standard conditions, pH 0)	0.000
Oxaloacetate + $2H^+ + 2e^- \rightarrow$ malate	−0.166
Pyruvate + $2H^+ + 2e^- \rightarrow$ lactate	−0.185
FAD + $2H^+ + 2e^- \rightarrow FADH_2$ (free solution)	−0.219
Glutathione dimer + $2H^+ + 2e^- \rightarrow$ 2 Reduced glutathione	−0.23
Lipoic acid + $2H^+ + 2e^- \rightarrow$ dihydrolipoic acid	−0.29
$NAD^+ + H^+ + 2e^- \rightarrow$ NADH	−0.320
$NADP^+ + H^+ + 2e^- \rightarrow$ NADPH	−0.324
Acetoacetate + $2H^+ + 2e^- \rightarrow$ β-hydroxybutyrate	−0.346
α-Ketoglutarate + $CO_2 + 2H^+ + 2e^- \rightarrow$ isocitrate	−0.38
$2H^+ + 2e^- \rightarrow H_2$ (pH 7.0)	−0.414

Table 1-2 Standard Reduction Potentials for Selected Biochemical Half-reactions

A complete redox reaction, with two half-reactions, can be written as follows:

$$A_{red} + B_{ox} \rightleftharpoons A_{ox} + B_{red} \tag{1-34}$$

This can be split into the two individual half-reactions, one written as a reduction and the other as an oxidation (subscripts indicate the state of the species, oxidized or reduced):

$$A_{red} \rightleftharpoons A_{ox} + 2e^-$$
$$B_{ox} + 2e^- \rightleftharpoons B_{red} \tag{1-35}$$

If we write a half-reaction as an oxidation, we must reverse the sign of the voltage associated with it. The change in emf, $\Delta E'^{\circ}$, for the overall reaction is simply the algebraic sum of the individual emf values for the half-reactions written so as to produce the overall balanced reaction equation:

$$\Delta E'^{\circ} = E'^{\circ}(B_{ox} \rightarrow B_{red}) - E'^{\circ}(A_{ox} \rightarrow A_{red}) \tag{1-36}$$

Note that if we write a half-reaction as an oxidation (as we did for compound A), we must reverse the sign of the voltage associated with it; this puts a minus sign in front of the term for compound A in this last equation.

The quantity $\Delta E'^{\circ}$ measures the overall tendency for the reaction to proceed as written under biochemical standard conditions, and it is closely connected to the standard biochemical state free energy change $\Delta G'^{\circ}$ for the reaction by the following relation:

$$\Delta G'^{\circ} = -nF\Delta E'^{\circ} \tag{1-37}$$

where n is the number of electrons transferred in the reaction, and F is the *Faraday constant,* equal to 96,480 Joules/volt-mole. For reactions that occur under nonstandard state conditions (mainly when the concentrations are not those of the standard state) we have

$$\Delta E' = \Delta E'^{\circ} - \frac{RT}{nF}\ln\left(\frac{[A_{ox}][B_{red}]}{[A_{red}][B_{ox}]}\right) \tag{1-38}$$

Also, for a single half-cell emf, we have

$$E' = E'^{\circ} - \frac{RT}{nF}\ln\left(\frac{[A_{ox}]}{[A_{red}]}\right) \tag{1-39}$$

Notice that the signs of $\Delta E'^{\circ}$ and of $\Delta G'^{\circ}$are opposite to each other. The more positive the emf or voltage difference, the greater the tendency for the reaction to proceed.

A good biochemical example is the reduction of pyruvate to lactate, as NADH (nicotinamide adenine dinucleotide; see Chapter 8) is oxidized to NAD^+. The two half-reactions and their standard emfs are

$$\begin{aligned} &\text{NADH} \rightleftharpoons \text{NAD}^+ + \text{H}^+ + 2\text{e}^- \quad && E'^{\circ} = +0.320 \text{ volt} \\ &\text{Pyruvate} + 2\text{H}^+ + 2\text{e}^- \rightleftharpoons \text{lactate} \quad && E'^{\circ} = -0.185 \text{ volt} \end{aligned} \tag{1-40}$$

(note the sign of the emf for oxidation of NADH) and the overall reaction is

$$\text{Pyruvate} + \text{NADH} + \text{H}^+ \rightleftharpoons \text{lactate} + \text{NAD}^+ \quad \Delta E'^{\circ} = +0.135 \text{ volt} \tag{1-41}$$

The standard biochemical reduction potential change here is +0.135 volt. The sign indicates that under standard conditions the reaction will be spontaneous. Using Equation 1-37, the standard biochemical free energy change for this reaction is −26.9 kJ/mol, which indicates a substantial tendency for the reaction to occur spontaneously under standard conditions.

Common Biochemical Conventions

Biochemists use a number of conventions in writing reaction equations, mainly for convenience and to emphasize points that are important in understanding the biochemistry. These conventions can differ from what regular chemists would write, because of the different views on what is important to represent in the equation.

- Biochemical equations (especially in diagrams) are often not balanced with respect to charge, and electrical charges on ionic species are often ignored.
- The complexation of certain species with metal ions (such as Mg^{2+}, Ca^{2+}, and Cl^-) is typically not shown, although it certainly occurs to an appreciable extent inside living systems.

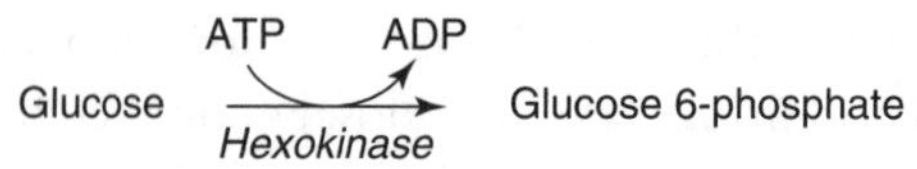

$$\text{Glucose} \xrightarrow[\textit{Hexokinase}]{\text{ATP} \quad \text{ADP}} \text{Glucose 6-phosphate}$$

Figure 1-8 Curved arrows show the participation of auxiliary species in a biochemical reaction.

- The state of titration of phosphate groups is often ignored; at pH values near 7, a mixture of different phosphate species occurs (e.g., PO_4^{3-}, HPO_4^{2-}, $H_2PO_4^-$), and the species is simply written as P_i (inorganic phosphate). The state of titration of phosphoryl moieties attached to organic compounds is likewise often ignored.
- Reactions often show a curved arrow to indicate the uptake and release of some auxiliary species. An example is the phosphorylation of the sugar glucose by the enzyme hexokinase, shown in **Figure 1-8**. Here adenosine triphosphate (ATP) enters the reaction and is converted to the diphosphate form ADP as its terminal phosphoryl group is transferred onto the glucose molecule.
- Because of the long names of many biochemicals, abbreviations are very often used (e.g., F for fructose, as long as it will not be confused with fluorine). These can be cryptic at times, but the context should help in deciphering what is meant by a particular abbreviation.

QUESTIONS FOR DISCUSSION

1. **Table 1-3** contains a list of chemical and physical processes for systems undergoing a change from an initial state to a final state. Decide whether the changes in the system are spontaneous. If they are spontaneous, explain the spontaneity in terms of entropy and order/disorder changes in the system. Also consider the questions contained in the table.
2. The formula for the free energy change in chemical equilibria, Equation 1-20, shows how the quantity ΔG depends on the concentrations of reactants and products. This formula can be adapted to physical processes, such as the transport of a solute over a difference in concentration between two regions:

$$\Delta G = RT \ln\left(\frac{C_f}{C_i}\right) \tag{1-42}$$

where C_f is the concentration in the final state, and C_i is the concentration in the initial state. Calculate the value of ΔG for glucose transport into a cell across the plasma membrane, where the glucose concentration is 5 mM outside (initial state) and 1 mM inside (final state). Why isn't there a term for ΔG° in this formula?
3. A total of 30.5 kJ/mol of free energy is needed to synthesize ATP from ADP and P_i under biochemical standard state conditions. The actual physiological concentrations of reactants and products are, however, not at 1 M. Calculate the free energy needed to synthesize ATP if the physiological concentrations are [ATP] = 3.5 mM, [ADP] = 1.50 mM, and $[P_i]$ = 5.0 mM.
4. Pyruvate can be reduced to lactate at the expense of oxidation of $FADH_2$ to FAD. Combine the two half-reactions to give a balanced spontaneous overall reaction, and then compute the biochemical standard-state free energy change for this reaction.

Initial State of System	Process	Final State of System
One gram of sucrose and a glass of 100 milliliters of water at room temperature	The sugar is poured into the glass of water.	A 1% solution of sucrose
An ice cube, weighing 20 grams, at $-10°C$; a benchtop at room temperature (25°C)	The ice cube is placed on the benchtop.	A puddle of 20 milliliters of water on the benchtop, at 25°C
A puddle of 20 milliliters of water on a lab benchtop, at 25°C	The puddle is allowed to stand.	A dry benchtop, and a slightly more humid lab atmosphere (Why?)
A fragile china cup on a benchtop, at room temperature (25°C)	The cup is pushed off the benchtop.	The cup hits the floor and breaks. The temperature of the cup fragments and the floor rises very slightly. (Why?)

Table 1-3 Chemical and Physical Processes for Question 1

5. The oxidation of malate to oxaloacetate can be coupled to the reduction of NAD^+ to NADH:

$$\text{Malate} + NAD^+ \rightarrow \text{oxaloacetate} + NADH + H^+$$

   a. Use Table 1-1 to verify that the biochemical standard-state free energy change here is approximately +29 kJ/mol.
   b. Mitochondrial concentrations of the reactants are as follows:

Oxaloacetate	5.0×10^{-6} mol/L
Malate	1.1×10^{-3} mol/L
NAD^+	7.5×10^{-6} mol/L
NADH	9.2×10^{-7} mol/L

   What is the free energy change in the mitochondrion for the reaction given earlier in this question?

6. The diet of a typical 70-kg adult human male in the United States may include a caloric intake of approximately 2500 Calories per day. The dietary Calorie (note the capitalization; 1 Cal is equal to 1000 calories) is equivalent to 4.185 kJ. Assume the efficiency of converting food energy to ATP is 50%. Calculate the weight of ATP synthesized by this adult per day (see Question 3 for the free energy needed to synthesize ATP). Compare this figure to the body weight and comment.

REFERENCE

G. G. Hammes. (2000). *Thermodynamics and Kinetics for the Biological Sciences*, Wiley-Interscience, New York.

CHAPTER 2

Carbohydrates

Learning Objectives

1. Define and use correctly the terms *aldose, ketose, pentose, hexose, diastereomer, enantiomer, pyranose, furanose, anomer, glycoside, starch, amylose, cellulose, glycosaminoglycan, proteoglycan, glycolipid, glycoprotein,* and *lectin.*
2. Recognize the structures of glucose, fructose, glucuronic acid, glucosamine, and *N*-acetylglucosamine.
3. Explain the D, L nomenclature system for simple carbohydrates; note that it does not predict the direction of rotation of plane polarized light.
4. Explain what is meant by the term *reducing sugar*. Distinguish between the reducing and nonreducing ends of a polysaccharide such as glycogen.
5. List several common biologically relevant modifications of simple sugars.
6. List three common disaccharides and their natural sources. Describe how they differ in structure.
7. Describe the structure of common simple polysaccharides such as starch, cellulose, and glycogen.
8. Describe the structure of common glycosaminoglycans such as hyaluronic acid, heparan sulfate, and chondroitin sulfate. Describe how they may be linked to proteins to form proteoglycans. Relate chemical features of these polysaccharides to the biological function of these polymers.
9. Describe the general biosynthetic pathway leading to mature proteoglycans, involving the endoplasmic reticulum and the Golgi apparatus.
10. List several common glycoproteins and give their function.
11. Explain how sugars are linked to proteins via asparagine and serine or threonine.
12. Describe differences in the glycolipids, especially the carbohydrate content, contributing to the different blood group antigens. Explain the biochemical basis for these differences.
13. Describe how elevated blood sugar can lead to hemoglobin glycosylation, and how quantitation of HbA_{1c} is used in following the effectiveness of treatment of diabetes.
14. Relate the release of heparan sulfate after tissue injury to its effects on blood clotting. Identify the differences between heparan sulfate and heparin.

Simple Sugars: Monosaccharides

Introduction

Carbohydrates (sugars and polymers made of sugars) are ubiquitous in biology and play many important roles. Here are just a few of the many ways carbohydrates are basic to biology:

- The simple sugar glucose is a principal source of metabolic energy for the cell. Cellulose, a polymer of glucose, strengthens the cell walls of plants.
- The cell uses carbohydrate chains to modify proteins and direct those proteins to their proper sites for function in the cell.
- In animals, the complex polymers known as glycosaminoglycans (chains of unmodified and modified sugars) lubricate and cushion joints; help form skin, hair, and feathers; help regulate blood clotting and assist the immune system; and help control cell-to-cell adhesion and interaction.

Basic Nomenclature

The formula for a carbohydrate, $(CH_2O)_n$, may be simple, but there is a great deal of complexity in the structures of such compounds. Inevitably, to properly describe this structural diversity, there is also a great deal of detailed nomenclature.

Conventionally, a monosaccharide is a carbohydrate that does not hydrolyze, while a disaccharide can be hydrolyzed to give two monosaccharides, a trisaccharide can be hydrolyzed to give three monosaccharides, and so on. A polysaccharide contains many monosaccharide units. Also, the smallest molecules regarded as carbohydrates have three carbon atoms; the exemplars here are glyceraldehyde and dihydroxyacetone (**Figure 2-1**). Compounds with only one or two carbons do not share extensive properties with those we regard as "sugars," so they are not regarded as saccharides.

The suffix "-ose" on a compound's name indicates a sugar. An *aldose* is a sugar derived from an aldehyde, and a *ketose* is derived from a ketone. A *triose* is a carbohydrate with three carbon atoms; a *tetrose* has four carbons; a *pentose* has five carbons; and a *hexose* has six carbons. These terms may be combined for a more complete specification of the compound. For example, an aldopentose is a sugar with five carbons and an aldehyde group.

Stereochemistry

A very important feature of sugars is the large number of isomers possible within the overall molecular formula, even for simple pentoses and hexoses. A quick review of some concepts and terminology from organic chemistry will help to keep matters clear.

- *Stereoisomers* are molecules that have the same molecular formula but differ in the way that the constituent atoms are oriented in space.

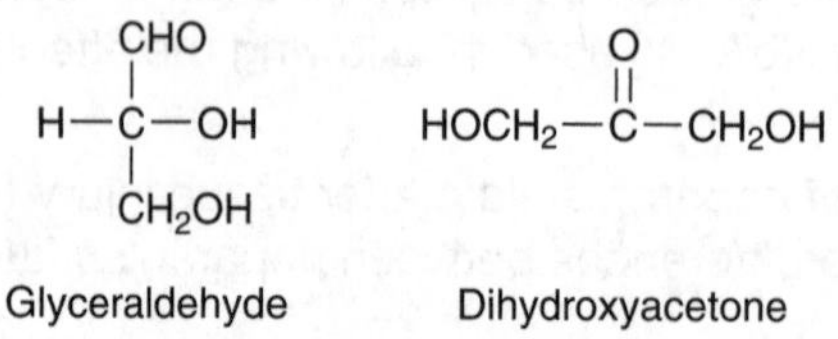

CHO
H—C—OH
CH_2OH
Glyceraldehyde

O
$HOCH_2—C—CH_2OH$
Dihydroxyacetone

Figure 2-1 The smallest saccharides, glyceraldehyde and dihydroxyacetone.

- *Enantiomers* are molecules that contain a center of asymmetry, usually a carbon atom known as a chiral ("handed") carbon. Enantiomers are mirror images of each other. They have the same physical properties, except they rotate polarized light in different directions. By convention, a + sign indicates rotation of the polarization to the right, while a − sign indicates rotation to the left. Because their physical properties are the same, it is often very difficult to physically separate enantiomers from each other.
- *Diastereomers* are stereoisomers that are not mirror images. Their physical properties differ, and this permits their physical separation. Note that a pair of stereoisomers that are not enantiomers must then be diasteromers.

Glyceraldehyde contains a chiral carbon, and there are two possible enantiomers of this compound. **Figure 2-2** illustrates these two forms using a Fischer projection. By convention, the C1 carbon is the aldehydic carbon, and it is drawn at the top of a vertical line of carbon atoms, C1 through C3. The chiral carbon is C2; the OH group is drawn to the right of the chiral carbon for what is denoted as the D isomer; the L isomer has this group drawn to the left side of this carbon.

In terms of visualizing the direction of bonds around C2, the vertically aligned bonds are imagined to be going into the plane of the drawing and away from the viewer, while the horizontally aligned bonds are directed upward, out of the plane of the drawing and toward the viewer. **Figure 2-3** presents the same structures using wedges in place of lines, to give a better sense of perspective on the direction of the bonds.

With respect to rotation of plane polarized light, the D isomer here rotates it to the right (the D originally indicated *dextro*, or right-handed, rotation and the L indicated *levo*, or left-handed, rotation). The D, L convention for stereoisomers can also be applied to other simple chiral compounds, such as amino acids. However, while many D monosaccharides do, indeed, rotate plane-polarized light to the right, this behavior is not universal. Instead, to indicate this particular physical property, as distinct from the configuration about the chiral carbon, it is preferable to use a prefix of + or −, with the + sign indicating right-handed rotation and the − sign indicating left-handed rotation.

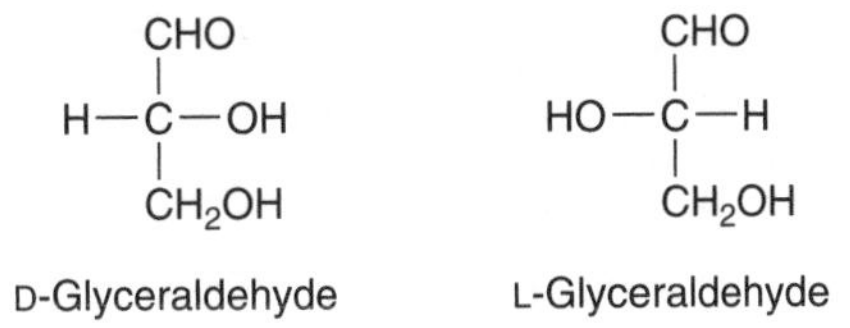

D-Glyceraldehyde L-Glyceraldehyde

Figure 2-2 D- and L-glyceraldehyde as Fischer projections.

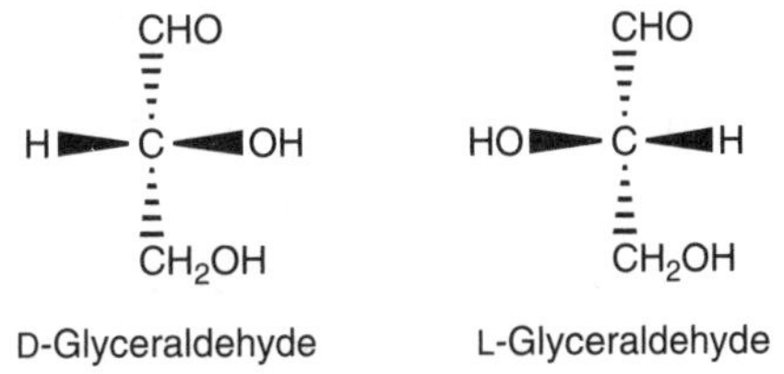

D-Glyceraldehyde L-Glyceraldehyde

Figure 2-3 D- and L-glyceraldehyde drawn using "wedge" bonds.

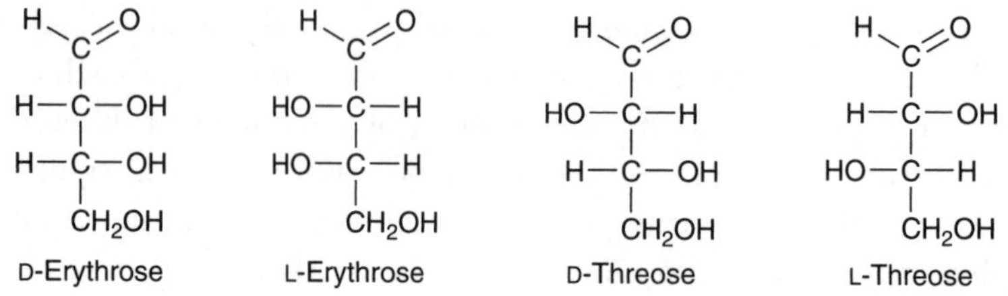

D-Erythrose L-Erythrose D-Threose L-Threose

Figure 2-4 Pairs of enantiomers for the aldotetroses: D- and L-erythrose, and D- and L-threose.

Tetroses have four carbons, two of which may be chiral. Consider first the possibilities for the aldotetroses. **Figure 2-4** shows erythrose and threose; there are mirror images for each of these compounds, so there are four stereoisomers overall—that is, two pairs of enantiomers. Note that either enantiomer of erythrose is a diasteromer of either enantiomer of threose. Either threose or erythrose can be tautomerized to a ketose, erythulose; D-erythrose gives D-erythulose, which in turn gives D-threose (**Figure 2-5**). A similar pattern holds for the interconversion of the L isomers.

With aldopentoses there are three chiral carbons, giving four different pairs of enantiomers: D and L forms for ribose, arabinose, xylose, and lyxose (**Figure 2-6**). There are also two ketopentoses, ribulose and xylulose, each with a D and an L form. The D isomers are the

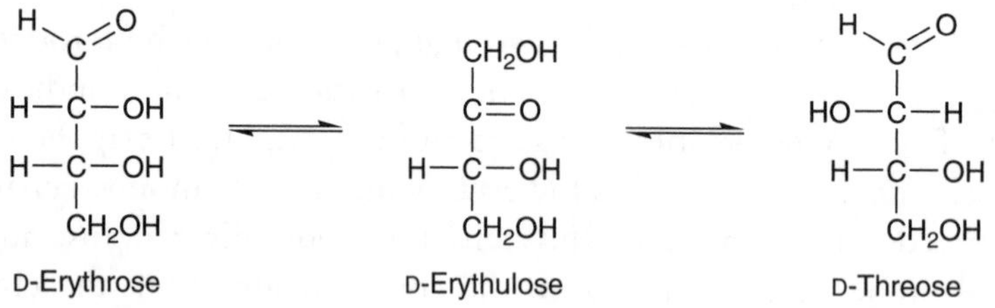

D-Erythrose D-Erythulose D-Threose

Figure 2-5 Tautomerization of D-erythrose to D-erythulose, and then to D-threose.

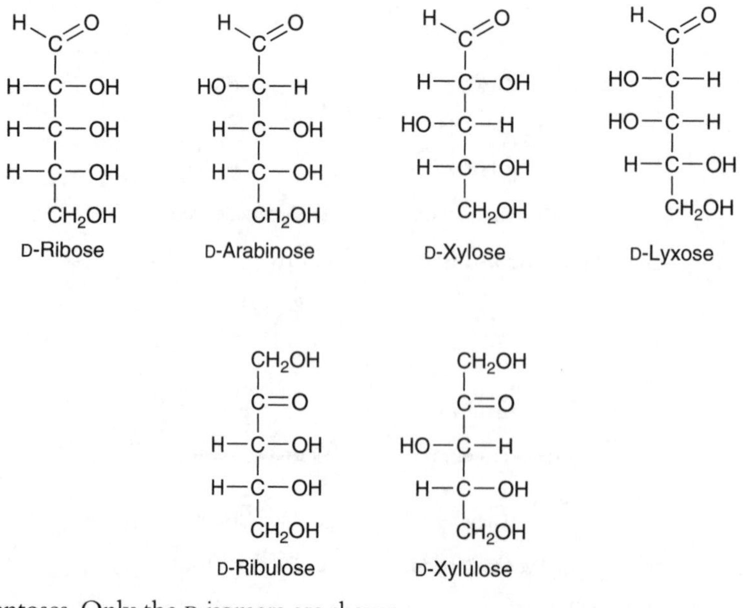

D-Ribose D-Arabinose D-Xylose D-Lyxose

D-Ribulose D-Xylulose

Figure 2-6 Pentoses. Only the D isomers are shown.

most important for biochemistry. Additionally, the important pentose derived from ribose, deoxyribose, is essential to the structure of DNA.

There are 4 chiral carbons for aldohexoses and 16 diastereomers. D-Glucose, D-mannose, and D-galactose are the most important for human biochemistry. There are also four ketohexoses, with D-fructose being the most important species. D-(+)-Glucose is sometimes referred to as dextrose, while levulose is D-(−)-fructose.

Cyclization

The aldopentoses and the hexoses show a strong tendency to cyclize in solution, forming rings with five or six members. These rings contain an oxygen atom as one of the members. Thus sugars with a five-membered ring resemble the compound furan, while those with a six-membered ring resemble pyran (**Figure 2-7**). This leads to the practice of designating the sugars in such conformations as *furanoses* and *pyranoses*, respectively. As a pyranose, glucose forms a hemiacetal (the product of a 1:1 reaction of an aldehyde with an alcohol; see **Figure 2-8**), which is relatively stable thanks to its cyclic structure. This reaction creates a new chiral center at C1 and leads to two new optically active forms, called *anomers*; C1 is referred to as the anomeric carbon in this case. The anomers are designated as α-D-glucopyranose and β-D-glucopyranose (**Figure 2-9**); these names are often abbreviated simply to α-D-glucose and β-D-glucose. Figure 2-9 shows these anomers in the stable "chair" conformation. Here the —OH groups at C2, C3, C4, and C5 are equatorial. However, notice that the —OH group at C1 may be either equatorial (the β anomer) or axial (the α anomer).

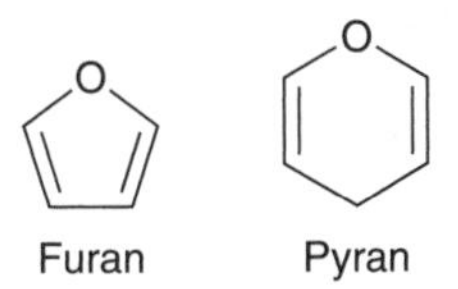

Furan Pyran

Figure 2-7 Furan and pyran.

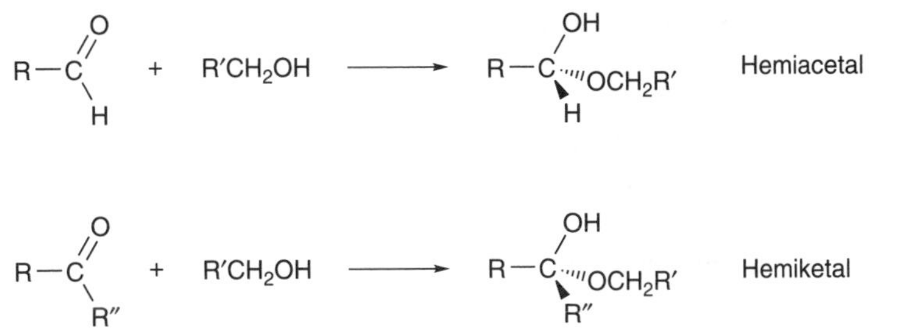

R—C(=O)—H + R′CH$_2$OH ⟶ R—C(OH)(H)—OCH$_2$R′ Hemiacetal

R—C(=O)—R″ + R′CH$_2$OH ⟶ R—C(OH)(R″)—OCH$_2$R′ Hemiketal

Figure 2-8 Hemiacetal and hemiketal formation.

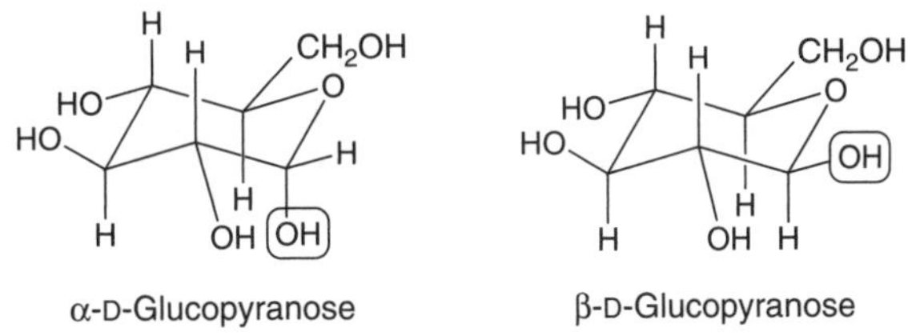

α-D-Glucopyranose β-D-Glucopyranose

Figure 2-9 Anomers of D-glucose. Some bond lengths have been extended to emphasized structural details and the —OH group attached to the anomeric carbon has been marked.

Fructose can cyclize to give either a furanose ring or a pyranose, through formation of a hemiketal (the product of a nucleophilic alcohol reacting with the carbonyl of a ketone). For either the pyranose or the furanose, two anomers are possible, α- and β-D-fructofuranose and α- and β-D-fructopyranose (**Figure 2-10**). In solution, the pyranose form predominates (approximately 60%) over the furanose form (approximately 40%), with a tiny amount of the open-chain form (much less than 1%). Ribose and deoxyribose (**Figure 2-11**) can also cyclize to form a furanose, with two anomers.

Reactivity and Common Derivatives

The hemiacetals and hemiketals formed in cyclizing pentoses and hexoses are still in equilibrium with the open-chain form of these sugars, although the equilibrium generally favors the cyclized form by a considerable margin. As a consequence, in solutions of these sugars, there will be small amounts of "free" aldehyde or ketone available for reaction. Aldehydes, such as aldoses, can be oxidized by mild agents. This behavior is the basis for the classic organic chemistry lab tests for an aldehyde, such as the silver mirror produced by Tollens' reagent, or the color changes produced by Benedict's solution or Fehling's solution. Because solutions of aldoses and ketoses will have small amounts of the "free" aldehyde or ketone, they can also react with these reagents. Sugars that give positive test results with these reagents are termed reducing sugars. The products of the oxidation of aldoses are called aldonic acids.

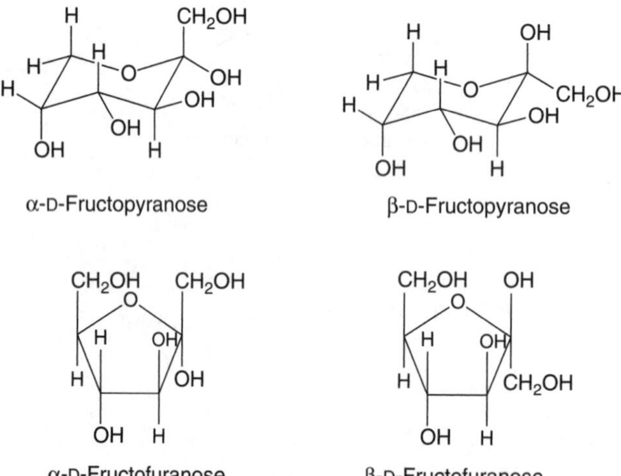

Figure 2-10 Anomers of D-fructose as a pyranose and furanose.

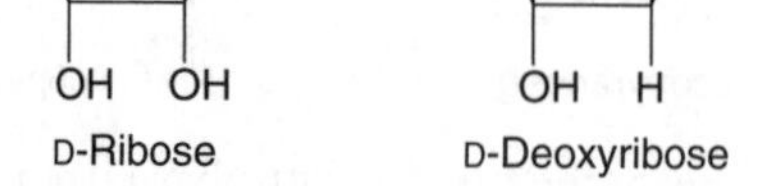

D-Ribose

D-Deoxyribose

Figure 2-11 D-Ribose and D-deoxyribose.

Conversely, the carbonyl group on aldoses and ketoses may be reduced to give the corresponding alcohol. **Figure 2-12** shows two important examples of this class of compounds. D-Sorbitol is also called D-glucitol. In the disease of diabetes mellitus, sorbitol accumulates in the lens of the eye and is associated with the formation of cataracts. The mechanism of cataract formation may possibly involve redox reactions in the formation of sorbitol from glucose and associated oxidative cross-linking of proteins through disulfide bridges.

Enzymes can oxidize monosaccharides to give a number of different products. Two important carboxylic acids that are derived in this way are *glucuronic acid* and *iduronic acid* (**Figure 2-13**). Note that iduronic acid is an epimer of glucuronic acid; an epimer is one of a pair of diasteromeric aldoses that differ only at the C2 position in their configuration.

Glycosides are formed from hemiacetals or hemiketals (that is, reducing sugars) by reaction with an alcohol. The product is a full acetal or full ketal (**Figure 2-14**). Glycosides are not reducing sugars. In naming these compounds, "glyc" is the general prefix for the combination

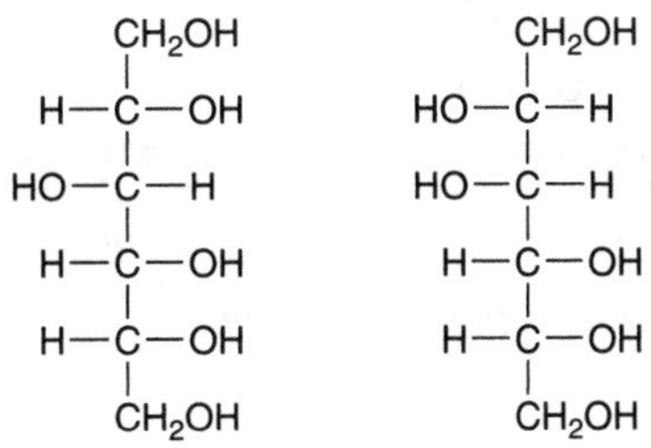

D-Sorbitol D-Mannitol

Figure 2-12 Sorbitol and mannitol are two important alditols, derived from the reduction of the corresponding aldoses.

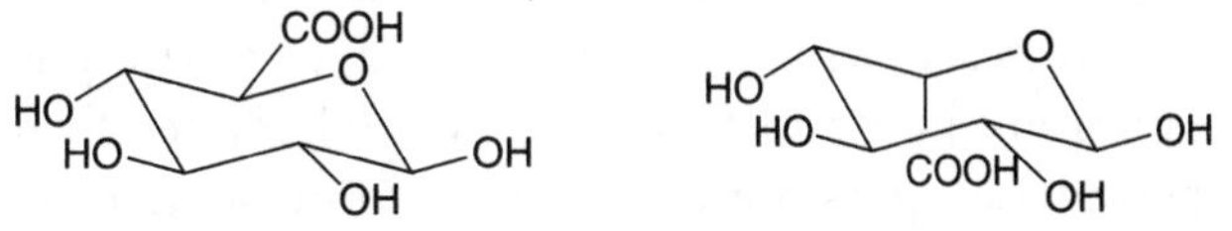

Glucuronic Acid Iduronic Acid

Figure 2-13 Uronic acids: glucuronic and iduronic acid.

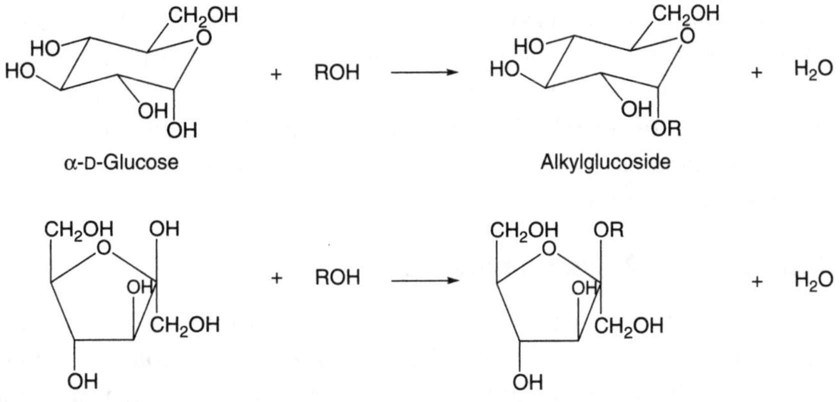

α-D-Glucose + ROH → Alkylglucoside + H_2O

β-D-Fructofuranose + ROH → Alkylfructofuranoside + H_2O

Figure 2-14 Glycoside formation, giving a full acetal or full ketal.

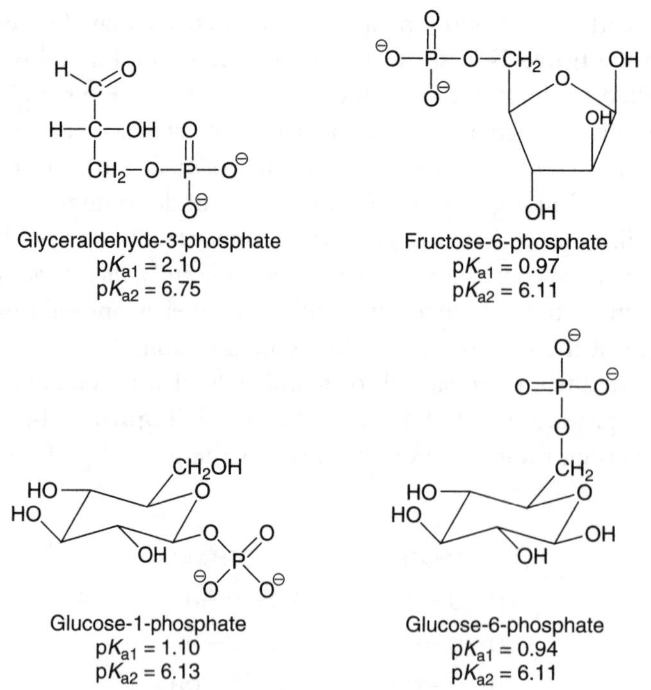

Glyceraldehyde-3-phosphate
$pK_{a1} = 2.10$
$pK_{a2} = 6.75$

Fructose-6-phosphate
$pK_{a1} = 0.97$
$pK_{a2} = 6.11$

Glucose-1-phosphate
$pK_{a1} = 1.10$
$pK_{a2} = 6.13$

Glucose-6-phosphate
$pK_{a1} = 0.94$
$pK_{a2} = 6.11$

Figure 2-15 Sugar–phosphate esters and their pK_a values.

of an unspecified sugar and alcohol. Thus reaction with methanol would give a methylglycoside, for example. If the sugar is specifically identified, one may have a glucoside (from glucose), a galactoside (from galactose), and so on. Glycosides are fairly stable and are not readily cleaved by hydroxide ion. However, the bond linking the alcohol and sugar can be cleaved by enzymes called glycosidases. Glycosides are widely distributed in plants and animals.

As alcohols, sugars can react with phosphoric acid to form phosphate esters. These compounds are quite important in the metabolism of carbohydrates, forming many important intermediates. Sugar–phosphate esters are acidic, even more so than orthophosphoric acid. **Figure 2-15** collects several important examples of carbohydrate phosphate esters that are important in energy metabolism. Hydrolysis of these compounds is thermodynamically favorable, a point that we will return to later (Chapter 9) as we discuss carbohydrate metabolism.

Natural polysaccharides may contain sugars that have been modified by sulfation or attachment of an amino group. Two common amino sugars are β-D-glucosamine and β-D-galactosamine (**Figure 2-16**). These amino sugars can be further modified by acetylation or other alterations. Also, in these natural polysaccharides, sulfate groups may be attached to sugars in a variety of ways (**Figure 2-17**). When dealing with these more complex compounds, it is convenient to use abbreviations for the monosaccharides and their derivatives. **Table 2-1** collects some of the most commonly used abbreviations.

Oligosaccharides and Polysaccharides

The terms "oligomer" and "polymer" are used to indicate molecules composed of linked units of simple constitution. The simple units are called monomers, and a molecule containing many monomers is called a polymer. An oligomer is essentially a short polymer; it contains two or more monomer units, but not as many as a polymer. The size difference between a polymer and an oligomer is not well defined. It is safe to say that a chain of 100 monomer units would

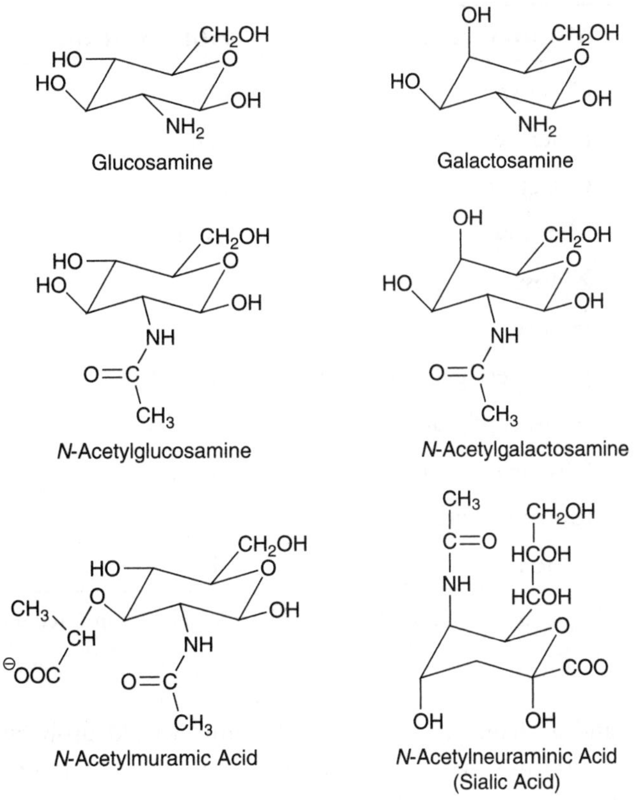

Glucosamine
Galactosamine
N-Acetylglucosamine
N-Acetylgalactosamine
N-Acetylmuramic Acid
N-Acetylneuraminic Acid
(Sialic Acid)

Figure 2-16 Amino sugars and their derivatives.

N-Acetylgalactosamine-4-sulfate
N-Acetylgalactosamine-6-sulfate
2-N-Sulfonato-3,6-bis-O-sulfonatoglucosamine

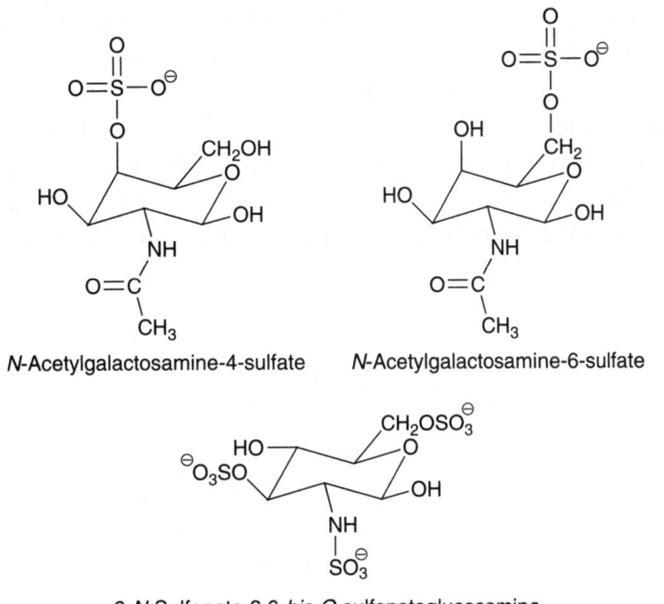

Figure 2-17 Sulfated sugars found in natural polysaccharides.

Monosaccharide	Abbreviation
Glucose	Glc
Fructose	Fru
Galactose	Gal
Mannose	Man
Xylose	Xyl
Fucose	Fuc
β-D-acetylgalactosamine	GalNAc
β-D-acetylglucosamine	GlcNAc
Glucuronic acid	GlcA
Iduronic acid	IdoA
Sialic acid	Sia

Table 2-1 Common Simple and Modified Monosaccharides Found in Glycosaminoglycans

qualify as a polymer, and a chain of only 10 or 20 units would probably be classified as an oligomer, but a chain of 50 units might in some cases be referred to as a polymer, and in other instances as an oligomer.

The prefixes "poly-" and "oligo-" can be combined with the name of the type of monomeric unit to specify the type of polymer or oligomer. For example, a long chain whose repeating monomeric units are all sugars would be regarded as a polysaccharide; a short chain of two or three nucleic acid units (nucleotides) might called an oligonucleotide, and so on.

Oligosaccharides

There are three common disaccharides: *sucrose*, *lactose*, and *maltose*. Sucrose, or common table sugar, is commercially prepared from sugar cane or sugar beets. It is widely found in plants. Sucrose itself is not a reducing sugar, so there are no "free" hemiacetal or hemiketal moieties in the disaccharide. Upon hydrolysis, sucrose gives D-(+)-glucose and D-(−)-fructose. These monomers are linked through the anomeric carbons, C1 of glucose and C2 of fructose (we shall abbreviate this as a 1 → 2 linkage), as shown in **Figure 2-18**, to form α-D-glucopyranosyl-β-D-fructofuranoside, which is both a glucoside and a fructoside.

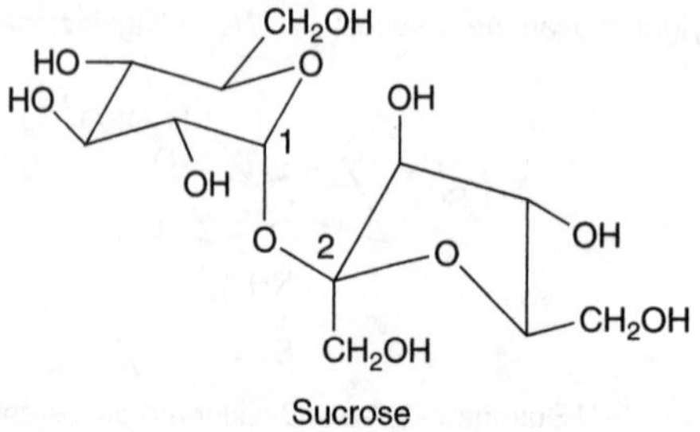

Figure 2-18 Sucrose: α-D-glucopyranosyl-β-D-fructofuranoside.

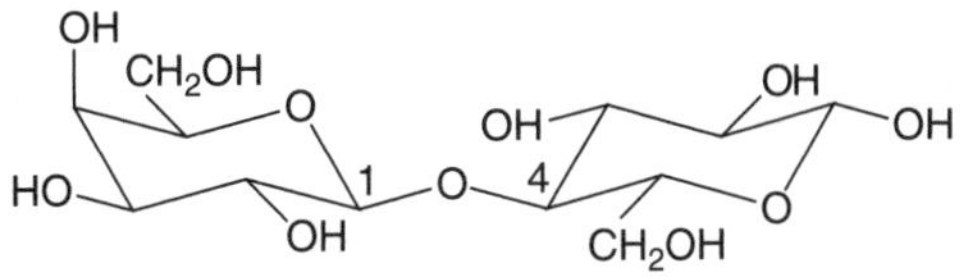

Lactose (β Anomer)

Figure 2-19 β-Lactose: 4-β-D-galactopyranosyl-D-glucopyranose.

Lactose is present in milk at approximately 5% concentration and is commercially prepared as a dairy by-product. A disaccharide of galactose and glucose, it is itself a reducing sugar, with the glucose attached to one of the oxygens of the galactose unit. This makes lactose technically a galactoside, not a glucoside; it is the glucose unit with its "free" hemiacetal that gives the disaccharide its character as a reducing sugar. Formally, lactose is 4-β-D-galactopyranosyl-D-glucose (**Figure 2-19**).

The breakdown of starch yields maltose. This disaccharide is a reducing sugar, which can be hydrolyzed to two molecules of glucose. The linkage is through an acetal, and there are two possible configurations of the anomeric carbon involved: α-maltose (4-α-glucopyranosyl-α-D-glucopyranose) or β-maltose (4-α-glucopyranosyl-β-D-glucopyranose). See **Figure 2-20**.

In later sections and chapters, we will usually drop the detailed specification of configuration and simply assume the configurations listed here.

Glucose Polymers

Starch is a plant storage form for glucose; it is a polymer of glucose. Acid hydrolysis converts starch to corn syrup. There are two main fractions: water-soluble *amylose* (about 20%) and water-insoluble *amylopectin* (about 80%). Amylose is a linear polymer of around 200 units of glucose with $\alpha(1 \rightarrow 4)$ linkages (**Figure 2-21**). Amylopectin is also a glucose polymer, but of

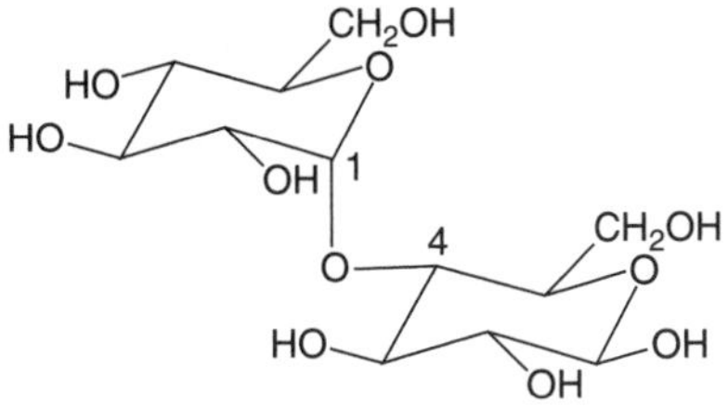

Maltose (α Anomer)

Figure 2-20 α-Maltose: 4-α-glucopyranoxyl-α-D-glucopyranose.

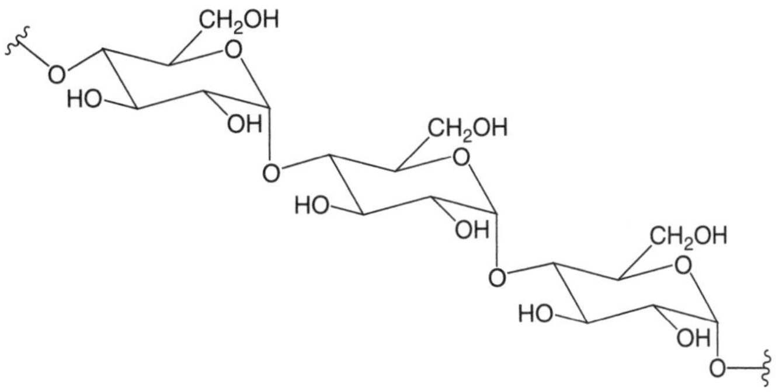

Figure 2-21 Amylose. Hydrogen atoms have been omitted for clarity.

higher molecular weight (at least 1000 glucose units per molecule), with occasional branches in the chain; most of the glucose residues are joined by $1 \rightarrow 4$ linkages, but the branches are formed using $\alpha(1 \rightarrow 6)$ linkages.

Glycogen is an animal polymer of glucose, similar to amylopectin, but with more branching. Its synthesis and breakdown are the subject of discussion in Chapter 9. Cellulose is the main polymer of the cell walls of plants; it forms woody structures. It is insoluble in water, unlike starch and glycogen. In cellulose, there are a few thousand glucose units per molecule. Although cellulose is a glucose polymer, it is not digestible by humans or by most animals. The glucose units are joined by $\beta(1 \rightarrow 4)$ linkages, unlike glycogen or starch (**Figure 2-22**), and animals generally do not make the enzyme needed to hydrolyze these bonds. Ruminant animals such as cattle and insects such as termites carry in their gut certain strains of bacteria that make the enzymes necessary to break down cellulose, enabling their animal hosts to digest cellulose.

As a part of the cell wall, the polymer chains of cellulose lie side-by-side, forming bundles; these bundles are twisted together to create strands and finally visible fibers. Wood contains lignin (cross-linked C9 aromatic units, related in structure and biosynthesis to the aromatic amino acids; **Figure 2-23**) embedded in cellulose fibers; the lignin gives the wood very high strength.

Glycosaminoglycans

Glycosaminoglycans (GAGs) are large linear polymers of repeating disaccharide units, commonly containing one or another amino sugar as one of the monomers in the disaccharide unit. Several types of glycosaminoglycans exist, including chondroitin sulfate, hyaluronan, heparan sulfate, and keratan sulfate; they differ in the type of disaccharide unit used in their synthesis. Glycosaminoglycans are found outside cells, on the cell surface, or as part of the extracellular matrix. They perform various roles, serving as mechanical support and cushioning joints, as cellular signals involved in cell proliferation and cell migration, and as inhibitors of certain key enzymes.

Glycosaminoglycans are often found attached to a protein core, forming what is called a *proteoglycan*. In the past, proteoglycans were called mucopolysaccharides.

Proteoglycans are more carbohydrate than protein, so their properties are mainly determined by the carbohydrate portion of the molecule. These carbohydrate moieties may contain

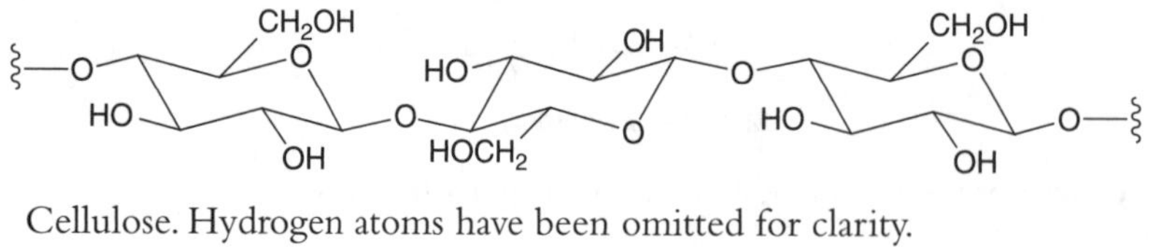

Figure 2-22 Cellulose. Hydrogen atoms have been omitted for clarity.

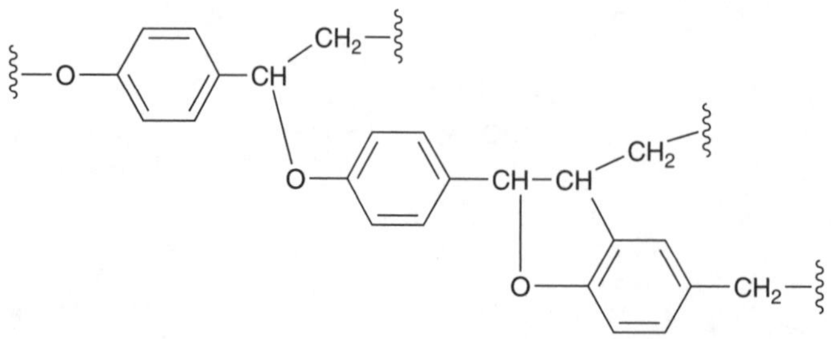

Figure 2-23 Lignin (partial structure).

carboxylic acids (uronic acids) or sulfated sugars, so generally the GAG chains carry a substantial negative charge. Charge repulsions will tend to drive the polysaccharide chains into an extended conformation. Additionally, the charges will help to attract water molecules, so the chains are highly hydrated. The typical proteoglycan is formed from multiple GAG chains on a single polypeptide chain. The overall structure might be described as "feathery"; see **Figure 2-24**.

Heparan sulfate (HS) is a sulfated polysaccharide, found as a component of cell-surface proteoglycans in mast cells, and on the surface of endothelial cells lining blood vessels. It is composed of repeating units of *N*-acetylglucosamine and uronic acids (either glucuronic or iduronic acids). Sulfation (sulfate ester formation) can be found at several positions on these residues; also, the acetyl group on *N*-acetylglucosamine may be replaced by a sulfate group (**Figure 2-25**). After an injury to tissue, oligosaccharides derived from this GAG are released and subsequently help to mediate the inflammatory response. Some of the released oligomers

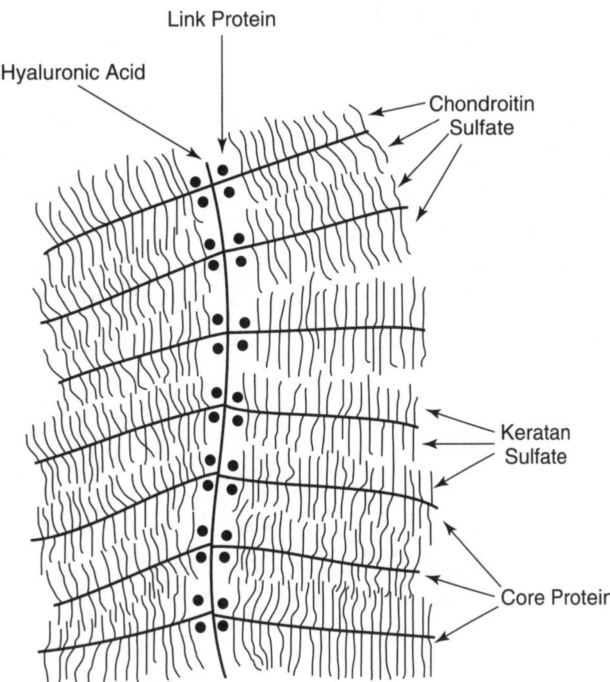

Figure 2-24 Proteoglycan structure. Core protein strands are heavily modified with keratin sulfate and chondroitin sulfate. The core protein strands are held in a complex with a strand of hyaluronic acid by link proteins.

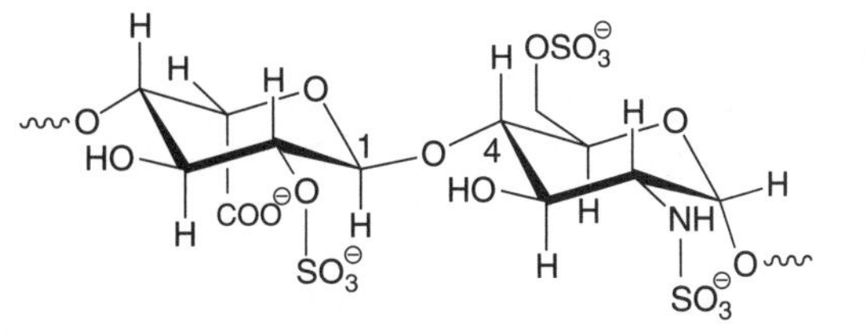

2-*O*-Sulfonato-iduronic acid 2-*N*-Sulfonato-6-*O*-sulfonato-glucosamine

Figure 2-25 Heparan sulfate.

promote activity by growth factors, chemokines, and cytokines; others are associated with recruitment of leukocytes to the injury site. A very important activity is the action of a particular pentasaccharide sequence as an anticoagulant. The fraction of heparan sulfate containing oligomers with this pentasaccharide sequence is designated as *heparin*. The pentasaccharide binds to and activates the enzyme antithrombin III. This enzyme is responsible for inhibiting thrombin, a protease involved in forming blood clots; this inhibition of thrombin, in turn, blocks blood clotting. Note that heparin is much smaller than heparan sulfate and that it is not linked to a protein core. Heparin is also more highly sulfated than the average random pentasaccharide sequence in heparan sulfate. A synthetic version of the key pentasaccharide is used clinically as an anticoagulant (see the discussion later in this chapter in connection with Figure 2-35).

Chondroitin sulfate (CS) is a relatively short polymer, consisting of alternating residues of glucuronic acid and galactose *N*-acetyl 4-sulfonate (**Figure 2-26**). *Dermatan sulfate* (DS) is a closely related GAG, which is composed of glucuronic acid and *N*-acetylgalactosamine. Chondroitin sulfate is found in the extracellular matrix. Its roles are mainly to lend mechanical support and flexibility to tissue; notably, it helps to form skin and cartilage. On membranes, CS and DS are involved in interactions with receptors for growth factors, where they may serve as cofactors for various growth factors.

Keratan sulfate (KS) is found in proteoglycans in three forms, two of which are branched. KS is found primarily in the cornea of the eye and in joint cartilage, where it serves mainly in a mechanical/structural role. It is formed from alternating units of galactose and sulfated *N*-acetylglucosamine (**Figure 2-27**).

Hyaluronic acid (HA; also called hyaluronate) is a long, linear polymer of alternating *N*-acetylglucosamine and glucuronic acid residues (**Figure 2-28**). It serves as a lubricant in joints in the form of synovial fluid; HA is also a principal constituent of the vitreous humor in the eye,

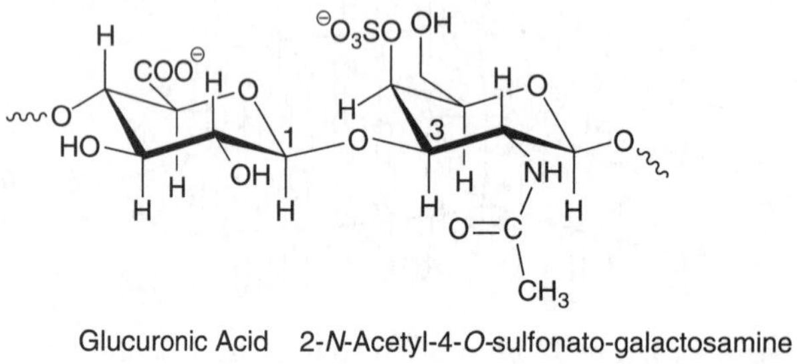

Glucuronic Acid 2-*N*-Acetyl-4-*O*-sulfonato-galactosamine

Figure 2-26 Chondroitin sulfate.

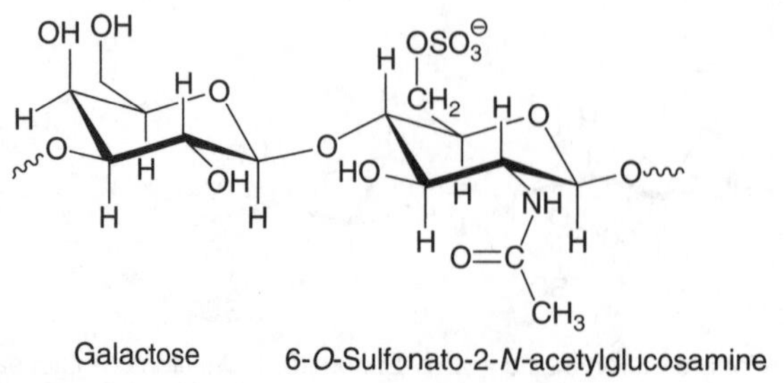

Galactose 6-*O*-Sulfonato-2-*N*-acetylglucosamine

Figure 2-27 Keratan sulfate.

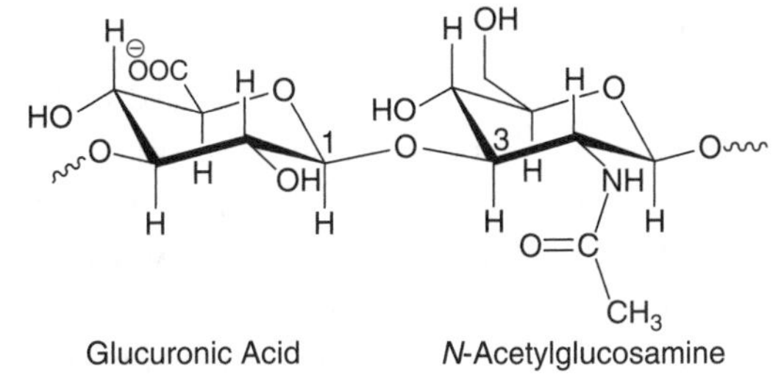

Figure 2-28 Hyaluronic acid.

and it helps to form cartilage. Unlike other GAGs, this polymer is neither sulfated nor attached to a protein core. It is secreted directly to the extracellular matrix. The degradation of HA that occurs after tissue injury releases smaller chains, which can participate in cell proliferation, migration, and differentiation; these degradation products also help to recruit leukocytes to the site of injury. Intra-articular injections of purified HA have been used therapeutically in cases of osteoarthritis.

Other Natural Polysaccharides of Interest

Agar is a linear polymer of sulfated and unsulfated galactose residues, prepared from marine algae; agarose (**Figure 2-29**) is derived from agar as the mostly unsulfated fraction. It is an alternating copolymer of galactose and 3,6-anhydro-galactose. This polymer is not a proteoglycan, but rather is purely carbohydrate. When dissolved in hot water and then cooled, it forms gels with suitable strength for lab use in electrophoresis; it is also used as a food additive to thicken liquid suspensions.

Chitin (Figure 2-29) is a polymer of *N*-acetylglucosamine units. The linkage between units is similar to that in cellulose; the main structural difference is that the C2 carbon now bears an amino group that is acetylated, instead of a hydroxyl group. Like cellulose, chitin is used for structural purposes; it forms the hard exoskeleton of arthropods (e.g., insects, spiders, and crabs).

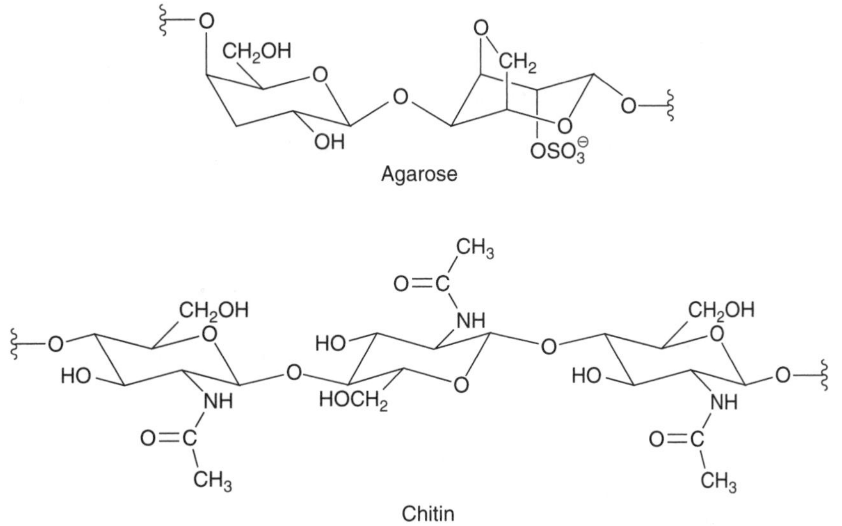

Figure 2-29 Agarose and chitin. Note the unusual ether bridge on the sulfated anhydrogalactose unit in agarose.

Biosynthesis of Proteoglycans

The biosynthesis of mammalian proteoglycans and the associated GAGs starts with the attachment of a xylose residue to the side chain of a serine on the core protein; two galactose residues and a glucuronic acid residue are then attached to the xylose (**Figure 2-30**). The pathways leading to the different GAGs diverge at this point, with different enzymes catalyzing the joining of the sugar residues and more enzymes modifying the residues after they are joined. Chain initiation takes place in the endoplasmic reticulum, and chain elongation and modification occur in the Golgi complex. The proteoglycans move to the cell surface and to the extracellular matrix, carried by vesicles that bud off the Golgi complex. This biosynthetic path is not applicable to hyaluronic acid, however, because this GAG is not attached to a protein but is instead extruded directly to the extracellular matrix.

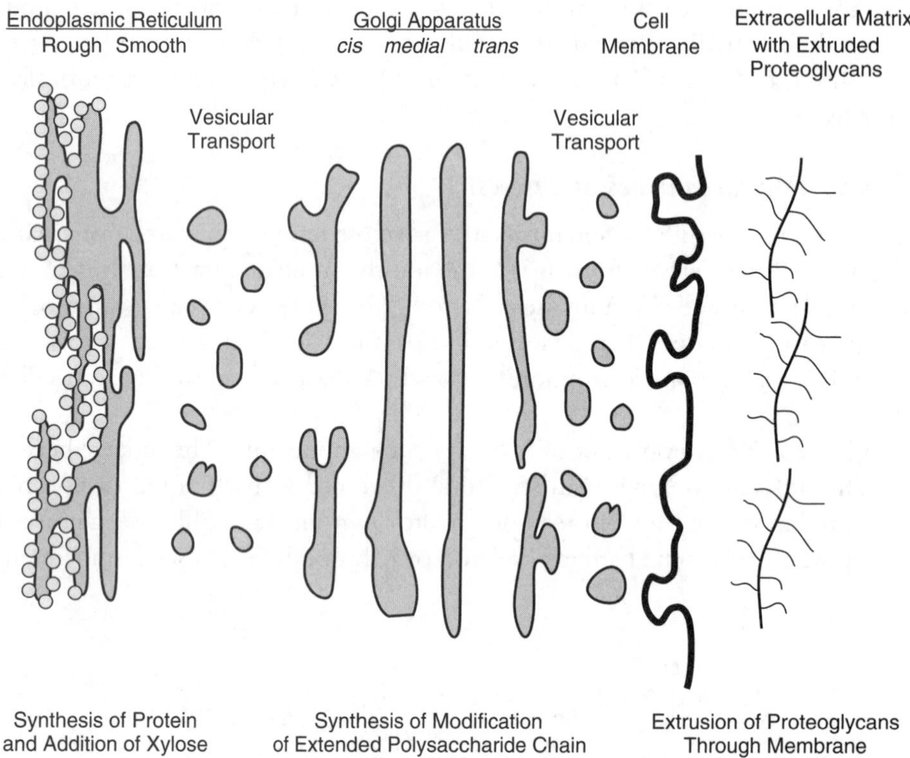

Figure 2-30 Biosynthesis pathway for mammalian proteoglycans and associated GAGs.

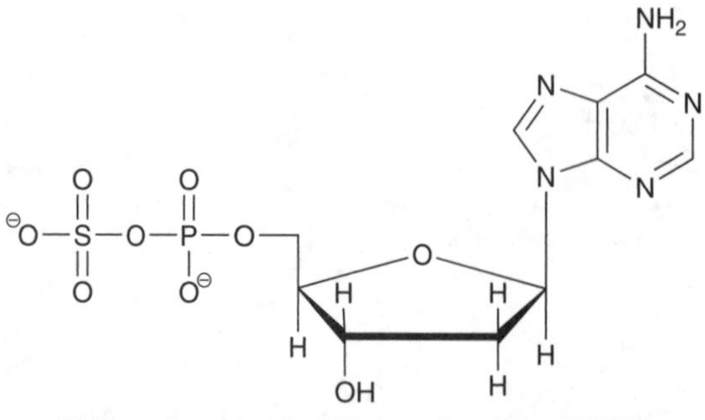

3′-Phosphoadenosine-5′-phosphosulfate (PAPS)

Figure 2-31 Structure of PAPS.

Sulfation reactions take place in both the endoplasmic reticulum and the Golgi complex. The donor of the sulfate group is a compound called PAPS, which is derived from ATP and sulfate (**Figure 2-31**). Sulfation reactions involving PAPS are also important in drug metabolism; the attachment of a sulfate improves the aqueous solubility of a drug or its metabolites, allowing for better excretion.

Other Glycoconjugates

As noted earlier, sugar molecules are attached to a wide variety of other biomolecules, playing roles in molecular recognition processes and stabilizing and perhaps protecting these other biomolecules. This section describes some of the most important classes of biomolecules where sugars are attached.

Glycolipids

Glycolipids, which consist of sugars attached to lipids, are found in biomembranes. Details of their structures are presented in Chapter 5. Sphingolipids are a general class of lipids that include a subclass (*glycosphingolipids*) in which sugars are attached to a ceramide molecule (**Figure 2-32**). A single sugar may be attached, or there may be longer chains, some with

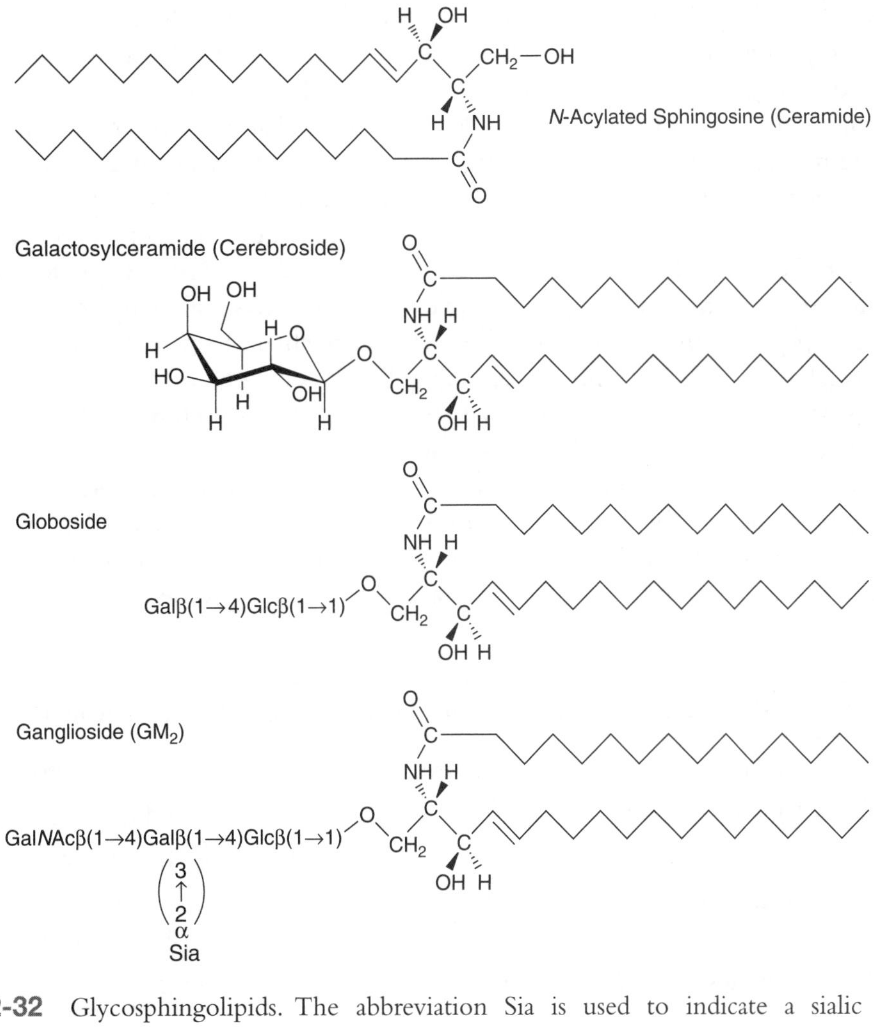

Figure 2-32 Glycosphingolipids. The abbreviation Sia is used to indicate a sialic acid, here *N*-acetylneuraminic acid.

branches. The combination of ceramide and a single sugar residue is called a cerebroside; a globoside is ceramide with a chain of a couple of sugars, and a ganglioside is ceramide with a rather complex sugar chain attached. Gangliosides are prevalent in the membranes of neurons. The sugar moiety or moieties of a glycolipid project outward from the surface of the cell's membrane, and these groups are frequently involved in cell–cell recognition.

Hexosidases are enzymes that break down cerebrosides and gangliosides, removing one sugar residue at a time. These enzymes are found in the lysosomal compartments of the cell. Defects in these enzymes can lead to serious pathologies (lipidoses), such as Tay-Sachs disease. **Table 2-2** lists several of these glycolipid storage diseases and identifies the enzyme deficiency involved in each.

Glycoproteins

Many cellular proteins are modified through the attachment of one or more carbohydrate chains; these are *glycoproteins*. Unlike proteoglycans, glycoproteins are mostly protein, with only a small fraction of their mass being carbohydrate. Also, the attached carbohydrate chains are generally shorter, contain more branching, and have more diversity in sugar sequence compared to the chains found in proteoglycans. In mammals, most cell-surface proteins are glycosylated. Glycoproteins may also be found as secreted proteins (in hormones such as thyroid-stimulating hormone and erythropoietin, in antibodies, and in lactalbumin). Soluble proteins in the cell may also be glycosylated; for example, ribonuclease B differs from ribonuclease A only in the attachment of a sugar chain to a particular asparagine on this enzyme.

Following protein synthesis, polypeptide chains in eukaryotes enter the lumen of the endoplasmic reticulum and later pass through the Golgi complex. During this passage, sugars may be attached to a nitrogen in the side chain of asparagine residues on the polypeptide (so-called *N*-linked carbohydrates) or to oxygens in the side chains of serine or threonine residues (so-called *O*-linked carbohydrates); see **Figure 2-33**. *N*-links are formed in the endoplasmic reticulum and in the Golgi complex, while *O*-links are formed only in the Golgi complex. Complex carbohydrate chains destined to be attached to asparagine are first assembled using a special lipid, dolichol phosphate, embedded in the membrane of the endoplasmic reticulum (**Figure 2-34**). The assembled chain is then transferred to the target protein. Simpler carbohydrate chains start with attachment of a single sugar residue to the target protein, and the chains are elongated by specialized enzymes. After processing in the endoplasmic reticulum, the glycoproteins may be further modified in the Golgi complex. Finally, these glycoproteins are sorted in the Golgi complex, to direct the proteins to their proper cellular locations—for example, the plasma membrane or internal organelles such as lysosomes.

Disease	Lipid Accumulated	Main Organs Affected	Enzyme Deficiency
Fabry	Ceramide trihexoside	Kidney	α-D-galactosidase
Gaucher	Glucocerebroside	Brain, liver, spleen	Glucosylceramide β-D-glucosidase
Krabbe	Galactocerebroside	Brain	Galactosylceramide β-D-galactosidase
Tay-Sachs	Ganglioside GM_2	Brain	β-D-Hexosaminidase A

Table 2-2 Glycolipid Storage Diseases

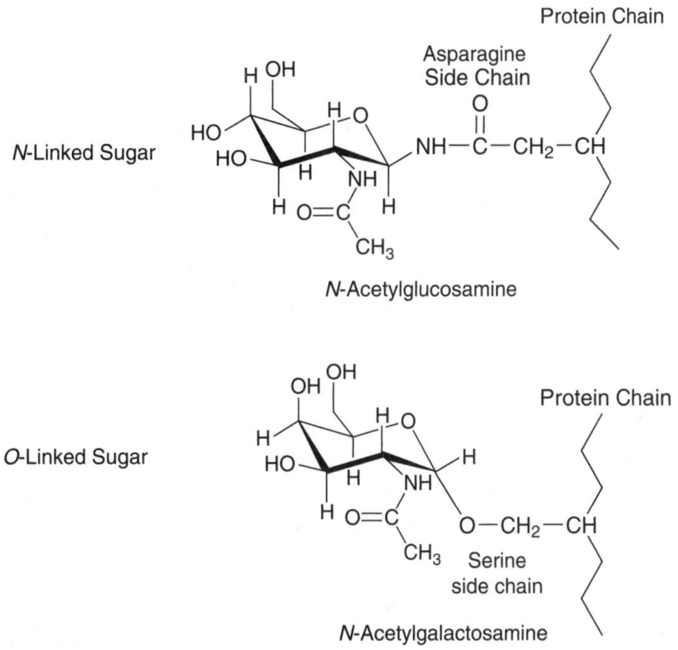

Figure 2-33 O- and *N*-linked sugars in proteoglycans.

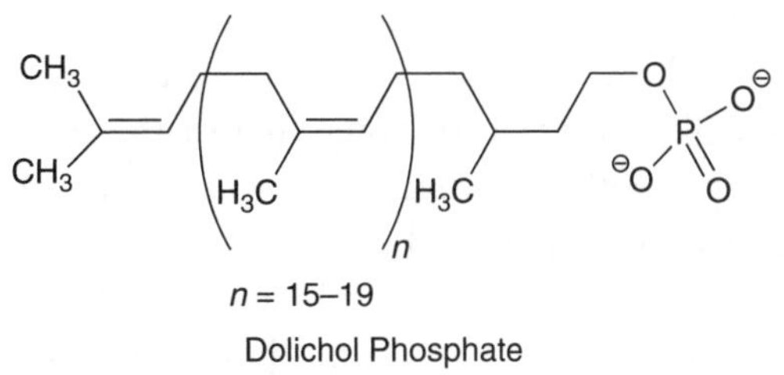

Figure 2-34 Dolichol phosphate.

Lectins

Lectins are proteins that specifically bind carbohydrate chains on the outside of cells to make particular cell-to-cell contacts. One class of lectins, C-type lectins, requires calcium ions to help form protein–carbohydrate complexes. Bacteria use lectins to adhere to epithelial cells in the gut, binding to oligosaccharides on the cell surface. Viruses enter cells by using the protein hemagglutinin to bind to sialic acid residues on glycoproteins embedded in the cell membrane. The "H" part of the designation of strains of influenza virus (e.g., the H1N1 strain of the influenza virus, commonly referred to as swine flu) refers to hemagglutinin; several different, but closely related forms of this viral protein exist. The "N" part of the nomenclature for the influenza virus refers to neuraminidase, another viral protein of which there are several variants. Neuraminidase is an enzyme that cleaves the glycosidic bond joining the sialic residue to the embedded protein after virus enters cell—an action that frees the virus for unpackaging and replication.

Clinical Applications

Clotting and Heparan/Heparin

Heparin is usually prepared from intestinal mucosa, which is rich in heparan sulfate proteoglycans. Heparin is a fraction of heparan. Its structure is that of a repeating disaccharide of glucosamine and iduronate, heavily sulfated. A pentameric sequence within this glycosaminoglycan has great affinity for antithrombin III, a plasma protein that inhibits proteases involved in forming blood clots. This pentasaccharide contains a rare 3-*O*-sulfated glucosamine (**Figure 2-35**). Complexation of heparin with antithrombin enhances the activity of antithrombin greatly, so heparin—and the pentasaccharide in particular—is used in anticoagulant therapy.

Blood Group Antigens

The membranes of red blood cells contain glycolipids that carry oligosaccharides recognized by the immune system. The lipid is a derivative of sphingosine (see Chapters 5 and 13 for more details on glycolipids). The oligosaccharide is composed of a glucose linked directly to the lipid, followed by a galactose residue, an *N*-acetylglucosamine residue, and then a galactose residue. There is usually a terminal L-fucose residue in a 1 → 2 linkage. The exact sequence of sugars, and the manner in which they are linked and branched by glycosyltransferase enzymes, determines the blood group type (**Figure 2-36**). One type of glycosyltransferase attaches a branching *N*-acetylgalactosamine to the galactose residue toward the end of the chain, giving the "A" blood type. Another type attaches galactose instead, giving the "B" blood type. In the "O" blood type, neither enzyme is active, and the chain is not branched. A rare blood type is produced by a deficiency in the enzyme that attaches the L-fucose; this is the "I" blood type. Other rare blood types are caused by linking the fucose in a 1 → 4 manner rather than a 1 → 2 linkage.

The immune system can produce antibodies against these various short oligosaccharides. People with A-type blood will have antibodies against the B-type oligosaccharides; conversely, people with B-type blood will produce antibodies against the A-type antigen. The antibodies can cause blood cells to clump together, leading to serious circulatory problems. For this reason, it is essential in blood transfusions to match the type of the blood donor to that of the blood recipient. People with the O-type antigens are called universal donors, in recognition of the fact that people with A- or B-type blood lack antibodies to the O antigen. Note, however, that people with O-type blood must receive that type in a transfusion, and not A- or B-type blood, because the A and B antigens would be recognized and attacked by the host immune system.

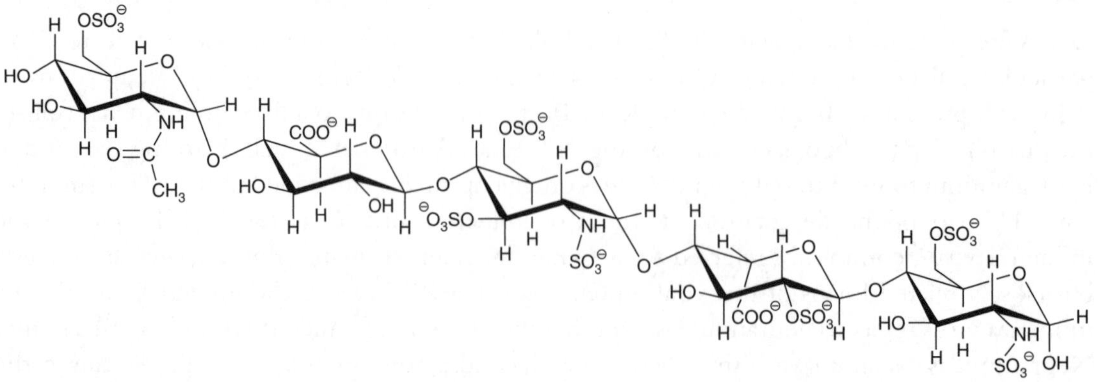

Figure 2-35 Heparin pentasaccharide.

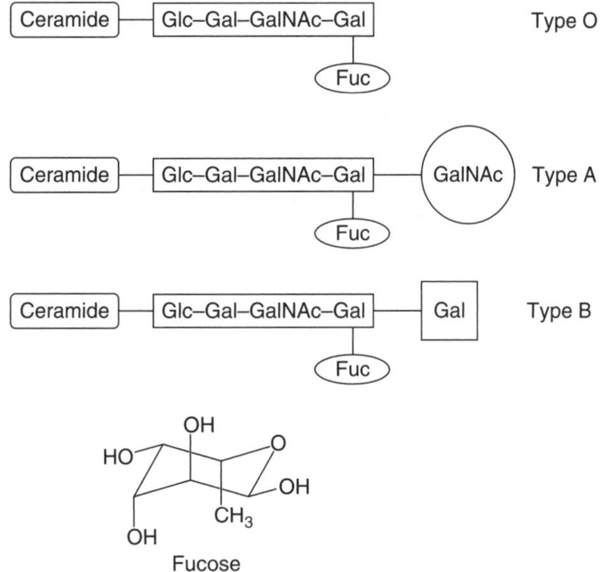

Figure 2-36 Glycolipids for the A-B-O blood types and the structure of fucose, an unusual sugar in these glycolipids.

Blood Glucose Levels, Hemoglobin Glycosylation, and Diabetes

The reducing sugar glucose has a free aldehyde when it is in the linear (not ring) form; this aldehyde is reactive with amino groups, so glucose can be covalently and nonenzymatically linked to a protein through the side-chain amino group of a lysine residue or the terminal $-NH_2$ of the protein chain. The extent of glycosylation of a common protein, such as hemoglobin (Hb) in circulating erythrocytes, depends on the concentration of free glucose. Glucose levels in blood are unusually high in the disease diabetes mellitus, so that Hb becomes glycosylated. Glycosylated Hb is denoted as HbA_1; the major sugar derivative comes from the reaction of glucose with the amino terminal group on the β subunit of Hb. This product, which is denoted as HbA_{1c}, can be detected and quantified using suitable clinical assays. The lifetime of a typical erythrocyte is 110 to 120 days, so the amount of glycosylated Hb is a record of the average level of glucose in the blood over the previous couple of months. A high level of HbA_{1c} indicates high blood glucose levels, signifying that blood glucose is not being well controlled; conversely, one check for satisfactory control of blood glucose in diabetes mellitus is the reduction in detected HbA_{1c}.

Action of Penicillin

A major component of bacterial cell walls is peptidoglycan, which is made of short peptide chains joined to a long heteropolysaccharide of alternating *N*-acetylglucosamine and *N*-acetylmuramic acid residues. The peptide chains are unusual in that they often contain a large proportion of D-amino acids, instead of the usual L-amino acids. These short peptide chains act as cross-links between polysaccharide chains. The cross-linking reaction is catalyzed by peptidoglycan transpeptidase. It is this enzyme that is the target of the antibiotic penicillin. Without a strong, intact cell wall, the bacteria cannot survive, and penicillin weakens the cell wall by inhibiting the cross-linking reaction.

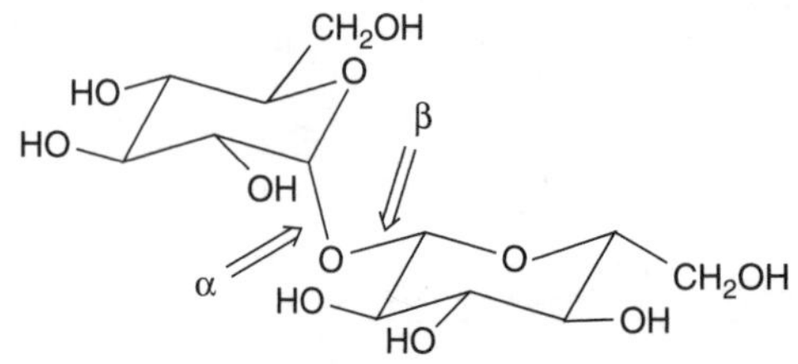

Figure 2-37 α, β-Trehalose. Arrows point to the α and β linkages.

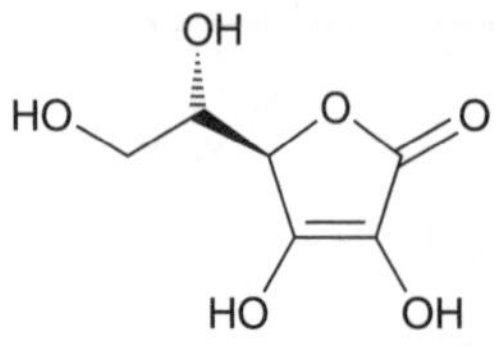

Figure 2-38 Vitamin C.

QUESTIONS FOR DISCUSSION

1. Is glycerol a carbohydrate? Is it a monosaccharide? What about acetone?
2. **Figure 2-37** gives the structure of trehalose. Predict the products of hydrolysis of this sugar. Is trehalose a reducing sugar? What about the products?
3. In solution, fructose exists about 60% in the pyranose form; of this 60%, 57% is the β-D-fructopyranose, and only about 3% is the α-D-fructopyranose. Why is the β anomer favored?
4. Suggest a structure for the product of the reaction of glucose with a primary amine (as in the N-terminal valine in the beta subunit of hemoglobin).
5. **Figure 2-38** presents a structure for ascorbic acid, vitamin C. Is vitamin C a carbohydrate?
6. Why does reduction of D-fructose give a mixture of D-sorbitol and D-mannitol? (See Figure 2-12.)
7. Heparin preparations have reportedly been contaminated with chondroitin sulfate (CS). Such contamination is quite serious, as it can lead to severe allergic reactions. The contaminating CS was oversulfated (to a degree not found naturally), and the presence of this contaminant was likely the result of deliberate adulteration by the supplier of the heparin. Compare the structures of heparin and CS, and comment on how CS could pass as heparin in cursory tests of the properties of the heparin preparation.

REFERENCES

C. G. Gahmberg and M. Tolvanen. (1996). "Why mammalian cell surface proteins are glycoproteins," *Trends Biochem. Sci.* 21:308–311.

R. T. Morrison and R. N. Boyd. (1992). *Organic Chemistry, 6th ed.*, Prentice-Hall, Englewood Cliffs, NJ.

M. Petitou, B. Casu, and U. Lindahl. (2003). "1976–1983, a critical period in the history of heparin: The discovery of the antithrombin binding site," *Biochimie* 85:83–89.

N. Sharon and H. Lis. (2004). "History of lectins: From hemagglutinins to biological recognition molecules," *Glycobiol.* 14:53R–62R.

K. R. Taylor and R. L. Gallo. (2006). "Glycosaminoglycans and their proteoglycans: Host-associated molecular patterns for initiation and modulation of inflammation," *FASEB J.* 20:9–22.

R. R. Yocum, D. J. Waxman, and J. L. Strominger. (1980). "Interaction of penicillin with its receptors in bacterial membranes," *Trends Biochem. Sci.* 5:97–101.

CHAPTER 3

Amino Acids and Proteins

Learning Objectives

1. Define and use correctly the terms *zwitterion, peptide bond, polypeptide, selenocysteine, ornithine, homocysteine, γ-aminobutyric acid, cystine, disulfide bridge, primary structure, secondary structure, tertiary structure, quaternary structure, α-helix, β-sheet, β-turn coiled coil, collagen helix, motif, domain, chaperone protein, molten globule, ubiquitin,* and *proteasome*.
2. Name and recognize the structures of the 20 common amino acids. Classify them into families according to physico-chemical properties. Recognize and use the common three-letter abbreviation for each of these amino acids.
3. Explain why 19 of the 20 common amino acids are optically active. Give the proper chemical structure and locate the chiral center(s) for each amino acid. Note that D isomers are uncommon, and give some examples where they occur.
4. Note that amino acids are high-melting solids and explain why they are moderately soluble in water. Recall and apply general rules on acidity and basicity of the ionizable or titratable groups present in the 20 common amino acids to explain titration curves.
5. List several of the less common amino acids, noting their characteristic biological roles.
6. Classify each of the 20 common amino acids into the appropriate one of the nine families of side chain properties.
7. Explain why the peptide group resists rotation around the C—N bond.
8. Recognize and use conventional representations of peptide chains, including representations of α-helices and β-sheets.
9. Distinguish fibrous and globular proteins by their characteristic properties, and give examples of each class of protein.
10. Distinguish among and recognize the four levels of protein structure.
11. Explain the basis for the flexibility of an extended polypeptide chain.
12. Outline the process of protein folding, noting the roles played by chaperone proteins, proline isomerase, and disulfide isomerase.
13. Compare protein folding to protein denaturation.
14. Explain the process of protein turnover, describing the two main paths for the process in eukaryotic cells. State reasons why turnover occurs.

Amino Acids

Amino acids have a wide variety of biological roles and, therefore, appear throughout biochemistry. Their characteristic chemical features help to determine these roles, and the common amino acids can be grouped, broadly speaking, into families on the basis of shared chemical features. There are 20 common amino acids, but there are also certain less common, yet still important amino acids to be recognized.

Roles of Amino Acids

Amino acids have several biological roles:

- They may be polymerized to form peptides, most notably proteins (polypeptides).
- They serve as precursors for other small biomolecules (e.g., purines, pyrimidines, porphyrins).
- They may be oxidized to serve as an energy source (fuel) for the cell.

Later chapters will discuss the synthesis of amino acids and their use as an energy source; we also defer to later chapters the connection of amino acids to other small biomolecules. This chapter focuses instead on the connection of amino acids to protein structure and properties.

General Features of Amino Acids

Amino acids contain two characteristic functional groups: an amino group and a carboxylic acid group.

- For amino acids used in proteins, these are attached to a central carbon atom, C_α, the alpha or α-carbon, to which are also attached a hydrogen atom and an organic side chain group R.
- The central carbon is a chiral center for 19 of the 20 common amino acids, and by far the common stereoisomeric form is the L isomer (**Figure 3-1**). Glycine has as its side chain a simple hydrogen atom, so it is not chiral. Proline has its side chain fused to the α-amino group, but it still has an asymmetric center in the α-carbon.
- D isomers of amino acids are found only rarely—for example, in bacterial cell walls and some short antibiotic peptides.

Some other important features of amino acids are as follows:

- Amino acids are characteristically isolated as white crystalline ionic solids with high melting points and poor solubility in organic solvents (they are moderately soluble in water).

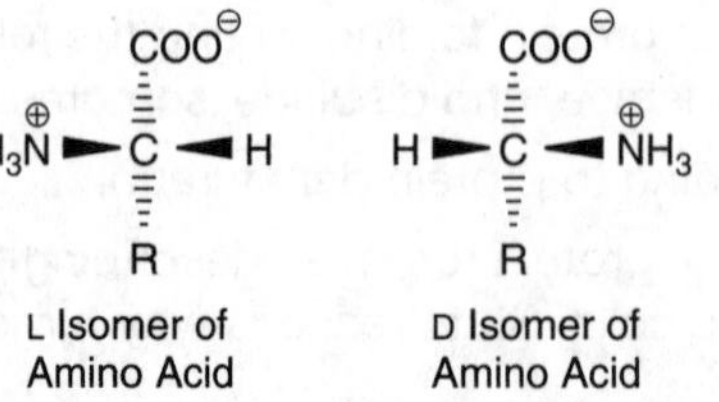

Figure 3-1 Stereochemistry of the two optical isomers of the common amino acids.

- Amino acids dissolve in water as dipolar ions, or *zwitterions*, due to ionization of the acid and amino groups (the side chains may also contain titrable groups and be ionized under physiological conditions).
- The α-carboxyl group typically has a pK_a around 2.0–2.4 and the α-amino group typically has a pK_a around 9.0–9.7.
- Titrable groups on the side chains vary considerably in their pK_a values (see **Table 3-1**).

Figure 3-2 shows the example of glycine and its titration behavior in water. Points to note here include the following:

- At acid pH, glycine is found mainly in the form of the cation; at alkaline pH, glycine is mainly in the form of the anion.
- At physiological pH, around pH 7, glycine exists mainly as the zwitterion, and only small amounts of the electrically neutral, cationic, or anionic species are present.
- At pH 6.1, there are equal (and relatively small) numbers of cations and anions, and the dominant species is the zwitterion.

The 20 Common Amino Acids

Table 3-1 collects the 20 common amino acids, showing their chemical structure, three-letter and one-letter abbreviations, and pK_a values for the α-carboxyl, α-amino, and side-chain functional groups. We will use the three-letter abbreviations freely from now on. Table 3-1 ignores ionization of the hydroxyl groups on the side chains of Ser and Thr because this occurs at quite unphysiological alkalinity (around pH 13). It includes the pK_a for the strongly basic side chain of Arg, at about pH 12.5; the positively charged guanidinium ion so formed will be present under most conditions. The side chains of Asp, Glu, and Lys have pK_a values are only slightly shifted from those typical of the isolated carboxylic acid or primary amino group. The shifts in pK_a are due to electrostatic interactions with the other ionized groups (the α-carboxyl and α-amino groups) on the molecule.

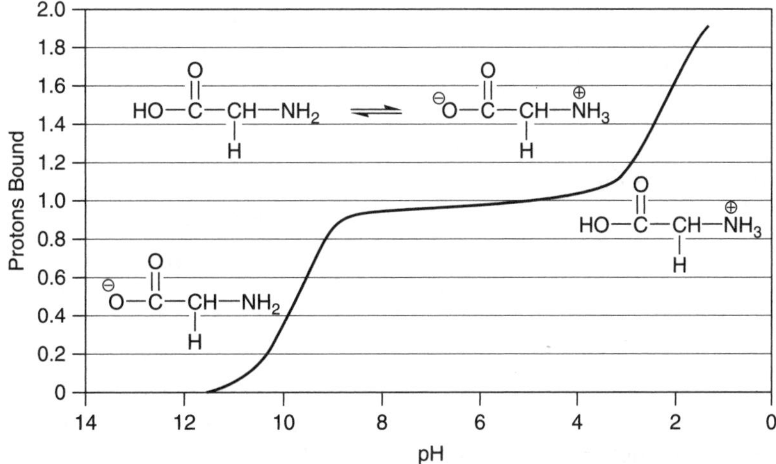

Figure 3-2 Titration curve of glycine (Gly), for pK_a values of 2.35 (carboxylic acid group) and 9.78 (amino group), showing structures of the dominant titrated species at acidic, neutral, and alkaline pH.

Amino Acid	Abbreviations		Structure	pK_a Values
	Three-Letter	One-Letter		
Alanine	Ala	A	O $H_2N-CH-C-OH$ CH_3	2.35 9.87
Arginine	Arg	R	O $H_2N-CH-C-OH$ CH_2 CH_2 CH_2 NH C=NH NH_2	1.83 8.99 12.48
Asparagine	Asn	N	O $H_2N-CH-C-OH$ CH_2 C=O NH_2	2.10 8.84
Aspartic acid	Asp	D	O $H_2N-CH-C-OH$ CH_2 C=O OH	1.99 3.90 9.90
Cysteine	Cys	C	O $H_2N-CH-C-OH$ CH_2 SH	1.92 8.35 10.46
Glutamic acid	Glu	E	O $H_2N-CH-C-OH$ CH_2 CH_2 C=O OH	2.10 3.07 9.47

Table 3-1 The 20 Common Amino Acids

Source: pK_a values taken from David A. Bender. (1985). Amino Acid Metabolism, 2nd ed., Wiley, New York.

Amino Acid	Abbreviations: Three-Letter	Abbreviations: One-Letter	Structure	pK_a Values
Glutamine	Gln	Q	$H_2N-CH(CH_2-CH_2-C(=O)-NH_2)-C(=O)-OH$	2.17 9.13
Glycine	Gly	G	$H_2N-CH(H)-C(=O)-OH$	2.35 9.78
Histidine	His	H	$H_2N-CH(CH_2-\text{imidazolyl})-C(=O)-OH$ (ring: N, NH)	1.80 6.04 9.76
Isoleucine	Ile	I	$H_2N-CH(CH(CH_3)-CH_2-CH_3)-C(=O)-OH$	2.32 9.76
Leucine	Leu	L	$H_2N-CH(CH_2-CH(CH_3)-CH_3)-C(=O)-OH$	2.33 9.74
Lysine	Lys	K	$H_2N-CH(CH_2-CH_2-CH_2-CH_2-NH_2)-C(=O)-OH$	2.16 9.18 10.79

Table 3-1 The 20 Common Amino Acids (Continued)

Amino Acid	Abbreviations: Three-Letter	Abbreviations: One-Letter	Structure	pK_a Values
Methionine	Met	M	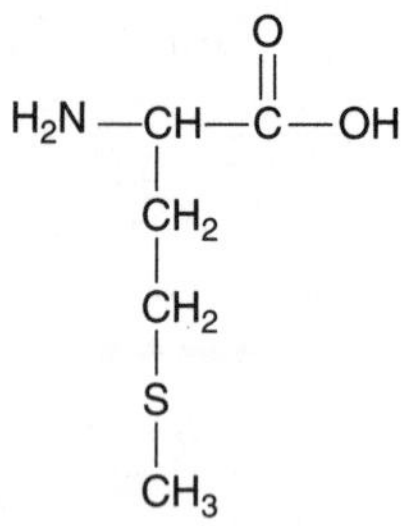 O H_2N—CH—C—OH CH_2 CH_2 S CH_3	2.13 9.28
Phenylalanine	Phe	F	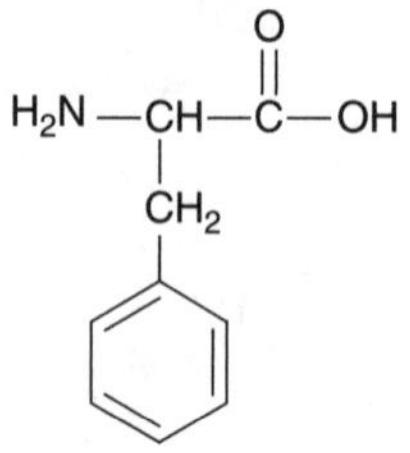 O H_2N—CH—C—OH CH_2	2.16 9.18
Proline	Pro	P	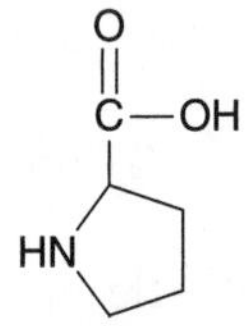 O C—OH HN	1.95 10.64
Serine	Ser	S	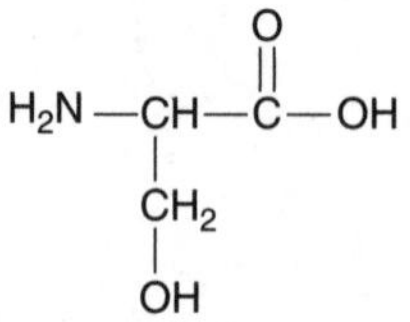 O H_2N—CH—C—OH CH_2 OH	2.19 9.21
Threonine	Thr	T	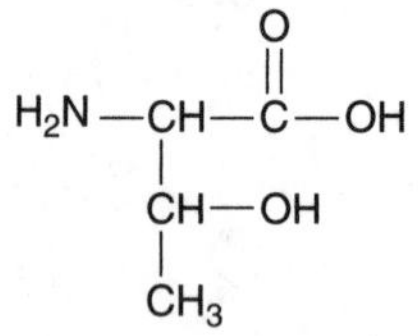 O H_2N—CH—C—OH CH—OH CH_3	2.09 9.10
Tryptophan	Trp	W	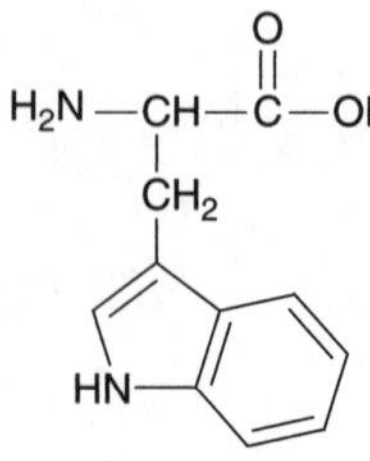 O H_2N—CH—C—OH CH_2 HN	2.43 9.44

Table 3-1 The 20 Common Amino Acids (Continued)

Amino Acid	Abbreviations		Structure	pK_a Values
	Three-Letter	One-Letter		
Tyrosine	Tyr	Y	$H_2N-CH(CH_2-C_6H_4-OH)-C(=O)-OH$	2.29 9.11 10.13
Valine	Val	V	$H_2N-CH(CH(CH_3)-CH_3)-C(=O)-OH$	2.29 9.74

Table 3-1 The 20 Common Amino Acids (Continued)

The potential for ionization of other side chains can be quite important in biological function.

- The phenolic group on Tyr is a weak acid and can be ionized to form a phenolate ion at pH values not so far from physiological, and its acid–base behavior may be important in catalytic mechanisms of some enzymes.
- The thiol group on the side chain of Cys is a weak acid and may also be ionized at a pH close to physiological; again, this can be important for acid–base behavior in certain enzyme catalytic mechanisms.
- The imidazole ring of His can accept or donate protons at pH values near neutral; this is an important factor in acid–base catalysis in many enzymes.

When the amino acids are polymerized into a polypeptide protein, the α-carboxyl and α-amino groups are joined in amide linkages and are effectively neutral as far as acid–base behavior is concerned. The side chains are another matter, however; the pK_a of the side-chain groups can shift toward either higher or lower pH values, depending on the local environment. Also, the terminal carboxyl and amino groups of a polypeptide chain retain their characteristic acid–base titration behavior, which can also be important for biological function.

Cysteine is notable for its ability to form disulfide bonds with adjacent thiols, especially Cys-to-Cys *disulfide bridges*, which are often important in stabilizing the folded tertiary structure of proteins. The combination of two Cys residues joined by such a bridge is the amino acid *cystine* (**Figure 3-3**). Bridge formation requires oxidation of the thiols on both participants; disruption of the disulfide bridge requires reduction.

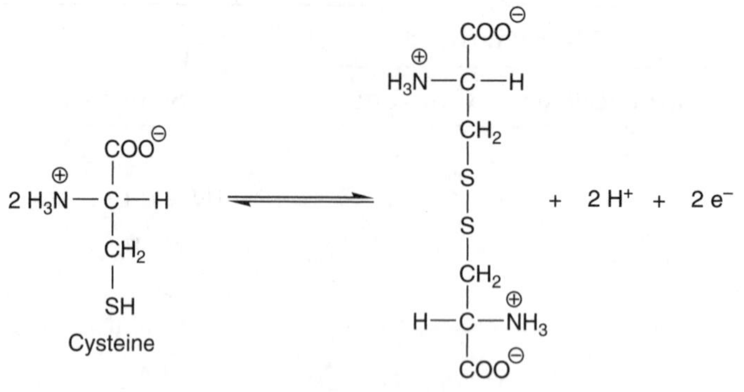

$$2\ H_3\overset{\oplus}{N}-CH(COO^{\ominus})-CH_2-SH \rightleftharpoons \ ^{\oplus}H_3N-CH(COO^{\ominus})-CH_2-S-S-CH_2-CH(COO^{\ominus})-\overset{\oplus}{N}H_3 + 2H^+ + 2e^-$$

Cysteine → Cystine

Figure 3-3 Oxidation of two Cys residues to form the amino acid cystine, containing a disulfide link.

Classification by Properties

The 20 common amino acids can be grouped by properties of the side chain into nine classes (**Table 3-2**). First, Gly, with its side chain of a simple hydrogen atom, is in a class by itself. The hydrogen atom presents the least steric hindrance to rotation or packing of neighboring groups in a protein, so Gly residues can contribute strongly to protein flexibility.

Second, there are the amino acids with alkyl side chains: Ala, Val, Leu, and Ile. The nonpolar character of the side chains of these amino acids makes their surface hydrophobic, and the packing of these side chains in the interior of proteins, away from exposure to water, helps to stabilize protein structures. The bulkiness of the side chains also contributes to forming specific shapes for binding sites on the surface of proteins.

Third, Pro is in a class by itself, due to its unique linkage of the side chain to both the α-carbon and the α-amino group. The short loop formed by the side chain constrains the conformation of this amino acid quite a bit, making the entire structure relatively rigid. The rigidity of Pro residues is an important factor in determining how a polypeptide chain will fold into its native protein structure.

Class	Members	Properties
1	Gly	Simple hydrogen atom side chain; nonpolar
2	Ala, Val, Leu, Ile	Aliphatic side chains; bulky and nonpolar
3	Pro	Side-chain loop connecting α-carbon and α-amino group; nonpolar and rigid
4	Phe, Tyr, Trp	Aromatic side chains; bulky, nonpolar
5	Cys, Met	Sulfur-containing nonpolar side chains; reactive thiol on Cys
6	Ser, Thr	Alcohols; hydrophilic and reactive hydroxyl groups
7	Glu, Asp	Carboxylic acids; anionic
8	Gln, Asn	Amides of carboxylic acids; polar, bulky
9	His, Lys, Arg	Basic side chains; cationic Lys and Arg, but titrable imidazole ring on His

Table 3-2 The Nine Classes of Amino Acids

The fourth class comprises the aromatic amino acids: Phe, Tyr, and Trp. The aromatic side chains are hydrophobic and bulky; like the aliphatic side chains of Ala, they affect protein packing. These side chains may also be used for molecular recognition in binding sites on protein surfaces.

The sulfur-containing amino acids Cys and Met form the fifth class. As noted earlier, two Cys residues can form a disulfide bridge (a cystine residue) and they can cross-link a peptide chain with itself or with another chain; this behavior can be quite important in stabilizing tertiary or quaternary protein conformations. The sulfur atom in Met is relatively polarizable and can contribute to molecular recognition in binding sites.

The sixth class is made up of the two amino acid alcohols, Ser and Thr. The hydroxyl group on the side chain is only very weakly acidic, but is an important site for protein modifications (e.g., phosphorylation and glycosylation) that can affect the overall functioning of the protein.

The seventh class includes the acidic amino acids Glu and Asp. The carboxyl groups of their side chains are ionized to anions under physiological conditions; this phenomenon contributes to the overall charge on a protein, important for its solubility and for recognition of binding partners.

The eighth class, containing Asn and Gln, is composed of the amides of the acidic amino acids. These amides are not titrable, but they are highly polar, and they participate in hydrogen bonding quite readily.

The ninth and last class collects the basic amino acids Lys, Arg, and His. We have already noted the importance of the acid–base behavior of His; the imidazole-ring nitrogens can also help bind metal ions. Lys has its amino group at the end of a relatively long chain, allowing flexibility in positioning the (usually positively charged) terminus in active sites, or for forming amide links to carboxyl groups of cofactors such as biotin. The positively charged guanidinium group on the side chain of Arg is often involved in especially strong ionic or hydrogen bonding interactions with negative ions such as carboxylates or phosphates.

Some Important but Less Common Amino Acids

Modified amino acids can be found in proteins and peptides, and certain other amino acids are not used in protein synthesis but are nonetheless important as signaling agents or as intermediates in biochemical pathways.

- Hydroxyproline and hydroxylysine (**Figure 3-4**) are found in the connective tissue protein collagen. The extra hydrogen-bonding opportunities offered by the presence of the extra hydroxyl group on these amino acids is a major factor in stabilizing collagen's characteristic left-handed helical conformation. Another common modification is phosphorylation (for Ser, Thr, and Tyr, on their hydroxyl groups; for Arg, on the guanidinium group).
- *Selenocysteine* appears in a few proteins, such as glutathione peroxidase (the enzyme that helps glutathione to detoxify harmful organic peroxides; see Chapter 12). Selenocysteine resembles Cys in structure, albeit with a selenium atom replacing the sulfur atom in the side chain.
- *Ornithine* (abbreviated as Orn) is similar to Lys, with an amino group at the end of its side chain. It is an important player in the urea cycle, to be discussed in detail in Chapter 14. It is also a precursor to arginine and to certain polyamines such as spermidine and spermine.
- *Citrulline* is derived from carbamoylation of ornithine on the side chain. Like ornithine, it is important in the urea cycle.
- *Homocysteine* is an intermediate in the catabolism of methionine, and it is closely connected to the functioning of the methyl-donor compound, *S*-adenosylmethionine. Chapter 14 describes its connection to the metabolism of folate and *S*-adenosylmethionine.

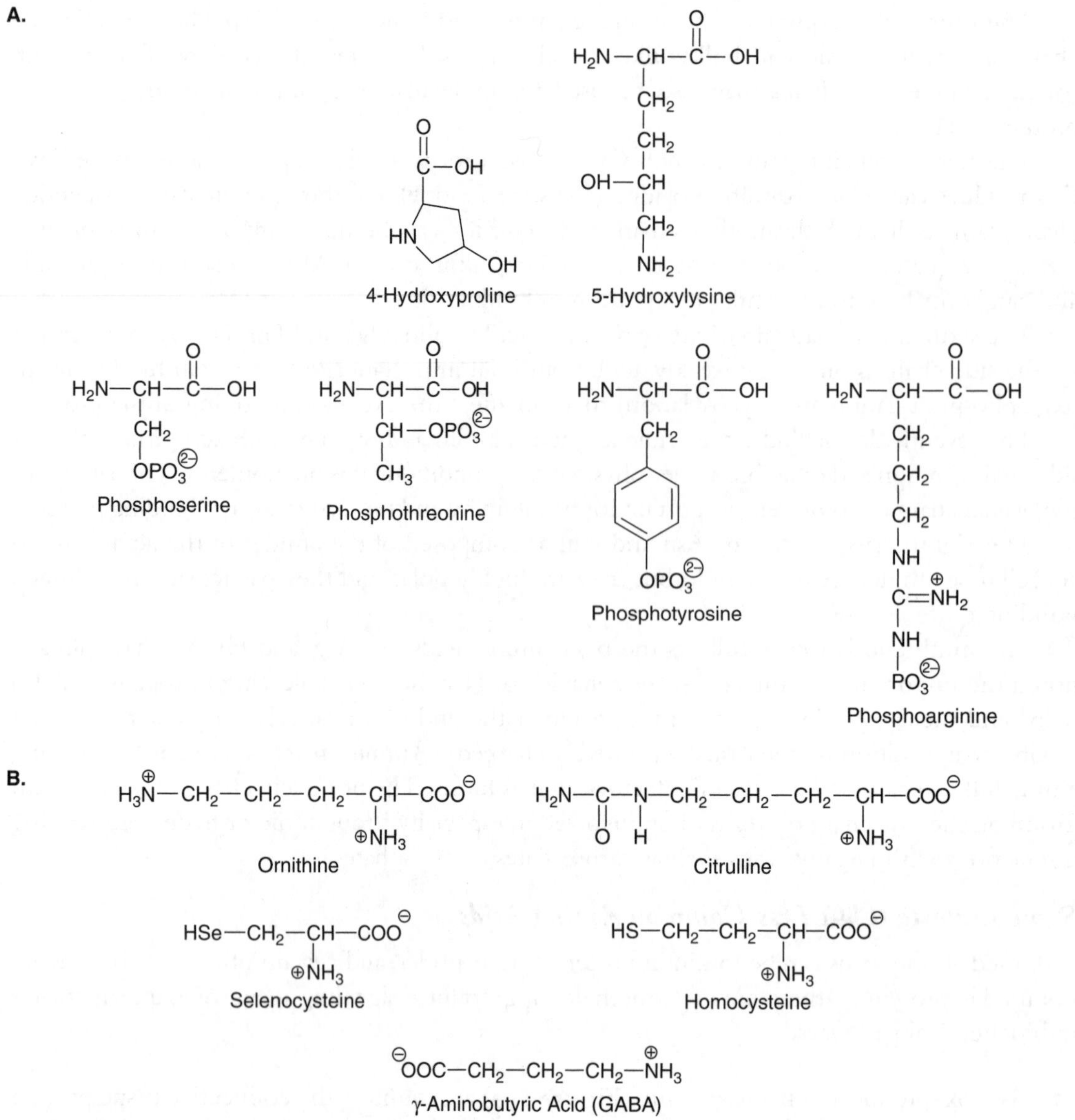

A.

4-Hydroxyproline

5-Hydroxylysine

Phosphoserine

Phosphothreonine

Phosphotyrosine

Phosphoarginine

B.

Ornithine

Citrulline

Selenocysteine

Homocysteine

γ-Aminobutyric Acid (GABA)

Figure 3-4 A collection of some less common, yet important amino acids. **A.** Common amino acids may be modified covalently. **B.** Certain amino acids are not commonly used in protein synthesis, but are important for other cell functions.

- *γ-Aminobutyric acid* (abbreviated as GABA) is an important neurochemical that inhibits neuronal action by binding to specific receptors (GABA receptors), both pre- and post-synaptically. Incidentally, the amino acids glycine and glutamate are also neurotransmitters, with glycine acting like GABA to inhibit neurotransmission and glutamate acting to excite neuronal action.

Polypeptides and Protein Primary Structure

Perhaps the most obvious biochemical role played by amino acids is as monomer constituents of proteins. Amino acids are covalently joined by special linkages that play an important role in the conformation that a polypeptide can adopt.

Amide Bonds and Peptide Linkages

In proteins, amino acids are joined by *peptide bonds*. A string of amino acids joined together by peptide bonds is called a *polypeptide*. (By convention, a polypeptide is considered a protein if its molecular weight is greater than several thousand g-mol^{-1} (say, 40–50 residues or longer), and the term *oligopeptide* is used to describe the shorter chains. See the comments in Chapter 2 on differentiating between oligomers and polymers.) Peptide bonds are amide linkages formed by the condensation of the α-carboxyl group of one amino acid with the α-amino group of another amino acid. The free energy of formation of a peptide bond is approximately +10 kJ/mol, so these bonds are thermodynamically unstable with respect to hydrolysis. However, the bonds are kinetically quite stable in neutral aqueous solution; the half-life for hydrolysis is on the order of a few hundred years.

Figure 3-5 shows the characteristic planarity of such a linkage. The planarity is due to the partial double-bond character of the C—N bond, involving resonance hybridization and the sharing of the lone pair of electrons on the amide nitrogen with the carbonyl carbon. This sharing of electrons makes the amide linkage more stable than, say, an ester linkage. Also, because the nitrogen's electrons are being shared, they are not readily available to bond to a proton from solution; hence amides resist titration and are essentially electrically neutral functional groups.

Rotation around the peptide bond is energetically restricted because of its partial double-bond character. This is not the case, however, for the carbon–carbon bond between C_α and the carboxyl group or for the nitrogen–carbon bond joining the amide group to the adjacent C_α. There is relatively free rotation possible around these single bonds, which leads to a great deal of possible conformational freedom for a polypeptide chain. Some conformations are lower in energy than others, however, which leads to the formation of certain characteristic folding patterns for polypeptides; this is the origin of the secondary and higher-order structure in proteins.

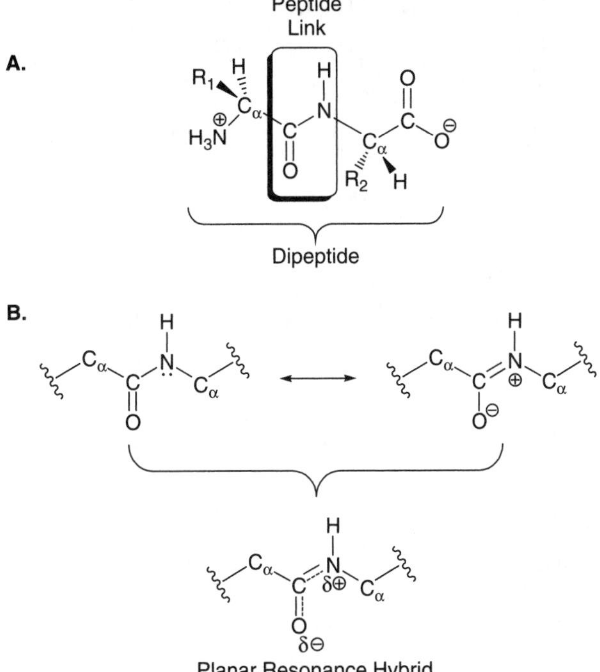

Figure 3-5 The peptide bond is an amide linkage between two amino acids. Its planar rigidity derives from its partial double-bond character. **A.** Amide bond linking two amino acids. **B.** Formation of planar resonance hybrid, showing partial double bonds.

Polymerization of amino acids into a polypeptide chain leaves one end of the chain with a free amino group (the N-terminus) and the other end with a free carboxylic acid group (the C-terminus). By convention, a polypeptide's sequence of amino acids is written starting with the N-terminus on the left and the C-terminus on the right. **Figure 3-6** shows such a representation of the tripeptide Gly-Ala-Phe, and **Figure 3-7** shows the more complicated structure of the peptide hormone oxytocin, which has a disulfide bridge. In the active hormone,

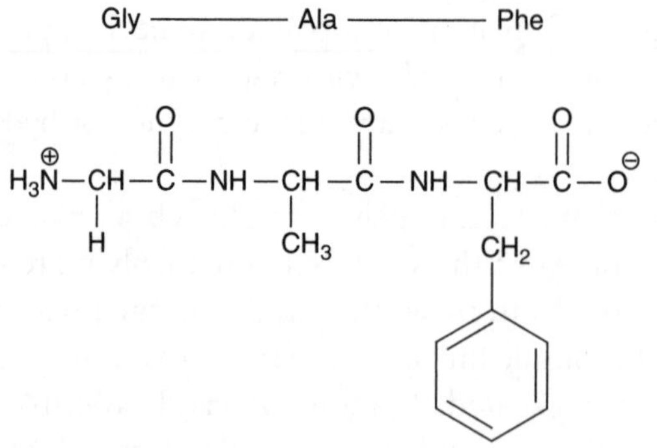

Gly —— Ala —— Phe

$H_3\overset{\oplus}{N}-CH(H)-C(=O)-NH-CH(CH_3)-C(=O)-NH-CH(CH_2C_6H_5)-C(=O)-O^{\ominus}$

Figure 3-6 Two representations of a typical short peptide, the first using common three-letter abbreviations and the second showing detailed atomic structure.

Cys–Tyr–Ile–Gln–Asn–Cys–Pro–Leu–Gly(NH_2) (S—S bridge between the two Cys residues)

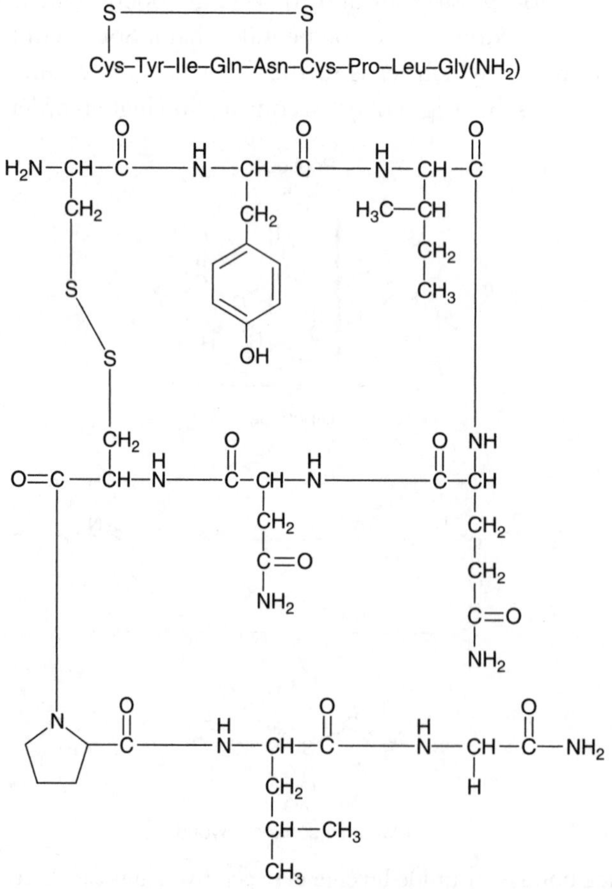

Figure 3-7 The peptide oxytocin has nine amino acids and a disulfide bridge. At this point, a detailed atomic structure becomes cumbersome and the compactness of the three-letter abbreviation system is an advantage.

the C-terminal glycine residue's carboxylate is modified to an amide instead—hence the special (NH_2) notation on this residue.

Amino acids are polymerized into polypeptides by ribosomes, which are complicated multisubunit assemblies of proteins and nucleic acids. The biosynthesis of polypeptides is discussed in depth in Chapter 16.

Protein Classification

Proteins may be classified by their structure. There are two major structural classes: globular and fibrous.

- Globular proteins have an overall spherical shape and are usually folded into a compact mass.
- Some are soluble in the aqueous cytosol, whereas others are embedded or otherwise closely associated with biomembranes.
- Examples of globular proteins are antibodies, many enzymes, and serum components such as albumin.
- Fibrous proteins tend to have an extended conformation, not spherical.
- Fibrous proteins are generally much less water soluble than globular proteins. Because of this lack of aqueous solubility, fibrous proteins are often found as aggregates.
- Examples of fibrous proteins include keratin, collagen, and silk fibroin.

Proteins may also be classified by their biological function. Following is a list of such functions with selected examples:

- Mechanical support and cushioning: collagen, elastin
- Mechanical work: actin, myosin, tubulin
- Catalysis: enzymes such as ribonuclease, hexokinase, DNA polymerase
- Transport and storage: hemoglobin, myoglobin, serum albumin
- Communication and defense: antibodies, peptide hormones, hormone and neurotransmitter receptors

Secondary and Higher-Order Structures

The *primary structure* of a macromolecule such as a protein or nucleic acid refers to the sequence of covalently bonded residues along the main chain of the polymer. Thus the sequence of amino acids in a polypeptide chains determines its primary structure. The *secondary structure*—the next higher level of macromolecular structure—refers to a regular spatial arrangement of the atoms along the chain backbone. The secondary structure is stabilized by weak, noncovalent interactions such as hydrogen bonds, hydrophobic interactions, and electrostatic attractions. Restriction of rotations about bonds in the covalently linked backbone limits the number of conformations a polypeptide chain can adopt, and for polypeptide chains there are two principal secondary structures, the α-helix and the β-sheet. Tertiary and quaternary levels of structure refer to yet higher levels of organization of polypeptide chains.

Secondary Structure

The α-Helix

The α-*helix* is formed from a single strand of polypeptide. It is stabilized by a characteristic pattern of hydrogen bonding of the carbonyl of one amide to the NH of another amide, four residues farther along the chain. **Figure 3-8** shows both a ball-and-stick model of a peptide

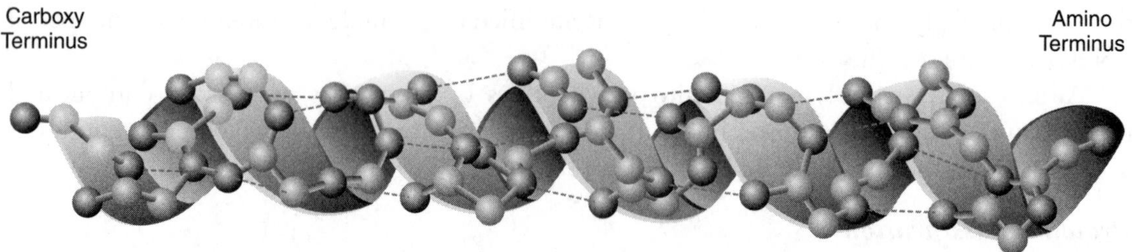

Figure 3-8 Hydrogen bonding in a polypeptide to form an α-helix, in a combined ball-and-stick/ribbon representation. The helical ribbon traces out the course of the polypeptide backbone. Hydrogen bonds are represented by dashed lines, joining the carbonyl of residue i to the NH group of residue $i + 4$. Side chains are not shown.

and a ribbon cartoon that traces the (idealized) curve of the polypeptide backbone. Dashed lines indicate the pattern of hydrogen bonding. These hydrogen bonds all point roughly in the same direction, parallel to the axis of the helix. All of the backbone carbonyl and NH residues are hydrogen bonded, except those near the ends of the helix.

The polypeptide backbone curls in space in a right-handed helix, the α-helix. (A left-handed helix is possible but disfavored because of potential steric interference between the polypeptide backbone and side chain groups.) There are 3.6 residues per turn of the helix, with one turn of the helix rising by 5.4 Å (a rise per residue of 1.5 Å). Because of the 1-to-4 pattern of hydrogen bonding, the helix brings close together residues along the chain that otherwise would be widely separated in space. Moreover, neighboring residues end up on opposite sides of the helix.

The side chains of the amino acids are exposed and project laterally away from axis of helix (not shown in Figure 3-8). All 20 of the common amino acids can fit into an α-helix, but some are found in α-helices more frequently than others. For example, Pro cannot participate in the normal hydrogen-bonding scheme and cannot rotate around the $N — C_\alpha$ bond; this will cause the helix to kink or bend at that point, so Pro is disfavored for inclusion in an α-helix. Gly residues lack a side chain and have considerably greater conformational freedom than the other amino acids; they have a much stronger tendency to form coiled structures and are also disfavored for inclusion in an α-helix. In contrast, some residues, such as alanine, have a high tendency to adopt the α-helical conformation. This is also true of other amino acids with nonpolar or bulky side chains, although (to avoid clashes between side chains) such residues are less likely to be nearest neighbors in the primary structure. Also, amino acids with oppositely charged side chains tend to be found three residues apart, such that the twist of the helix brings together their opposite charges for strong favorable interactions.

The β-Sheet

The β-*sheet* structure is formed from two or more strands of amino acids. The strands are extended, and there is a roughly coplanar alignment of backbone atoms across the strands. Like the α-helix, the β-sheet uses hydrogen bonding between backbone carbonyl and amino groups on the strands. However, the hydrogen bonds are not in the 1-to-4 pattern of the α-helix, but instead go across the strands, at right angles to the general direction of the component strands. **Figure 3-9** illustrates hydrogen bonding and two senses of direction possible for adjacent strands: aligned parallel to one another or in an antiparallel orientation.

The "sheet" description is taken from the coplanarity of the backbone atoms for the participating strands. A "pleated sheet" describes the pattern of alternation of C_α atoms above and below the plane of the sheet. In real proteins, the sheets generally are not precisely planar,

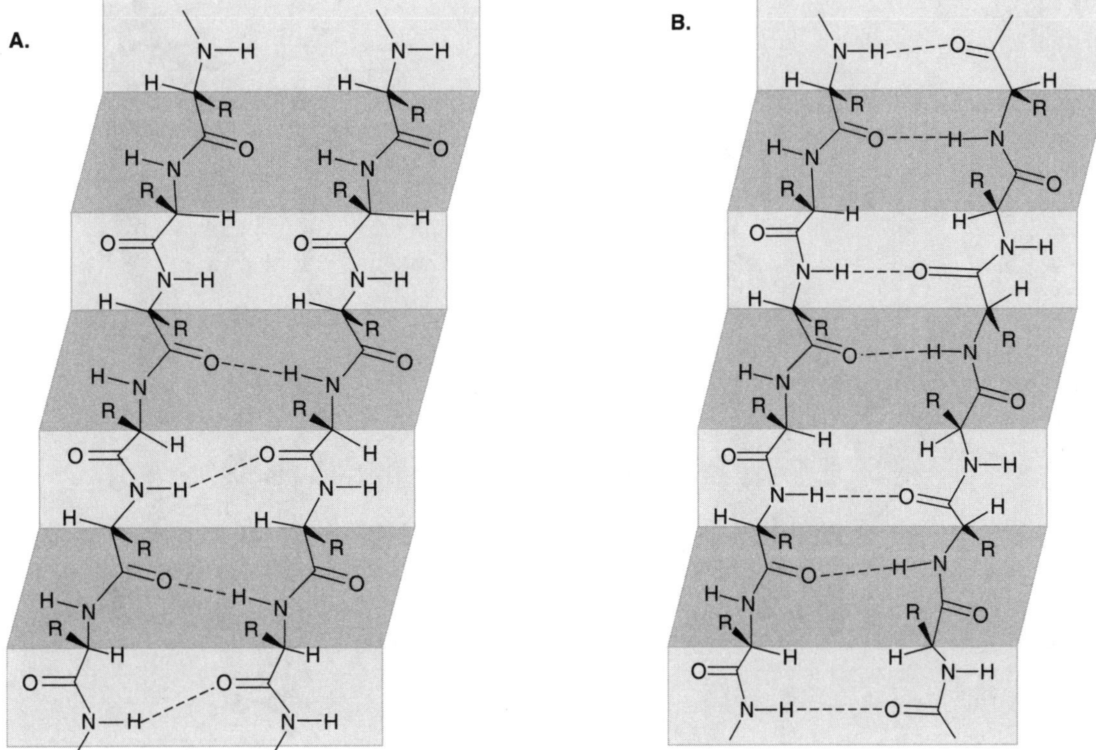

Figure 3-9 Hydrogen bonding in β-sheet structures, emphasizing the "pleating" induced by the planarity of the peptide linkages. **A.** Parallel strands. **B.** Antiparallel strands.

but instead tend to have a right-handed twist. The side chains of the constituent amino acids project above and below the plane of the sheet. **Figure 3-10** uses structures from real proteins and superimposes the common ribbon representation of the sense of direction for the backbone onto the conventional ball-and-stick atomic representation for the two types of β-sheets.

The β-Turn

A high proportion of residues in tightly folded proteins are involved in turns of the backbone. These turns may flexible loops of a few amino acids, serving to join different stretches of secondary structure, or they may be quite sharp turns that reverse the chain direction. One common structural element found in connection with antiparallel β-sheet structures is the β-*turn*. A few variations on this type of turn exist; **Figure 3-11** shows the two most common ones in which residue i is hydrogen-bonded to residue $i + 3$. This structure uses four amino acids to effect a 180° turn in chain direction. Gly and Pro are often found in β-turns, with Gly contributing its conformational flexibility to the turn, and Pro adopting a *cis* conformation to tighten the turn.

Tertiary Structure

The *tertiary structure* of a macromolecule refers to a larger-scale organization of the polymer chain than is seen at the level of the secondary structure. For proteins, this arrangement includes how elements of the secondary structure are linked to and packed against one another. The tertiary structure is stabilized principally by noncovalent interactions, although the covalent linkages provided by disulfide bonds between cysteine residues can be an important factor

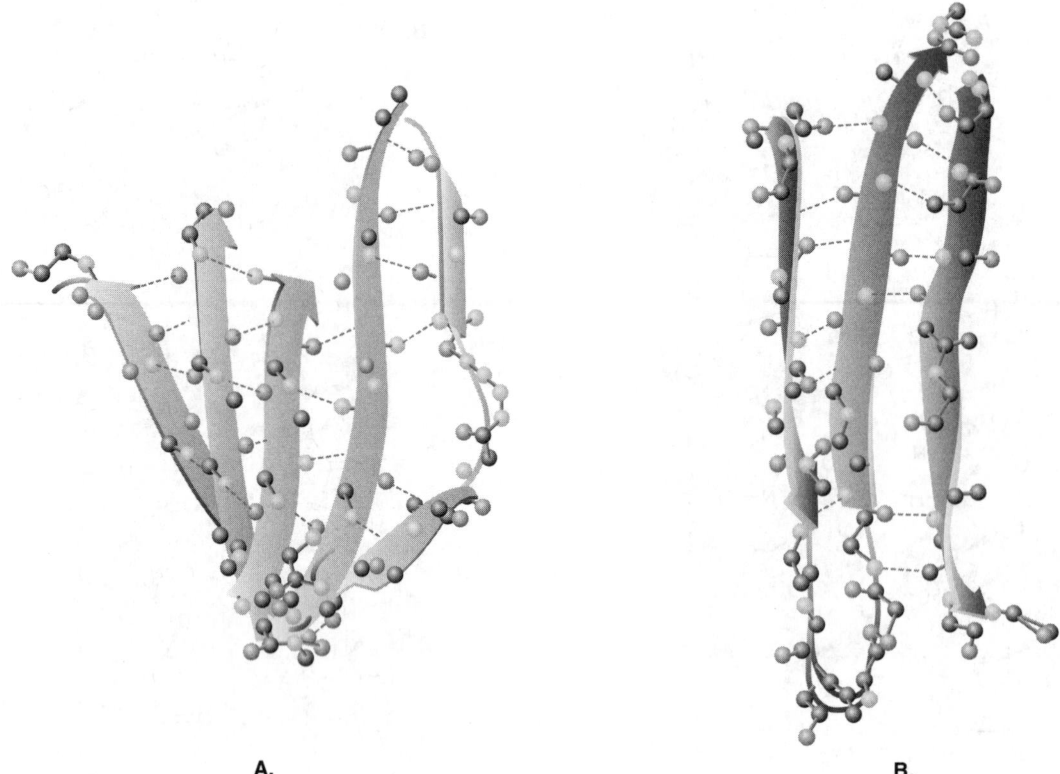

Figure 3-10 Combined ball-and-stick/ribbon representation of β-sheet structures found in actual proteins. The ribbons trace out the course of the polypeptide backbone. Note the curvature of the ribbons; real β-sheet structures are rarely perfectly flat. **A.** Parallel β-sheet (from flavodoxin, PDB entry 3KAP). **B.** Antiparallel β-sheet (from superoxide dismutase, PDB entry 1CB4).

as well. Two main types of proteins, *fibrous* and *globular*, can be distinguished by their tertiary structures as well as by certain chemical properties.

Different proteins may share a common packing scheme or folding pattern for two or more secondary structural elements. Such a folding pattern is called a *motif*. A motif may be a small region of the protein, or it may dominate the overall packing and folding of a relatively large region. Motifs are usually formed from adjacent chain segments, rather than from segments that are distant from each other along the polypeptide backbone. Generally, motifs are not independently stable. If isolated from the rest of the protein structure, they tend to unfold. Several structural motifs are shown in **Figure 3-12.**

Fibrous Proteins

Fibrous proteins tend to have extended tertiary conformations, which well suit their roles in mechanical support and flexibility in tissues. Collagen is a typical fibrous protein, with many subtypes, that is involved in skin structure and in connective tissue. It has a high proportion of Gly, Ala, Pro, and hydroxyproline residues in its polypeptide chains. Collagen has a distinctive secondary structure, that of a triple helix.

- The chains are arranged in a right-handed triple-stranded helix, which is quite distinct from the α-helix (**Figure 3-13**).

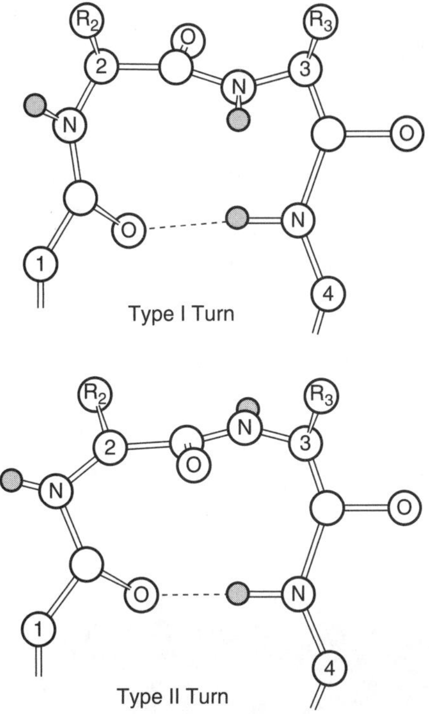

Figure 3-11 The two main types of β-turns, in a ball-and-stick representation. The carbonyl oxygen of the first amino acid is hydrogen-bonded to the amide NH of the third amino acid. The numbers indicate the α-carbon atoms of the four amino acids involved in the β-turn; the relative positions of the side-chain groups R2 and R3 are shown for two of these carbons.

- The primary structure of these strands is also unusual, containing many repeating tripeptide units that have the sequence Gly-X-Y, where X is typically Pro and Y is typically hydroxyproline. The absence of a bulky side chain on Gly permits the backbones of the three chains to be packed close together.
- The restricted conformations of the Pro and hydroxyproline residues lead to sharp turns in the polypeptide backbone.
- Together, the repeating tripeptide units help wind the three strands into a rodlike bundle. This bundle is quite resistant to mechanical extension (i.e., it has great tensile strength).
- In connective tissue, collagen triple helices are packed together into fibrils, which are then cross-linked by covalent bonds between Lys residues and hydroxyprolines or prolines. The result is a very stable and strong pad of connective tissue.

The collagen triple helix is also found as a structural element in many other proteins, particularly those of the complement system of proteins in the immune system. The characteristic rodlike structure may participate in higher-order structures in these proteins, and it may serve as a distinct, recognizable feature for interaction with other proteins.

Another typical fibrous protein is keratin (not to be confused with the polysaccharide keratan sulfate). Keratin is used to build hair, nails, and claws, and it also stiffens and supports the skin; its secondary and tertiary structures contribute directly to the necessary mechanical properties for these uses. Keratin has a high proportion of a characteristic structure (a structural motif) called a *coiled coil*.

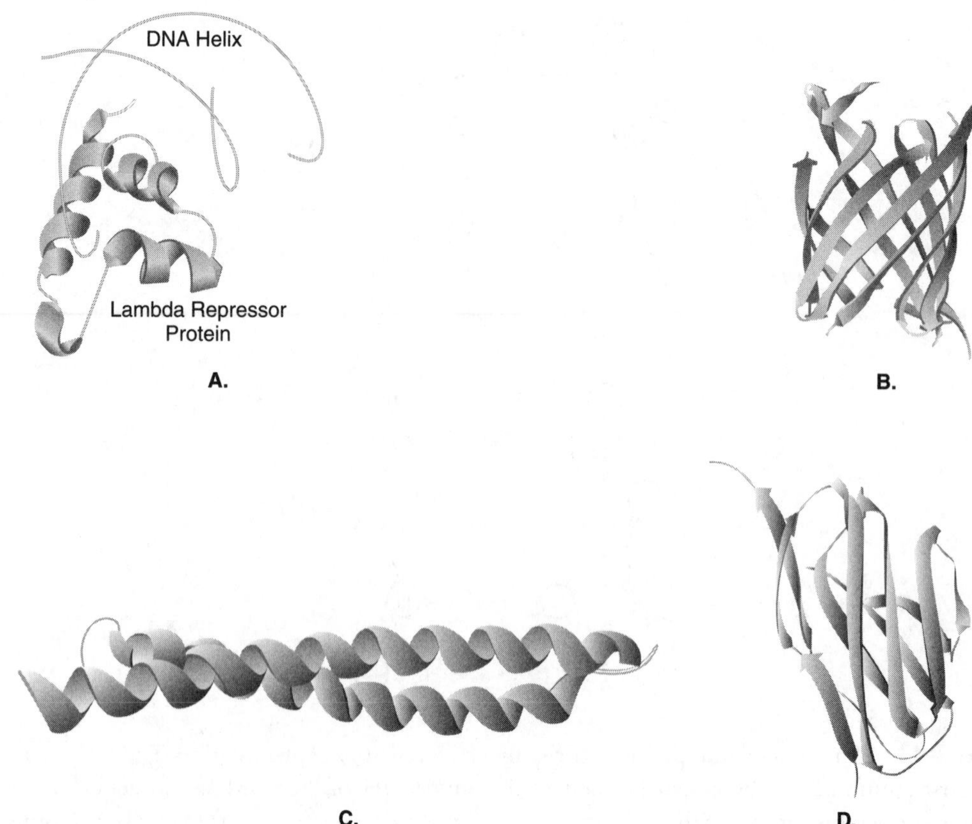

Figure 3-12 Four structural motifs in protein folding, using ribbon representations. **A.** Helix–turn–helix motif of α-helices in the lambda repressor protein (from PDB entry 1LMB; DNA helix is sketched as a coil). **B.** β-Barrel in the green fluorescent protein of the jellyfish *Aequorea victoria* (from PDB entry 1EMA). **C.** Coiled coil motif of α-helices in apolipoprotein E (from PDB entry 1LPE). **D.** Two plies of the β-sheet in the VL chain domain of immunoglobulin G (immunoglobulin fold; PDB entry 1IGT).

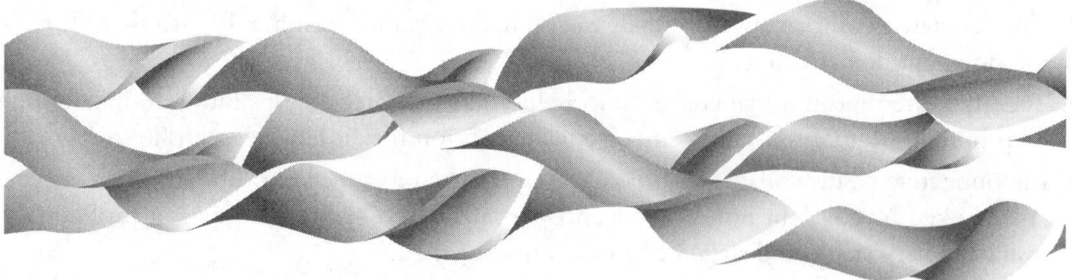

Figure 3-13 Collagen triple helix (from PDB entry 1CGD). Polypeptide backbones are traced as a coil.

- The coiled coil is built from α-helices, with the α-helices being wound around each other in a left-handed helix (recall that the α-helix is itself a right-handed helix). Characteristically a coiled coil involves two polypeptide strands, as found in keratin; three- and four-stranded structures have been found in other proteins. See Figure 3-12, panel C.
- The left-handed, low-angle twist of the strands around each other permits interlocking of side chains, typically with a nonpolar side chain inserted into a cavity formed from the side chains of four residues on the other strand. Winding of the α-helices around each other

promotes rigidity and strength in this tertiary structure, just as winding the strands of a rope make it stronger.

Further strengthening is gained through the occasional disulfide cross-links between the strands.

Globular Proteins

As the name implies, globular proteins are roughly spherical in shape. The surfaces of such proteins, however, may be relatively rough, not smooth, with ridges and valleys, some of which may be quite deep (this is often a characteristic of enzymes and their catalytic sites, for example). Amino acids with nonpolar side chains generally are found to populate the interior of the protein. In contrast, amino acids with polar and ionic side chains predominate on the protein's surface. In this way, the polar and ionic side chains help to solvate the protein, while the nonpolar, hydrophobic side chains are kept buried away from contact with water.

Globular proteins are generally compactly folded and have very little vacant space in their interiors. A single, properly folded polypeptide strand may have several α-helices and/or several β-sheets, tightly packed together to form the overall globular shape. The regularity in packing the secondary structural elements is what is meant by tertiary structure in these proteins. Turns in the backbone (as in β-sheet structures) tend to be found on or near the surface of the protein; flexible loops of polypeptide strands connecting different secondary structures also tend to be located on the protein's surface.

A large protein may contain two or more regions of the polypeptide chain that individually have a compact folded structure, called *domains* (**Figure 3-14**). Like motifs, domains are composed of secondary structural elements; also like motifs, they are formed from neighboring segments of the polypeptide chain. Domains differ from motifs in being more stable (they may fold as independent units).

Quaternary Structure

Many proteins are built up with subunits, or independently folded polypeptide chains that fit together with complementary surfaces. *Quaternary structure* refers to this multisubunit structure; the term may also refer to the association of protein chains with nucleic acids, as in ribosomes or nucleosomes. The subunits may be identical or nonidentical polypeptide chains; if identical, the subunits may be called monomers. The simplest quaternary structure is a dimer, but more complicated assemblages are common (**Figure 3-15**). A familiar example is that of hemoglobin, which has four subunits of two different types (α and β). These form a tetramer with the stoichiometry $\alpha_2\beta_2$, with a roughly tetrahedral shape overall. Subunits may be arranged in symmetric patterns, especially if the subunits are identical. Extended filamentous structures, composed of hundreds of monomer units, are also possible, as in the protein tubulin.

Flexibility of the Polypeptide Chain

Unfolded polypeptide chains are quite flexible. For all of the common amino acids except Pro, it is relatively easy to rotate around the $N—C_\alpha$ and C_α—carbonyl bonds, so the backbone can adopt many different conformations. Additionally, multiple rotational conformations are possible for each of the side chains. Larger structural changes that are short of unfolding are also feasible. Even when the polypeptide chain is folded into its final tertiary structure, there is still a great deal of rapid, local fluctuation in atomic positions within the protein. These variations can range from individual amino acids moving against their neighbors, to motions of entire domains sliding and rotating past one another.

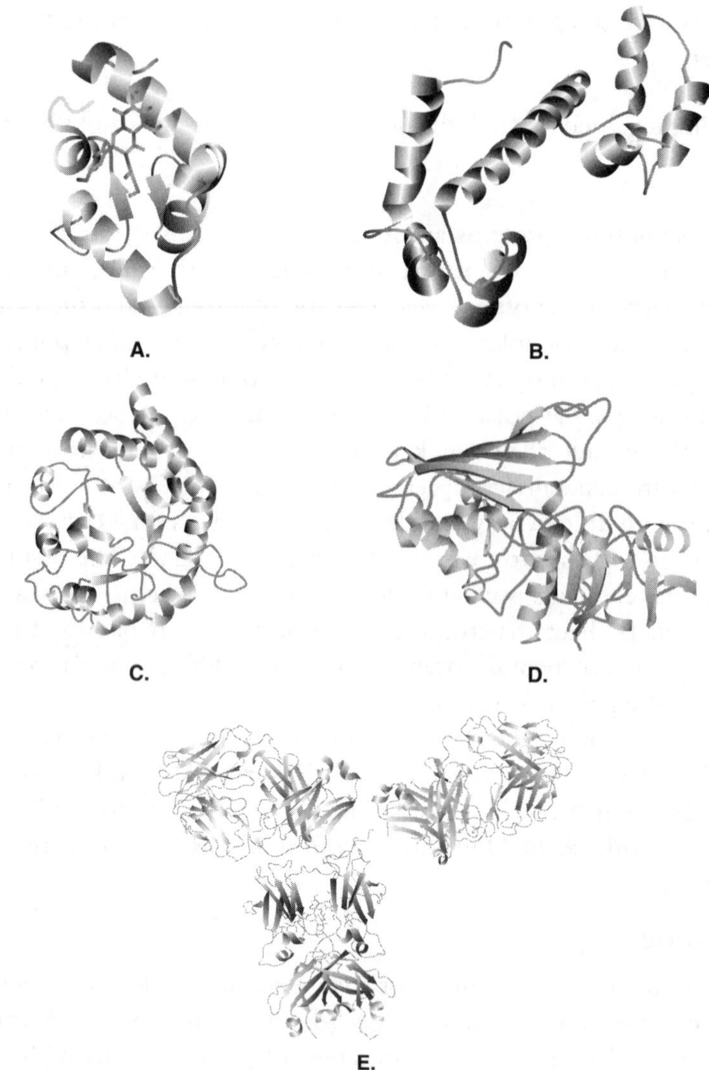

Figure 3-14 Examples of protein domains. **A.** Troponin C α-helices (PDB entry 4TNC). **B.** Calmodulin α-helices and calcium ion binding domains (PDB entry 1CLL). **C.** β-Barrel in triose phosphate isomerase (PDB entry 2JK2). **D.** Nicotinamide binding site in glyceraldehyde-3-phosphate dehydrogenase (PDB entry 3E5R). **E.** Immunoglobulin folds in immunoglobulin G (PDB entry 1IGT).

- Rotation of methyl groups on these side chains will occur on the picosecond (10^{-12} sec) time scale.
- Segments of the polypeptide backbone will twist and flex over a few tenths of a nanometer, with frequencies on the order of 10^9 to 10^{10} sec^{-1}.
- Larger-scale motions, involving whole domains or polypeptide chains, are also possible, and they can be very important in the functioning of the protein.

The large-scale motions may be slow, taking seconds to occur, or they may be very fast, taking as little as a few hundredths of a nanosecond (10^{-9} sec). They can involve quite substantial displacements of whole domains. For example, during activation of the multisubunit enzyme aspartate transcarbamoylase, the whole enzyme expands by approximately 11 Å, with rotations

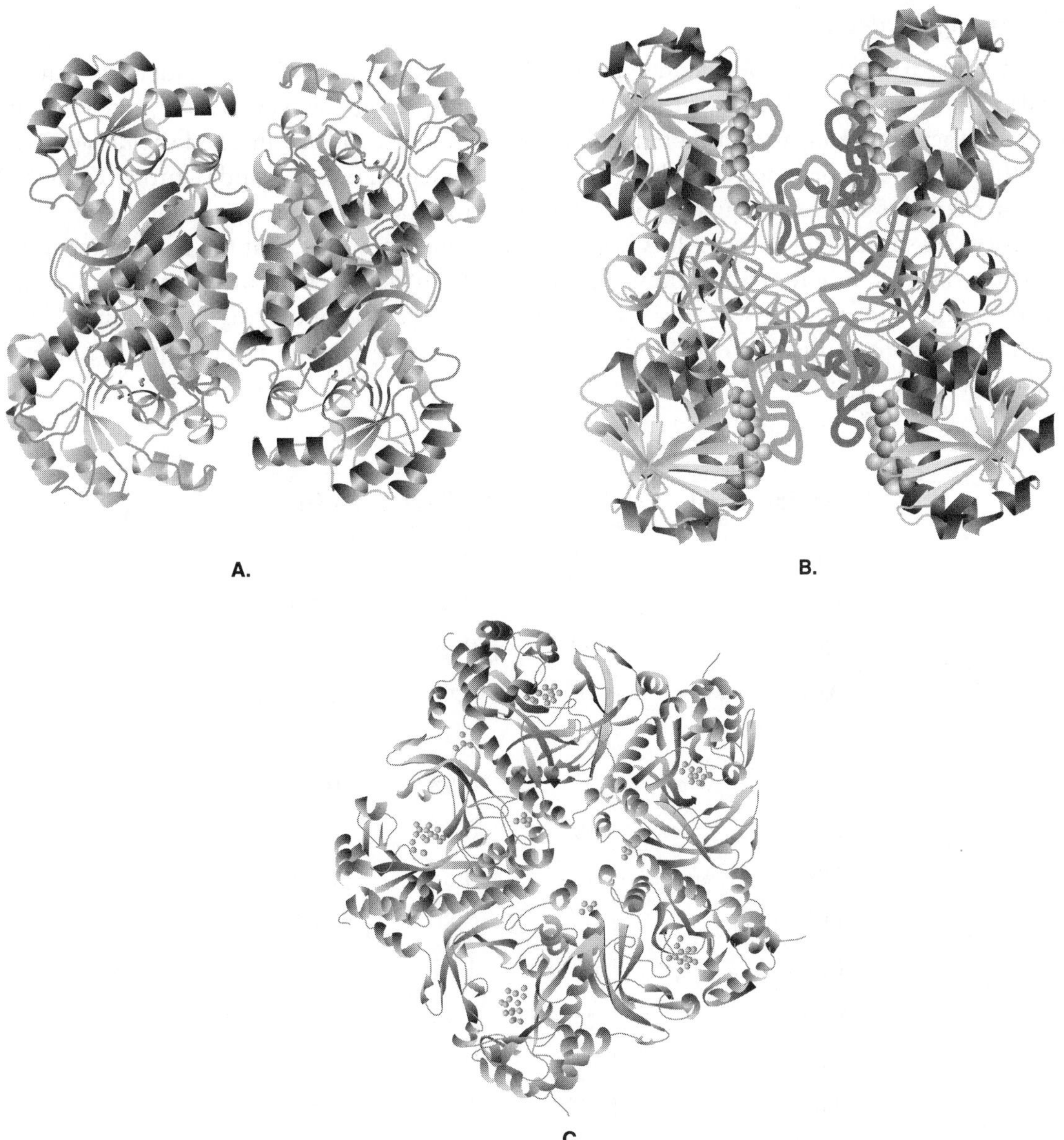

Figure 3-15 Examples of multimeric proteins, using ribbon representations. **A.** Hemoglobin, a tetramer of two kinds of subunits, α and β, with the stoichiometry $\alpha_2\beta_2$ (PDB entry 2HHB). **B.** Glyceraldehyde-3-phosphate dehydrogenase, a tetramer of 4 identical subunits (PDB entry 3E5R). **C.** Glutamine synthetase (human; PDB entry 2OJW), a pentamer of identical subunits.

of subunits of 10° to 15°. Many enzymes and related proteins contain two major domains or lobes, connected by a flexible "hinge" region, that form a binding site for a small molecule. In these proteins, recognition and binding of the proper small molecule typically involves movement of the two lobes together; in some cases this closure can cause shifts in the two lobes of up to 35°. The changed conformation is still well organized, however, with a recognizable structure. Such changes in conformation can be important in the functioning of a protein, and will be further discussed in Chapter 6, where we take up the concepts of allosterism and cooperativity.

Folding of Proteins

The folding pattern of a polypeptide chain is determined primarily by its sequence of amino acids. Certain amino acids have a greater propensity for forming one type of secondary structure over another; this tendency was noted earlier for the α-helix and alanine, and the *collagen helix* and the Gly-X-Y tripeptide, but it also holds for preferences in β-sheets and β-turns. **Table 3-3** summarizes the relative frequency of occurrence for the 20 common amino acids across α-helices, β-sheets, and β-turns. It is important to realize, however, that the local polypeptide sequence is not the only factor in how a protein folds. In fact, packing of secondary structural elements into the tertiary structure can bring into contact amino acids from quite widely separated regions of the sequence, and these contacts may be highly important in stabilizing the tertiary structure.

Amino Acid	α-Helix	β-Sheet	β-Turn
Ala	1.41	0.72	0.82
Arg	1.21	0.84	0.90
Asp	0.99	0.39	1.24
Asn	0.76	0.48	1.34
Cys	0.66	1.40	0.54
Gln	1.27	0.98	0.84
Glu	1.59	0.52	1.01
Gly	0.43	0.58	1.77
His	1.05	0.80	0.81
Ile	1.09	1.67	0.47
Leu	1.34	1.22	0.57
Lys	1.23	0.69	1.07
Met	1.30	1.14	0.52
Phe	1.16	1.33	0.59
Pro	0.34	0.31	1.32
Ser	0.57	0.96	1.22
Thr	0.76	1.17	0.90
Trp	1.02	1.35	0.65
Tyr	0.74	1.45	0.76
Val	0.98	1.87	0.41

Table 3-3 Relative Frequencies of Occurrence of Amino Acids in Elements of Protein Secondary Structure

Tabulated values are the frequencies of finding the specified residue in the specified conformation, divided by the average frequency of residues in that conformation.

Source: Data from R.W. Williams, A. Chang, D. Juretic, and S. Loughran. (1987). "Secondary structure predictions and medium range interactions," *Biochim. Biophys. Acta* 916:200–204.

The folding of proteins is nonrandom and proceeds through intermediates, first with accumulation of secondary structures, then with tertiary structures. For some proteins, this process may be preceded by a general collapse of the extended, unfolded polypeptide chain into a more compact globular structure with much hydrophobic interaction between side-chain residues. This *molten globule* then accumulates secondary and tertiary structural elements and finally achieves the full tertiary structure. In general, folding in the cell is rapid, occurring within seconds in vivo.

Protein folding, particularly for large proteins with complicated folding patterns, is often assisted by *chaperone proteins*. The chaperones are large multisubunit complexes that perform several roles in connection with protein folding:

- They assist newly synthesized chains to fold properly.
- They aid in the movement of proteins across membranes to target organelles or for secretion to the cell's exterior.
- They help misfolded proteins to unfold and refold correctly, particularly after heat shock or other stresses to the cell.
- They help to block the aggregation of misfolded proteins, and they assist in resolubilizing and refolding aggregated proteins.
- They assist in the assembly of multimeric protein structures.
- They are components of some signal transduction pathways in the cell.

It appears that these chaperones recognize and bind to misfolded proteins through exposed hydrophobic segments that would otherwise be buried in the protein's interior. The chaperones then promote correct refolding, in processes whose details are not yet well understood.

Two additional systems assist proteins in reaching the proper tertiary structure. These systems operate specifically on Cys and Pro residues.

- Proteins with multiple disulfide bridges have the potential for multiple mispairings of the contributing cysteine residues, which would likely block formation of the correct tertiary structure. The cell contains enzymes—namely, protein disulfide isomerases—that specialize in exchanging disulfide bond partners, so that the correct cysteine pairings and tertiary structure is achieved.
- Proline residues mostly have the *trans* geometry, but to facilitate formation of β-turns, the *cis* geometry is preferred (**Figure 3-16**). The cell contains proline isomerases that specifically isomerize proline residues from *trans* to *cis* geometry for this reason.

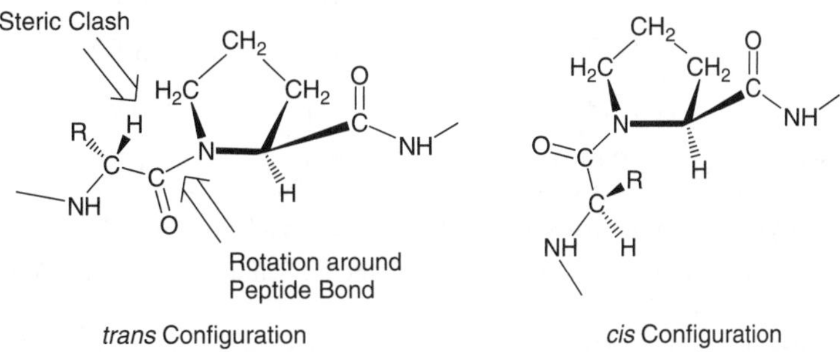

Figure 3-16 Proline: *trans* and *cis* isomers.

Protein Unfolding

Unfolding of a protein is called denaturation. It is not quite the reverse of folding. Unfolding is sometimes reversible for small proteins, but for large ones it tends to be irreversible. Disulfide bridges are often important in reestablishing the proper chain contacts and alignments for forming secondary structures and packing them together into the proper tertiary structure. Heat and reducing agents can "scramble" these linkages, making the transition irreversible. Some further characteristics of protein unfolding are outlined here:

- Denaturation results in loss of function for the protein, and may target it for destruction by cellular machinery (see the material on protein turnover later in this chapter).
- The unfolding process can be monitored spectroscopically by changes in protein absorbance or fluorescence, by heat absorption (calorimetry), or by changes in solution viscosity as the chain expands.
- Unfolding can be provoked by extremes of pH or temperature; also, certain solutes (e.g., urea, detergents, and organic solvents like methanol) can destabilize proteins and cause them to unfold. These solutes tend to disrupt the hydrophobic interactions in the interior of the folded protein, thereby destabilizing it.
- The unfolded form is not tightly packed but rather has an extended chain structure. Generally much more flexible, it leads to a loss of recognizable pattern for polypeptide backbone conformation.

The folded protein structure is only marginally stable. Free energy changes for denaturation at room temperature of some typical small globular proteins are summarized in **Table 3-4**. These values are scaled by the number of residues in the protein, but it is clear that on a per-residue basis, the values for ΔG are only slightly positive, at a few hundred J/mol. Values for larger globular proteins containing multiple domains tend to be similar because the domains often denature independently.

Even at room temperature, hydrogen bonds and other weak noncovalent interactions that stabilize the folded form of a protein transiently break and re-form. Such fluctuations can be important for the proper functioning of the protein. For example, these small conformational changes may allow it to bind small molecules securely, or to fit together with other proteins in larger assemblies.

Protein	Molecular Weight	ΔH (298 K)	ΔS (298 K)	ΔG (298 K)
Ribonuclease	13,600	2.37	6.70	0.37
Lysozyme	14,300	2.02	5.52	0.38
Myoglobin	17,900	0.04	−0.80	0.64
Carbonic anhydrase	29,000	0.80	1.76	0.28

Table 3-4 Thermodynamics of Denaturation of Selected Small Proteins

ΔH is in kJ per mole of amino acid residue; ΔS is in J/K per mole of amino acid residue; ΔG is in kJ per mole of amino acid residue.

Source: Data from P. L. Privalov and S. J. Gill. (1988). "Stability of protein structure and hydrophobic interaction," *Adv. Protein Chem.* 39:101–234.

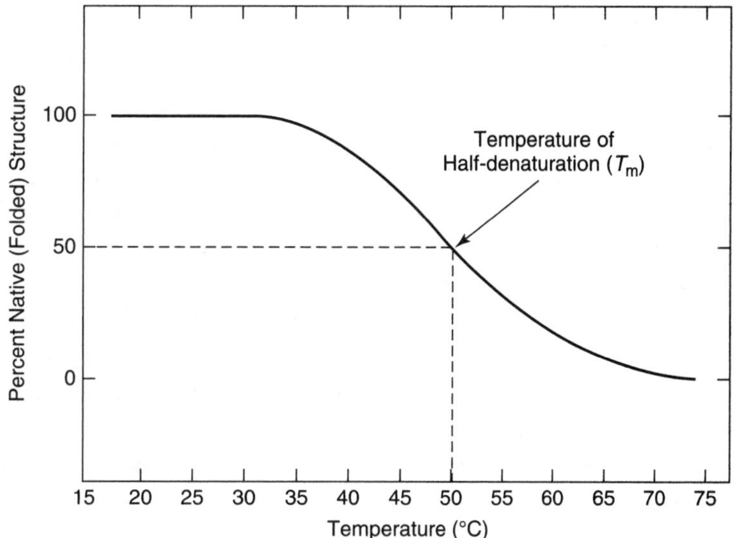

Figure 3-17 Thermal denaturation of a protein. The temperature of the midpoint of the transition from native to unfolded conformation is denoted as the T_m.

Raising the temperature causes more thermal fluctutations in a protein's structure as more of these weak interactions are disrupted. Finally, a critical loss of stability occurs when there is sufficient weakening of the structure; with only a slight further rise in temperature, first the tertiary structure and then the secondary structure of the protein are lost. This loss of structure resembles that occurring in a solid-to-liquid phase transition, like the melting of ice into liquid water; it can be loosely described as "melting" the protein. It can be monitored using a variety of techniques, such as changes in optical absorbance or fluorescence, or changes in solution viscosity (**Figure 3-17**). A similar order-to-disorder transition is seen with nucleic acids and their secondary structure; see Chapter 4.

Protein Turnover

Protein *turnover* is the process of recycling proteins into their constituent amino acids, for reuse by the cell. Turnover is necessary for many reasons:

- To eliminate misfolded or damaged proteins before they aggregate and interfere with cell processes
- To regulate the cell cycle by breaking down in a timely fashion proteins used transiently during the cell cycle
- In the immune system, to provide the necessary cleavage of foreign antigenic proteins for presentation to and recognition by other immune system cells

A polypeptide chain is kinetically stable but thermodynamically unstable; thus digestive enzymes generally do not need any exogenous energy source to break down polypeptides into the constituent amino acids. However, this process must be controlled because uncontrolled proteolysis would be dangerous to the cell.

Two main systems are used for protein degradation in mammalian cells: the lysosomal system (involving specialized cellular vesicles called lysosomes and associated transport systems) and a ubiquitous, cytosolic system involving a polypeptide called *ubiquitin* and a multisubunit enzyme assembly, the *proteasome*.

The Lysosomal System

Lysosomes are membrane-bound cytoplasmic organelles that form the major degradative compartment in the cell. The lysosomal system is responsible for the nonspecific degradation of organelles (especially damaged organelles), selective degradation of cellular proteins, and the breakdown of "foreign" materials that the cell contacts. These substances include proteins, nucleic acids, and even whole bacteria that have been taken in or that have invaded the cell. Materials may reach the lysosome through several principal routes: endocytosis, autophagy, and chaperone-mediated autophagy. These processes are described in Chapter 5.

Lysosomes are extremely acidic, with a pH in the range 3.8–5.0, which promotes denaturation of proteins and nucleic acids. Lysosomes also contain numerous hydrolytic enzymes that operate under these acidic conditions to break open bacterial cells, digest lipids, and break down the backbone bonds in the protein and nucleic acid polymers, reducing them to their constituent amino acids and nucleic acid. These building-block molecules can then be passed out of the lysosome for recycling by the cell.

The Ubiquitin/Proteasome System

The ubiquitin/proteasome system is mainly responsible for turnover of the cell's own proteins, but it also contributes to the breakdown of foreign proteins. *Ubiquitin* (Ub) is a 76-residue polypeptide that can be linked to other proteins to mark them for degradation. This linkage occurs through a special amide bond, an isopeptide bond, using the C-terminal Gly residue of Ub and the ε-amino group of a Lys in the target protein (**Figure 3-18**). The linkage process is tightly controlled:

- Ub is first activated for this conjugation by an enzyme that couples ATP hydrolysis to formation of a thioester bond of the C-terminal Lys of Ub and the thiol on the side chain of a key Cys residue on the enzyme.

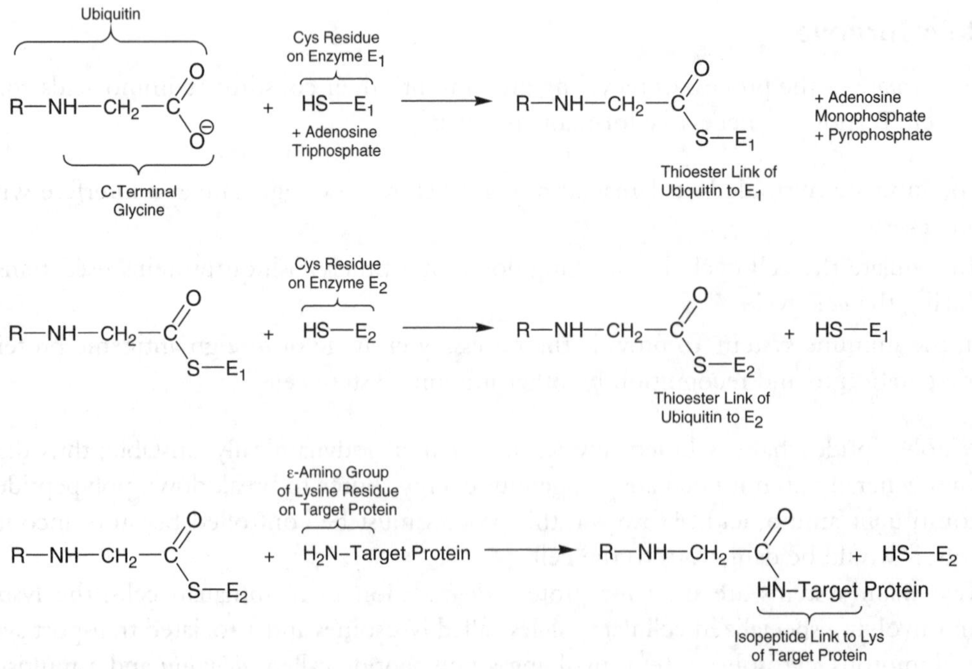

$$R{-}NH{-}CH_2{-}C({=}O)O^{\ominus} + HS{-}E_1 \xrightarrow{+\text{ Adenosine Triphosphate}} R{-}NH{-}CH_2{-}C({=}O){-}S{-}E_1 + \text{Adenosine Monophosphate} + \text{Pyrophosphate}$$

Ubiquitin; C-Terminal Glycine; Cys Residue on Enzyme E_1; Thioester Link of Ubiquitin to E_1

$$R{-}NH{-}CH_2{-}C({=}O){-}S{-}E_1 + HS{-}E_2 \longrightarrow R{-}NH{-}CH_2{-}C({=}O){-}S{-}E_2 + HS{-}E_1$$

Cys Residue on Enzyme E_2; Thioester Link of Ubiquitin to E_2

$$R{-}NH{-}CH_2{-}C({=}O){-}S{-}E_2 + H_2N{-}\text{Target Protein} \longrightarrow R{-}NH{-}CH_2{-}C({=}O){-}HN{-}\text{Target Protein} + HS{-}E_2$$

ε-Amino Group of Lysine Residue on Target Protein; Isopeptide Link to Lys of Target Protein

Figure 3-18 Forming an isopeptide linkage of ubiquitin to the ε-amino group of a lysine on a protein, marking the protein for degradation.

- The Ub group is then transferred to a second enzyme, again using a cysteine residue on that protein.
- In a third step, the Ub group is transferred to the target protein in a reaction catalyzed by yet another enzyme.

The target proteins may receive one or several Ub moieties attached to them. Also, chains of Ub moieties may be attached to a single Lys on the target. The target is recognized for marking with Ub through certain characteristic amino acid sequences, of which several exist. Some require modification (e.g., by phosphorylation) or interaction with other proteins before they are recognized by the ubiquitin system.

Proteins with multiple Ub groups are recognized by the *proteasome*, the second major component of this degradation system. The proteasome is a very large, multisubunit protein assembly that degrades protein chains into short oligopeptides. ATP is used in the unfolding process, but the details of its participation are not yet clear.

Overall the proteasome has a cylindrical shape, with one or two protein caps on the ends of the cylinder. The central cylinder is composed of a stack of four rings, as shown in **Figure 3-19**. Each ring has seven subunits, either α or β (actually, the β subunits are not completely identical to one another, and differ slightly in their amino acid sequences). The caps serve as regulatory units and are thought to help unfold Ub-marked proteins. The central cylinder of the proteasome contains a hollow central chamber, in which multiple proteolytic activities take place that are associated with the β subunits. A targeted polypeptide chain enters through the end of the cylinder past the cap; the cap drives the chain into an extended unfolded conformation, with exposed amides that can be attacked by enzymes in the central chamber of the proteasome. This attack results in cleavage of the polypeptide into oligopeptides of various sizes; the majority are short chains containing seven to eight amino acids. These oligopeptides leave the chamber and enter the cytosol, for further breakdown and recycling of the amino acids.

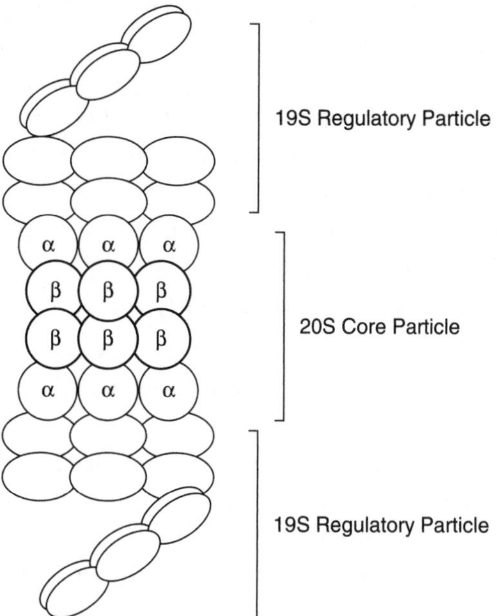

Figure 3-19 The 26S proteasome, showing 19S regulatory units attached to a central 20S cylindrical core. (19S, 20S, and 26S refer to the sedimentation coefficient, a measure of how rapidly a particle is separated via sedimentation in a centrifuge; the sedimentation coefficient increases with the molecular mass of the particle but decreases with frictional resistance or buoyancy of the particle.)

QUESTIONS FOR DISCUSSION

1. Classify hydroxyproline, hydroxylysine, selenocysteine, and ornithine into one or another of the nine classes listed in Table 3-2 for the 20 common amino acids. Explain your reasoning.
2. How would the pK_a of a lysine side-chain amino group shift if the group were surrounded by nonpolar groups? What would happen if the amino group were next to an ionized carboxylic acid?
3. The proteolytic hydrolysis in vivo of peptides containing only the D-isomers of the constituent amino acids is greatly reduced compared to the hydrolysis of the same peptides that contain only the L-isomers. Why?
4. The industrial polymer "nylon-11" is polymerized 11-aminoundecanoic acid. This polymer resists swelling when exposed to water, and resists degradation by hydrocarbons. It is used in natural gas pipelines and in fuel tanks. What is the structure of the polymer? What is the basis for its high resistance to water and to hydrocarbons?
5. Residues with aromatic side chains are often found to be separated by three residues in an α-helix. Why?
6. The cosmetic treatment of "permanent" waves in hair depends on some chemistry involving the disulfide linkages in keratin α-helices. The first step in getting a "perm" involves stretching the hair while it is moist and heated; this will tend to unravel the α-helices in the keratin and bend the hair into the desired shape. The hair is then treated with a reducing agent, typically under alkaline conditions, for a brief period, while maintaining the tension. Then a neutralizing and mildly oxidizing solution is applied, which is rinsed away, leaving the hair with the desired curl. Which residues in keratin would likely be affected by reducing or oxidizing agents? (Hint: Think about disulfide linkages.) Would the "perm" work if the order of treatment were reversed? Why or why not?
7. The enzyme lactate dehydrogenase has four subunits of identical or nearly identical proteins. Two different genes code for these protein subunits; the two types of subunits that result (call them type H and type M) differ slightly in their properties, but each readily associates with the other subunit type. How many different types of tetramers will this lead to? What are their subunit stoichiometries?
8. How would an isopeptidase (cleaving ubiquitin from ubiquitylated proteins) help to stabilize proteins that otherwise might experience rapid turnover in the cell?
9. Proline has a low frequency of occurrence in β-sheets. Why?
10. What would be the effect of replacement of Gly residues in collagen by bulkier amino acids such as Glu or Trp? Also, which substitution would be less destabilizing, Ala or Val? Ala or Asp?
11. Table 3-4 reports the ΔG, ΔH, and ΔS values for denaturation per residue, for several proteins. Ribonuclease has 124 amino acid residues. Calculate ΔG, ΔH, and ΔS for denaturation of the entire protein, at 298 K. Is the overall free energy change for denaturation of this protein dominated by enthalpy or entropy changes? If ΔH and ΔS remained constant as the temperature rose, at what temperature would the free energy of denaturation go to zero?

REFERENCES

T. E. Creighton. (1993). *Protein Structure and Molecular Properties*, 2nd ed., W. H. Freeman, New York.

N. J. Darby and T. E. Creighton. (1993). *Protein Structure*, IRL Press, Oxford, UK.

E. S. Kempner. (1993). "Movable lobes and flexible loops in proteins," *FEBS Lett.* 326:4–10.

J. S. Richardson. (1981). "The anatomy and taxonomy of protein structure," *Adv. Protein Chem.* 34:167–339.

A. Varshavsky. (1997). "The ubiquitin system," *Trends Biochem. Sci.* 22:383–387.

CHAPTER 4

Nucleic Acids

Learning Objectives

1. Define and use correctly the terms *gene, genome, intron, exon, mRNA, rRNA, tRNA, ribonucleoside, ribonucleotide, deoxyribonucleoside, deoxyribonucleotide, pyrimidine, purine, cytosine, thymine, adenine, guanine, uracil, Watson–Crick pairing, primary structure, secondary structure, tertiary structure, quaternary structure, oligonucleotide, inverted repeats, hairpin, triplex, quadruplex, G-quartet, palindrome, supercoiling, cruciform, ccc DNA, topoisomerase, nucleosome, helix-coil transition,* T_m, and *hybridization.*
2. List five major roles of nucleotides in the cell.
3. Describe important structural features of pyrimidine and purine nucleotides. Relate these features to the chemical and physical properties of those molecules, including solubility and hydrogen-bonding capability.
4. Relate keto–enol tautomerization of the bases to the formation of Watson–Crick base pairs.
5. Explain the origins of the stability of the DNA double helix, and list factors that can destabilize this structure. Explain how DNA denaturation is reversible.
6. List the major species of RNA found in the cell, and briefly describe their functions.
7. Recognize and compare the structures of the different secondary and tertiary structures adopted by nucleic acids, including A-, B-, and Z-form double helices, as well as cruciforms, triplexes, and quadruplex structures.
8. Explain how duplex DNA can be supercoiled. Distinguish between the two main types of supercoiling, plectonemic and solenoidal. Explain the importance of topoisomerases as targets for antibiotic action.
9. Describe the secondary and tertiary structure of a typical tRNA molecule, listing important structural features.
10. Recognize the special modifications, known as the "cap" and "tail," to the 3′ and 5′ ends of a mRNA molecule.
11. Describe the structure of a nucleosome. Explain its importance for the packaging of DNA in eukaryotic cells.

Introduction

Deoxyribonucleic acid (DNA) and ribonucleic acid (RNA) are large polymers composed of deoxyribonucleotides and ribonucleotides, respectively. DNA is the central repository of genetic information, storing and transmitting it from generation to generation. RNA helps in the expression of this information, functioning as an intermediary between DNA and the synthesis of proteins; it has several other important roles in the cell as well.

Genes are segments of DNA that specify particular proteins or particular species of RNA that are used in structural or catalytic roles by the cell. A chromosome is a single DNA molecule carrying a set of genes. Although DNA in viruses and bacteria is characteristically organized as a single chromosome, eukaryotes typically carry multiple chromosomes of different sizes. Humans have 23 pairs of chromosomes. A *genome* is the complete genetic complement of a cell. A simple organism such as the bacterium *Escherichia coli* might have a genome of 4000 genes; humans are thought to have approximately 30,000 distinct genes. In eukaryotes, genes are often organized with regions coding directly for peptide sequences (expressed regions, or *exons*), interspersed with stretches of DNA that do not code for anything (intervening regions, or *introns*); a single gene may be divided into several exons and introns (see **Figure 4-1** for an example).

In addition to gene sequences, some DNA regions help to control the expression of genes. Moreover, eukaryotic cells contain large amounts of DNA that do not directly code for a polypeptide gene product. In fact, only 30% of the human genome actually specifies genes (including both exon and intron sequences), and only 1% of the human genome is finally expressed as protein gene products (that is, present as exon sequences). A large proportion (approximately 45%) of the human genome is formed of transposable sequences (transposons), which can move from one site to another in the genome; many of these, however, are inactive. Another appreciable fraction of human genomic DNA plays a structural role in organizing chromosomes with centromeres and telomeres. Centromeres are complexes of DNA and proteins that, during mitosis, help to direct the segregation of chromosomes into daughter cells. Telomeres are DNA regions at the ends of chromosomes that stabilize and protect the chromosome from degradation.

RNA molecules in cells are significantly smaller than chromosomes. **Table 4-1** compares the sizes of DNA and RNA molecules as isolated from cells. The stored genetic information is transcribed from DNA into RNA as messages (messenger RNA or *mRNA*), and the information from the mRNA is, in turn, translated to direct the synthesis of polypeptide chains (proteins); we return to this process in Chapter 16. In addition to its role as a messenger in conveying genetic instructions, RNA forms part of the protein synthesis machinery of the cell, the ribosome. RNA molecules help to organize the structure of the ribosome, and a portion of RNA even participates directly in the ribosome's catalytic process of forming polypeptides. In both bacteria and higher organisms, smaller RNA species, known as transfer RNA (*tRNA*) molecules, convey amino acids to the ribosome for assembly into polypeptides. Another class of small RNA molecules is involved in base modification reactions of ribosomal

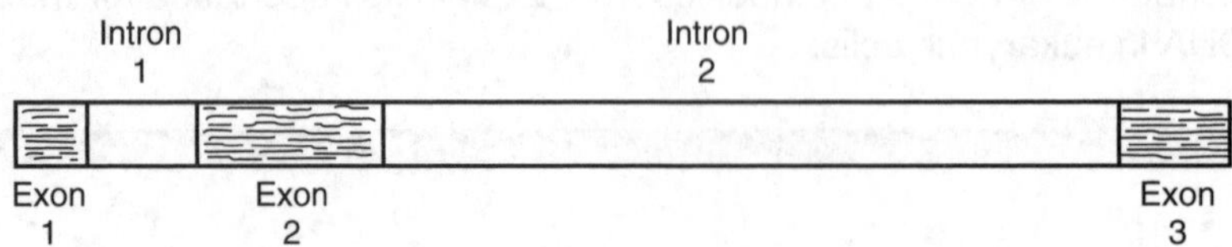

Figure 4-1 Intron/exon structure of the β-globin gene.

Small interfering RNAs (siRNA)	21–23 bases
Yeast $tRNA^{Phe}$	76 bases
Human 5S rRNA	120 bases
Human 18S rRNA	1900 bases
Human 28S rRNA	4700 bases
SV40 DNA	5243 base pairs
Adenovirus DNA	36,000 base pairs
E. coli chromosome	4.6×10^6 base pairs
Human chromosome 1	220×10^6 base pairs
Human chromosome 21	33×10^6 base pairs

Table 4-1 Sizes of Selected RNA and DNA Molecules

RNA. Additionally, in higher organisms, yet another class of RNA is involved in the enzyme complexes that protect the ends of chromosomes against degradation, and another class of small double-stranded RNA molecules is involved in suppressing gene expression (small interfering RNAs or siRNA). Also in higher organisms, some small RNA molecules possess catalytic activity and are important in processing mRNA; these are called ribozymes.

The molecular basis of many diseases, such as sickle cell anemia, phenylketonuria, and Lesch-Nyhan syndrome, can now be traced back to differences at the level of single genes in DNA. Additionally, variations in drug absorption and metabolism across patient populations can often be traced back to diversity in genes that code for the proteins responsible for those functions. Many diagnostic tools for diseases of genetic origin, as well as for certain viral and bacterial infections, have emerged from researchers' discoveries about nucleic acid structure and function. New therapies involving nucleic acids are being developed, including agents that may block replication of viruses and drugs that focus on controlling and perhaps repairing or replacing aberrant genes that are expressed in cancer or other genetic diseases. The recent success in obtaining the nucleotide sequence of the entire human genome has the potential to spur further advances in diagnosis and therapy.

Major Roles of Nucleotides

Both DNA and RNA are built from nucleotides. Besides serving as precursors for RNA and DNA, nucleotides are ubiquitous in cellular processes:

- Adenosine triphosphate (ATP) is used as a free energy carrier for reactions, transport, work, and other activities.
- Nucleotides are components of many important enzymatic cofactors.
- They serve in activating intermediates in metabolic reactions—for example, by activating glucose in sugar metabolism.
- They often function as metabolic regulators or signaling agents; for example, cyclic adenosine monophosphate (cAMP) serves as a "second messenger" in hormonal signaling, and the general sensitivity of the body's metabolism to the cellular energy stores is connected to levels of adenosine nucleotides.

Later chapters elaborate on these processes and the roles of nucleotides in them. Chapter 8 provides several examples of nucleotides as a part of important enzymatic cofactors; Chapter 11 covers the biosynthesis of the energy carrier, ATP; and the uses in energy metabolism of nucleotides and their derivatives appear throughout Chapters 8 through 16. Furthermore, Chapter 15 explores nucleotide metabolism in detail and relates that metabolism to drug action important in the treatment of, for example, cancer. Chapter 16 gives details on the biological synthesis of DNA, RNA, and proteins. To prepare for this material, this chapter emphasizes the structure and function of the polymerized nucleotides, DNA and RNA; surveys their roles in the synthesis of proteins; and relates their structures and functions to diagnostic and therapeutic approaches involving those polymers.

Bases, Nucleosides, and Nucleotides

The four bases in DNA responsible for encoding genetic information are *thymine, adenine, cytosine,* and *guanine.* The bases guanine and adenine belong to the family of *purines* (**Figure 4-2**). Some other notable members of the purine family include caffeine and theobromine (found in chocolate), and the anticancer agent 6-mercaptopurine. In RNA, the thymine base is replaced by *uracil,* which lacks the methyl group of thymine. The bases thymine, uracil, and cytosine belong to the *pyrimidine* family; the powerful anticancer agents 5-fluorouracil and cytarabine are members of this family as well (**Figure 4-3**).

Purines and pyrimidines are weakly basic because they have $-NH_2$ groups. In acidic solution these groups can be protonated and can introduce a positive charge on the base. In alkaline solution, a proton on the N3 nitrogen of a pyrimidine, or on the N1 nitrogen of a purine, can dissociate; the base then acts functionally as a weak acid (**Figure 4-4**). Additionally, bases can tautomerize, with the ring nitrogens accepting a proton (**Figure 4-5**). Alternatively, a proton can shift from a nitrogen to the oxygen of a carbonyl group on the base. For purines and pyrimidines the keto form dominates this keto–enol tautomerization.

In solution, nucleotides can hydrogen bond with one another and can stack their heterocyclic rings on top of one another, enjoying a hydrophobic interaction. **Figure 4-6** shows several schemes for association of various nucleotide bases by hydrogen bonding. The most famous

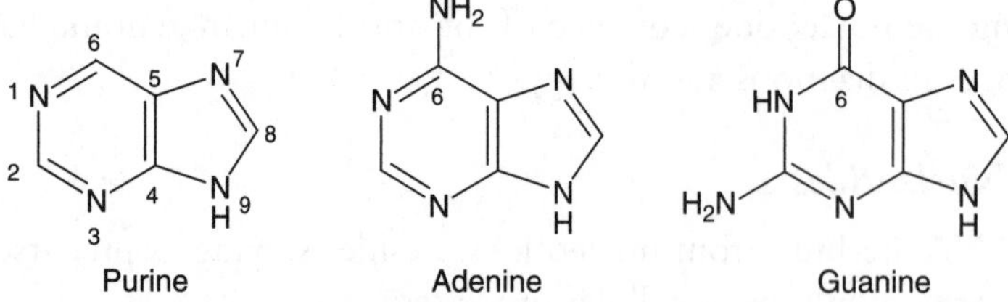

Figure 4-2 Purine bases. The ring position numbering is shown for reference.

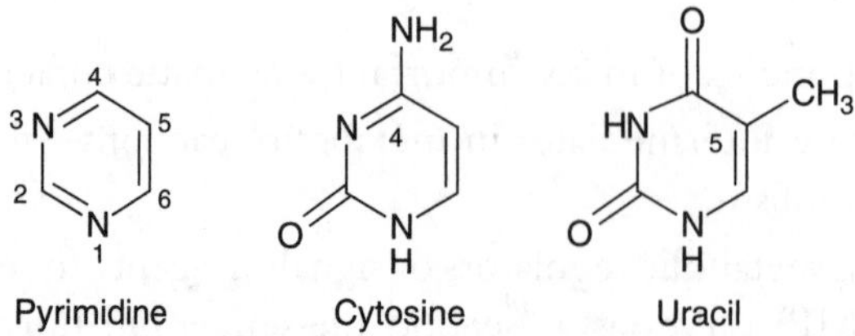

Figure 4-3 Pyrimidine bases. The ring position numbering is shown for reference.

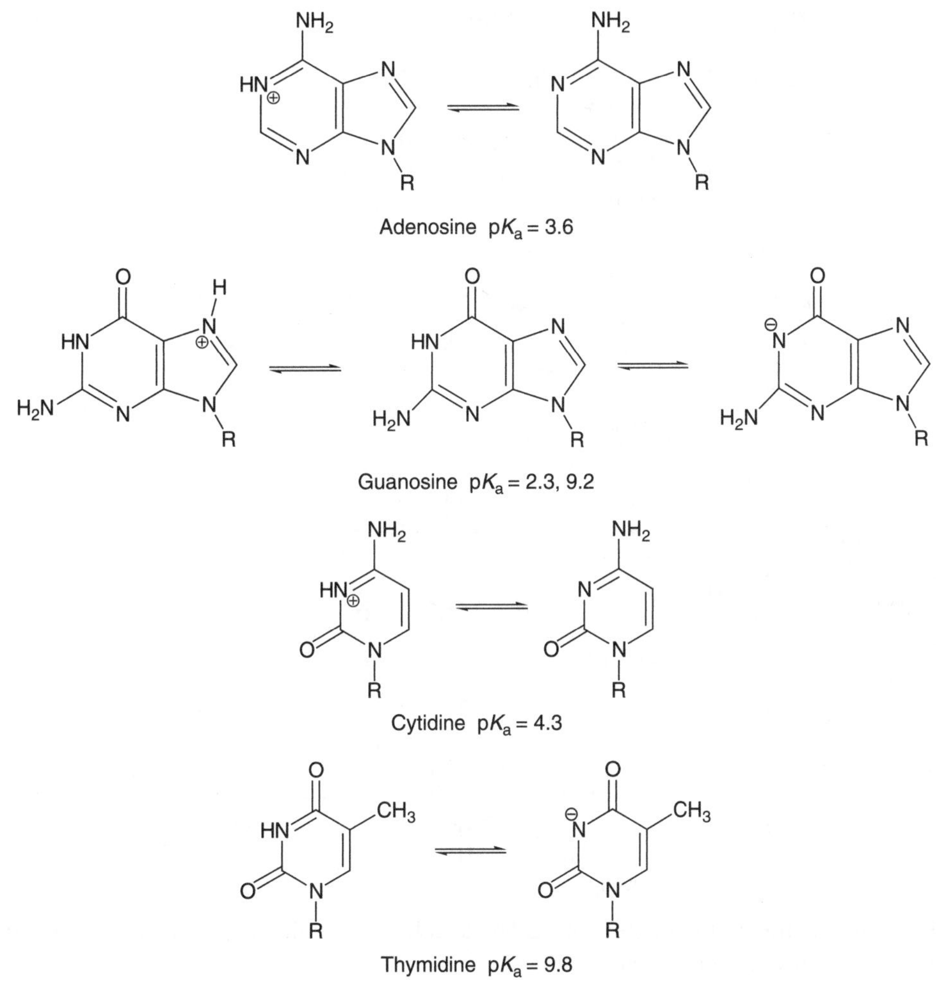

Adenosine pK_a = 3.6

Guanosine pK_a = 2.3, 9.2

Cytidine pK_a = 4.3

Thymidine pK_a = 9.8

Figure 4-4 Titration sites and pK_a values for nucleosides.

of these is that proposed by James Watson and Francis Crick, resulting from their discovery of the DNA double helix, in which adenine pairs with thymine, and guanine pairs with cytosine. The keto tautomers of purines and pyrimidines form the base-to-base hydrogen bonds that are important for Watson–Crick base pairing. This type of base pairing is highly important for the association of polymerized strands of nucleic acid. Interestingly, however, in an aqueous solution of free single nucleotides there is very little Watson–Crick pairing; instead, the bases associate by stacking and by alternative hydrogen-bonding patterns.

Uracil and the other pyrimidine bases are, by themselves, not very water soluble. Purine is itself fairly water soluble, but the derivatives adenine and guanine are much less so. Addition of a polar sugar moiety, and of ionic phosphoryl groups, significantly improves the aqueous solubility of both purines and pyrimidines.

Two pentose sugars are important here, *ribose* and *2-deoxyribose* (**Figure 4-7**). The latter lacks the hydroxy group of ribose at the C2 position. Covalent linkage of the sugar to pyrimidine bases is from the C1 carbon of the sugar to the N1 nitrogen of the pyrimidine base, a glycosidic link. For purines, the glycosidic link is from the C1 carbon to the N9 nitrogen of the purine. The combination of sugar and base is referred to as a *nucleoside*.

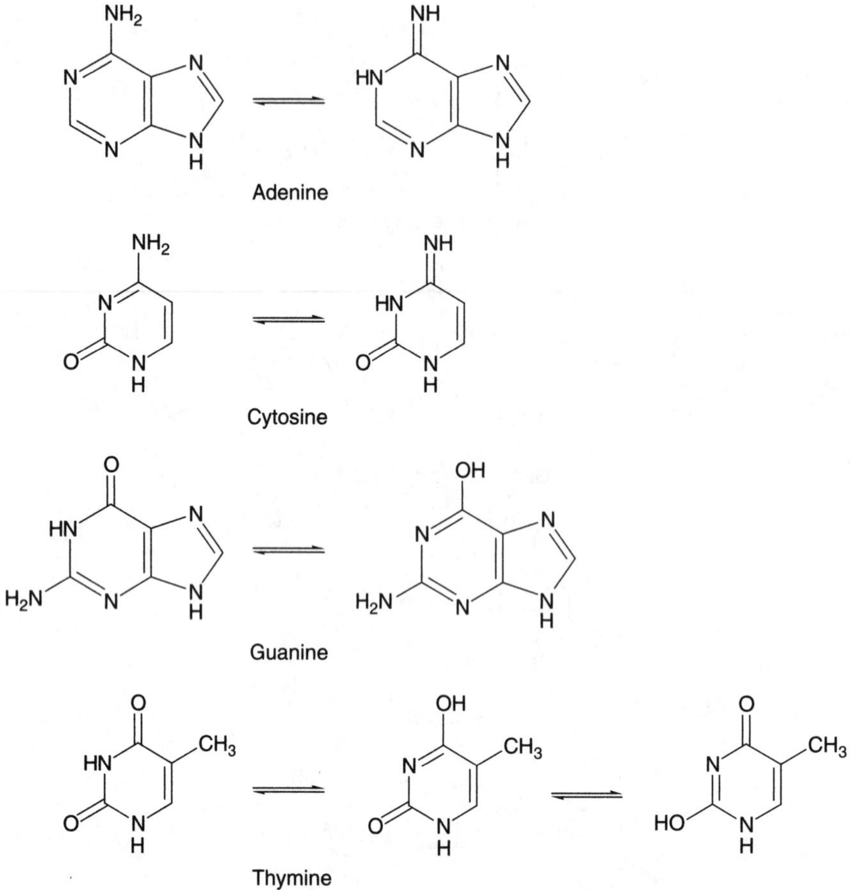

Figure 4-5 Imino and enol tautomers of nucleic acid bases. Dominant forms are on the left; minor (imino and enol) forms are on the right.

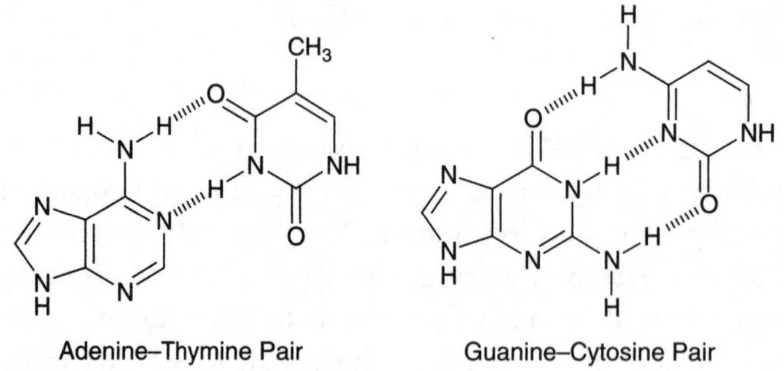

Adenine–Thymine Pair

Guanine–Cytosine Pair

Figure 4-6 Base pairing schemes in DNA.

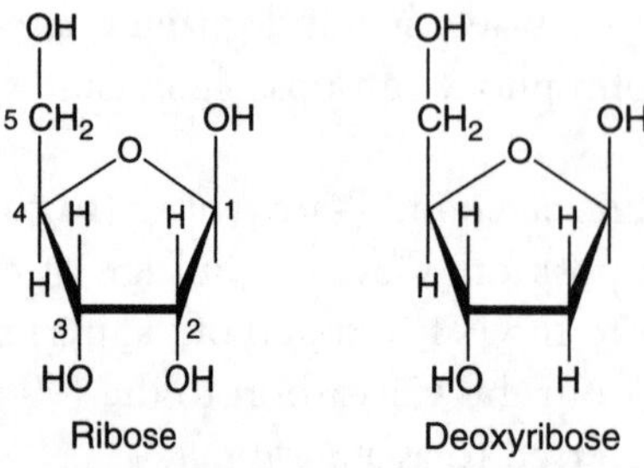

Figure 4-7 Ribose and deoxyribose.

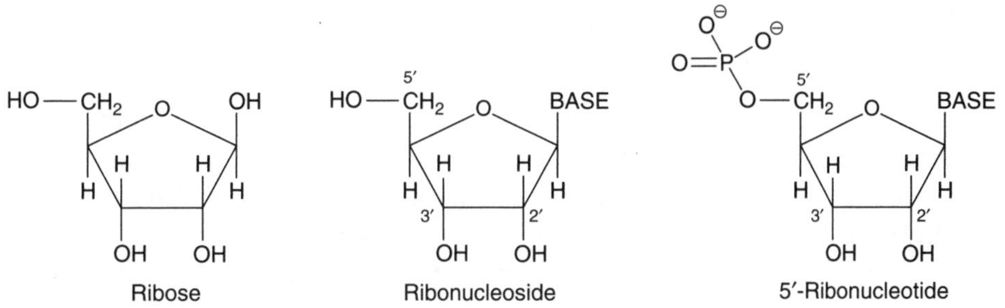

Figure 4-8 General structures of nucleosides and nucleotides.

The sugars may be phosphorylated, and in the polymers of DNA and RNA the sites of phosphorylation are the 3′ and 5′ positions on the sugars. By convention, the prime indicates positions on the sugar instead of the base (this convention distinguishes, for example, C-5 on uracil from C-5′ on ribose). When a nucleoside is phosphorylated, the result is a *nucleotide*. Thus the same compound could be described as either a nucleoside 5′-phosphate or as a 5′-nucleotide, for example (**Figure 4-8**).

Deoxyribonucleotides are synthesized from ribonucleotides through the action of ribonucleotide reductase (see Chapter 15). By convention, when naming nucleosides and nucleotides, the "d" prefix indicates the 2′-deoxyribose sugar in abbreviated forms; the absence of "d" in the name implies that ribose is present instead. **Table 4-2** summarizes these points of nomenclature.

Nucleotides carry a negative electrical charge, due to ionization of the phosphates. The precursor of these ions, phosphoric acid (H_3PO_4), is itself a strong acid, with three dissociable protons. When incorporated into a nucleotide the monophosphate, diphosphate, and triphosphate groups will ionize. For example, adenosine triphosphate (ATP) has four dissociable protons, with pK_a values for three of these below pH 5, while the fourth has a pK_a of approximately 6.9. In solution at physiological pH, a solution of ATP will, therefore, have molecular species in several different titrated forms carrying three or four negative charges.

Base	**Ribonucleoside**	**Ribonucleotide (5′-Monophosphate)**
Uracil	Uridine	Uridylic acid (uridylate) or UMP
Cytosine	Cytidine	Cytidylic acid (cytidylate) or CMP
Adenine	Adenosine	Adenylic acid (adenylate) or AMP
Guanine	Guanosine	Guanylic acid (guanylate) or GMP
Base	**Deoxyribonucleoside**	**Deoxyribonucleotide (5′-Monophosphate)**
Thymine	Deoxythymidine	Deoxythymidylic acid (deoxythymidylate) or dTMP
Cytosine	Deoxycytidine	Deoxycytidylic acid (deoxycytidylate) or dCMP
Adenine	Deoxyadenosine	Deoxyadenylic acid (deoxyadenylate) or dAMP
Guanine	Deoxyguanosine	Deoxyguanylic acid (deoxyguanylate) or dGMP

Table 4-2 Nomenclature for Nucleic Acid Bases, Nucleosides, and Nucleotides

Primary Structure of DNA and RNA

The sequence of nucleotide residues, when covalently linked together in a linear chain in a polynucleotide, is called the *primary structure* of the polynucleotide. The covalent linkage between the nucleotide units is through phosphodiesters, with one phosphate group bonded to two successive sugars, using the 3′ —OH group of one sugar and the 5′ —OH group of another (**Figure 4-9**). **Figure 4-10** shows a common abbreviated representation of such structures. The sugars and phosphate groups are not shown explicitly. Single-letter abbreviations are used for the bases, and the lowercase "d" indicates that the sugar is deoxyribose (the absence of the "d" implies the sugar is instead ribose, although this convention is often ignored when the context makes it clear that the polymer is DNA and not RNA). The lowercase "p" represents the 5′ phosphate group; the existence of the 3′ —OH group is not shown explicitly but is only implied. By convention, for single-stranded DNA or RNA, the 5′ terminus of the chain is written on the left, the 3′ terminus on the right; that is, the base sequence is written 5′ → 3′.

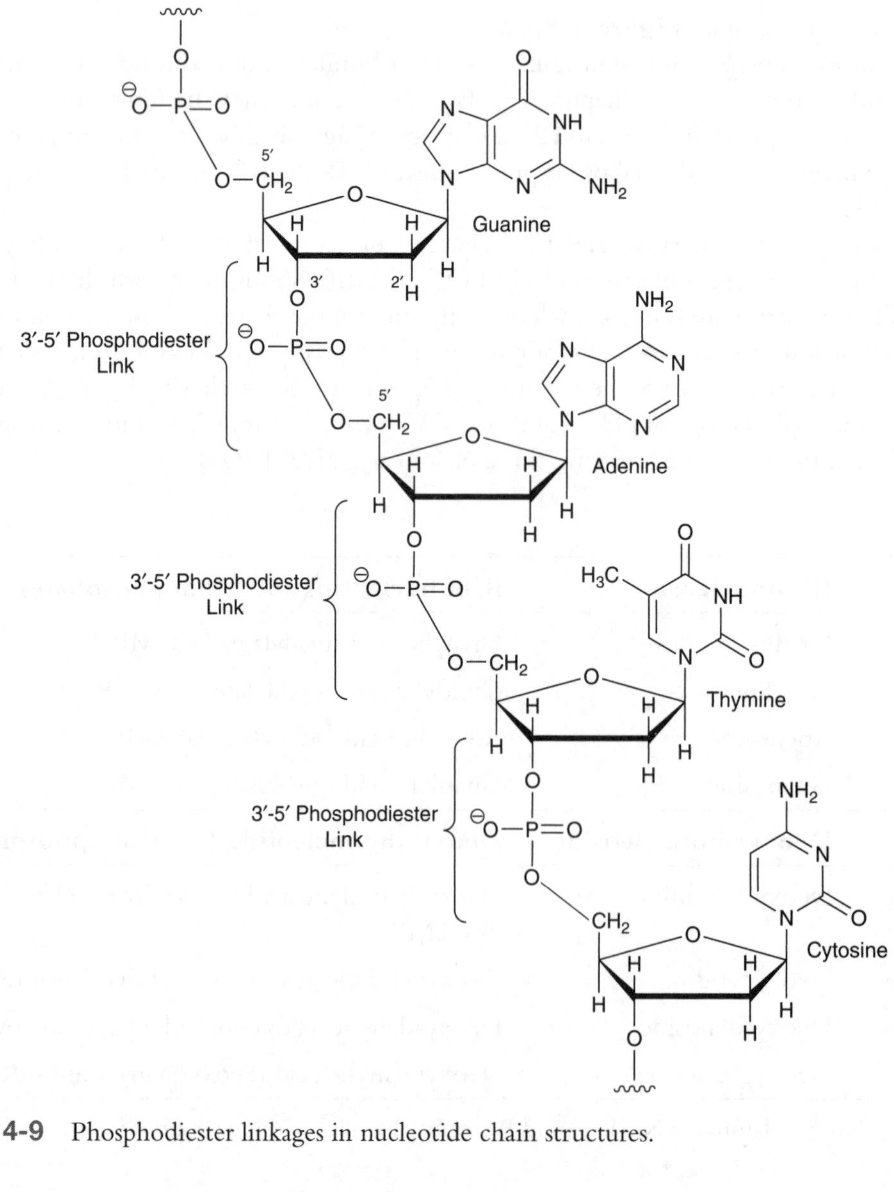

Figure 4-9 Phosphodiester linkages in nucleotide chain structures.

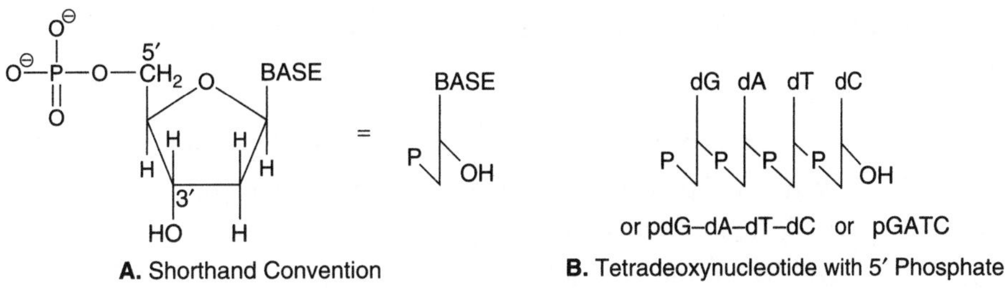

BASE = BASE (P, OH)

A. Shorthand Convention

dG dA dT dC

P P P P OH

or pdG–dA–dT–dC or pGATC

B. Tetradeoxynucleotide with 5′ Phosphate

Figure 4-10 Conventions for abbreviations in the oligonucleotide chain structure.

Secondary Structure

Secondary structure refers to the stable, repeating conformational pattern in a polymer. DNA and RNA both have highly distinctive secondary structures, deriving from the properties of their constituent nucleotides.

DNA Secondary Structure

The DNA Double Helix

The stable solution conformation of DNA is the famous double helix (**Figure 4-11**): two polynucleotide chains wound around each other, with complementary pairing of the bases in

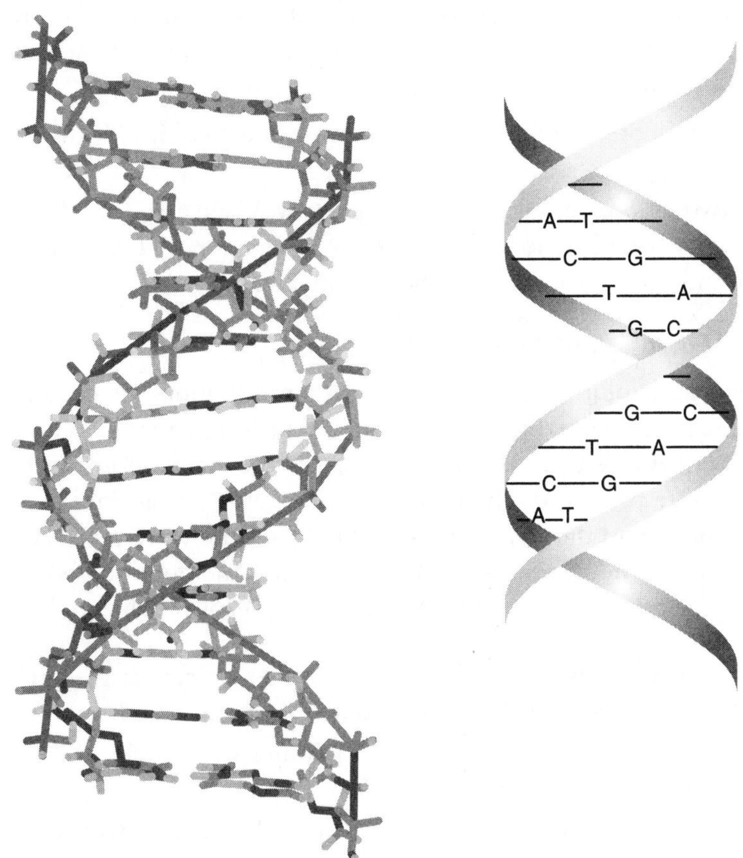

Figure 4-11 Representations of the B-form DNA double helix: a "stick" model and a "ribbon" model.

a scheme proposed by James Watson and Francis Crick. Notable features of the double helix include the following:

- The bases lie to the interior of the helix, where their planar faces are hidden from solvent.
- The bases are stacked on top of one another, such that the plane of each base is nearly perpendicular to the long axis of the helix.
- The sugar–phosphate backbone is largely exposed to solvent.
- The helix has a right-handed twist. It makes a complete turn every 3.4 nm, or about 10.5 residues. The overall diameter of the helix is approximately 2.0 nm.
- The strands are antiparallel; one strand runs $3' \rightarrow 5'$ while the other runs $5' \rightarrow 3'$.
- There are two grooves (major and minor) in the helix, where the edges of the bases are exposed to solvent.
- Overall, the double helix behaves mechanically like a semi-flexible rod. Long molecules can be bent such that their ends may be covalently joined to form a closed, circular molecule with two strands.

Another highly important feature is the joining of the two strands by *Watson–Crick complementary base pairing* (see Figure 4-6):

- Adenine is paired with thymine; guanine is paired with cytosine.
- The base pairs are joined by hydrogen bonds, with two hydrogen bonds joining adenine and thymine, and three hydrogen bonds joining guanine and cytosine.
- The hydrogen bonding enforces the coplanarity of the two paired bases.
- The base pairs stack on top of one another in overlapping fashion, with the stack resembling the treads in a spiral staircase.
- Because the two strands complement each other by base pairing, the base sequence of one strand necessarily specifies the sequence of the other strand. This has major consequences for the replication and repair of the genetic material.

DNA Can Also Form a Left-Handed Helix

Under certain unusual solution conditions (high concentrations of certain salts or organic cosolvents), duplex DNA can twist into an alternative helical form, the Z-form helix. Here the bases still form Watson–Crick complementary pairs, with the sugar–phosphate backbone exposed to solvent and the base pairs in the helix interior. The base pairs are still nearly perpendicular to the axis of the helix, and the strands are still antiparallel. However, the most striking feature of the Z-form is that the helix has a left-handed twist, just the opposite from the B-form helix (**Figure 4-12**). Some other notable differences from the B-form helix are highlighted here:

- There are 12 base pairs per turn of the helix, and one turn covers a length of about 4.4 nm, as opposed to 10 base pairs per turn, and about 3.4 nm per turn for the B-form helix.
- The phosphodiester backbone traces a zig-zag course (the origin of the "Z" designation), not a smooth curve as in the B-form.
- The helix is somewhat slimmer than the B-form helix, with a diameter of approximately 1.8 nm.
- The major groove is much shallower, and the minor groove is much deeper and narrower, than in the B-form helix.

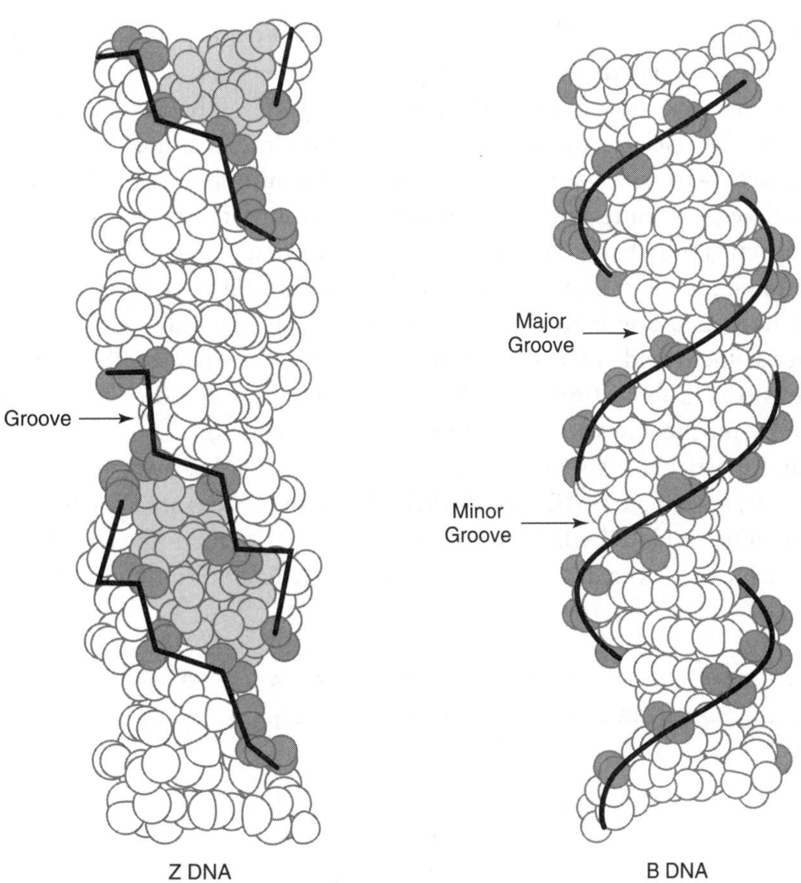

Figure 4-12 Comparison of space-filling models of DNA double helices. The Z-form helix is left-handed, while both the B-and A-form helices are right-handed. Note the zig-zag structure of the polynucleotide backbone in the Z-form helix. With permission from A. Rich, A. Nordheim, and A.H.-J. Wang. (1984). *Annu. Rev. Biochem*. 53:791. Copyright 1984 Annual Reviews, Inc.

It is thought that the vast majority of duplex DNA in solution is in the B-form, interrupted only rarely with runs of the Z-form helix. Tracts of Z-form helix may, however, be important for regulating gene expression.

Under other rather artificial conditions (e.g., alcoholic solutions that dehydrate the polymer), DNA can adopt an A-form helix. This right-handed, double-stranded helix contains antiparallel strands, similar to the B-form helix described earlier. There are, however, very noticeable differences in this A-form helix. The minor groove becomes shallower, while the major groove deepens. Also, the twist of the helix is more pronounced: The rise per base pair is only 0.26 nm, not the gentler rise of 0.34 nm per base pair found in the B-form helix. The base pairs are also tilted more sharply than in the B-form helix, and the sugar ring has a different puckering. Under in vivo conditions, where the DNA is well hydrated, it is unlikely that the A-form helix will be formed, so it is probably not important in the functioning of the cell.

Unusual DNA Structures

Inverted repeated sequences (*inverted repeats*) occur throughout genomic DNA. These sequences have a two-fold symmetry such that the sequence along a given strand is self-complementary and can be paired to form a double *hairpin* or *cruciform* structure. In duplex DNA, these inverted repeats are *palindromes,* DNA sequences that read the same on both strands when read in the same direction (e.g., 5′ → 3′). **Figure 4-13** illustrates the possible folding of a palindromic sequence into a cruciform with two hairpins.

Nucleic acids can also form triple helices or *triplexes*—that is, structures with three strands held together by stacking of the bases and extra hydrogen bonds to accommodate the third strand. **Figure 4-14** shows some possible triplex-forming hydrogen-bonding schemes. Thanks to the multiple possibilities for hydrogen bonding around the bases, the standard Watson–Crick pairs can accept a third base to form a triplex. Notice that the acid–base behavior of pyrimidines is involved here, as the cytosine residue of the third strand is protonated at the N3 position to form two hydrogen bonds to a guanine residue. Such structures are limited by pH, however, and are not stable outside of acidic conditions. Notice also that the third base attaches itself to a purine; thus triplex formation generally requires that one strand of a duplex have an extended series of only purine bases, to which the third strand can attach.

Certain unusual DNA sequences have the ability to fold back on themselves repeatedly to form a *quadruplex* structure (**Figure 4-15A**). These sequences are enriched in guanine bases. In fact, the guanine residues hydrogen-bond to each other to form the four-base structure, known as a *G-quartet*, which contains a monovalent ion coordinated to the four bases (**Figure 4-15B**).

A.

5′G—A—G—G—C—A—A—T—C—C—A—A—A—A—A—G—G—A—T—T—G—C—T—G—C 3′

3′C—T—C—C—G—T—T—A—G—G—T—T—T—T—T—C—C—T—A—A—C—G—A—C—G 5′

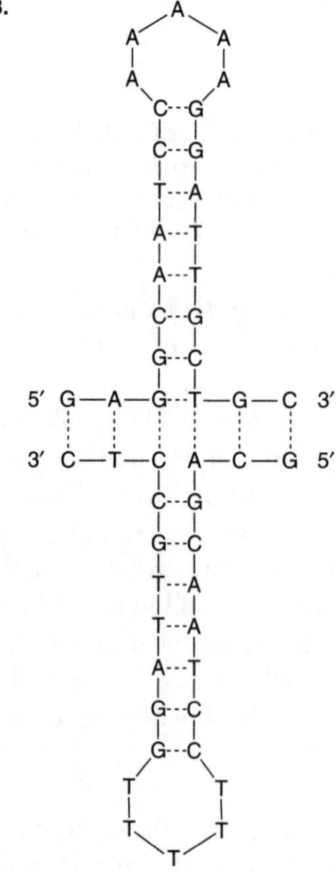

Figure 4-13 **A.** Palindromic (inverted repeated) sequence. **B.** Cruciform structure folded from inverted repeated sequence.

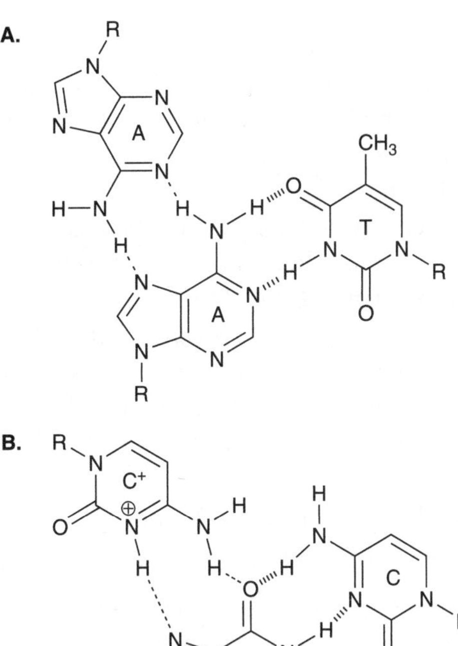

Figure 4-14 Hydrogen bonding schemes in base triplets. Thicker dashed lines show canonical hydrogen bonds, as found in Watson–Crick base pairs. Thinner dashed lines indicate noncanonical hydrogen bonds used to attach the triplet base. **A.** AAT triplet. **B.** C$^+$G C triplet. Note the protonation at N3 of the third cytosine here.

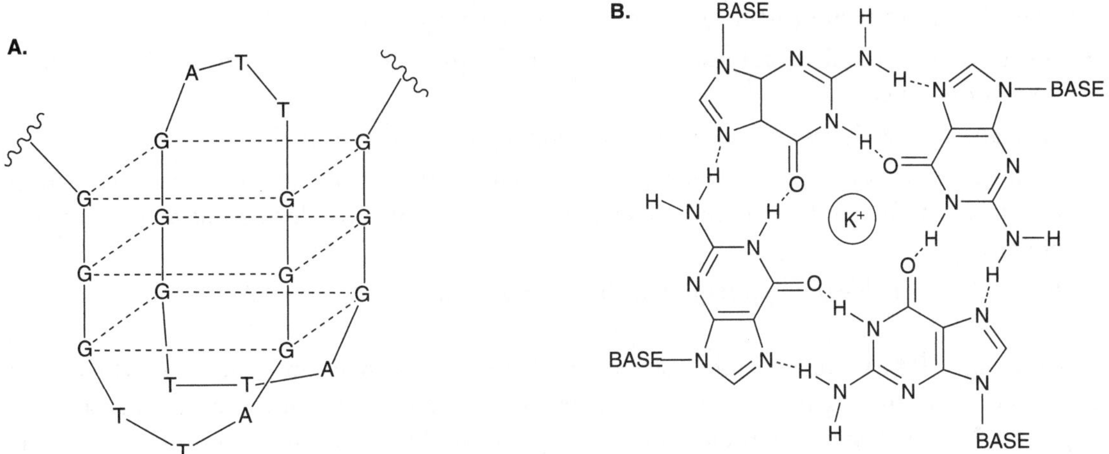

Figure 4-15 **A.** One possible folded structure involving G-quartets. **B.** A G-quartet formed around a central potassium ion.

To fold the strand back and forth as shown in Figure 4-15, the runs of guanine residues must be interrupted by other base sequences that will form the joining single-stranded loops. G-quartets and quadruplex structures are important structural features of telomeres, the protein–DNA complexes that lie at the end of eukaryotic chromosomes. Chapter 16 covers telomeres and their function in more depth.

RNA Secondary Structure

RNA is generally found as single chains, whereas DNA naturally occurs as a duplex of two separate chains. The base uracil replaces thymine in RNA, and in duplex forms there is complementary pairing of uracil with adenine. This base pair is stabilized by two hydrogen bonds, just like the adenine–thymine pair.

In RNA, because of complementary base pairing, the chain can frequently be folded back on itself, forming right-handed double-helical regions in which the strands are arranged in antiparallel fashion. As in the B-form helix of DNA, the bases are paired in complementary fashion, and the planar base pairs are stacked on one another. The phosphodiester backbone remains on the exterior of the helix, while the paired bases are located to the interior. The RNA double helix differs from the B-form helix of DNA in several ways, however—for example, forming instead of the A-form helix described earlier for DNA.

- The diameter of the RNA helix is thicker, at 2.6 nm.
- The base pairs are tilted at an appreciable angle to the axis of the helix (approximately 20°).
- A complete turn of the helix requires 11 base pairs, and occurs over a helical run of length 2.9 nm.
- The major groove is narrower and deeper, and the minor groove wider and shallower, than in the B-form helix.

The extra —OH group on ribose, versus deoxyribose, changes the puckering of the sugar and the overall hydration of the residues, leading to these differences from the B-form helix.

The secondary structures of tRNA molecules resemble a cloverleaf (**Figure 4-16**). Notable features here include the following characteristics:

- Several (four to five) short helical runs of four to six base pairs each
- Several single-stranded regions, some forming loops at the ends of runs of helix (called stem-loop structures)
- Several modified bases and sugars, often involving modification by methylation
- A short stretch of single-stranded RNA—a bulge—that is not involved in a stem-loop structure, in the middle of the molecule (Not all tRNA molecules have this feature, however.)
- An exposed single-stranded region at the 3′ end of the RNA molecule

Messenger RNA can also fold back on itself to form stem-loop structures, which may play a role in controlling gene expression. In eukaryotes, the 5′ end of the molecule carries a "cap" of a 7-methylguanine residue, attached to the chain by an unusual 5′ phosphoryl group, rather than through the usual 3′ linkage (**Figure 4-17**). Additionally, at its 3′ end the mRNA often carries a long run of up to 200 adenylate residues (a poly A "tail"). These modifications are thought to protect the mRNA against degradation, and the cap structure plays a role in recognition of the mRNA by ribosomes.

Like the smaller tRNA molecules, ribosomal RNA molecules fold back on themselves, forming multiple short runs of helix, stem-loop structures, and bulges. Also like the tRNA molecules, these rRNA molecules are often modified to carry unusual bases.

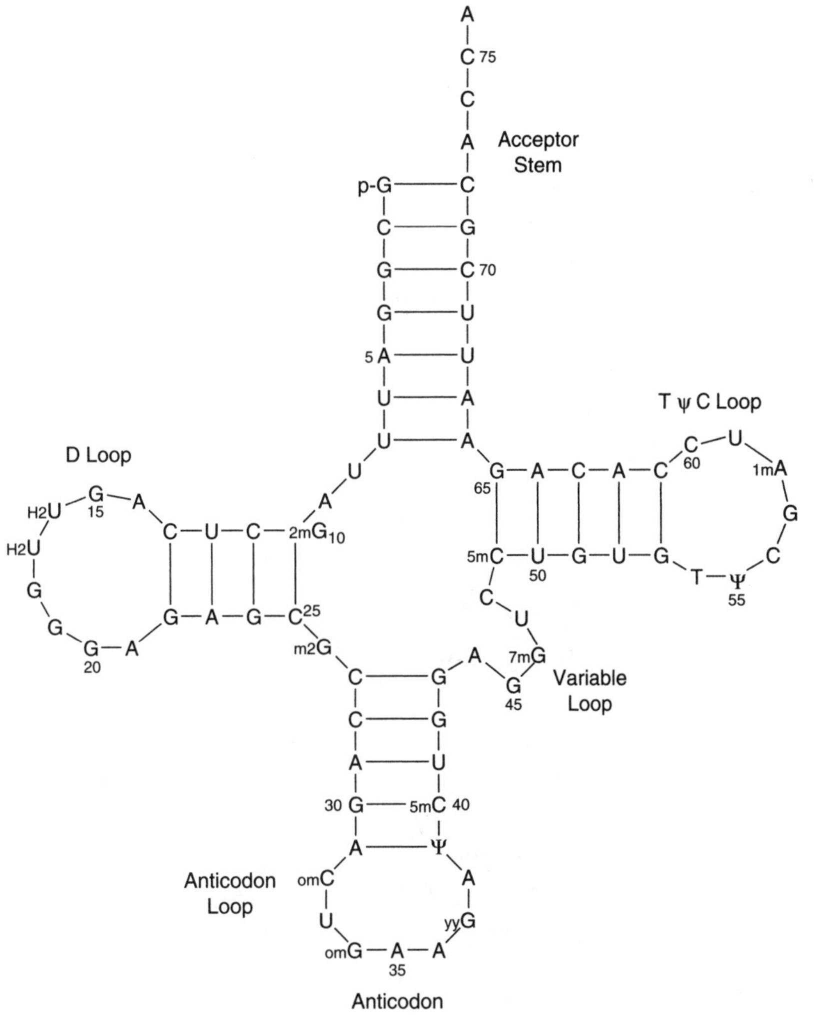

Figure 4-16 Two-dimensional structure of yeast phenylalanine tRNA, showing a base pairing scheme and the characteristic stem-loop structures. Several nucleosides have been modified, as indicated: 2mG, ^{2}N-methylguanosine; h2U, 5,6-dihydrouridine; m2G, ^{2}N-dimethylguanosine; omC, *O*2′-methylcytosine; omG, *O*2′-methylguanosine; yyG, a heavily modified guanosine; Ψ, pseudouridine; 5mC, 5-methylcytidine; 7mG, ^{7}N-methyl-8-hydroguanosine; 5mU, 5-methyluridine (thymidine); 1mA, 6-hydro-1-methyladenosine.

Tertiary and Quaternary Structure

The tertiary structure of a biopolymer refers to a characteristic repeating structure in three dimensions for a single molecule. The quaternary level of structure refers to the characteristic spatial arrangement of two or more different polymer chains. Here we are concerned with the folding of nucleic acids and the association of nucleic acids with proteins. Chapter 3 has already given examples of tertiary and quaternary structures of proteins composed of multiple subunits.

Tertiary Structure of tRNA

For nucleic acids, the tertiary level of structure includes the packing of helices, bulges, and single-stranded coils into a stable and more or less compact body. A good example here is

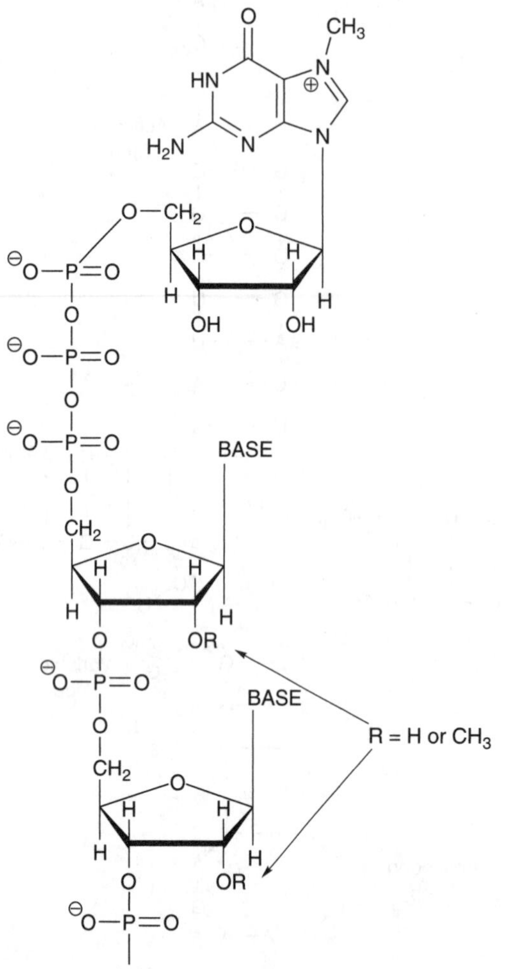

Figure 4-17 "Cap" structures found on eukaryotic mRNA. Note the terminal 7-methylguanine residue and the possible methylation of two neighboring sugars.

the tertiary structure of tRNA. **Figure 4-18** shows the tertiary structure of a typical tRNA molecule. Note how a single strand of RNA is folded back on itself, then how the stem-loop structures are packed, with exposure of the single-stranded loops and the single-stranded region at the 3′ end of the chain.

DNA Supercoiling

Linear pieces of DNA in solution have, on average, one turn of the B-form helix every 10.5 base pairs. Because DNA is flexible, however, long molecules can bend enough so that their ends may be covalently joined to form a continuous, circular double-stranded molecule, without disturbing the number of helical turns. This circular DNA molecule could be laid flat without straining it. DNA in this form is described as relaxed, and the molecule so produced is a covalently closed, circular DNA (*ccc DNA*). The covalent joining of the strands fixes the number of times one strand winds around the other; mathematically, this is a constant for that molecule.

We could, however, twist the DNA before joining it covalently, which would change the number of times the strands wound around or crossed each other. The twist could go in either

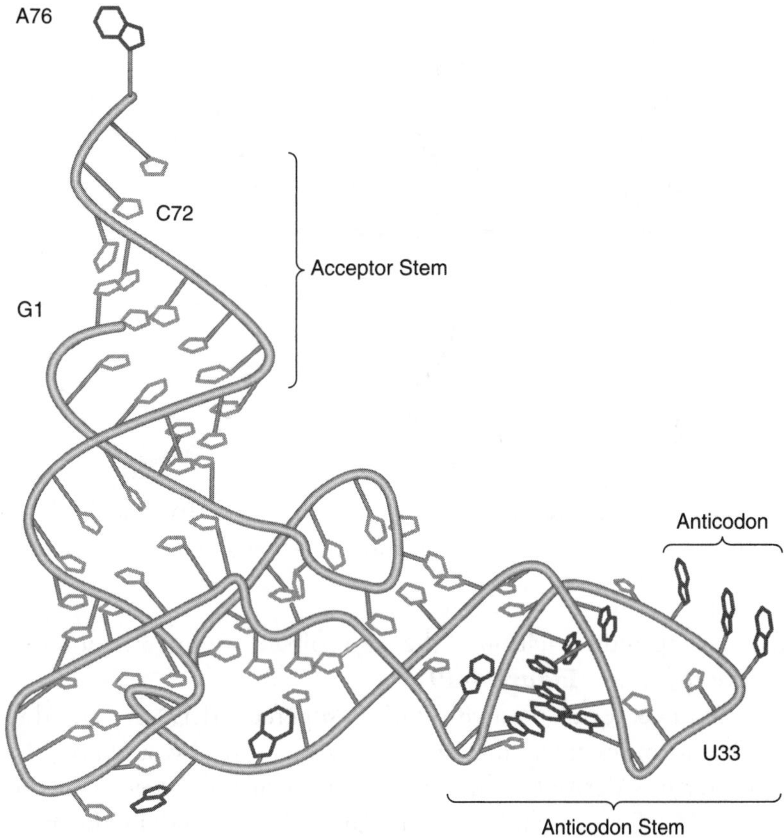

Figure 4-18 Ribbon representation of the three-dimensional structure of a folded tRNA, showing the characteristic packing of helices and the overall molecular shape resembling the letter L. From PDB entry 1EHZ.

direction, to overwind or underwind the helix. Also, the twist would have to be introduced as complete revolutions of one strand around the other (an integer number, in other words), to match up the strands before covalently closing them. The strain from this twisting is distributed along the length of molecule, producing small changes at each base pair from the relaxed B-form helix. These perturbations redirect the axis of the helix through space in a manner that promotes an overall winding of the helical coil around itself, a coiling of the coil. The DNA is now *supercoiled*, a tertiary level of DNA structure. Depending on whether the ccc DNA is underwound or overwound in comparison to relaxed DNA, we have a molecule with either positive or negative supercoiling. Underwinding could arise if the original relaxed helical molecule has a "bubble," a region where the bases are unpaired and the strands separated. Such an open region might arise during transcription or some other enzymatic process operating on the DNA. If a DNA molecule with such a bubble is allowed to reform an intact helix, with the bases fully paired, then the entire stretch of DNA will be underwound. This arrangement produces a negatively supercoiled molecule.

The strain of such negative supercoiling can be relieved if the DNA contains palindromic sequences. The molecule can extrude a cruciform, using the self-complementary sequences of the palindrome to form two stem-loop structures. The extrusion absorbs the underwinding, so that the helical regions are no longer twisted into supercoils. Cruciform structures may be important for DNA replication, for genetic recombination, and for gene regulation.

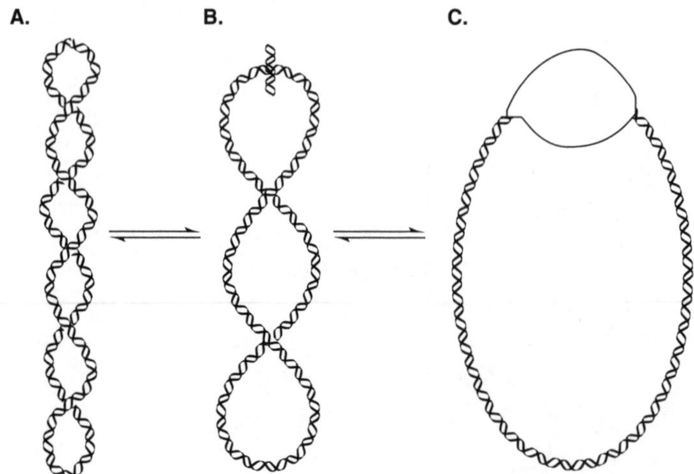

Figure 4-19 Supercoiling of DNA **(A)** can extrude a cruciform **(B)** if an inverted repeat sequence is present; alternatively, a part of the DNA can denature to relax the supercoiling **(C)**.

Alternatively, unpairing and separation of the base pairs in a limited region of the double helix can help to relieve the strain (**Figure 4-19**).

Apart from negative versus positive twisting, supercoiled DNA can adopt either of two general forms. One form resembles that which a twisted thread would take; this is plectonemic supercoiling (the term is derived from a combination of the Greek words for "twisted" and "thread"). The second form resembles a tubular coil, as found in the wiring of electrical apparatus such as electromagnets; this is solenoidal supercoiling (**Figure 4-20**).

The long chromosomes of eukaryotic DNA are separated by attached proteins into distinct domains in which the ends of the DNA are not free; rather they are constrained by the attached protein. The DNA in such domains may be supercoiled. Solenoidal supercoiling, combined with nucleosome formation (discussed later in this section), allows for greater compaction of DNA than does plectonemic supercoiling, and is important in packaging such chromosomal DNA into forms that can be accommodated inside the nucleus.

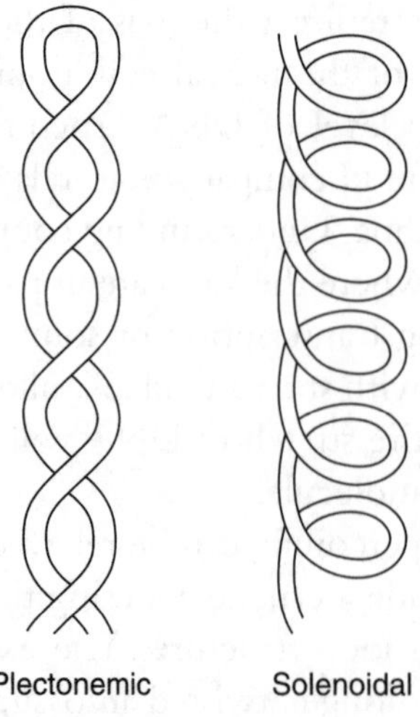

Figure 4-20 Plectonemic and solenoidal supercoiling.

Clinical Application

The topology of a DNA molecule refers to the strand winding discussed in this section. Molecules with different degrees of supercoiling are referred to as topoisomers, meaning isomers differing in their topology, which here refers specifically to the amount and type of supercoiling. *Topoisomerases* are enzymes that can change the winding of the DNA helix and thus interconvert DNA topoisomers. In general, two types of topoisomerases are distinguished. Type I topoisomerases operate by first cleaving one strand, then rotating that strand around the other, and finally reclosing the strand at the site of cleavage. Type II enzymes cleave both strands, pass another double-stranded portion of the same molecule through the point of cleavage, and reseal the strands at the point of cleavage. Blockage of topoisomerase action would interfere with gene expression and cell replication; these processes are closely connected to winding and unwinding of DNA and hence to the supercoiling of DNA. Some notable anticancer agents that block the action of type I topoisomerases include the natural product camptothecin and its derivatives topotecan and irinotecan (**Figure 4-21A**). Other anticancer drugs (e.g., etoposide and teniposide; **Figure 4-21B**) poison type II topoisomerases complexes with DNA. Furthermore, the bacterial forms of the topoisomerase enzymes are sufficiently different from the eukaryotic enzymes that antibiotics targeting bacterial topoisomerases are quite effective. The quinolones are an excellent example of a class of type II topoisomerase inhibitors with such specificity (e.g., nalidixic acid and derivatives; see Chapter 16 and Figure 16-27).

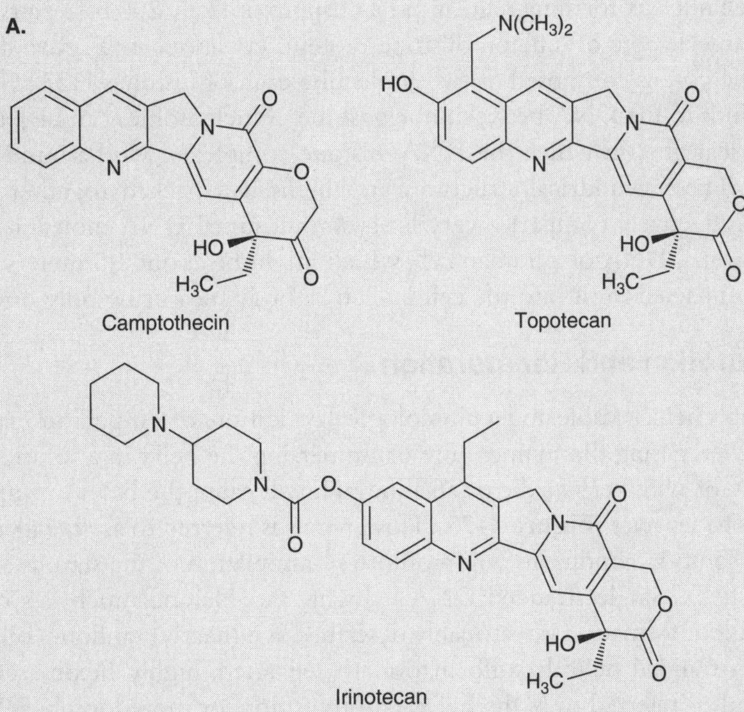

Figure 4-21 Anticancer agents that inhibit topoisomerases. **A.** Inhibitors of type I topoisomerases: camptothecin and its derivatives topotecan and irinotecan. **B.** Inhibitors of type II topoisomerases: etoposide and teniposide.

(Continued)

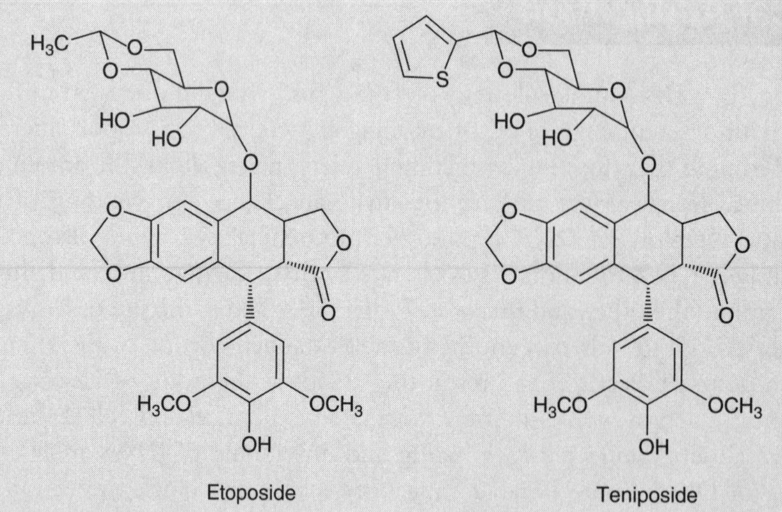

Figure 4-21 Anticancer agents that inhibit topoisomerases. **A.** Inhibitors of type I topoisomerases: camptothecin and its derivatives topotecan and irinotecan. **B.** Inhibitors of type II topoisomerases: etoposide and teniposide. (Continued).

Nucleosomes

Histones are basic proteins that bind strongly to DNA. They help to organize and compact DNA in the cell nucleus, forming regular units of approximately 200 base pairs of DNA wound around an octameric core of different histone proteins (a *nucleosome*; **Figure 4-22**).

The histone core is composed of two molecules each of histones H2A, H2B, H3, and H4. Histone H1 binds to the DNA between nucleosomes. Nucleosomes can be packed together to form a cylindrical fiber in which the DNA–histone complexes wind around it in the fashion of a solenoid. These cylindrical structures are themselves packed together in higher-order structures that effectively compact a very long chromosomal DNA molecule. In this way, the entire chromosomal DNA of a human cell, which might be about 1.5 meters in length if fully extended, is compacted to fit into the cell nucleus, a body measuring only micrometers across.

DNA Denaturation and Renaturation

The DNA double helix is stable under physiological conditions of temperature, salt concentration, and pH. However, raising the temperature or immersing the helix in a solution with very low amounts of salt, or with very acidic or alkaline pH, will cause the bases to unpair and unstack, and the strands to separate (**Figure 4-23**). This process is referred to as *denaturation* of the DNA. Reversing the solution conditions will promote re-association of the strands and re-formation of the double helix. Single-stranded DNA is highly flexible and much less ordered than the duplex helix; its conformation is reasonably described as a (nearly) random coil. The conversion from a double-stranded helical conformation to separated, highly flexible conformations of the single strands is referred to as the helix–coil transition, or more loosely as "melting" of the DNA double helix. The ability of the DNA double helix to open and close in this fashion is highly important for several fundamental cell processes, including replication of DNA, gene expression, and repair of damaged DNA (see Chapter 16). This process occurs over a limited temperature range, and the midpoint of the transition is where half of the nucleotides are

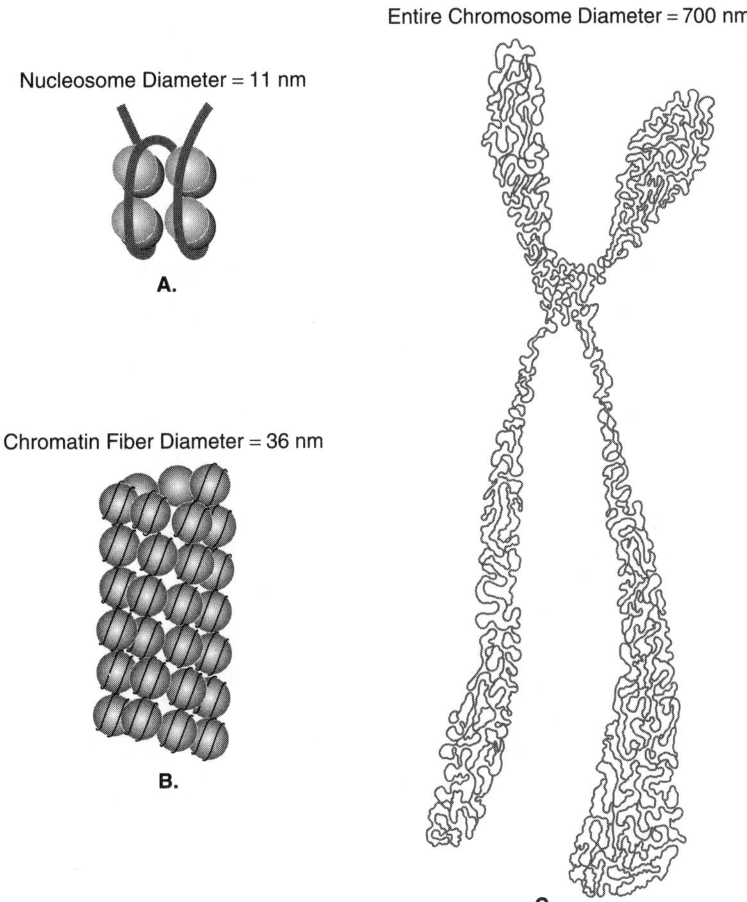

Figure 4-22 Structure of a nucleosome and packing of nucleosomes into chromatids. **A.** Single nucleosome, showing double-stranded DNA in a left-handed solenoidal winding around a histone octamer. **B.** Packing of nucleosomes in a fiber of chromatin; six to seven nucleosomes are packed per turn, in a left-handed solenoidal winding. **C.** Metaphase chromosome with packed chromatin fibers.

unpaired and unstacked. The temperature at which this occurs is denoted as T_m, called the melting temperature or—more formally—the transition midpoint temperature.

When nucleic acid bases are stacked on one another, electronic interactions between the bases decrease their optical absorbance compared to an unstacked conformation. Conversely, when a polynucleotide helix is heated, the optical absorbance increases as the bases unpair and unstack. The largest change in optical absorbance occurs around 260 nm. This change in absorbance allows for easy monitoring of the helix–coil transition by UV absorbance measurements (**Figure 4-24**).

Major thermodynamic factors affecting helix stability include the following phenomena:

- Coulomb repulsions along backbone, from the charged phosphates, and the attraction of counterions to those phosphates
- Hydrogen bonds between the base pairs
- The entropically favorable release of waters solvating individual nucleotides as the helix forms

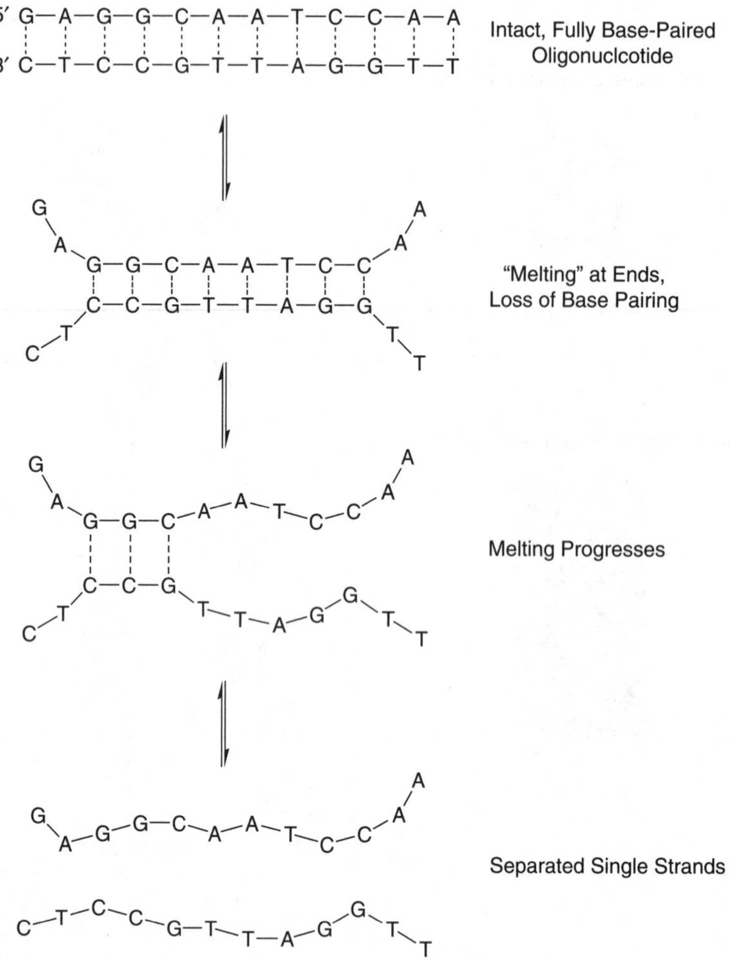

Figure 4-23 Helix unpairing and strand separation.

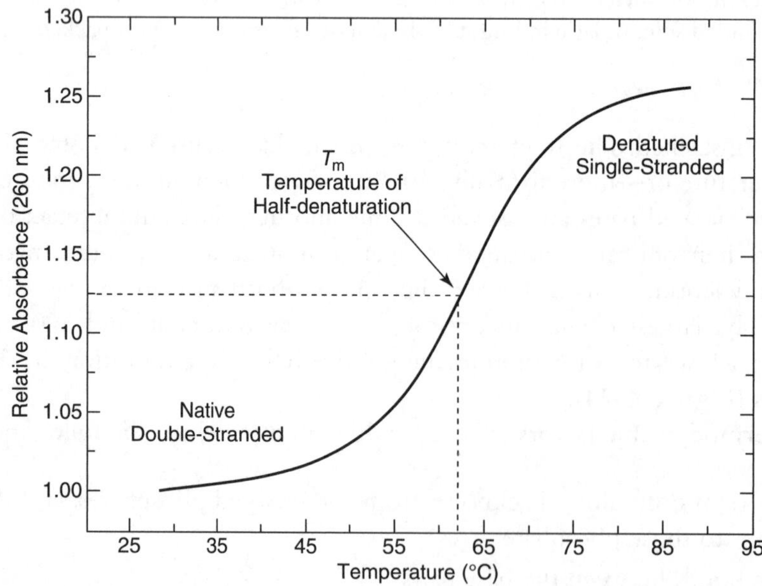

Figure 4-24 Typical oligonucleotide melting curve, showing the increase in absorbance as the folded double-stranded structure is lost.

- The relative entropic favorability of a less organized, "melted" state for the polynucleotide strands
- Stacking interactions between neighboring bases and base pairs

Obviously, favorable and attractive interactions must outweigh the repulsive ones, or a helix would not form. Generally, longer helical molecules are more stable than shorter ones. Short double helices tend to "fray" from the ends relatively easily, while end-fraying is relatively less important for the longer molecules. These longer molecules instead tend to denature through the formation and enlargement of internal single-stranded regions, or "denaturation bubbles."

It is possible to reduce the unfavorable Coulomb repulsions along the phosphodiester backbone by adding more salt to solution, which helps stabilize the helix. Solution pH can also affect helix stability; some groups on the bases are capable of accepting protons in acidic solution or giving them up in basic solution, which may affect hydrogen bonding and Coulomb interactions between the nucleotides. Adding alcohols to the solution tends to destabilize the helix by reducing the amount of stabilizing interactions with water; at high enough concentrations, alcohols and similar organic compounds may denature or even precipitate DNA.

Base pairs do not contribute equally to stability of DNA double helix. G-C pairs contribute more to stability, mainly thanks to the three hydrogen bonds in a G-C pair versus two hydrogen bonds for A-T pairs. The T_m varies almost linearly with the total mole content of guanine and cytosine residues in a double helix. For example, in 0.2 M salt, the transition temperature in °C is given fairly accurately by the formula $T_m = 69.3 + 0.41(G + C)$, where $(G + C)$ is the mole fraction of guanine plus cytosine in the polymer.

The thermodynamic contribution to stability from base stacking depends on details of the interaction between stacked, neighboring base pairs. Thus base sequence—not just base percentage composition—affects stability and melting temperature. Generally, stacking G-C (or C-G) base pairs on top of similar G-C/C-G pairs is more favorable than stacking A-T/T-A pairs on other A-T/T-A pairs. At 37°C, in 1 molar NaCl solution at pH 7, the average $\Delta G°$ for extending an oligonucleotide helix by one base pair would be about -6 kJ/mol; the average enthalpy change would be -33 kJ/mol; and the average entropy change would be -88 J/mol-K.

It is possible to form a double helix of complementary base pairs with one strand made entirely of DNA and the other made entirely of RNA. The helix so formed resembles the A-form helix. This hybridization of DNA and RNA strands is especially important in gene expression and the action of the enzyme RNA polymerase in synthesizing RNA molecules whose sequence is determined by a DNA sequence.

It is also possible to accommodate non-Watson–Crick base pairs in either a DNA or RNA double helix. For example, G-U or G-T pairs can fit into either type of helix, because the overall size of such a mismatched pair matches that for a proper Watson–Crick pair. Some loss of stability to the helix occurs upon introducing such mismatches because of the loss of stabilizing hydrogen bonding; some subtle perturbations of stacking interactions may also arise. The mismatch instability results in a somewhat lower melting temperature T_m for the helix with one or more mismatches, compared with a helix whose two strands are precisely complementary, with no mismatches.

Forming a double helix from two oligonucleotide strands can be relatively rapid. The kinetics are second order, with a rate constant at room temperature of approximately 1×10^6 M^{-1} s^{-1}. Dissociation of a double-stranded oligonucleotide is likewise rapid, occurring within milliseconds after switching to a high temperature. For long polynucleotides, while the initial base unpairing is still rapid, the dissociation process can become much slower, as it can take minutes or longer for the two single-stranded molecules to unwind from each other. Likewise, formation of a long helical molecule from two long, complementary, single-stranded molecules may take place very slowly due to the difficulty in aligning all base pairs properly and due to the hydrodynamic resistance to rewinding the long strands around each other.

Clinical Application

One very important biotechnological application of the ability of DNA to form self-complementary helices is in studies of gene expression using microarray technology. This technique enables researchers to detect and quantitate changes in mRNA production (e.g., gene expression) due to disease states, drug treatment, genetic mutations, changes in environmental variables, and so on.

With this technique, the researcher first extracts mRNA from some biological source (e.g., a whole organism, a selected tissue type, or a culture of a particular type of cell). This extract will, of course, contain many species of mRNA, all differing in sequence and in abundance. Each RNA molecule is then labeled with, for example, a fluorescent dye molecule. Alternatively, before labeling the researcher may take some intermediate preparatory steps in which the RNA molecules are copied into DNA, forming so-called cDNA, and then the copies are enzymatically "amplified" by a special enzymatic technique, the polymerase chain reaction. The result is still a mixture of many species of polynucleotides, differing in sequence according to the gene from which they were derived; they also still differ in their relative abundance, which represents the different levels of expression of the corresponding genes in the biological source.

The next step is to prepare a microarray. The microarray is a solid substrate material (e.g., glass or plastic) on which are deposited spots containing well-defined single-stranded oligonucleotides, one species of oligonucleotide to a spot. The oligonucleotides are covalently attached to the substrate material. With suitable technology, the spots may be placed quite close to one another, with thousands occupying each square millimeter of substrate. The sequences of the oligonucleotides (referred to as "probes") should be carefully chosen so as to match those of the genes or RNA transcripts of interest (the "target sequences"), while avoiding sequences that will tend to fold up on themselves in a hairpin structure, or that would match too closely unrelated, nontarget sequences.

Next, the microarray is bathed in a solution of the (possibly amplified and converted) mRNA targets under conditions of temperature, pH, and salt concentration that promote the proper pairing of sequences on the targets with the probes. This step may require some time, to allow for dissociation of improperly matched target–probe pairs, and formation of the more stable, properly paired matches. The formation of the target–probe pairs is called hybridization.

At this point, the microarray is washed with buffer to remove unhybridized target molecules. What remains are presumably only the most stable, and therefore correctly paired, matches of target and probe molecules. These pairings are then detected by the presence of the label adhering to the microarray substrate surface. The presence of the label in a particular spot indicates that that probe sequence (or rather its complementary sequence, as target molecule) was present in the original biological sample. The intensity of the label within a spot indicates the abundance of that particular sequence in the original sample and, therefore, the relative degree of expression of the corresponding gene in the cell, tissue, or organism.

In addition to studies of gene expression, microarray technology has many other applications. For example, it is used for the detection and characterization of genetic mutations, the detection and characterization of microbial pathogens, and DNA sequencing.

QUESTIONS FOR DISCUSSION

1. There are 10, not 16, distinct dinucleotide base-pair sequences. Thus the dinucleotide sequence (5′) G-T (3′) on one strand is equivalent to the sequence (5′) A-C (3′) on the other. What are the other 9 distinct dinucleotide base-pair sequences?
2. The bacterial virus λ has about 48,000 base pairs in the form of a single double helix of DNA.
   a. Assuming the DNA to be in the B-form helix, how long is this molecule?
   b. How many helical turns does it have?
   c. If the bases G, A, T, and C occur with equal frequency in this DNA, how many times will the specific sequence GATC occur in the molecule?
3. Suppose that the phosphodiester backbone of DNA was replaced by amide linkages between the sugars. How might this change affect the stability of the duplex? (Consider charge repulsions and chain flexibility.)
4. Which process would take place more rapidly: folding a self-complementary single-stranded molecule into a hairpin structure or joining two separate, complementary strands into a duplex? Assume that the same number of base pairs are formed in the two cases and that the concentration of strands is equal in both cases.
5. Using inverted repeated sequences, design an oligonucleotide sequence of DNA that will fold into a cloverleaf/cruciform structure.
6. Consider the effect of methylation of bases on pairing possibilities in duplex DNA for 5-methylcytosine, and N6-methyladenine. Would 5-methylcytosine be able to participate in triplex formation?
7. Which would be more sensitive to changes in salt concentration: melting of a duplex DNA or melting of a triplex? Why?
8. Recognition of DNA sequences by gene-regulatory proteins often involves specific hydrogen-bonding contacts between the protein and the DNA. Which features on duplex DNA might be recognized by a protein? To distinguish particular base sequences, would it be better for the protein to probe for contacts via the major groove or the minor groove? Why?

REFERENCES

R. L. P. Adams, J. T. Knowles, and D. P. Leader. (1992). *The Biochemistry of the Nucleic Acids*, 11th ed., Chapman and Hall, London, UK.

P. Belmont, J.-F. Constant, and M. Demeunynck. (2001). "Nucleic acid conformation diversity: From structure to function and regulation," *Chem. Soc. Rev.* 30:70–81.

C. M. Niemeyer and D. Blohm. (1999). "DNA microarrays," *Angew. Chem. Int. ed.* 38:2865–2869.

Y. Pommier, E. Leo, H.-L. Zhang, and C. Marchand. (2010). "DNA topoisomerases and their poisoning by anticancer and antibacterial drugs," *Chem. Biol.* 17:421–433.

J. SantaLucia, Jr., H. T. Allawi, and P. A. Seneviratne. (1996). "Improved nearest-neighbor parameters for predicting DNA duplex stability," *Biochemistry* 35:3555–3562.

R. B. Stoughton. (2005). "Applications of DNA microarrays in biology," *Annu. Rev. Biochem.* 74:53–82.

I. Tinoco, Jr. (1996). "Nucleic acid structures, energetics, and dynamics," *J. Phys. Chem.* 100:13311–13322.

K. M. Vasquez and P. M. Glazer. (2002). "Triplex-forming oligonucleotides: Principles and applications," *Q. Rev. Biophys.* 35:189–107.

S. A. Wasserman and N. R. Cozzarelli. (1986). "Biochemical topology: Applications to DNA recombination and replication," *Science* 232:951–960.

CHAPTER 5

Lipids and Biomembranes

Learning Objectives

1. Define and use correctly the terms *fatty acid, sterol, sphingolipid, triglyceride, phosphatidate, lysophosphatidic acid, phosphoglyceride, inositide, cardiolipin, phosphatidylcholine, phosphatidylserine, phosphatidylethanolamine, lecithin, cholesterol, ceramide, sphingosine, sphingomyelin, cerebroside, ganglioside, sulfatide, eicosanoid, arachidonic acid, amphiphile, lipid bilayer, bilayer vesicle, integral membrane protein, peripheral membrane protein, fluid mosaic model, lipid raft, mediated diffusive transport, active transport, symport, antiport, cyclo-oxygenase (COX),* and *NSAID.*
2. List the five major lipid classes and the four major biochemical roles of lipids.
3. Use proper chemical nomenclature to describe various fatty acids. Distinguish among pertinent isomers of fatty acids.
4. Recognize the structures of palmitate, stearate, oleate, linoleate, and linolenate.
5. Relate features of chemical structure of lipids to their physical behavior (e.g., aqueous solubility, melting temperature, effect on membrane fluidity).
6. Describe what is meant by "essential" fatty acid. Name the essential fatty acid (for humans), and be able to recognize its structure.
7. Recognize the structure of cholesterol. List biochemical roles for cholesterol and outline its biosynthesis, noting the role of HMG CoA reductase and the importance of this enzyme as a drug target.
8. Recognize the structure of sphingosine. List several common sphingolipids and identify their biochemical roles. Relate these sphingolipids to the diseases called lipidoses.
9. Recognize the structure of arachidonic acid. Relate it to the formation of prostaglandins, leukotrienes, and thromboxanes. List the general biological roles played by these compounds.
10. Describe the hydrophobic effect and give a qualitative explanation for its origin.
11. Describe the spontaneous assembly of amphiphilic molecules into aggregates such as micelles and bilayers. Qualitatively explain amphiphilic preferences for forming micelles versus bilayers, based on simple molecular packing constraints.
12. List the principal biomembrane structures found in a mammalian cell, and briefly describe their functions.

13. Describe the various ways in which proteins can be associated with a biomembrane.
14. Describe how solutes can pass through membrane barriers. Distinguish among passive diffusion, mediated passive diffusion, and active transport across biomembranes. List sources of free energy that drive active transport.
15. Using appropriate equations and data, calculate free energy changes for solute transport involving gradients of concentration across membranes. For transport of charged solutes, include the effects of membrane potentials or voltage differences as well.
16. Relate the action of aspirin and other nonsteroidal anti-inflammatory agents to the functioning and inhibition of cyclo-oxygenases. Recognize the structure of aspirin.
17. Relate the action of leukotrienes to the disease of asthma. Describe two mechanisms by which the inflammatory effects of leukotrienes may be reduced or blocked.
18. Describe the general structure of the lipid A endotoxin from *E. coli* that is responsible for toxic shock syndrome.

Overview

Classes and Biological Roles of Lipids

Lipid Classes

For convenience, lipids may be categorized into five different classes (**Table 5-1; Figure 5-1**), based on their structure:

- *Fatty acids* are distinguished by their terminal carboxylic acid moiety and long saturated or unsaturated carbon chains.
- Glyceryl esters are built from fatty acids esterified to the trihydric glycerol molecule; *phosphoglycerides* (or glycerophospholipids) are formed from fatty acids and glycerol 3-phosphate, and *triglycerides* are formed from a glycerol molecule esterified with three fatty acids.
- *Sphingolipids* are built up from fatty acids and sphingosine, a long-chain alcohol carrying an amine group.
- *Sterols* have a characteristic structure of four fused rings (the steroid nucleus).
- Isoprene units (2-methyl-1,3-butadiene) are joined in a regular head-to-tail way to make up the class of natural products called *terpenes*. Terpenes include vitamins A, E, and K; biological pigments such as β-carotene; and the many essential oils derived from plants that are used as perfumes or flavoring agents.

Lipid Roles

Lipids serve in major amounts in four primary roles:

- To form phospholipids and glycolipids, which are components of biomembranes
- As hormones and second messengers inside cells, for communication and regulation
- As fuel molecules and as a way for cells to store energy

Lipid Class, with Selected Examples	Function
1. Fatty acids	Metabolic fuel, precursors to other lipids
Palmitic, stearic, oleic, arachidonic acids;	Components of triglycerides, membrane lipids
prostaglandins; leukotrienes	Hormones and intracellular modulators
2. Glyceryl esters	Storage and structure
Acylglycerols,	Fatty acid storage, metabolic intermediates
phosphoglycerides	Membrane structure
3. Sphingolipids	Membranes, intracellular modulators
Sphingomyelin,	Membrane structure
glycosphingolipids	Membranes, surface antigens
4. Sterol derivatives	Structure, digestion, and signaling/ regulation
Cholesterol,	Membrane, lipoprotein structure
cholesteryl esters,	Storage and transport
bile acids,	Lipid digestion and absorption
steroid hormones,	Metabolic regulation
Vitamin D	Calcium and phosphorus metabolism
5. Terpenes	Vitamins, signaling/regulation
Vitamin A	Vision, epithelial integrity
Vitamin E	Lipid antioxidant
Vitamin K	Blood coagulation

Table 5-1 The Five Major Classes of Lipids

- As "molecular recognition" features, in the acylation of proteins, for targeting of proteins to membranes and organelles

Not to be overlooked is the service of lesser amounts of certain lipids as protective antioxidants (e.g., vitamin E), as pigments and odorants, and as enzyme cofactors (e.g., vitamins A and K).

Fat as a Fuel

Fatty acids are an important energy source and storage reserve; they represent a major alternative to carbohydrates as fuel for the cell and body. They have a high caloric value—approximately 38 kJ/g versus approximately 17 kJ/g for glycogen or starch. Fatty acid oxidation provides at least half of the oxidative energy in major organs and tissues. Fatty acid breakdown produces acetyl-CoA, as does the degradation of glucose and of many amino acids. The structure and biochemistry of acetyl-CoA, a common intermediate in energy metabolism, are discussed in more detail in Chapter 8, which examines the general metabolic strategy of funneling metabolic reactions to a common intermediate.

Energy Storage

Fatty acids are the major constituent of triglycerides and phospholipids (**Figure 5-2**). In triglycerides, three fatty acid chains are attached to a common backbone molecule of glycerol to form a triacyl glycerol; the linkages are all common oxy–ester links. In phospholipids, two fatty acids are esterified to a molecule of glycerol, with a sugar–phosphate esterified at the third carbon of the glycerol. The major storage form of fatty acids is as triglycerides.

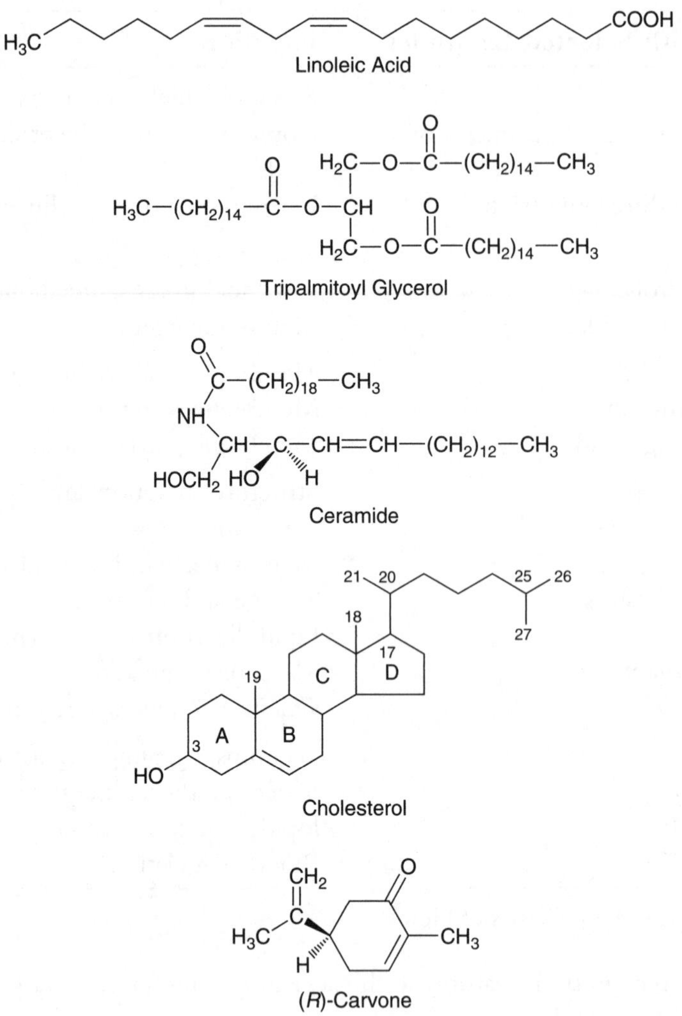

Figure 5-1 A sampling of biological lipids, with examples from each of the five major classes: a fatty acid (linoleic acid), a glyceryl ester (a triglyceride, tripalmitoyl glycerol), a sphingolipid (ceramide), a sterol (cholesterol), and a terpene [(*R*)-carvone].

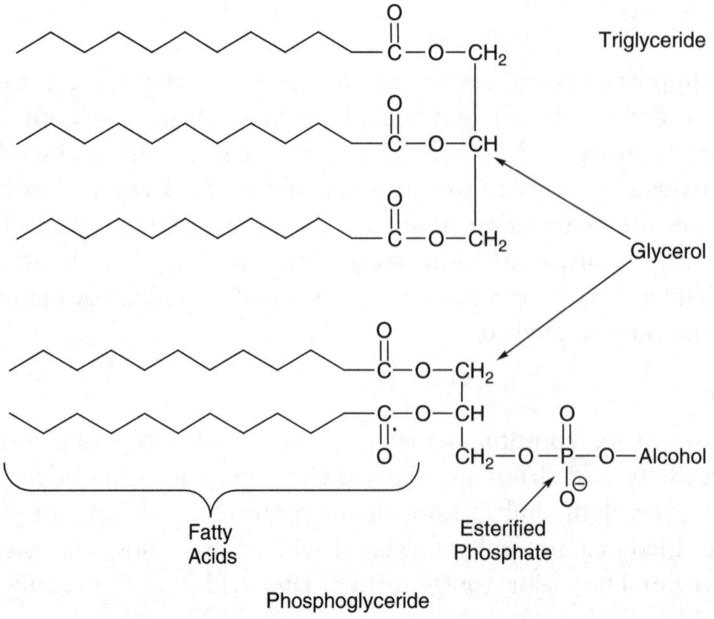

Figure 5-2 Triglyceride and phosphoglyceride structure comparison.

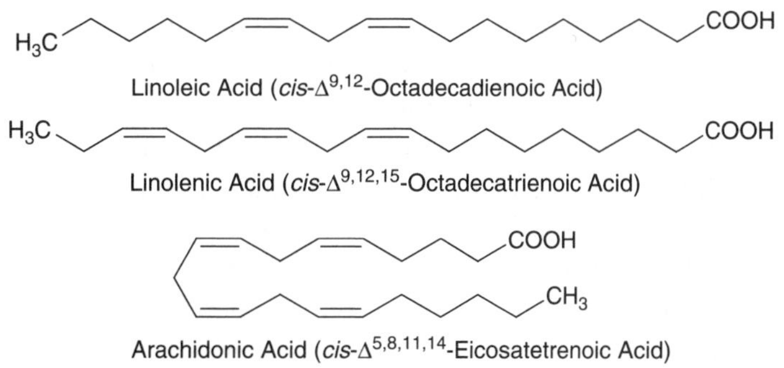

Figure 5-3 Linoleic acid (the essential fatty acid) and two related fatty acids, linolenic acid and arachidonic acid.

The metabolism of fatty acids is compartmentalized, with oxidation occurring in the mitochondrion and synthesis in the cytosol. As with glycolysis versus gluconeogenesis, the pathways are different and involve different enzymes.

Why not store energy as carbohydrate? The energy density for fat is higher than that for glucose polymers by approximately 2.5 times. As a consequence, the body, with only $\frac{2}{5}$ the storage mass (and volume), can store the same amount of energy. This is a good survival and competitive strategy for animals; they can move quickly because they can move smaller masses faster. Plants, by contrast, are sessile. Without the need to move about, they store energy as carbohydrate in stalks and tubers. Seeds are exceptions to this rule, containing lots of fatty acids and oils. The lower mass/volume ratio achieved by using fatty acids instead of carbohydrates favors seeds' wide dispersal and the survival of the plants generating them.

Essential Fatty Acids

One fatty acid, *linoleic acid*, is classed as *essential* for humans. The body is unable to synthesize linoleic acid, yet it serves as a precursor to most of the eicosanoids (see below). Linoleic acid must be provided in the diet. (See the structures in **Figure 5-3**.)

Linolenic acid is not considered to be essential, but a derivative of it (docosahexaenoic acid) is abundant in retinal photoreceptor membranes, so adequate dietary intake of linolenic acid is advisable. Fortunately, plants synthesize linoleic and linolenic acid, and a balanced diet with an adequate amount of vegetables supplies the necessary amounts.

Additionally, arachidonic acid is considered by some authorities to be an essential fatty acid, although it is synthesized from linoleic acid and thus is not absolutely required in the diet. Arachidonic acid is a precursor to leukotrienes, prostaglandins, and thromboxanes.

Chemical Features of Fatty Acids and Acyl Glycerols

The naming of fatty acids can be confusing, but the location of carbon–carbon double bonds in fatty acid chains is quite important metabolically, so it is necessary to have conventions for describing fatty acid structures in a compact way. The presence in a fatty acid of the carboxylic acid is important in forming triglycerides and membrane lipids, while the association and packing of the nonpolar aliphatic chains in these molecules is important in how they are stored and used in biomembranes.

Nomenclature

The names of fatty acids are derived from the corresponding alkane, with *-oic* replacing *-e*.

Saturated fatty acids have only single bonds between the carbon atoms; examples include acetic acid, butyric acid, myristic acid, and palmitic acid. Unsaturated fatty acids have one or more carbon–carbon double bonds in the alkyl chain. The monounsaturated fatty acids have only one carbon–carbon double bond, while polyunsaturated fatty acids have two or more. The double bonds are almost always *cis* double bonds.

So-called trans fats are derived from polyunsaturated natural fats (e.g., soy oil) by an industrial hydrogenation process that leaves some double bonds in the *trans* geometry. The trans fats have been widely used in the food industry because of their low cost and physical properties that are suitable for cooking. High dietary intake of trans fats has a high correlation with coronary heart disease, however, and there is now a general trend away from their use.

To indicate the position of carbons in the fatty acid chain, multiple conventions may be used. The carbon atoms may be numbered, starting from the carboxylate end under the Δ-numbering convention. Alternatively, numbering may start at the opposite end. Also, Greek letters may be used; carbons 2 and 3 (in the Δ-numbering convention) usually are denoted as α and β, respectively (this is similar to the convention used for carbon atoms in amino acids). The terminal methyl group is usually denoted as ω. **Figure 5-4** shows these various conventions for lauric acid, a 12-carbon saturated fatty acid.

Multiple conventions are also used for denoting the location of the double bonds. For example, the position of a double bond may be indicated by Δ with a superscript that indicates the distance from the carboxylate end. As an example, *cis*-Δ^9 means a *cis* double bond between carbons 9 and 10.

In a second convention, the chain length and number of double bonds are noted systematically, using a numerical shorthand notation. Some examples are provided here:

- C_{16} FA without any double bonds—16:0 (e.g., palmitic acid)
- C_{18} FA with two double bonds—18:2 (e.g., linoleic acid, but note that this doesn't specify the location of the two double bonds)
- C_{18} FA with three double bonds at positions 9, 12, and 15—18:3(9,12,15) (e.g., linolenic acid)

In a third convention, the distance from the terminal methyl group (the ω carbon) is given as a superscript. For example, oleic acid is an ω^9 unsaturated fatty acid (but is also a Δ^9 unsaturated fatty acid). Another way of representing the location of the double bond would be to write ω-9 instead of ω^9.

This convention is where the term "omega-3" comes from, for fish oils. Fish oil in the diet is cardioprotective, anti-inflammatory, and anti-carcinogenic. So-called omega-3 fatty acids are major constituents of fish oil, and are thought to be the compounds responsible for these body-protective

	ω-Terminus										Carboxyl Terminus	
	CH_3–	CH_2–	CH_2–	CH_2–	CH_2–	CH_2–	CH_2–	CH_2–	CH_2–	CH_2–	CH_2–	COOH
Δ-Numbering	12	11	10	9	8	7	6	5	4	3	2	1
n-or ω-Numbering	1	2	3	4	5	6	7	8	9	10	11	12
Greek Letter Designation	ω									β	α	

Figure 5-4 Conventions for designating the carbon atoms in fatty acids, applied to lauric acid, a C12 fatty acid.

activities. These fatty acids actually originate from phytoplankton and are passed up the food chain until they reach humans. Such polyunsaturated fatty acids (PUFAs) have their "first" point of unsaturation three carbons in from the methyl terminus. Two common omega-3 fatty acids are eicosapentaenoic acid (EPA), which has 20 carbons in the chain and 5 double bonds, and docosahexaenoic acid (DHA), which has 22 carbons and 6 double bonds (**Figure 5-5**).

Table 5-2 lists some of the most important fatty acids found in mammalian tissue. Acetic acid is related to the common metabolic intermediate acetyl-CoA. Palmitic, stearic, and oleic acids are prevalent in phospholipids and triglycerides, and are common in biomembranes and in adipose tissue deposits of fat. Linoleic, linolenic, and arachidonic acids are minor constituents of phospholipids, so are mainly associated with biomembranes.

Table 5-3 shows a number of dietary sources—both animal and plant—of fatty acids. Notice that animal fats tend to have a higher proportion of saturated and long-chain fatty acids than do plant oils. An exception is coconut oil, which has a high proportion of the shorter-chain saturated, fatty acids (lauric and myristic acids).

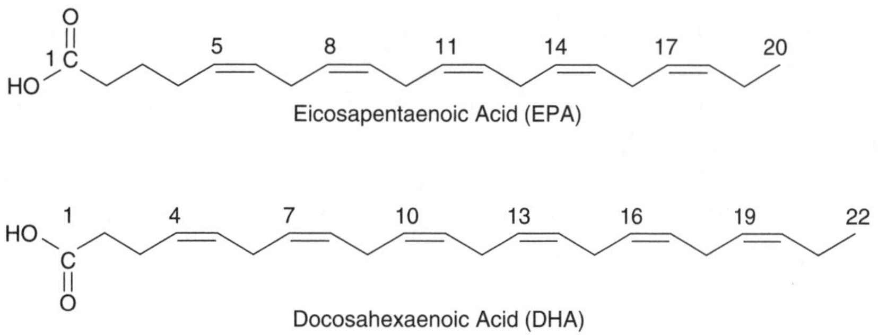

Figure 5-5 Two important ω-3 fatty acids found in fish oil: eicosapentaenoic acid (EPA) and docosahexaenoic acid (DHA).

Descriptive Name	Systematic Name	Carbon Atoms	Double Bonds	Position of Double Bonds*
Acetic	Ethanoic	2	0	
Myristic	Tetradecanoic	14	0	
Palmitic	Hexadecanoic	16	0	
Stearic	Octadecanoic	18	0	
Oleic	Octadecenoic	18	1	9
Linoleic	Octadecadienoic	18	2	9, 12
Linolenic	Octadecatrienoic	18	3	9, 12, 15
Arachidonic	Eicosatetraenoic	20	4	5, 8, 11, 14

Table 5-2 Important Fatty Acids in Mammalian Tissues

*Position of the double bonds listed according to the Δ numbering system. In this numbering system, only the first carbon of the pair is listed: 9 means between carbons 9 and 10, starting from the carboxyl end.

Fatty Acid	Tallow	Butter	Lard	Coconut Oil	Olive Oil	Cottonseed Oil	Soybean Oil	Safflower Oil
Lauric	—	3	—	54	—	—	—	—
Myristic	3	11	2	18	—	—	—	—
Palmitic	26	31	25	8	11	20	10	5
Stearic	25	14	15	2	2	2	4	2
Oleic	36	30	45	5	79	18	24	17
Linoleic	2	2	9	1	7	60	54	76
Others	5	6	1	12	1	—	8	—

Table 5-3 Approximate Percentage Fatty Acid Composition of Some Edible Fats

Other Important Chemical Features of Fatty Acids

Fatty acids are carboxylic acids. The pK_a is approximately 4.8 for most fatty acids. Under physiological conditions (near neutral pH), most of the carboxylate groups are ionized (more than 99% deprotonated).

Fatty acids have long nonpolar "tails" that reduce their solubility in water (**Figure 5-6**). If the carboxylate group is ionized, most fatty acids are slightly soluble in water; in contrast, if the group is protonated (and hence electrically neutral), the aqueous solubility drops to negligible levels. The nonpolar tail, of course, improves fatty acids' solubility in nonpolar media (e.g., solvents such as hexane).

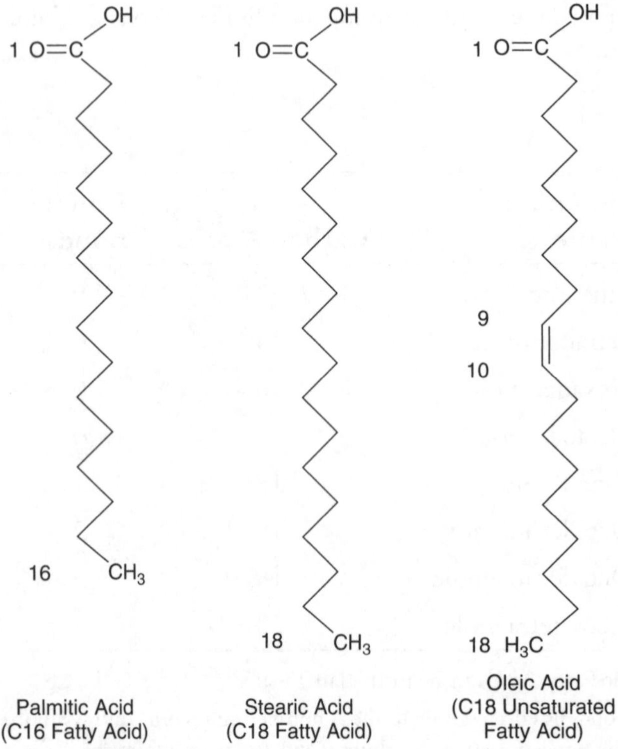

Figure 5-6 Comparison of three common long-chain fatty acids, two of which are saturated (palmitic and stearic) and one of which is unsaturated with a *cis* double bond (oleic acid).

The presence of one or more double bonds in the tail, and the geometry (*cis* versus *trans*) of the double bond, can lower the melting point of the free fatty acid. This is due to steric interference in the packing of tails by the bends or kinks in the tail caused by the *cis* geometry of the double bond(s). This factor has implications for the temperature dependence of the fluidity of biomembranes: Unsaturated fatty acids (e.g., phospholipids, discussed later in this chapter) can modulate the close packing of tails in the lipid bilayer of membrane, thereby changing the local fluidity or viscosity. This, in turn, may alter the activity of membrane-embedded enzymes and transport systems.

Compare the structure of oleic acid (C18:1) with stearic acid (C18:0) in Figure 5-6, and notice how the *cis* double bond in the oleic acid would block close, side-by-side packing of these fatty acids. Packing of oleic acid molecules would lead to open spaces between neighbors, a very unfavorable arrangement (**Figure 5-7**). By comparison, with stearic acid the molecules are easily packed side-by-side without any open spaces, a much more stable arrangement. This difference explains the higher melting point of the saturated fatty acids over the unsaturated fatty acids and the greater rigidity of membranes containing saturated fatty acids as constituents of the phospholipids.

Triacylglycerols (Triglycerides; Neutral Fats)

Triglycerides (triacylglycerides; triacylglycerol) are esters of glycerol in which all three positions are esterified with a fatty acid (see Figures 5-1 and 5-2). It is possible to have a different fatty acid species esterified at each of the three positions on glycerol. Because of the ester linkage, these are not acidic compounds, so do not ionize; they are electrically neutral. The triglycerides are stored as oil droplets in adipose tissue.

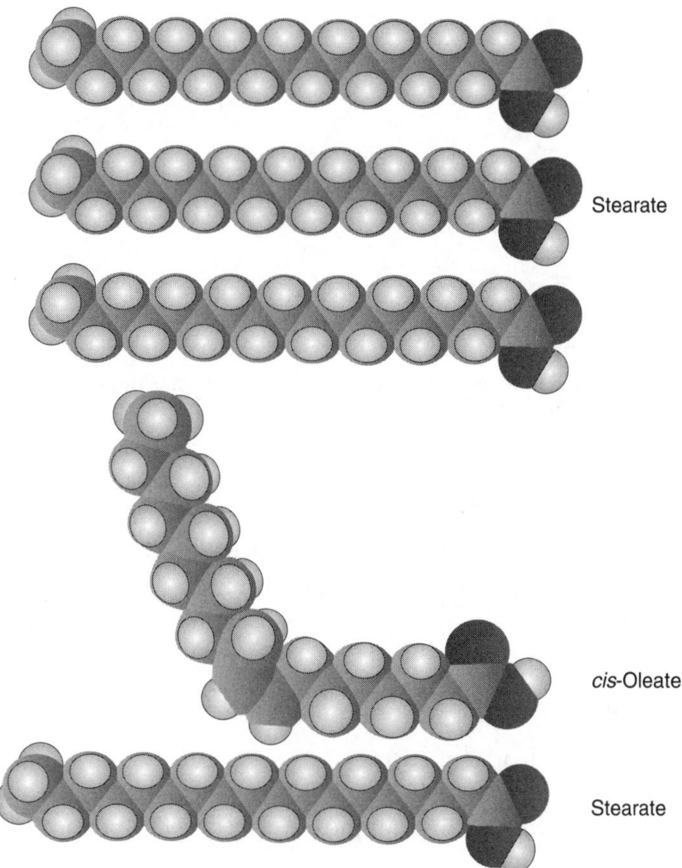

Figure 5-7 The *cis* double bond in oleate disrupts the close packing of stearate chains.

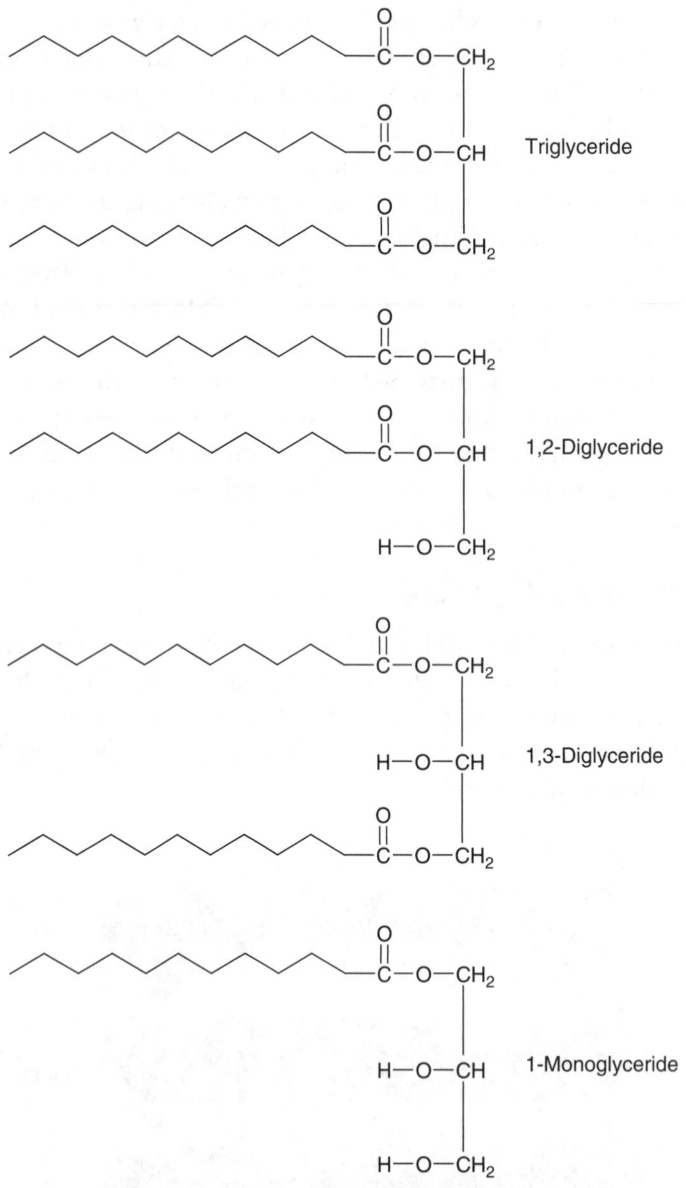

Figure 5-8 Neutral fat is primarily composed of triglycerides—that is, three fatty acids esterifying a single molecule of glycerol. Diglycerides have two fatty acid chains, and the glycerol can be either 1,2-diacylated or 1,3-diacylated.

Monoglycerides (monoacylglycerides) and diglycerides have one or two fatty acids, respectively, attached to glycerol (**Figure 5-8**). Monoglycerides have some slight solubility in water; triglycerides usually do not. Note that monoglycerides or diglycerides may appear with the acyl groups at positions 1, 2, or 3 of the glycerol backbone.

Phospholipids

Major Biological Functions

Phospholipids have several primary functions:

- As membrane components: Phospholipids are a predominant constituent of most biomembranes.

- In surfactant action: Dipalmitoyllecithin in the lung serves to reduce surface tension in alveoli and allow free expansion and contraction of lung tissue. Phosphatidylcholine acts as a detergent and solubilizing agent in bile, to dissolve and transport cholesterol.
- For communication: Phosphatidylinositol 4,5-*bis*-phosphate plays a central role in one of the major signal transduction pathways.

Structure and Nomenclature

The general structure for a phospholipid is based on esterification of glycerol, with acyl groups (fatty acids) attached at the 1 and 2 positions on the glycerol (a 1,2-diacylglycerol), and the 3 position esterified with phosphoric acid or a derivative thereof, such as a phosphate diester bridge to another alcoholic group (**Figure 5-9**). The fatty acid in the typical phospholipid usually has an even number of carbon atoms (14 to 24). The fatty acid may be unsaturated, with *cis* geometry across the double bond. The position of attachment of the fatty acid to the glycerol backbone is indicated by number. Various biological alcohols may be attached to the phosphate group, including serine, ethanolamine, and choline (**Figure 5-10**). Thus one can speak of *phosphatidylcholine, phosphatidylserine*, and so on. Phosphatidylcholine is also known as *lecithin*.

Inositides are phospholipids in which inositol is the attached alcohol. Inositides play an important role in biological signal transduction and in anchoring glycoproteins to the plasma membrane of the cell.

Note the attachment of an alcohol to the phosphate group in these phospholipids. Without the alcohol, the compound is called a *phosphatidate*. If only one fatty acid is attached to the glycerol backbone, it is called a *lysophosphatidate*. Lysolecithin is 1-acylglycerophosphorylcholine (**Figure 5-11**); notice that the fatty acid chain (the acyl group) is not specified. The "lyso" part of the name comes from the detergent action of this compound, which readily solubilizes biomembranes and causes cell lysis.

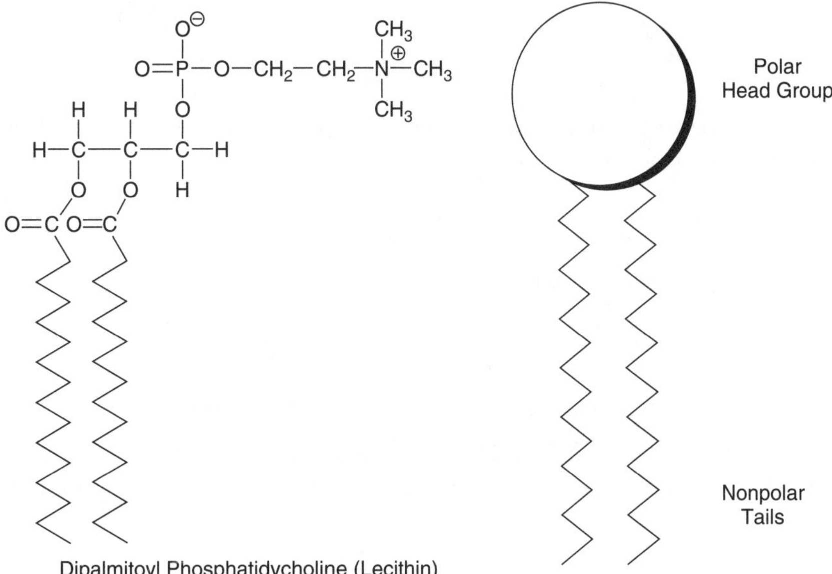

Figure 5-9 Basic structure of a phospholipid: two fatty acid chains and a phosphate moiety esterifying a glycerol, with the phosphate at the third position on the glycerol, to form a phosphatidate. Frequently the phosphate is further attached to an alcohol ("alcohol" here includes a wide variety of compounds with a free —OH group; see Figure 5-10). **A.** Chemical structure. **B.** Schematic representation emphasizing the polar head and nonpolar tails.

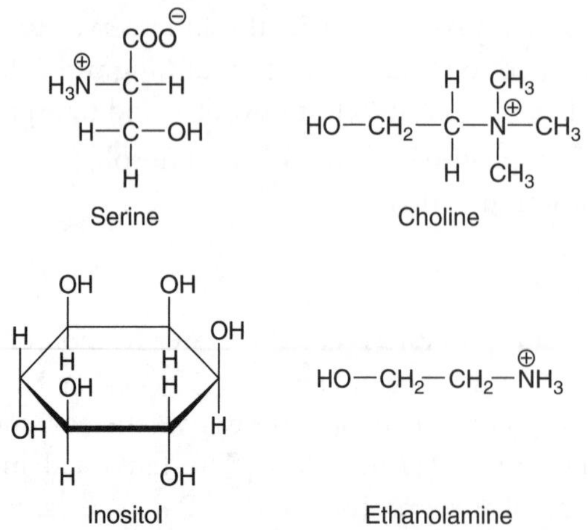

Figure 5-10 A selection of "alcohols" commonly found in phospholipids, attached to the phosphate moiety.

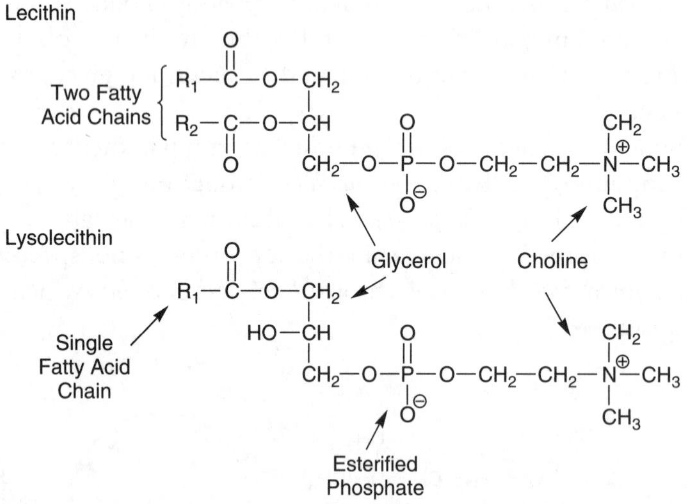

Figure 5-11 Structures of lecithin and lysolecithin (lysophosphatidylcholine). Lysolecithin has only one fatty acid chain and can act as a detergent to lyse cells.

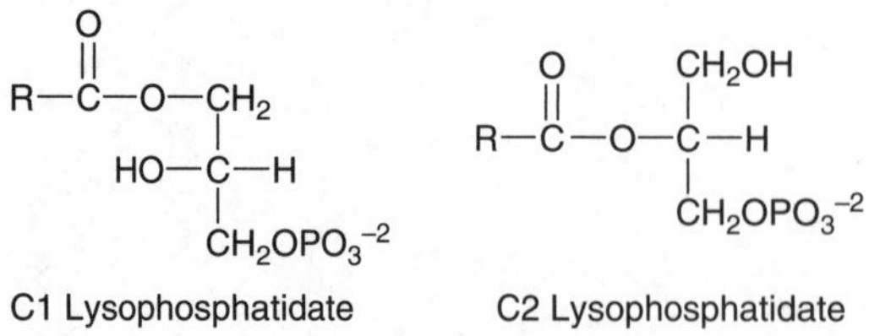

Figure 5-12 Lysophosphatidates have a single fatty acid chain and lack the alcohol attached to the phosphate group. The fatty acid chain can be attached at either the C1 or C2 position of the glycerol backbone.

Lysophosphatidate (lysophosphatidic acid) is a monacylglycerol phosphate (**Figure 5-12**). The acyl group may be attached to either C1 or C2 of the glycerol backbone. Saturated fatty acids usually are found esterified to the C1 position of the glycerol, while unsaturated fatty acids tend to be found at the C2 position.

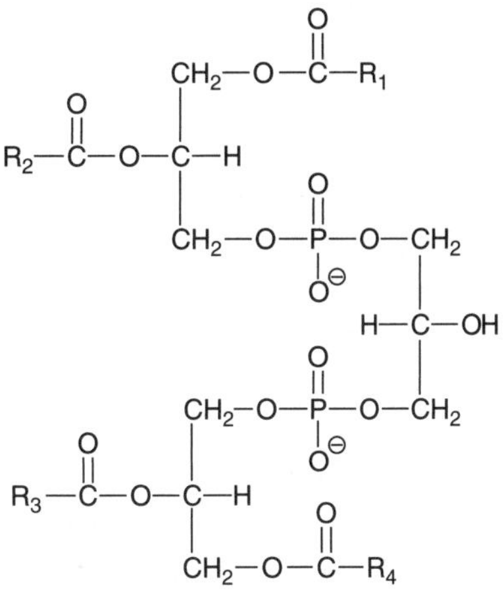

Figure 5-13 Cardiolipin is a complex phosphoglyceride.

Cardiolipin is a complex phosphoglyceride in which glycerol appears not only in the "backbone" but also as the biological alcohol esterified to the phosphate group (**Figure 5-13**). It may help to stiffen certain biological membranes.

Cholesterol

Biological Roles

Cholesterol and related compounds have a number of important roles to play in the cell:

- Cholesterol is a precursor to digestive and solubilizing agents—for example, the bile acids, such as cholic acid, or conjugates with glycine or taurine.
- Cholesterol is a precursor to the steroid hormones, such as the gonadal hormones estradiol and testosterone, and the adrenocortical hormone hydrocortisone (cortisol).
- The vast bulk of cholesterol in the body serves as a membrane constituent that helps to stiffen neighboring acyl groups and reduce their flexibility, thereby overall reducing membrane fluidity.
- Cholesterol and sphingolipids (see the next section) can associate to form recognizable domains (termed "lipid rafts"; discussed in a later section) in the outer leaflet of the lipid bilayer of a biomembrane.

Structure and Chemical Properties

Cholesterol has a characteristic structure with four fused rings. The numbering and ring-lettering system is presented in **Figure 5-14.** The presence of only one polar functional group makes cholesterol quite nonpolar, with characteristically low aqueous solubility and high lipid solubility. Cholesterol has only a single hydroxyl "head group" but several nonpolar groups—for example, two methyl groups, a single double bond, and attached branched alkyl chain of 8 carbons. Cholesterol can be esterified with fatty acids (e.g., with palmitic or linoleic acid), resulting in greater hydrophobicity. Approximately 70% of plasma cholesterol is esterified.

The normal range for serum cholesterol in humans is 3.9 to 6.2 mmol/L, or 150 to 240 mg/dL. This high value (despite the fact that cholesterol has only very limited aqueous solubility) is due to much of the cholesterol being bound by plasma lipoproteins.

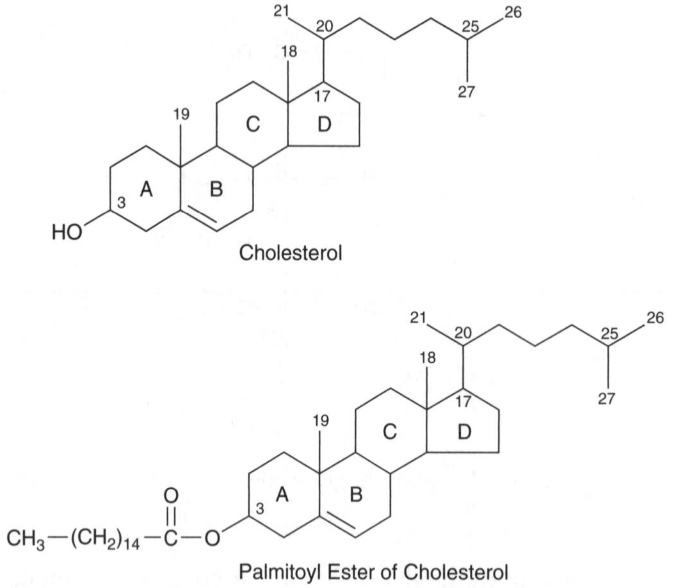

Cholesterol

Palmitoyl Ester of Cholesterol

Figure 5-14 Cholesterol may be acylated with fatty acids; compare cholesterol to the palmitoylated form.

Sphingolipids

Biological Roles

Sphingolipids are derivatives of *sphingosine* (**Figure 5-15**). Roles for sphingolipids are diverse:

- Certain sphingolipids act intracellularly as second messengers in signal transduction pathways, helping to regulate cell division, differentiation, migration, and apoptosis (programmed cell death).
- As membrane components, they tend to rigidify or stiffen the lipid bilayer and to reduce diffusibility of integral membrane components.
- With carbohydrate modifications, sphingolipids in cell membranes act as points for biological recognition, as in the human blood group types (see Chapter 2).

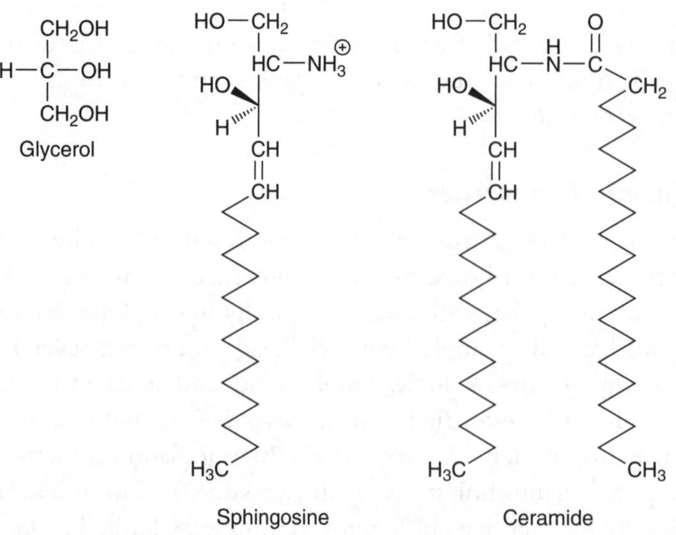

Figure 5-15 Like glycerol, sphingosine can be esterified with a fatty acid chain. Ceramide is a derivative of sphingosine and a precursor to the sphingolipids.

Structures

Sphingosine is derived from palmitoyl-CoA and serine, in a series of reactions not covered here. Note the single "tail," the C-C double bond, and the amino group that can be used for forming amide linkages. In the human body, there is virtually no free sphingosine; instead, this lipid is immediately derivatized, primarily through the intermediate ceramide. Ceramide is then used to make *sphingomyelin, cerebrosides*, and other compounds that are important constituents of the myelin membranes of nerve cells.

Ceramide is the *N*-acyl derivative of sphingosine; the fatty acid here is often behenic acid (a saturated C22 fatty acid), but other fatty acids may be used instead. Ceramide itself is only an intermediate and is not an important membrane constituent. Its reaction leads to sphingomyelin (**Figure 5-16**) and the cerebrosides galactosylceramide (Gal-Cer) and glucosylceramide (Glc-Cer). Glc-Cer then acquires hexose residues to form *gangliosides*. Sulfation reactions on the hexoses produce the *sulfatides*; the donor here is 3′-phosphoadenosine-5′-phosphosulfate (PAPS; **Figure 5-17**).

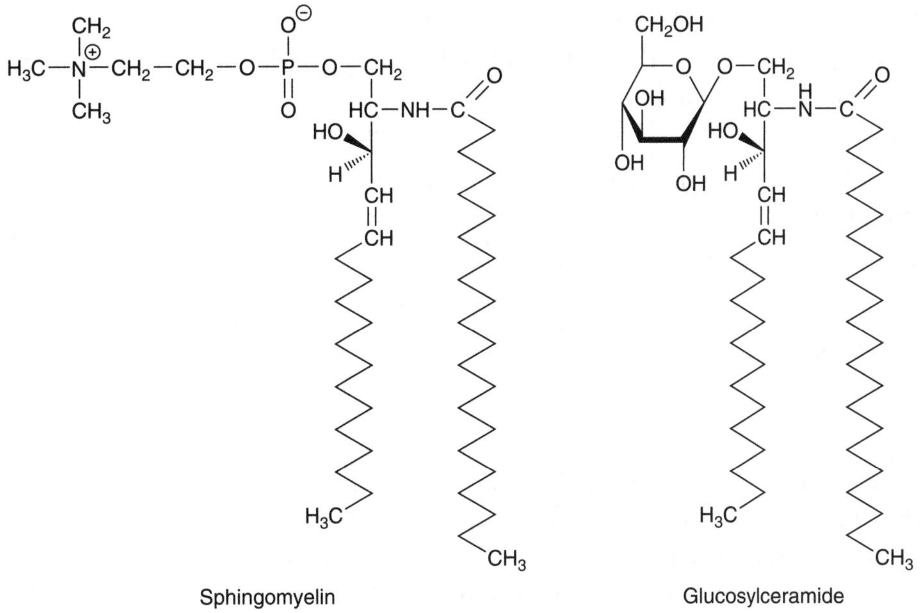

Sphingomyelin

Glucosylceramide

Figure 5-16 Two sphingolipids commonly found in biomembranes: sphingomyelin and glucosylceramide.

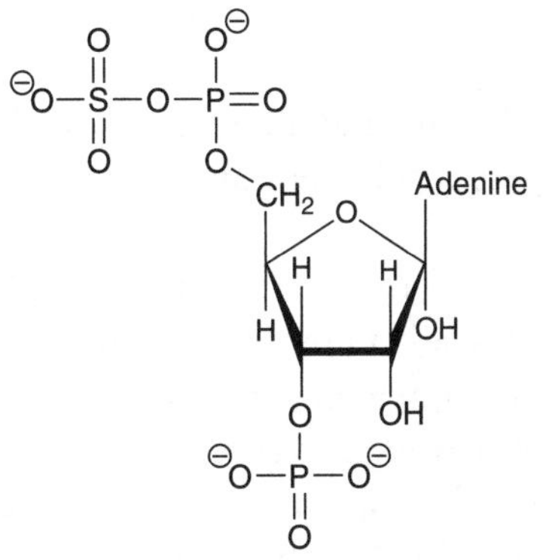

Figure 5-17 3′-Phosphoadenosine 5′-phosphosulfate (PAPS) is a common donor of sulfate groups in biological sulfation reactions.

Disease	Lipid Accumulation	Enzyme Deficiency	Primary Organs Involved
Gaucher	Glucocerebroside	Glucosylceramide β-glucosidase	Liver, spleen, brain
Niemann-Pick	Sphingomyelin	Sphingomyelinase	Brain, liver, spleen
Krabbe	Galactocerebroside	Galactosylceramide β-galactosidase	Brain
Fabry	Ceramide trihexoside	α-galactosidase	Kidney
Tay-Sachs	Ganglioside GM_2	β-Hexosaminidase A	Brain
Wolman	Cholesterol esters and glycerides	Not well characterized	Liver, kidney
Cholesterol ester storage disease	Cholesterol esters and triglycerides	Cholesteryl ester hydrolase	Liver, spleen, lymph nodes, elsewhere
Cerebro-tendinosus xanthomatosis	Dihydrocholesterol (cholestanol)	Sterol hydroxylase in bile acid synthetic pathway	CNS, eyes, tendons
β-Sitosterolemia and xanthomatosis	Plant sterols	Not well characterized	Tendons, skin, circulatory system
Refsum	Phytanic acid	Phytanic acid hydroxylase	CNS, skin, bone

Table 5-4 Lipidoses

Sphingomyelin is broken down by removal of the phosphorylcholine moiety, carried out by the enzyme sphingomyelinase. Hexosidases break down cerebrosides and gangliosides, removing one sugar residue at a time. These enzymes are found in the lysosomal compartments of the cell. Defects in these enzymes can lead to serious pathologies (lipidoses; see **Table 5-4**).

Eicosanoids

Structure and Functions

Eicosanoids (20-carbon fatty acids) include prostaglandins, leukotrienes, and thromboxanes. These molecules act as messengers inside cells and between neighboring cells; they are local hormones (**Figure 5-18**).

Conventional representations of these molecules emphasize the folding back of the carbon chain on itself. For the prostaglandins and thromboxanes, this arrangement is a natural consequence of the five- and six-membered ring structures in these molecules. For arachidonate and the leukotrienes, the conformation as written resembles that adopted by the molecules in the active sites of the enzymes that operate on them. When arachidonate is incorporated into biomembranes (discussed later in this chapter), it will naturally adopt a more extended conformation.

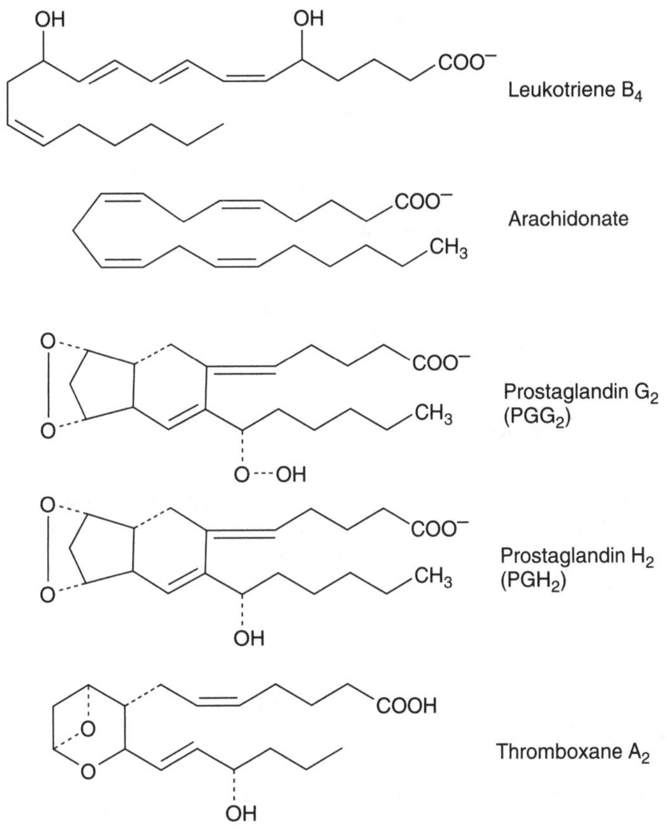

Figure 5-18 Eicosanoids are fatty acids with 20 carbons in the chain. Arachidonic acid is the precursor to the leukotrienes, the prostaglandins, and the thromboxanes.

Arachidonic Acid

An important precursor to the eicosanoids is *arachidonic acid*, a 20:4 FA. It is derived, as arachidonyl-CoA, from linoleoyl-CoA. The pathway involves chain lengthening (by two carbons, from 18 to 20) and the introduction of two additional C–C double bonds.

A dietary deficiency in linoleic acid would block biosynthesis of arachidonic acid. Because arachidonic acid is a precursor for prostaglandins, leukotrienes, thromboxanes, and prostacyclin, such a deficiency can have serious consequences for maintenance of blood pressure, the ability of platelets to aggregate, the inflammatory response, and many other physiological systems.

Derivatives of Arachidonic Acid

Arachidonic acid is incorporated into the phospholipids of the cell membranes. It is released by the action of phospholipase A_2, and then undergoes reactions that convert it to prostaglandins, prostacyclins, thromboxanes, and leukotrienes (**Figure 5-19**).

Prostaglandins have a five-membered ring generated through prostaglandin synthase action. They serve as local hormones and can affect a wide array of biological processes. Some mediate the process of inflammation; others can inhibit platelet aggregation in the blood-clotting cascade. Prostaglandins can also inhibit gastric acid secretion. Prostaglandins also play a role in reproduction; PGE_2 and PGF_2 can induce parturition.

Leukotrienes are produced through the action of lipoxygenase and other enzymes. They characteristically have (at least) three conjugated double bonds. They, and the related

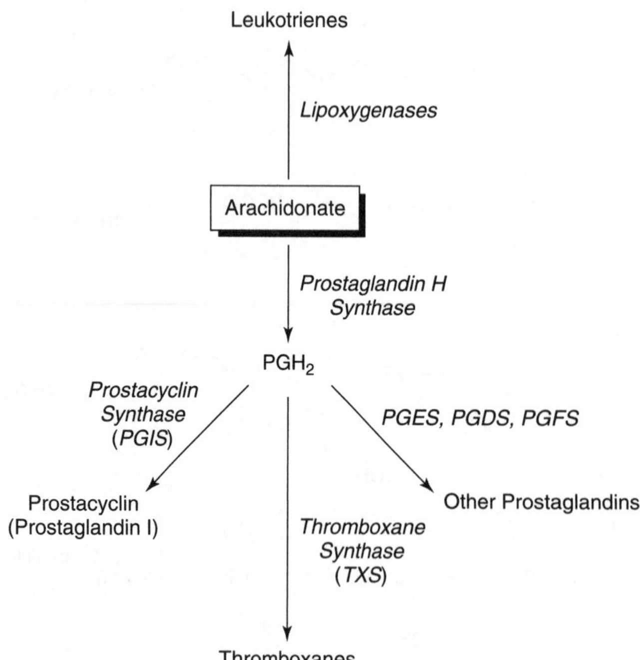

Figure 5-19 Distinct biosynthetic pathways lead from arachidonic acid to the leukotrienes, the prostaglandins, and the thromboxanes.

hydroxyeicosatetraenoic acids (HETEs), have diverse actions; not much is known about the exact mechanisms. Some leukotrienes are involved in regulating neutrophil and eosinophil function. Others promote smooth muscle contraction and constriction of the airways, and trachea. An important clinical point is that leukotrienes are involved in the bronchoconstriction and inflammation that arises in asthma and anaphylactic shock.

Thromboxanes are made from prostaglandin H_2 by the enzyme thromboxane synthase. Thromboxane synthase is related to the cytochrome P450 enzymes. Thromboxane A_2 stimulates platelet aggregation; prostacyclin opposes this action.

Prostaglandin H Synthase

The enzyme prostaglandin H synthase has two enzymatic activities: a *cyclo-oxygenase* (COX) activity and a hydroperoxidase activity. The cyclo-oxygenase incorporates two molecules of oxygen into arachidonic acid and forms a cyclopentane ring, leading to prostaglandin G_2. The hydroperoxidase converts this compound to prostaglandin H_2 (PGH_2).

After PGH_2 is synthesized, it is acted upon by a variety of enzymes (synthases), leading to production of prostacyclin, thromboxanes, and other prostaglandins. These products serve as local hormones that stimulate a variety of cellular responses.

Lipoxygenases are not the same as cyclo-oxygenases; lipoxygenases are responsible for the synthesis of the leukotrienes. Several different lipoxygenases exist and are responsible for the diversity in leukotrienes. These enzymes, which are mixed-function oxidases, are found in leukocytes, the spleen, the liver, the heart, and the brain.

Biomembranes

A major distinguishing characteristic of the cell is the presence of biomembranes, first to separate the contents of the cell from the "outside," and second to form interior compartments for diverse biochemical functions. Biomembranes are stable assemblies yet are dynamic and flexible. Their basic structure is that of a lipid bilayer, but they often contain surprisingly large amounts of protein. They pose a barrier to the passage of matter, but together with their associated proteins, they play an essential role in concentrating certain chemical species for use by the cells.

Lipid Bilayers

The Hydrophobic Effect

The poor aqueous solubility under ambient conditions of many nonpolar compounds, especially drugs, is well known to biochemists and medicinal chemists. Also well known is the tendency of nonpolar compounds to self-associate and to segregate into a separate nonaqueous phase; we just have to think of oil and water to be reminded of this property. This tendency is summarized as the *hydrophobic effect*. Certain compounds, mostly nonpolar ones, seem to "fear" contact with water and, therefore, are described as "hydrophobic."

The hydrophobic effect is ubiquitous throughout biochemistry. It is often a major factor in the binding of drugs to receptors or of substrates or inhibitors to enzymes, in the folding of proteins and nucleic acids into their characteristic secondary structures, and more. In the context of lipid biochemistry, it is largely responsible for the self-assembly of lipid molecules into micelles and bilayers.

Under typical cellular conditions the enthalpy change ΔH for solvation of nonpolar compounds in water tends to be fairly large and favorable ($\Delta H < 0$). The entropy change, however, tends to oppose this; ΔS is large and negative (unfavorable) for aqueous solvation of small nonpolar compounds. The net result is that the free energy change ΔG for solvation is typically large and positive—that is, highly unfavorable. These thermodynamics principles underlie the general observation that nonpolar organics tend not to dissolve in water.

The reasons for the large, favorable ΔH for solvation of nonpolar organics are not entirely clear. Perhaps an enhancement of hydrogen bonding occurs among the water molecules in the shell of hydration around the organic solute. Favorable van der Waals interactions of the solute with the surrounding water molecules will occur as well. In forming a hydration shell around a (small) nonpolar molecule, the water molecules can arrange themselves to maintain—or at least not sacrifice much of—their water-to-water hydrogen bonding (they, of course, cannot form hydrogen bonds to the nonpolar surface of the solute).

The reasons for the large and unfavorable entropy changes upon dissolving nonpolar solutes are not entirely clear either. This kind of entropy change does, however, seem to be connected with a net ordering of the waters in the first one or two layers around the solute. These waters apparently lose some of their freedom of movement (rotation and translation); they may also be somewhat more compressed than their neighbors in the bulk aqueous phase. The result is an entropic resistance to forming lots of individually solvated nonpolar molecules dispersed throughout the aqueous phase. For dissolving nonpolar molecules in water the term $-T\Delta S$ outweighs the term ΔH in the free energy relation $\Delta G = \Delta H - T\Delta S$, and as a result we have an overall unfavorable free energy change; nonpolar organics dissolve poorly in water.

When two nonpolar small molecules meet and bind to each other in an aqueous environment, some of the water of hydration at the junction of their nonpolar surfaces is released into the bulk aqueous phase (**Figure 5-20**). This water thereby gains more freedom and becomes less ordered than when it hydrated the nonpolar molecule. Although the two nonpolar molecules are now associated with one another and are in a more ordered state, because many more waters are released and become disordered, the net result is an overall increase in the system's entropy; ΔS is favorable for this process. The enthalpy change also tends to be negative and favorable, so

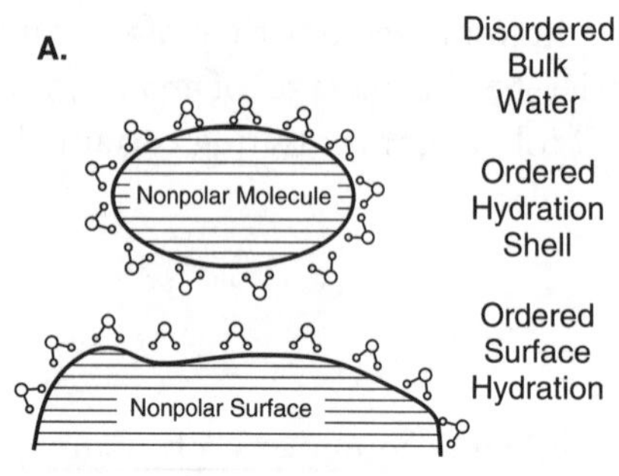

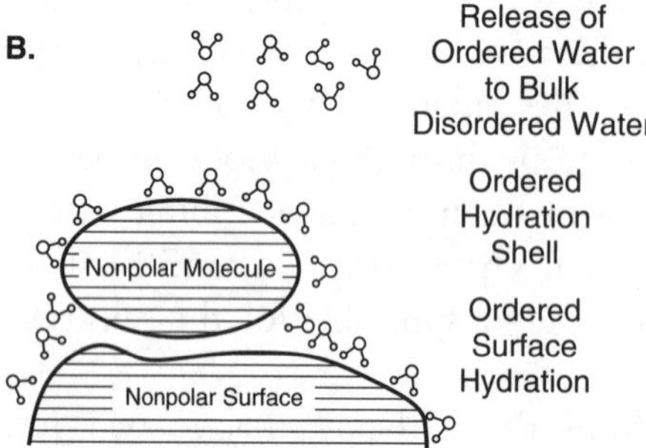

Figure 5-20 The hydrophobic effect drives the association of nonpolar surfaces in water. **A.** Both nonpolar molecular surfaces have a layer of ordered water. **B.** Juxtaposition of the surfaces releases water to the bulk phase, where it becomes more disordered, producing a favorable entropy change.

that the free energy change for the association of nonpolar molecules in aqueous solution tends to be quite favorable.

A warning is needed here: A large heat capacity change is associated with the hydrophobic effect. Increasing the temperature can lead to large changes in ΔH, ΔS, and ΔG. At temperatures much above 37°C (310 K), the sign of the entropy change can reverse and cause ΔG to change sign as well. The discussion presented here assumes conditions of temperature, salt, and pressure similar to those in the human body.

Amphiphile Self-Assembly

Amphiphiles are molecules with separate polar and nonpolar regions. In aqueous solution, they have a tendency to have their polar region oriented toward the aqueous phase, to interact favorably with water, and to have their nonpolar region segregated away from contact with water. Thus, in solution, these molecules tend to self-assemble into aggregates like those shown in **Figure 5-21.** Also, at an air–water interface, a monolayer of amphiphiles assembles with their nonpolar tails oriented toward the (nonpolar) air phase.

The type and shape of aggregate formed by an amphiphile depend strongly on the packing of the polar head and nonpolar tails in the aggregate. Single-tailed amphiphiles (e.g., detergents, lysophosphatidates) have a molecular shape resembling a cone, with the polar head group at the wide base of the cone and the nonpolar alkyl tail leading to the pointed tip of the cone. Molecules with this shape can be packed together, avoiding gaps on the surface and internal voids in the nonpolar region, to form spherical or globular micelles. Depending on the exact nature of the headgroup, the tail, the species of added salt and other factors, the micelle may resemble a football more than a sphere; extended cylindrical structures are even possible. Although some dispersion in the size of the aggregate occurs, clearly the length of the amphiphile tail, the area

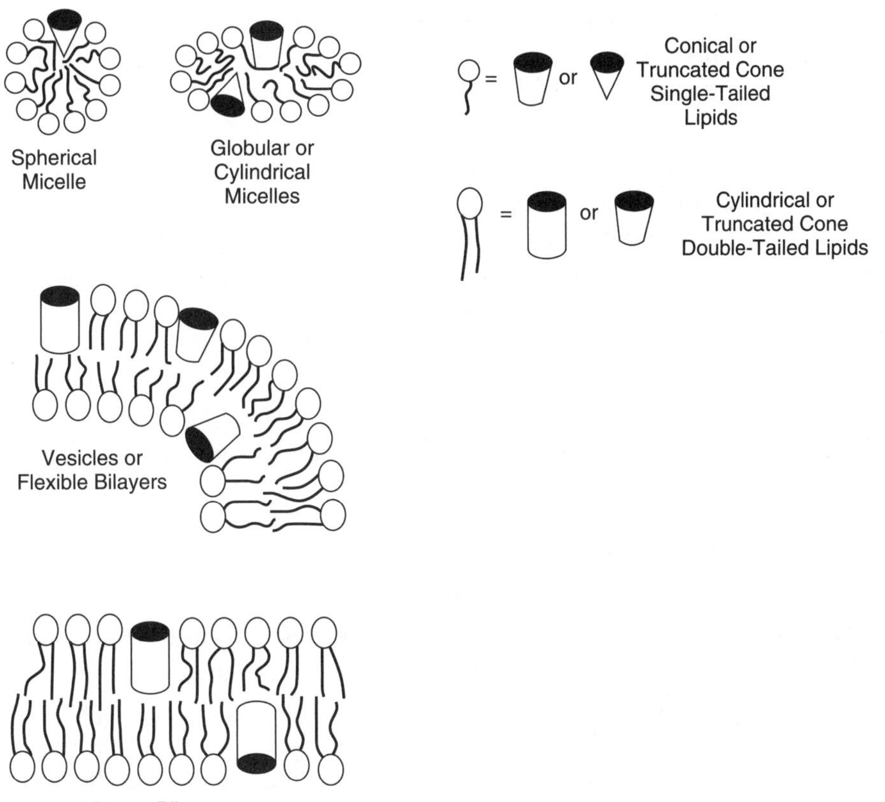

Figure 5-21 Amphiphiles will spontaneously self-assemble into aggregates. The type of aggregate depends strongly (though not exclusively) on molecular packing considerations. Amphiphiles with conical molecular shapes tend to pack into micelles, whereas those with cylindrical shapes tend to pack into bilayers, which can be folded into vesicles.

of the head group, and the volume of the entire molecule constrain the number of amphiphile molecules per aggregate, typically to less than a few hundred molecules per (globular) micelle.

Lipid Bilayers

Double-tailed amphiphiles have structures that resemble cylinders, again with the polar head group at one end and the two nonpolar tails filling up the body of the cylinder. The cylindrical shape is not easily packed into a spherical shape. Instead, simple packing constraints lead to a flat or planar assembly (a monolayer or sheet). Even so, there is a need to remove the nonpolar tails from contact with water. It is satisfied by adding a second sheet, in opposite orientation, to the first sheet. Such a bilayer structure can be extended laterally almost without limit, unlike the globular micelles, which have a definite constraint on their size. Monolayer "leaflets" in a lipid bilayer can be peeled away from one another by freeze-fracturing, and the (frozen) structure can be visualized by electron microscopy. The thickness of the bilayer depends on the type of lipid incorporated into it, especially the length of the alkyl tails of the fatty acids attached to the phospholipids and sphingolipids. Roughly speaking, a typical phospholipid bilayer has a thickness of approximately 6–7 nm, with the phospholipid head groups each occupying an area of approximately 0.7 nm^2.

Bilayers can be bent or folded, as seen in organelles like the endoplasmic reticulum or Golgi apparatus, or in the inner membrane of a mitochondrion. It is also possible to roll a bilayer into a closed, spherical surface, with the interior containing some aqueous solution; such a structure is called a *bilayer vesicle*. The budding of vesicles from biomembranes, and their merger with the same, is an important mechanism for transporting material about in the cell. The stiffness or resistance to folding of a bilayer depends on the type of lipid incorporated into the bilayer and on the presence of small ions (e.g., Ca^{2+}) and associated proteins. Small ions such as Ca^{2+} may neutralize negative charges on the head groups and allow these groups to approach one another more closely, thus affecting their relative packing and perhaps promoting curvature in the bilayer. Proteins may insert into the bilayer and act as "wedges" to promote curvature; proteins with positively charged regions apposed to the bilayer may also neutralize Coulomb repulsions between head groups, thereby affecting packing and bilayer curvature.

Bilayers enriched in cholesterol or sphingolipids tend to be stiffer than those composed mainly of phospholipids. Also, the longer and more saturated the nonpolar fatty acid tails on the lipids are, the more difficult it is to bend the bilayer. Conversely, if the amphiphiles have unsaturated tails, they may not pack together so closely, and the interstitial vacancies that result will tend to increase the flexibility of the bilayer.

Bilayer Transitions and Fluidity

At low temperatures, the tails of the fatty acids in a bilayer tend to align and pack together to maximize contacts and van der Waals attractions. Under these conditions, the bilayer becomes less and less flexible, and much less lateral motion of the individual lipid molecules is noted. The bilayer resembles a sort of two-dimensional crystal or gel, with long-range ordering of the individual lipid molecules and little motion permitted to those molecules. As the temperature increases, the thermal agitation of the lipid tails increases, as does their disorder (**Figure 5-22**). The lateral motion of the molecules increases greatly as well.

Because the molecules are so closely packed and interact so intimately, the transition from the ordered, tightly packed gel state of the bilayer to the disordered, fluid-like state occurs over a very small rise in temperature; the transition is highly cooperative. This change resembles the process seen in ordinary solid-to-liquid phase transitions (e.g., ice to water), so it is referred to as a "melting" transition. For most biomembranes the transition temperature is relatively low, so that in vivo the membrane is "fluid-like." Generally, proteins and other biomolecules associated with a biomembrane are relatively free to move about laterally, within the plane of the bilayer, with the bilayer offering a lateral viscosity comparable to that of, say, olive oil. Individual lipid molecules within a leaflet can interchange position on a time scale of approximately 10^{-7} seconds (they are not so free to exchange from one leaflet to the other, so this movement occurs much more slowly, on a time scale of approximately 10^5 seconds).

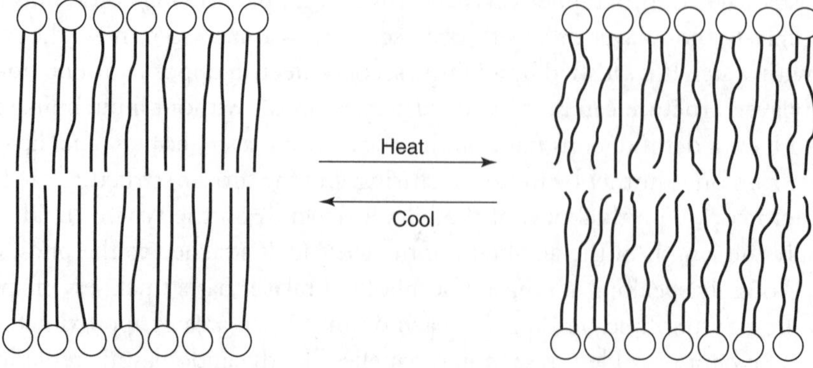

Figure 5-22 The gel-to-fluid phase transition for a lipid bilayer, emphasizing the increase in disorder and flexibility of the nonpolar tails of the lipids upon heating.

The type of alkyl tail in the amphiphiles making up the bilayer will have a definite influence on the midpoint temperature ("melting temperature") for the gel-to-fluid transition. Long, saturated alkyl tails will pack together well and, therefore, will resist thermal agitation. Shorter chains or those with unsaturation or with short branches (e.g., methyl groups) that block close packing will have weaker cohesion and will undergo the transition at a lower temperature.

Biomembrane Structure

Biomembranes are an essential constituent of living cells. Their primary function is to act as a barrier, blocking passage of water and dissolved solute molecules; biomembranes also block invasion by pathogens, such as bacteria or viruses. The plasma membrane of a typical eukaryotic cell enables the cell to maintain a consistent internal environment compatible for life processes, with the proper pH, concentration of small ions, amounts of nutrients, and so on. A biomembrane barrier also provides a way for the cell to separate itself from dangerous or toxic waste products, which can be expelled to the exterior. Inside the cell, biomembranes form compartments for the separation and regulation of myriad biochemical processes. Thus opposing biochemical reactions can take place simultaneously but in different compartments. For example, in one compartment a cell can break down damaged proteins, while synthesizing replacement proteins in another compartment.

Because biomembranes separate different biochemical processes, they are typically asymmetric: They have distinct "faces" or sides, with an unequal distribution of lipids, carbohydrate modifications, and membrane-associated proteins, that provide distinctly different biochemical activities. The asymmetry in lipid composition can result in different degrees of fluidity in one leaflet versus the other, which may influence the activity of the associated proteins or the degree and direction of folding of the membrane bilayer. Differences in the distribution of charged lipids between leaflets can result in development of an electrical potential across the membrane, which may be important for transport of charged solutes across membrane (discussed later in this section).

The asymmetry of a biomembrane is a persistent feature. A fairly strong barrier prevents any transverse motion of a lipid or membrane-associated protein from one leaflet to the other. Lipids do not readily "flip" from one leaflet to the other, nor do proteins freely tumble in the bilayer. Membrane-associated proteins generally are oriented in the lipid bilayer, so they project distinct functional domains to one side versus the other. For example, the insulin receptor is a protein that has an extracellular domain that specifically binds insulin molecules, a domain that spans the bilayer, and an internal cytoplasmic domain that interacts with other proteins to convert the signal of a "bound insulin" into a set of chemical reactions that alters the cell's physiology. Carbohydrate modifications to the lipids and proteins of the plasma membrane are also asymmetrically distributed, with the great majority being directed to the exterior of the cell. Indeed, mammalian cells are typically surrounded by a coat of sticky sugar chains.

Eukaryotic cells are distinguished from prokaryotes by the presence of organelles, membrane-bound internal compartments that are not found in prokaryotes. Several different kinds of organelles exist, and not all eukaryotic cells have all possible types of organelle. **Figure 5-23** shows a hypothetical mammalian cell with a selection of the most common types of organelles.

Major compartments and functions of the organelles are as follows:

- The plasma membrane is the outer cell membrane, whose major function is the control of entry and exit of materials from the cell. Secondarily, it forms and maintains contacts and communication with other cells and conducts electrical impulses (for a nerve or muscle cell).

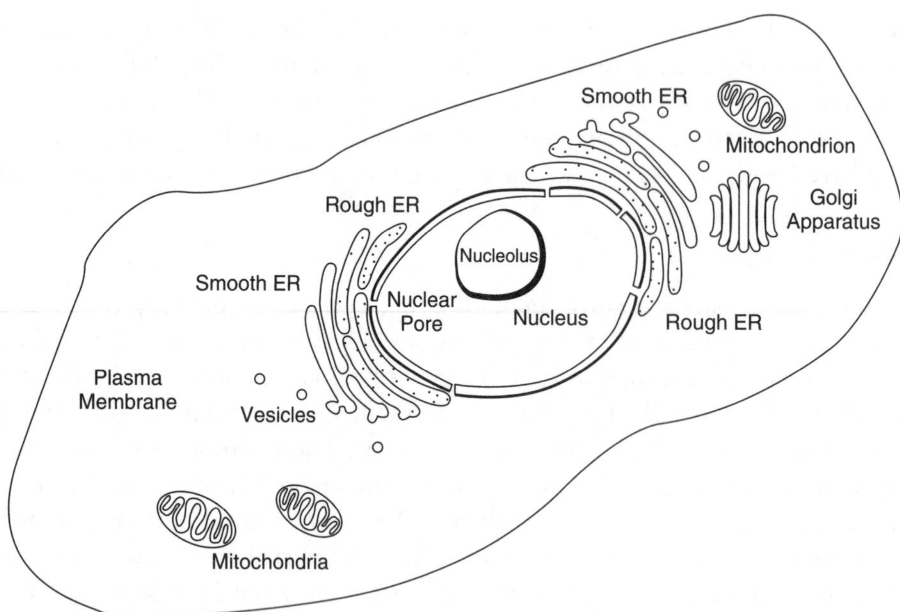

Figure 5-23 Biomembrane structures in a hypothetical mammalian cell, showing important organelles.

- The nuclear compartment has a double-membrane structure. It is the central repository for genetic material consisting of DNA in the form of chromatin. Gene transcription and RNA synthesis occur in an inner structure called the nucleolus. Nuclear pore complexes control the movement of proteins and RNA into and out of the nucleus.
- The endoplasmic reticulum (ER) is a continuous network of folded sac-like and tube-like membranes, running from the nucleus outward, with many interior channels and vestibules. It can be divided into two general regions. The rough ER, located near the nucleus, has ribosomes bound to the membranes, giving them the "rough" appearance in electron micrographs. The smooth ER, located farther away from the nucleus, does not have ribosomes and so appears smooth by comparison. The ER is responsible for protein synthesis and folding, along with various modification reactions of proteins, especially in the attachment of carbohydrate chains; it is also involved in the production of membrane lipids.
- The Golgi apparatus is a set of flattened sac-like structures that is often found close to the ER. It receives and acts on proteins and membrane lipids to further modify them, and then passes those substances on to other parts of the cell through the budding of vesicles.
- Lysosomes are digestive vesicles containing enzymes that degrade proteins and nucleic acids. They help to break down foreign bodies, such as ingested bacteria.
- Mitochondria have a double-membrane structure, in which the outer membrane has many large pore complexes and the tightly sealed, highly involuted inner membrane contains a very high proportion of embedded proteins (more than 70% of this inner membrane is protein, by weight). These organelles are the central energy-generating structures for the cell; the mitochondria are where carbohydrates, fats, and amino acids are thoroughly oxidized to drive the synthesis of ATP for the cell.

Biomembranes as Heterogeneous Lipid Mixtures

Bilayer structure in biomembranes is complicated by the wide variety of lipid constituents and proteins associated with the membrane. The situation with respect to membrane-associated proteins is quite complex. Different tissues, and the organelles within the cells of those tissues, of course, vary widely in terms of their biological function. Because a wide variety of proteins are needed to mediate these functions, large differences in protein species and overall protein content of these various biomembranes are inevitable.

The situation is only somewhat less complicated for the lipid composition of biomembranes. **Table 5-5** presents data on the phospholipid composition of membranes found in rat liver cells. At least nine species of lipids were detected (only trace amounts of some were found), not including cholesterol. Table 5-5 shows quite striking differences in the relative amounts of these phospholipids, depending on their cellular location. For example, only the mitochondrion has significant amounts of diphosphatidylglycerol, and the plasma membrane is enriched for sphingomyelin and phosphatidylserine, by comparison to the other membranes assayed. Presumably these differences in composition are related to the differences in function associated with the membranes.

An important feature of these lipid mixtures is the range of temperatures amenable to the gel-to-fluid transition. Biomembrane lipid mixtures have a broader phase transition compared to bilayers prepared with just one lipid species, and they tend to start to melt at a somewhat lower temperature. In higher organisms, this characteristic helps to keep the transition temperature below body temperature, promoting bilayer flexibility and fluidity where needed for different membrane functions. The temperature and breadth of the transition can be modulated by changes in lipid composition. As a consequence, one internal membrane may be relatively stiff and gel-like, to provide a rigid container, while another membrane may be fluid and flexible, for motion of associated enzymes and transporters—all at the same temperature.

Lipid–lipid association in bilayers is relatively nonspecific, due mainly to the hydrophobic effect and the van der Waals attractions of the nonpolar lipid tails for one another. Almost any two bilayer membranes can be fused together to form a larger, continuous bilayer. This facility permits, for example, certain membrane-enveloped viruses to merge with the plasma membrane of target cells and infect them. It also allows laboratory manipulation of different cell lines to fuse two cells from different sources and create a daughter hybrid cell; creation of such hybrid cells has become a major tool in investigating cell biology. Of course, this capability also forms the basis of vesicular traffic between different organelles and membranes in the cell.

Phospholipid	Mitochondrial Membrane	Endoplasmic Reticulum	Plasma Membrane	Golgi Membrane
PE	34.6	21.8	23.3	23.5
PC	40.3	58.4	39.3	54.0
SPH	0.5	2.5	16.0	7.8
DPG	17.8	1.1	1.0	1.0
PI	4.6	10.1	7.7	8.6
PS	0.7	2.9	9.0	3.0
LPC	n.d.	9.5	1.0	0.4

Table 5-5 Lipid Composition of Rat Liver Organelles

Abbreviations used: PE, phosphatidylethanolamine; PC, phosphatidylcholine; SPH, sphingomyelin; DPG, diphosphatidylglycerol; PI, phosphatidylinositol; PS, phosphatidylserine; LPC, lysophosphatidylcholine; n.d., not determined.

Data expressed as a percentage of total phospholipid phosphorus.

Source: Adapted from F. Zambrano, S. Fleischer, and B. Fleischer. (1975). *Biochim. Biophys. Acta* 380:357–369.

Biomembranes do not necessarily have a symmetric distribution of lipids, either laterally or between the two leaflets. Given that different types of lipids will have different biological roles, there will be asymmetry in lipid distribution across the leaflets as well as laterally within a leaflet. In general, in mammalian cells the outer leaflet of the plasma membrane will be enriched in glycolipids, especially sphingolipids with attached carbohydrate chains. The glycolipids are important for recognition by the immune system and in forming cell–cell contacts.

Types of Membrane-Associated Proteins

Proteins form associations with lipid bilayers in several ways, which creates different classes of membrane-associated proteins (**Figure 5-24**).

- *Peripheral membrane proteins* bind to the surface of the bilayer, primarily through ionic attractions and hydrogen bonding. Generally they are free to move about laterally. Although they may deform the bilayer locally, they do not penetrate into the bilayer to any extent. These proteins can also be detached from the bilayer relatively easily.
- *Integral membrane proteins* have a substantial portion of their body inserted into the bilayer; they may penetrate only one leaflet of the bilayer, or they may extend completely through the second leaflet. These proteins are very firmly attached to the bilayer, and generally can be removed only through the action of detergents.
- Acylated proteins may be attached to the face of a bilayer through the immersion of a nonpolar acyl "tail" in the bilayer leaflet; the acyl tail acts here as a sort of anchor to hold the protein on the surface of the bilayer. The acyl chains are commonly derived from myristic or palmitic acids, and are linked covalently to the protein. Here the body of the protein is outside the bilayer. These proteins can be released from the membrane through the action of enzymes that cleave the linkage joining the anchor to the protein.
- An important subclass of this last group are those proteins carrying a glycosylphosphatidylinositol (GPI) anchor (**Figure 5-25**). The GPI anchor provides two acyl tails to hold the protein close to the face of the bilayer. The enzyme phospholipase C can release such proteins from the membrane.

The membrane-embedded portions of integral membrane proteins generally consist of amino acids with nonpolar side chains. In some cases, the secondary structure of the embedded region may be an embedded β-barrel structure in the bilayer, creating a pore in the membrane. Pores may also be formed by the association of two or more polypeptide chains that fold into a

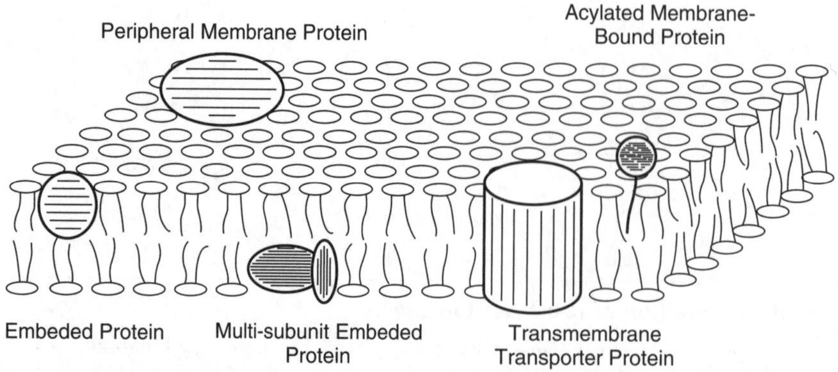

Figure 5-24 Cartoon representation of protein–membrane associations.

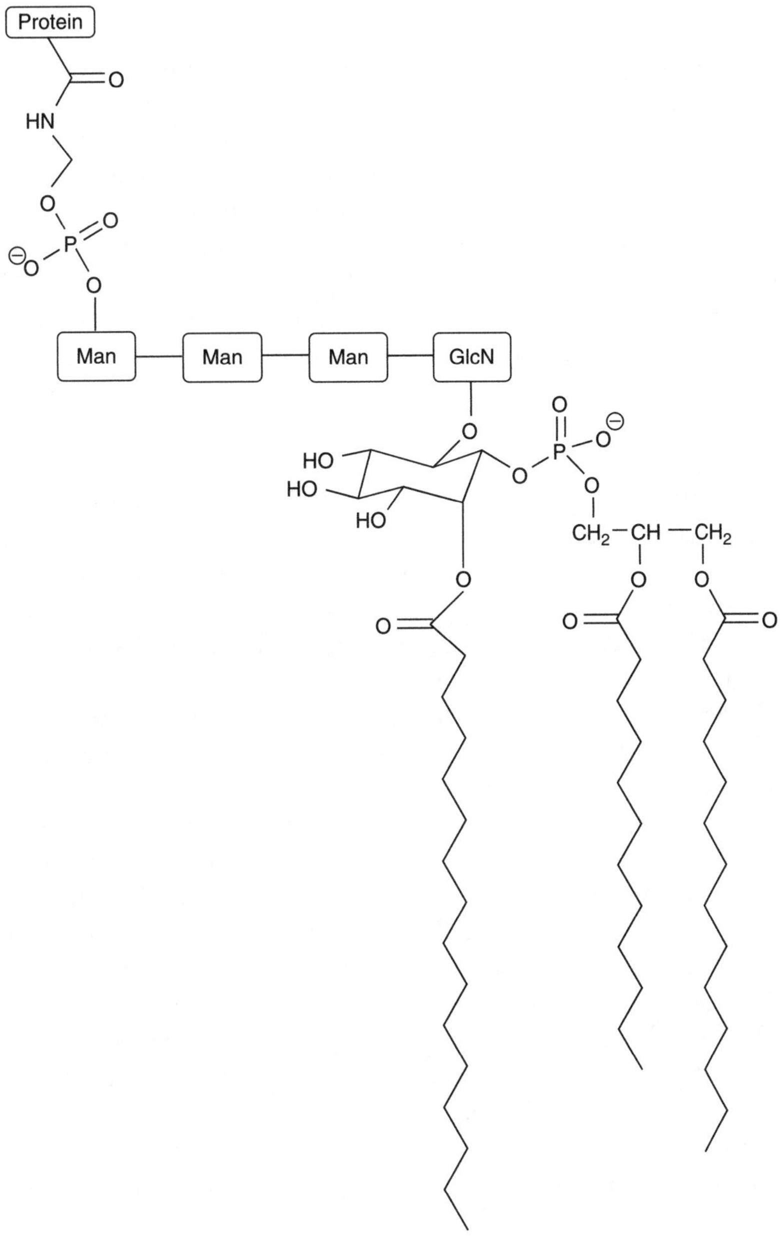

Figure 5-25 GPI anchor structure. Fatty acid chains are embedded in a bilayer leaflet, while the sugar chain acts as a tether to hold the protein in close proximity to the face of the membrane. Man = mannose, GlcN = glucosamine.

β-barrel; for example, the maltose transporter protein of *E. coli* is a trimer of identical subunits that form an extended β-barrel, to admit the passage of large, hydrated sugar molecules.

A common structural motif for integral membrane proteins is an α-helix or a bundle of α-helices. In the latter case, the backbone of the polypeptide chain may cross and recross the bilayer several times (many membrane-bound drug receptors will have such a structure). For transmembrane proteins, the embedded segment is generally oriented so that the axis of the helix or helices is roughly perpendicular to the plane of the bilayer. Recall that in the α-helix, the side chains extend laterally away from the axis of the helix. The nonpolar character of the embedded side chains favors their interaction with the nonpolar interior of the lipid bilayer; in this way, they help to firmly anchor the protein in the membrane.

Fluid-Mosaic Model of Biomembranes

In architecture and the fine arts, a mosaic is a two-dimensional pattern of tiles, glass pieces, or small stones inlaid in a surface. A biomembrane bears a certain resemblance to such a mosaic: There is a two-dimensional surface (the lipid bilayer) with a variety of objects embedded in that surface (proteins, glycolipids, and the like). Unlike in a tile or stone mosaic, however, the pattern in a biomembrane is not necessarily fixed in place; often there is considerable lateral motion of the embedded pieces, not to mention the inherent fluidity of a phospholipid bilayer itself. In other words, a biomembrane can be thought of as a *fluid mosaic*, with the embedded pieces moving around, either at random or perhaps with some sense of directed motion. The lipid bilayer provides a sort of two-dimensional solution that dissolves the associated proteins and permits their lateral motion (see Figure 5-24).

Lipid Rafts

Because of the relative freedom of lateral motion within a bilayer, one might expect the mixture of lipids there to be relatively homogeneous. Perhaps surprisingly, the evidence indicates that biomembranes actually do have some lateral organization, which has implications for the biological functioning of the membrane. Studies of detergent-resistant fragments of plasma membranes and the membranes of some subcellular organelles found them to be enriched in sphingolipids and cholesterol, forming so-called *lipid rafts* (**Figure 5-26**). The current view of biomembrane structure envisions biomembranes as having phase-separated regions: one that is fluid-like and enriched for phospholipids, and the other that is more rigid and ordered, containing a high proportion of cholesterol and sphingolipids.

The carbohydrate moieties attached to the heads of sphingolipids are thought to help promote their lateral association. At the same time, a sphingolipid head group occupies a substantial interfacial area—more than would be simply subtended by the nonpolar tails. This mismatch between the area occupied by the head group and the volume occupied by the tails leaves packing voids in the interior of the bilayer leaflet, which tend to be filled by cholesterol molecules. Cholesterol may also function to fill voids at the interface between leaflets. Regions enriched in sphingolipids and cholesterol tend to be less fluid and more ordered than neighboring regions that are rich in (disordered) phospholipids. This lateral segregation of lipid domains can be important for the functioning of membrane-embedded proteins (cross-membrane transporters and channels, enzymes, and various receptors) and for cellular processes such as cell division, vesicle formation and fusion, or phagocytosis.

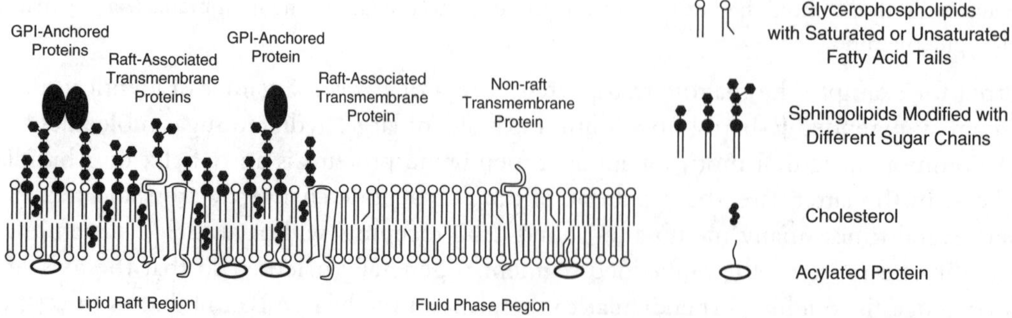

Figure 5-26 Cross-section of a biomembrane showing the fluid-phase and lipid raft regions. Lipid rafts are enriched in sphingolipids and cholesterol, and have a different protein composition than fluid-phase regions.

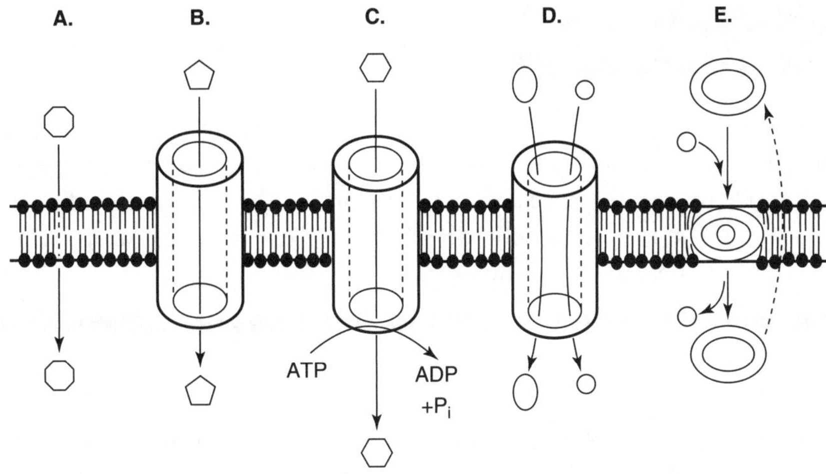

Figure 5-27 Transmembrane transport mechanisms. Proteins are schematized as hollow cylinders for simplicity in visualizing transport; the actual structures are much more complicated. **A.** Simple passive diffusion. **B.** Mediated diffusive transport. **C.** Active transport, at the expense of ATP hydrolysis. **D.** Cotransport of two solutes (symport is shown). **E.** Mediated transport by a small lipid-soluble carrier.

Transport Across Membranes

While lipid bilayers are relatively permeable to water, dissolved gases, and small nonpolar organic compounds, they form a significant barrier to the passage of large molecules such as proteins or DNA, or to any small molecule with a polar or ionic nature. Several biochemical mechanisms facilitate the transport of such materials across a biomembrane, as shown in **Figure 5-27**.

Passive Diffusion

First, consider transport of a solute down a concentration gradient. In terms of free-energy changes, this *passive diffusion* is a spontaneous process. As noted, small nonpolar solutes can simply diffuse across the bilayer, with net transport occurring in the direction of lower concentration of that solute. This mechanism is how oxygen crosses from red blood cells into actively working muscle cells, for example.

Mediated Diffusive Transport

The activation barrier to crossing a lipid bilayer tends to slow the process, so some assistance may be needed to accomplish transport of materials in a timely way for the cell. To increase the rate of transfer of solutes across a membrane, special carrier or transporter molecules may be used. Especially for larger molecules or those with some polar or ionic nature, the solute needs help crossing the bilayer.

One common mechanism for transport of such solutes is for the solute to pass through a pore or channel that crosses the bilayer (*mediated diffusive transport*). These pores or channels are made of one or more bilayer-embedded protein chains, with the chains folded to project nonpolar amino acid side chains into the interior of the bilayer, while polar side chains are projected into the lumen of the pore or channel. This arrangement of the side chains stabilizes the proteins in the bilayer while providing an attractive polar environment for the polar solute. In some cases, conformational changes in the embedded protein are needed as a part of the transport mechanism. For example, a transporter protein that spans the membrane may envelope the solute, binding it selectively and tightly, and then undergo a conformational change that expels the solute to the other side of the bilayer.

Clinical Application

In the case of some ionic solutes, such as potassium ions or protons, there exist specialized small molecules that combine the ability to bind the ionic solute with the ability to dissolve in, and cross, the lipid bilayer. An example is the antibiotic valinomycin, an unusual macrocycle made by the microorganism *Streptomyces fulvissimus*, which binds K^+ ions and carries them across biomembranes.

Active Transport

To perform transport against a concentration gradient, a source of free energy must be found because movement of solute up a concentration gradient is not spontaneous by itself. It is necessary to couple the unfavorable transport up a concentration gradient to some other biochemical process that itself is intrinsically favorable and that—when combined with the unfavorable uphill transport process—will yield an overall spontaneous process. The coupling is mediated by specialized embedded proteins (really, embedded enzymes) that can perform this process of *active transport*. There are several ways in which this process can be carried out.

One possibility is to harness the free energy of hydrolysis of adenosine triphosphate (ATP). Under cellular conditions, ATP hydrolysis is a spontaneous process, so coupling it to the nonspontaneous transport up a concentration gradient can make the overall process spontaneous, with a favorable free energy change. The transporter protein would bind and hydrolyze ATP, using this free energy release to drive conformational changes that carry the solute across the membrane to a region of higher concentration. An important example of such a mechanism is found in the antiport of Na^+ and K^+ ions in animal cells by the Na^+-K^+ pump, a membrane-embedded enzyme that expels Na^+ ions from the cell and imports K^+ ions. For each ATP molecule hydrolyzed, approximately three Na^+ ions are pumped outward and two K^+ ions are passed inward. This process results in a cellular milieu that is depleted in positive charges and establishes a transmembrane voltage difference (which can be itself exploited for active transport of other solutes, as discussed later in this section). Another important ion pump is responsible for maintaining a low internal concentration of Ca^{2+} ions; this system also hydrolyzes ATP, and it involves the antiport of protons as calcium ions are expelled.

A second possibility for moving a solute against its concentration gradient is to couple this process to the transport of a different solute species down its own concentration gradient. Like coupling to ATP hydrolysis, such a system may provide enough free energy to carry the first solute up its concentration gradient. The direction of (spontaneous) transport of the second solute may be in the same direction (*symport*) or in the opposite direction (*antiport*) as that of the first solute. An important example here is the cotransport of sodium ions with glucose by cells in the small intestine. The low intracellular concentration of Na^+ (maintained by the ion pump discussed earlier) provides a favorable free energy change for symport of a sodium ion with a molecule of glucose, even though the glucose may be more concentrated inside the cell than outside.

A third possibility is to exploit the electrical potential that may be present across a membrane. Differences in the distribution of charged lipid head groups across a bilayer will result in the formation of an electrical field and an associated voltage gradient across the bilayer; also, the ion gradient established by ion pumps such as the Na^+-K^+ ATPase pump (described earlier) will create a voltage difference. Positively charged solutes will be attracted to the side of the membrane with the lower or more negative electrical potential (voltage); transfer of such a solute in this direction will have a negative free energy contribution from this electrostatic interaction. The following expression applies to the free energy of transfer of a charged solute from region 1 to region 2, taking account of differences in concentration and electrical voltage between the two regions:

$$\Delta G = RT \ln\left(\frac{C_2}{C_1}\right) + zF(V_2 - V_1) \tag{5-1}$$

Here z is the electrical charge on the solute (complete with its sign and magnitude, such as $+1$ for Na^+ or -2 for SO_4^{2-}), F is the Faraday constant, C_1 and C_2 are the concentrations of solute in the two regions, and V_1 and V_2 are the voltages in the two regions. Notice that the two terms contributing to ΔG could have opposite signs; the concentration term could be positive (for transfer to a higher concentration), while the voltage term could be negative (for transfer to a lower potential state). If the transmembrane voltage difference were large enough, this term could outweigh the unfavorable contribution from moving the solute up a concentration gradient, making the overall process favorable. In Chapter 11 we will see that the transmembrane potential across the inner mitochondrial membrane is highly important in the generation of ATP by the mitochondrion.

Other sources of free energy that may drive active transport are the absorption of light (by specialized pigmented cells, such as those found in the retina) and the transfer of electrons in redox reactions. This latter source will be discussed in more detail in Chapter 11 in connection with oxidative phosphorylation.

Proteins that perform mediated diffusive or active transport strongly resemble enzymes (discussed in the next two chapters). Whether or not they catalyze a chemical reaction, these proteins share with enzymes three important characteristics: their high specificity or selectivity (they transport only one or a few chemically related species); the property of saturability (there is a maximum rate of transport that depends on the number of such proteins working in the membrane); and their inhibition by specific compounds (particularly competitive inhibition and irreversible inhibition; see Chapter 7).

Additionally, cycles of vesicle formation and fusion with biomembranes afford cells another major means by which to transport solutes, macromolecules, and other materials from one cellular compartment into another.

Clinical Applications

Cyclo-Oxygenases and Their Inhibition

The Two Types of Cyclo-Oxygenase

In humans, two different cyclo-oxygenase enzymes are involved in eicosanoid metabolism, catalyzing the same type of reaction: the formation of a peroxide and a cyclopentane ring on arachidonic acid. The enzymes also act on other long-chain, polyunsaturated fatty acids such as those found in fish oil. Currently, much research is exploring the pharmacological effects of these other reaction products.

COX-1 is distributed throughout the body; it is always present (a "constitutive" activity). Primarily it makes hormones (prostaglandins) to keep the stomach lining intact and the kidneys functioning properly.

COX-2 also makes prostaglandins, whose release leads to inflammation, pain, and fever. While some tissues express COX-2 constitutively, most do not. For this reason, COX-2 activity was historically classified only as "inducible," meaning that some external stimulus had to affect the cells or tissue for copies of the enzyme to be made.

Action of Aspirin and Other Nonsteroidal Anti-Inflammatory Drugs

Aspirin and other nonsteroidal anti-inflammatory drugs (*NSAIDs*) reduce inflammation, block clotting, and reduce pain. How do these drugs work?

Aspirin acetylates a specific residue at the active site of the cyclo-oxygenase activity of prostaglandin synthase (**Figure 5-28**). This reaction irreversibly blocks the enzyme from acting on arachidonic acid to synthesize PGH_2. Without PGH_2, the synthesis of other prostaglandins stops, and the messengers that incite inflammation are reduced, affording relief from pain, swelling, redness, and other discomfort. Also, thromboxanes are no longer made. In particular, no TXA_2—a potent aggregator of platelets—is made. Hence, clotting is reduced. The covalent attachment of the acetyl group in the enzyme's active site permanently blocks the enzyme from functioning; restoration of COX activity will come only with the synthesis of new copies of the enzyme.

Ibuprofen, naproxen, and some other anti-inflammatory medications (**Figure 5-29**) bind noncovalently and inhibit the enzyme, thereby producing relief from inflammation. Because they are not permanently attached to the enzyme, however, eventually they leave the active site and are excreted, allowing the enzyme to become active once more.

There is currently much interest in the development of inhibitors that are specific for COX-2 because these drugs would be more selective than aspirin for targeting the "inducible" COX activity. The hope is that by targeting COX-2, mainly the inflamed tissue would be specifically affected to reduce pain, swelling, and redness, without the harmful side effects associated with aspirin (e.g., loss of blood clotting activity, loss of protection of the gastric lining). Such agents would be useful in treating osteoarthritis, for example, whereas prolonged aspirin use is well known to produce nose bleeds, gastric upsets, and even ulcers.

Two recently controversial prescription drugs, celecoxib and rofecoxib (**Figure 5-30**), are potent inhibitors of cyclo-oxygenase activity. Rofecoxib, but not celecoxib, shows at least a 10-fold selectivity for COX-2 over COX-1, but the ratio seems to depend on assay conditions, with different enzyme sources and preparations giving different selectivity ratios. Unfortunately, use of rofecoxib has been linked to an increased incidence in adverse cardiovascular events, such as stroke and heart attack. While celecoxib is still marketed (with due cautions on its use), rofecoxib has been withdrawn from the U.S. market.

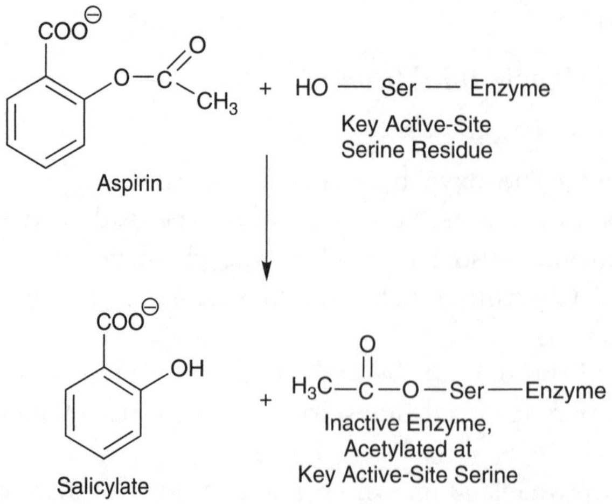

Figure 5-28 Aspirin acetylates a key serine residue in the active site of the prostaglandin H synthase, and irreversibly inhibits the enzyme.

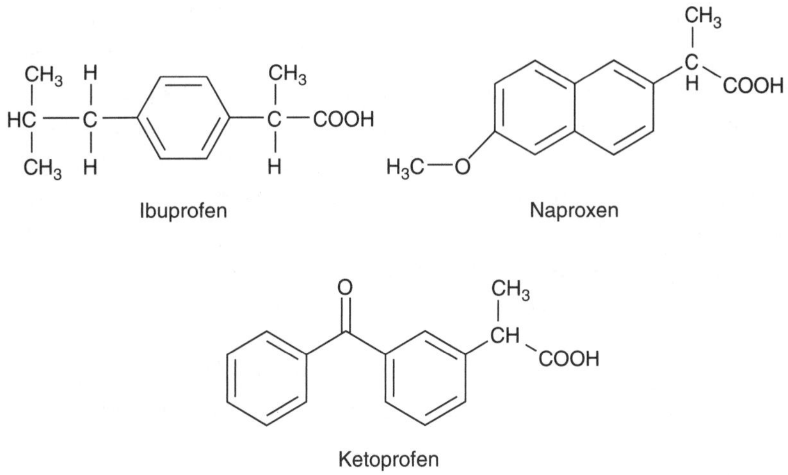

Figure 5-29 Three common nonsteroidal anti-inflammatory drugs (NSAIDs): ibuprofen, naproxen, and ketoprofen. All are reversible inhibitors of the prostaglandin H synthase.

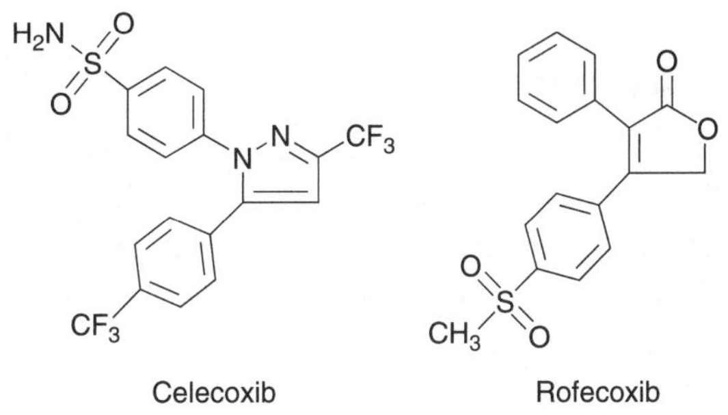

Figure 5-30 Two prescription NSAIDs. Rofecoxib has been withdrawn from the market.

Lipidoses

Certain genetic diseases result in derangements of lipid storage. These so-called lipid storage diseases, or *lipidoses*, are caused by a defect in the activity of one or another of several catabolic enzymes, notably those involved in sphingolipid and sterol metabolism (see Table 5-4).

All lipidoses are rare, with Gaucher disease being the one most commonly seen in the clinic. Several of these diseases have multiple subtypes, and the severity can vary with the subtype. Treatment for many lipidoses is only supportive, and there may be no specific therapy (enzyme replacement therapies for Gaucher disease and Fabry disease are available now, however). Some are associated with particular ethnic groups; for example, Tay-Sachs and Gaucher disease are associated with Jewish families.

Leukotrienes and Treatments for Asthma

Asthma is a pathological condition involving edema and constriction of the airway. It can be induced by allergens, exercise, and exposure to cold temperatures. Leukotrienes play a critical role in its pathology.

Leukotrienes are made primarily by inflammatory cells, such as macrophages, mast cells, and polymorphonuclear leukocytes (the "leuko" part of the name "leukotriene" stems from the original isolation of these compounds from leukocytes). They are synthesized from arachidonic acid by the enzyme 5-lipoxygenase (abbreviated as 5-LO), a non-heme iron dioxygenase, and further acted on by various specialized enzymes.

Leukotrienes exert their action by binding to and stimulating specialized leukotriene receptors that are coupled to G-proteins; several types of leukotriene receptors are known. There are hints that leukotrienes may also act at other types of receptors.

The 5-LO enzyme also acts on other long-chain polyunsaturated fatty acids, making analogs of leukotrienes called lipoxins. Lipoxins are themselves potent messengers. They are currently the subject of research for their potential in fighting inflammation and resolving pathophysiological processes.

By blocking either the enzymes responsible for leukotriene synthesis or the receptors for leukotrienes, it is possible to alleviate the symptoms of asthma.

- Zileuton (trade name Zyflo) inhibits 5-LO inside mast cells, macrophages, and other cells. This action blocks the synthesis of leukotrienes directly, thereby reducing their inflammatory effects.
- Montelukast (trade name Singulair), pranlukast (Onon, Altair), and zafirlukast (Accolate) act at the CysLT1 receptor for leukotrienes (this receptor is thought to be responsible for most of the symptoms of asthma). These agents are competitive antagonists for the leukotrienes C4 and E4, which act at this receptor.

Lipopolysaccharides: Endotoxins

Gram-negative bacteria such as *E. coli* have an outer membrane that is largely covered by lipopolysaccharides (LPS). LPS has a central moiety, called lipid A, to which is attached an elaborate polysaccharide chain, the details of which will vary across bacterial species and strains within species. If the immune response to LPS is excessive ("toxic shock"), the result can be a severe inflammation that leads to death.

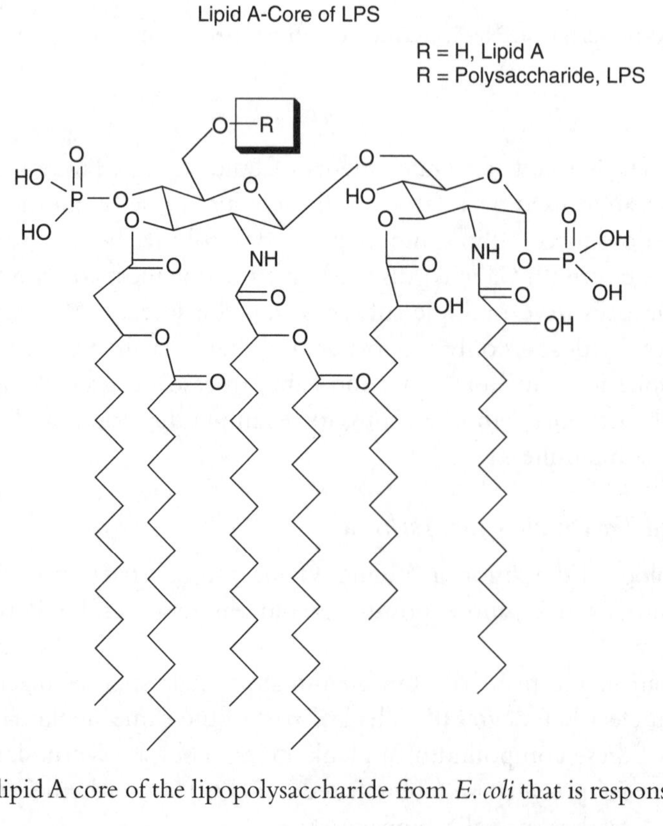

Lipid A-Core of LPS

R = H, Lipid A
R = Polysaccharide, LPS

Figure 5-31 The lipid A core of the lipopolysaccharide from *E. coli* that is responsible for toxic shock syndrome.

Lipid A is the primary immunostimulatory fragment of LPS (**Figure 5-31**). Injection of very small quantities of lipid A, without any live bacteria, can produce fever and inflammation in mammals. Interestingly, a precursor of lipid A, in which two of the fatty acid chains are not yet added, is in humans an antagonist to LPS; however, in mice this precursor is an agonist.

QUESTIONS FOR DISCUSSION

1. Elaidic acid (*trans*-9-octadecenoic acid) is a stereoisomer of which common dietary fatty acid? Would dietary consumption of elaidic acid tend to promote or hinder the fluidity of cellular membranes? Why?
2. From Figure 5-32, deduce how many isoprene units are used to form:
   a. Vitamin A_1 (also known as retinol, the precursor to the visual pigment 11-*cis*-retinal)
   b. Camphor (with its characteristic penetrating odor)
   c. (*R*)-Carvone (the compound contributing the characteristic flavor of spearmint)
3. Jasmonate (**Figure 5-32**) is a signaling compound used by plants. Which class of animal signaling agents does it resemble?
4. In extracting vitamins E and K from tissue (**Figure 5-33**), biochemists use ethyl ether, chloroform, or benzene. However, phospholipids are more effectively extracted using ethanol or methanol. Both sets of biological lipids are nonpolar, so why are they not extracted using the same solvents?
5. One treatment for Gaucher disease is to inhibit glucosylceramide synthase. How would inhibiting this enzyme help to reduce the pathology of the disease?
6. With its single fatty acid "tail," lysolecithin forms globular micelles, whereas lecithin (with two such tails) much prefers to form planar bilayers instead. Also, lysolecithin is much more effective than lecithin as a solubilizing agent for other lipids. Consider the packing of phospholipids (especially the nonpolar "tails") into spherical micelles versus planar bilayers, and propose an explanation for the effectiveness of lysolecithin versus lecithin in solubilizing other lipids.

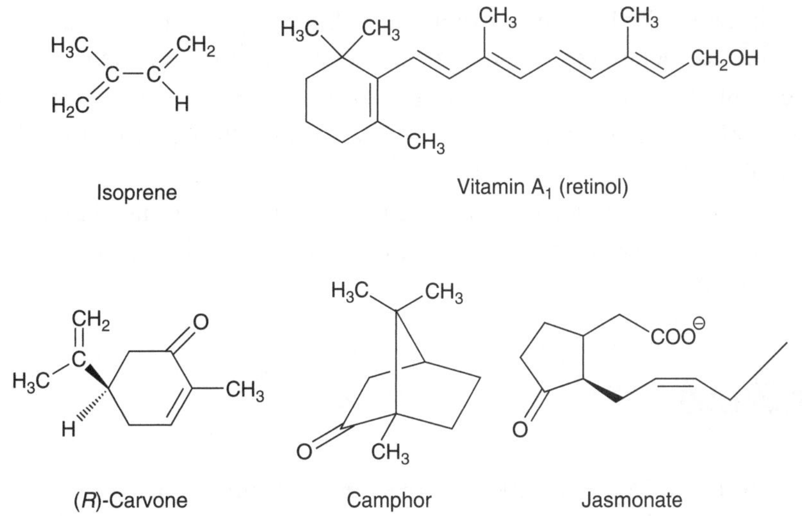

Figure 5-32 Terpenes are natural products made from a five-carbon building block, isoprene.

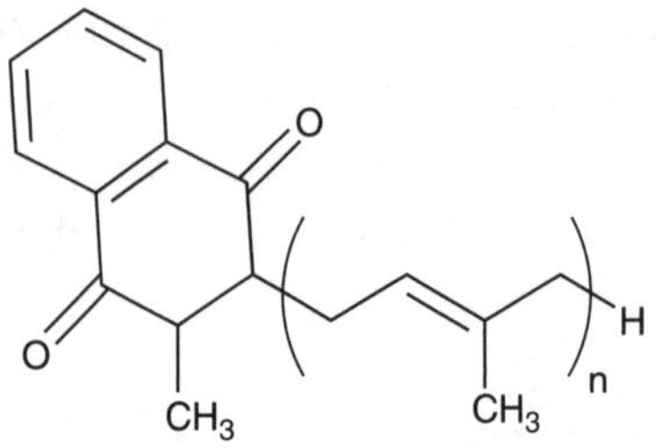

Vitamin K
(n = 4, 5)

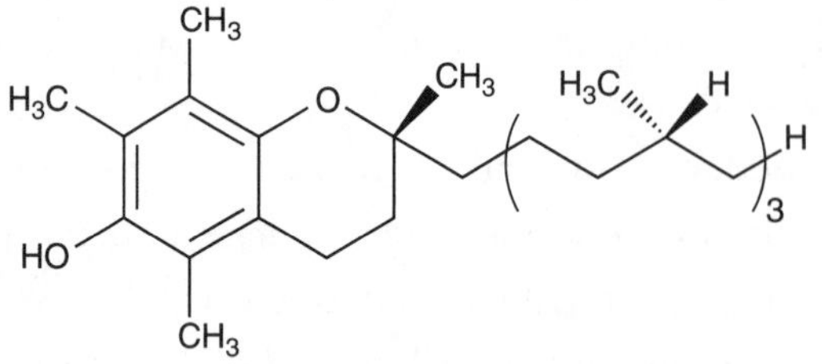

Vitamin E
(Only α-Tocopherol is Shown)

Figure 5-33 Vitamin K and vitamin E are both actually groups of related compounds, all of which are lipid soluble.

7. Olestra is a dietary fat substitute in which six to eight fatty acids are esterified to a central molecule of sucrose. It is used in food preparation to replace normal fat, or triglycerides, because it has much the same physical–chemical characteristics as regular triglycerides. Unlike triglycerides, Olestra is not digested by intestinal lipases, and it passes through the digestive tract unchanged. Hence, its use in food preparation (especially for fried foods) can reduce fat calories taken in the diet.
   a. Given that the ester linkages of the fatty acids to the sucrose are chemically the same as those joining fatty acids to glycerol in triglycerides, why can't the body's lipases break down Olestra?
   b. Fried snack foods prepared with Olestra have been fortified with vitamins A, D, E, and K. Why might such fortification be advisable?
8. Microorganisms isolated from hot springs in Yellowstone National Park tend to have longer saturated alkyl chains in their phospholipids than do related species growing under more temperate conditions. Propose an explanation for the difference.
9. The hydrophobic interaction as A and B form a complex is typically accompanied by release of water. Why would formation of electrostatic/ion-pairing interactions between A and B also tend to release water?
10. Explain qualitatively how alkyl chain stiffness in an amphiphile aggregate would affect the equilibrium between vesicles and planar bilayers. Which form is favored by stiff chains, and why?

REFERENCES

A. L. Blobaum and L. J. Marnett. (2007). "Structural and functional basis of cyclooxygenase inhibition," *J. Med. Chem.* 50:1425–1441.

W. Blokzijl and J. B. F. N. Engberts. (1993). "Hydrophobic effects: Opinions and facts," *Angew. Chem. Int. Ed. Engl.* 32:1545–1579.

C. D. Funk. (2001). "Prostaglandins and leukotrienes: Advances in eicosanoid biology," *Science* 294:1871–12875.

J. N. Israelachvili, S. Marcelja, and R. G. Horn. (1980). "Physical principles of membrane organization," *Q. Rev. Biophys.* 13:121–200.

K. Jacobson, E. D. Sheets, and R. Simson. (1995). "Revisiting the fluid mosaic model of membranes," *Science* 268:1441–1442.

D. Lingwood and K. Simons. (2010). "Lipid rafts as a membrane-organizing principle," *Science* 327:46–50.

D. Mozaffarian et al. (2006). "Trans fatty acids and cardiovascular disease," *New Engl. J. Med.* 345:1601–1613.

Y. Shibata, J. Hu, M. M. Kozlov, and R. A. Rapoport. (2009). "Mechanisms shaping the membranes of cellular organelles," *Annu. Rev. Cell Dev. Biol.* 25:329–254.

S. J. Singer and G. L. Nicolson. (1972). "The fluid mosaic model of the structure of cell membranes," *Science* 175:720–731.

CHAPTER 6

Enzyme Mechanisms and Regulation

Learning Objectives

1. Define and use correctly the terms *enzyme, substrate, catalytic power, substrate specificity, cofactor, coenzyme, prosthetic group, apoenzyme, holoenzyme, active site, induced-fit, lock-and-key, rate of reaction, rate law, rate constant, order of reaction, molecularity of reaction, unimolecular, bimolecular, general acid–base catalysis, transition state, catalytic triad, serine protease, acyl-enzyme intermediate, metallo-enzyme, metalloprotease, allosteric effector, allosteric protein, cooperativity, T/taut state,* and *R/relaxed state*.
2. List and describe the six general types of reactions catalyzed by enzymes; list at least one enzyme for each type of reaction.
3. Describe the salient characteristics of active sites in enzymes.
4. Explain the origin of the catalytic power of enzymes; list and apply the basic physico-chemical factors that contribute to catalysis.
5. State what a cofactor is, and distinguish between coenzymes and prosthetic groups. Explain why cofactors are needed for certain enzyme reactions.
6. Describe the substrate specificity of the following enzymes: RNase A, chymotrypsin, trypsin, elastase, carboxypeptidase A, and aspartate transcarbamoylase.
7. Describe, with appropriate diagrams or sketches, the catalytic mechanisms for the enzymes RNase A, chymotrypsin, and carbonic anhydrase.
8. Describe the physiological roles of the enzymes chymotrypsin, carbonic anhydrase, and aspartate transcarbamoylase.
9. Describe the enzymatic conformational changes that occur during catalysis by the enzyme aspartate transcarbamoylase. Relate these to the concerted model and induced-fit model of enzyme action.
10. List different mechanisms by which enzyme activity may be regulated. Differentiate between noncovalent and covalent mechanisms. Note the importance of phosphorylation and of proteolysis, and the possibility of many other types of covalent modification.

Introduction

General Importance of Enzymes

Enzymes are biological catalysts that act to speed up biochemical reactions. Many biochemical reactions need catalysis to occur on a suitable time scale for physiology. If not catalyzed, these reactions may be far too slow for a cell to make use of them.

Most enzymes are proteins composed of one or more polypeptide chains. In addition, some very special species of RNA can catalyze reactions and are regarded as enzymes in their own right (so-called ribo-enzymes, or ribozymes). For the most part, however, when we speak of enzymes, we mean proteins that catalyze reactions.

Of medical interest is the fact that (at least) 71 enzymes are drug targets, and more than 300 drugs on the market are enzyme *inhibitors*. Inhibitors block the catalytic activity of the enzyme. An enzyme-inhibitory drug acts to reduce or eliminate the product of the reaction(s) catalyzed by the enzyme; this inhibition is intended to lead to a therapeutic effect.

Enzymes generally must operate under very mild conditions (room or body temperature, pH near 7, aqueous solution, modest amounts of salts present), and they perform their reactions quickly and relatively efficiently. These properties are very unlike those of the catalysts so often used in organic chemistry laboratories or in industrial processes, which typically require organic solvents and high temperatures, and which frequently involve long reaction times and the production of unwanted by-products or contaminants. Enzyme catalytic activity is also controllable, being stimulated or inhibited by relatively modest changes in cellular conditions.

The compounds acted on by enzymes are called *substrates*. The usual abbreviation for substrate is the letter S; that for the enzyme is the letter E. Some enzymes may have just one substrate, whereas others may have two or more. Many drugs that target an enzyme will resemble the natural substrate of that enzyme, while other drugs may target an enzyme through their resemblance to the transition state of the reaction catalyzed by the enzyme.

Catalytic Power and Specificity of Enzymes

The *catalytic power* of an enzyme refers to the acceleration of the reaction rate over that for the noncatalyzed reaction. Reaction rates can be accelerated by orders of magnitude. Millionfold accelerations are not uncommon. **Table 6-1** presents some examples.

Enzyme	Catalytic Action	Rate Enhancement
Lysozyme	Hydrolyzes bacterial cell wall	Acceleration factor of 1× over the non-enzyme-catalyzed reaction
Lactate dehydrogenase	Oxidizes lactate to pyruvate	Factor of approximately 1000×
Carbonic anhydrase	Hydrates CO_2 to give bicarbonate	Factor of $7.7 \times 10^6 \times$
Orotidine decarboxylase	Removes carboxyl from orotidine 5′-monophosphate to give uridine 5′-monophosphate	Factor of $1.4 \times 10^{17} \times$, one of the greatest rate enhancements ever seen for an enzyme

Table 6-1 Selected Enzymes: Catalytic Activities and Rate Accelerations

The *substrate specificity* of an enzyme refers to its action on a limited set of substrates. Most enzymes act on only one or a few chemically related compounds, and they perform only one or a few closely related types of chemical catalysis. For example, among the various enzymes secreted in the process of food digestion, one enzyme class specializes in breaking down carbohydrate polymers, while another class of enzyme acts on dietary lipids to break them down for absorption and uptake from the gut. Both classes are "digestive" enzymes, aiding in extracting nutrients from food, but their specific chemical targets are quite different kinds of compounds—sugar chains versus lipids.

Enzymes can be highly sensitive to what may seem to be minor chemical differences in candidate targets. This extends to selectivity in action on stereoisomers, geometric isomers, or even anomeric differences in the way bonding of two moieties is made. For example, in animal cells, the enzymes responsible for the synthesis of fatty acids with carbon–carbon double bonds (unsaturated fatty acids) generate such bonds with the *cis* geometry, not the *trans* geometry. As noted in Chapter 2 on carbohydrates, polysaccharide chains of glucose, in the form of cellulose, are virtually indigestible for humans, because humans do not make enzymes that can hydrolyze the $\beta(1 \rightarrow 4)$ linkages in this polysaccharide. In contrast, humans can readily digest starch molecules, glucose polymers with $\alpha(1 \rightarrow 4)$ linkages, because humans do make enzymes that recognize and can act on this slightly different sort of linkage.

Cofactors in Enzyme Catalysis

The protein nature of enzymes imposes limitations on their catalytic abilities. A good deal of enzyme catalysis is based on using the side chains of amino acids as acids or bases, or as nucleophiles or electrophiles. Amino acid side chains may also serve to neutralize electrical charges on incoming substrates, or they may provide hydrophobic patches or hydrogen-bonding groups by which to hold the enzyme substrate. Not all types of chemical reactions can be catalyzed by amino acid side chains alone. An example here is a redox reaction: None of the 20 common amino acids has a side chain that readily acts as a reducing or oxidizing agent. Enzymes often use small organic or inorganic molecules (*cofactors*) for assistance in performing these other types of reactions.

There are two main subcategories of enzyme cofactors: prosthetic groups and coenzymes. A *prosthetic group* is a tightly bound cofactor (often covalently bound). Examples include various flavins, heme groups, and biotin. A *coenzyme* (sometimes called a co-substrate) is distinguished by its relative freedom: It is typically held only loosely by the enzyme, and can be released and taken up again relatively freely. A good example is nicotinamide-adenine-dinucleotide (NAD^+), which participates in redox reactions.

Vitamins and minerals provide the precursors for these cofactors. The body processes the vitamin or mineral into a form that can be used by the enzyme. One vitamin may provide more than one cofactor; an example is vitamin B_2 (riboflavin), which is used in making flavin mononucleotide (FMN) and flavin adenine dinucleotide (FAD).

The complete complex of a protein with all necessary small organic molecules, metal ions, and other components is termed the *holoprotein* or *holoenzyme*; when the non-proteinaceous part is stripped away, the remaining protein is termed the *apoprotein* or *apoenzyme*. Thus myoglobin that has lost its heme group would be termed apomyglobin; a molecule of the enzyme carbonic anhydrase that has lost its zinc cofactor would be referred to as being in the apoenzyme form.

Active Sites of Enzymes

The *active site* of an enzyme is the region that binds substrates, cofactors, prosthetic groups, and so on, and contains the residues that help to hold (bind) the substrate or that directly participate in the reaction. Active sites are generally small, typically occupying less than 5% of the total

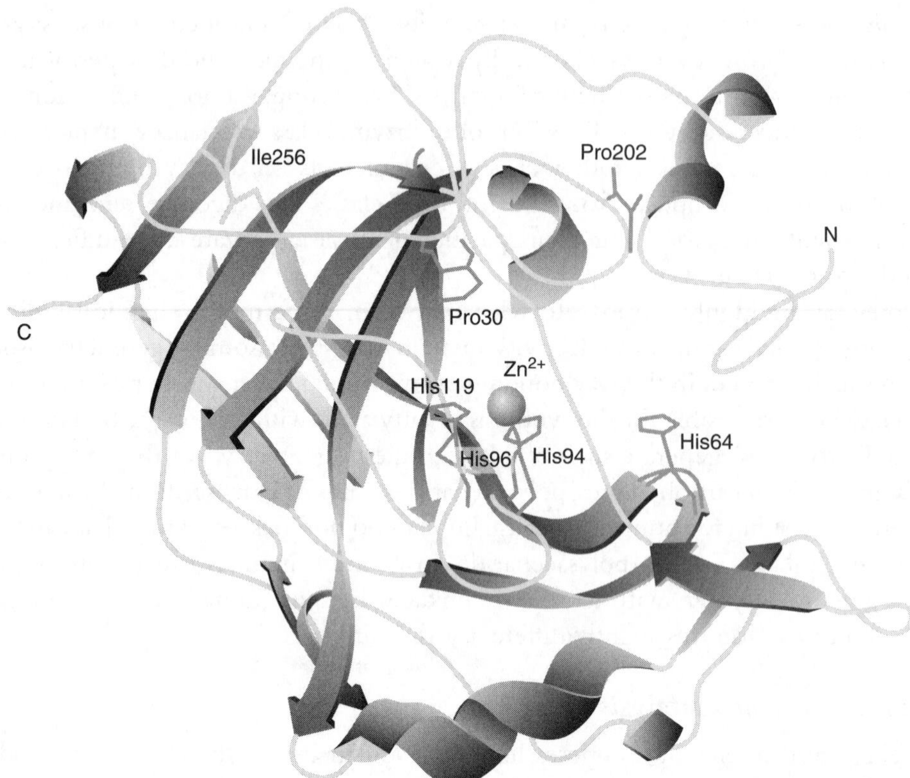

Figure 6-1 Ribbon representation of the backbone of carbonic anhydrase II, with key residues indicated along with the zinc ion cofactor. The active site here is a deep pocket with the zinc ion at the bottom.

Source: Adapted with permission from V.M. Krishnamurthy et al. Carbonic anhydrase as a model for biophysical and physical-organic studies of proteins and protein-ligand binding (2008). *Chem. Rev.* 108:946–1051. Copyright 2008 American Chemical Society.

surface area of an enzyme. They tend to form the largest cleft or crevice on the surface of the protein (**Figure 6-1**) and, therefore, have a three-dimensional character; they are not simply flat patches on a protein's surface. Active sites are often formed by groups from widely separated amino acids (in terms of polypeptide chain sequence); this feature is related to the folding of the enzyme to form its characteristic secondary and tertiary levels of structure. Precise protein folding aligns functional groups in the active site for specificity in binding substrate and then in catalyzing the reaction.

The microenvironment around the site (e.g., local electric fields, polarizability of the surroundings, solvent accessibility) may change the properties of functional groups. For example, the pK_a of a carboxylic acid group may shift to favor the ionized form if there is a nearby positively charged group. Also, the redox potential of a prosthetic group held by the enzyme has been noted to depend on its exposure to solvent, its state of titration, and the local electrostatic environment; such a group may be a highly powerful oxidizing agent in one environment, but may be a considerably less powerful agent if it is located at a different site in the enzyme.

Only a few residues in the active site participate directly in catalytic action. Typically these are the polar side chains of certain amino acids. The peptide backbone, with its hydrogen-bonding capabilities and electric dipoles, may help here as well. In contrast, the binding of substrate may involve several different chemical groups, both polar and nonpolar, and the region involved in binding may be more extensive than the space occupied by the few catalytically active groups.

The polar residues participate in hydrogen-bonding and electrostatic interactions and, of course, in short-range van der Waals interactions. Nonpolar side chain residues may help in binding and aligning the substrate and cofactor(s), and can help in the enzyme's recognition and acceptance or rejection of potential substrate molecules, just on the basis of molecular shape.

The substrate is bound by multiple, weak noncovalent interactions: van der Waals, ionic, and hydrogen bonds; dipole and multipole electrostatic interactions; and so on. As a consequence, the free energy change ΔG for binding is relatively small, typically ranging from -10 to -50 kJ/mol, well below that for forming a covalent bond. The corresponding binding constant K_{bind} is relatively small as well, ranging from 10^2 to 10^8 M^{-1}. If the binding were too tight, then the substrate or product might never be released in time for the cell to use it. If the binding were too loose, there might not be a high enough concentration of substrate to fill a sufficient number of enzyme active sites for the amount of product needed. In vivo, typical substrate concentrations are 10^{-3} M or less, and given these concentrations the binding constant must be at least 10^3 M^{-1} to achieve 50% occupancy.

Conformational Change: Induced-Fit Versus Lock-and-Key Models

Proteins are flexible, and the binding of substrate, inhibitor, or other effectors of activity can cause either small or large conformational changes in an enzyme. These changes may be local changes, limited to the region immediately surrounding the substrate or inhibitor. In some cases, however, the displacements can be propagated over large distances through the protein, and can even pass from one polypeptide subunit to a neighboring subunit, to affect the latter unit's conformation as well. Particular examples of this—for example, hemoglobin and the enzyme aspartate transcarbamoylase—will be discussed later.

Two idealized versions of the role of enzyme conformation in substrate selectivity and catalysis are the *lock-and-key* model and the *induced-fit* model.

Lock-and-Key Model

The lock-and-key model (**Figure 6-2**) was based on early work on the highly specific action of enzymes on their substrates. The basic notion is that the substrate must fit into the active site of the enzyme precisely, just as a key fits into a specific lock, so that functional groups align properly and there is a good steric fit. The matching of complementary molecular shapes and functional groups on the enzyme and the substrate would explain the selectivity of the enzyme. The lock-and-key model is often interpreted to mean that the enzyme does not need to change shape or conformation to catalyze the reaction.

Induced-Fit Model

In the induced-fit model (**Figure 6-3**), the functional groups may have to be moved into position for correct alignment, and there is not necessarily a good steric fit initially. The enzyme changes

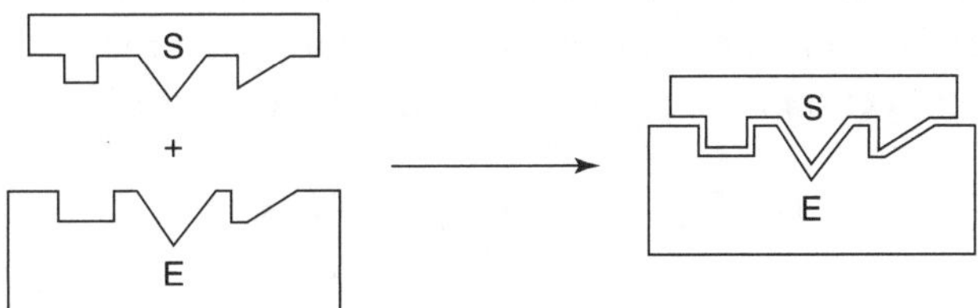

Figure 6-2 The lock-and-key mechanism. The enzyme and substrate have preexisting complementary shapes.

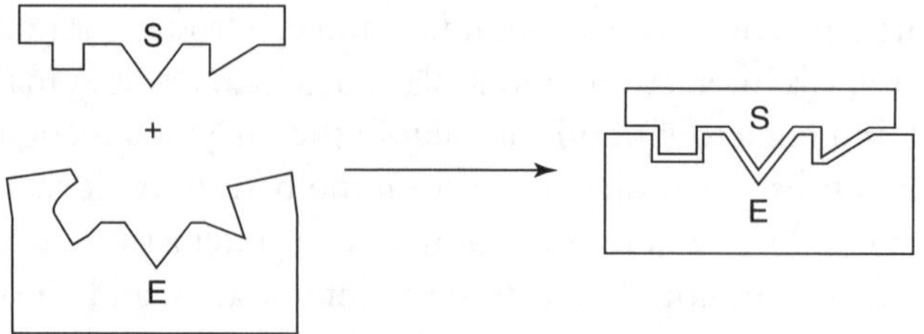

Figure 6-3 The induced-fit mechanism. Binding of substrate induces the enzyme to change its shape to match that of the substrate.

shape upon binding substrate, which in turn aligns the functional groups and allows for good steric fit. In other words, the binding site is complementary in shape to S only *after* S is bound.

Real enzymes often tend to use an induced-fit mechanism, at least to a small degree; enzymes are rarely completely rigid. Part of the active site may be relatively rigid, while another portion of the site may be mobile. The shape change around the binding site may call for conformational changes elsewhere in the protein as well. Furthermore, the substrate itself may be flexible in free solution, at least to a limited degree, and the binding reaction by the enzyme may simply select those substrate molecules that are already in a conformation that matches the surface of the enzyme's binding site (this is essentially the selection of an appropriate substrate conformation by the enzyme). Also, there may be distortion of the conformation of the substrate as it fits into the active site, which could aid in catalysis.

Enzymatic Catalysis

The progress of an enzyme-catalyzed reaction can be analyzed using fundamental concepts of chemical kinetics. The type of reaction catalyzed by an enzyme permits its classification into one of six broad categories. Enzymes use a variety of chemical mechanisms to accomplish catalysis; some of these mechanisms will be quite familiar from organic chemistry, other less so. Enzymes often use two or more types of mechanism in performing catalysis, which can make it more difficult to understand their mechanism of action.

Short Review of Basic Chemical Kinetics Concepts

The *rate of a chemical reaction* is defined as the change in concentration, over time, of a selected chemical species. The rate is often given the symbol v, short for "velocity." The rate is expressed mathematically as the derivative of concentration with respect to time of the selected chemical species—for example, $v = d[\mathrm{A}]/dt$. This quantity has the dimensions of concentration over time; typically, it has the units of molarity/seconds.

A *rate constant* is a quantity expressing the proportionality of the rate and some function of chemical concentrations. Usually the rate constant is given the symbol k, often with subscripts attached that indicate a direction or a particular step in a mechanism. The dimensions and units for k will depend on the particular function of chemical concentrations.

A chemical *rate law* is a mathematical expression connecting the rate of reaction and some function of chemical concentrations. As an example, for the reaction

$$\mathrm{NH_4^+ + NO_2^- \rightarrow N_2 + 2H_2O} \tag{6-1}$$

the rate law is

$$\mathrm{Rate} = k[\mathrm{NH_4^+}][\mathrm{NO_2^-}] \tag{6-2}$$

The two quantities surrounded by square brackets form the function of chemical concentrations for this rate law.

The *order* of a reaction is the sum of the powers (exponents) of the concentrations in the rate law. In the preceding example, the overall reaction is second order; it is first order with respect to either NH_4^+ or NO_2^-.

The *molecularity* of a reaction refers to the number of particles (molecules, ions, atoms) altered in a reaction. The reaction $A \rightarrow P$ is *unimolecular*, while the reaction $A + B \rightarrow P$ is *bimolecular*.

Figure 6-4 shows schematically the progress of a reaction from reactant A to product B. The product is shown to have a lower Gibbs free energy than the substrate, so the reaction is thermodynamically favorable. The reaction must pass over a high energetic barrier, represented by $\Delta G^\ddagger$, to reach the final product state. This barrier slows the reaction; the rate of reaction is determined by the highest point along the reaction progress coordinate. This highest point represents the *transition state*, a highly unstable species that is intermediate in bonding and conformation between reactant and product. The transition state is present only for a very brief time, perhaps the duration of a single molecular vibration (approximately 10^{-13} sec), and then it falls apart, back to reactant or forward to product.

The theory of chemical kinetics says that for passage through the transition state, the rate constant is proportional to the exponential of the free energy change $\Delta G^\ddagger$ involved in reaching that transition state:

$$k = \text{constant} \times \exp(-\Delta G^\ddagger/RT) \tag{6-3}$$

where R is the gas constant and T is the absolute (thermodynamic) temperature. The larger the barrier, the greater is $\Delta G^\ddagger$ and the smaller k becomes (that is, the slower the reaction occurs). Enzymes basically achieve their catalytic power through a reduction in the height of the barrier $\Delta G^\ddagger$.

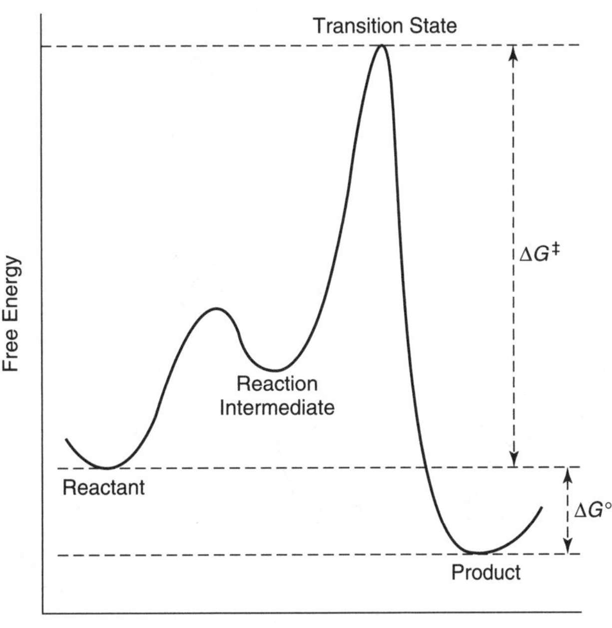

Figure 6-4 Reaction progress diagram, showing the thermodynamic favorability of the reaction (the free energy of the product is lower than that of the reactant) and the high kinetic barrier to the reaction. Also present is an unstable reaction intermediate, distinct from the transition state.

Enzymatic Binding to the Transition State and Rate Acceleration

The reduction in the barrier to reaction is achieved by enzymes through their stabilization of the transition state. Let us compare an enzyme catalyzing a one-substrate reaction to that same reaction but without any enzyme catalyst to aid it. **Figure 6-5** presents the two reaction schemes. The upper reaction scheme shows enzyme in the presence of substrate $(E + S)$, forming first an $E \cdot S$ complex, which we will assume is more stable than the state for the free enzyme and free substrate. This complex then passes through a transition state, which we denote as $(E \cdot S)^{\ddagger}$; then product is released, and the free enzyme is ready for another cycle of catalysis. The lower reaction scheme B shows the corresponding reaction for substrate going through a transition state $S^{\ddagger}$ and on to product; the enzyme is present but only as a spectator, not as a catalyst, in this scheme.

Figure 6-6 depicts the relative free energies of the various states for these two reaction schemes. In the uncatalyzed reaction, there is a free energy change on passing from the reactant state $(E + S)$ to the (substrate-only) transition state $(E + S^{\ddagger})$, which is $\Delta G^{\ddagger\circ}(S^{\ddagger})$. This barrier slows the uncatalyzed reaction. A drop to the final product state $(E + P)$ then occurs. The pathway for the enzyme-catalyzed reaction is similar, except that we introduce an initial free energy drop in binding substrate by the enzyme, represented by $\Delta G^{\circ}_{\text{bind}}(S)$. Then there is a rise

$$E + S \rightleftharpoons E \cdot S \rightleftharpoons (E \cdot S)^{\ddagger} \rightleftharpoons E + P$$

$$E + S \rightleftharpoons E + S^{\ddagger} \rightleftharpoons E + P$$

Figure 6-5 Kinetic reaction schemes for enzyme-catalyzed conversion of S to P, and the uncatalyzed reaction of S to P.

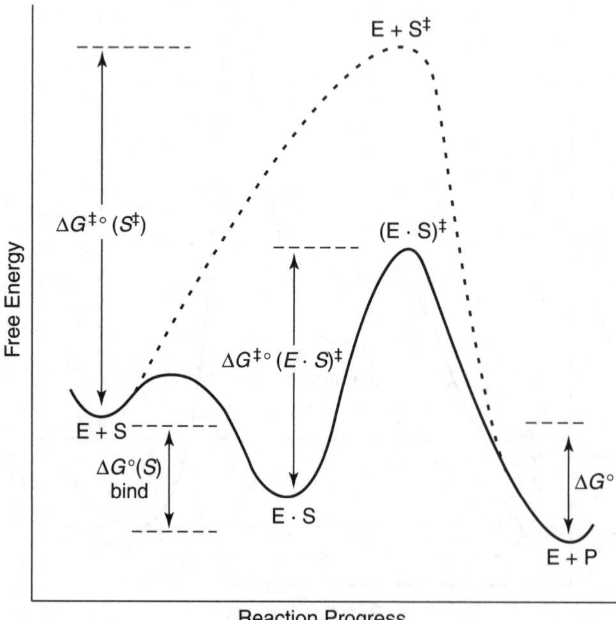

Figure 6-6 Reaction progress diagrams for the two kinetic schemes in Figure 6-5. The dashed line indicates the path for the uncatalyzed reaction; the solid line traces the path for the enzyme-catalyzed reaction. See the text for definitions of the symbols.

to the transition state, with free energy change $\Delta G^{\ddagger\circ}(E \cdot S^{\ddagger})$, and a final drop to the product state $(E + P)$. The overall free energy change for the reaction, ΔG°, is the same for either reaction; the enzyme does not affect the equilibrium thermodynamics of the reaction, only the kinetics.

Although there are two paths starting from the same state $(E + S)$ and leading to the same product $(E + P)$, the barrier to reaction is significantly lower when the enzyme binds substrate and stabilizes the transition state. Notice that we measure the height of the activation barrier for the enzyme-catalyzed reaction from the most stable state on the reactant side of the diagram to the top of the barrier, the transition state. Even with the initial drop in free energy to the E · S complex, the activation free energy for the enzyme-catalyzed reaction is lower than that for the uncatalyzed reaction. With a lower barrier, the rate of the catalyzed reaction is faster. In many cases, the increase in rate due to enzyme catalysis is extremely large—in some cases, as large as a factor of 10^{17}.

From the basic thermodynamic relation $\Delta G = \Delta H - T\Delta S$, we have the counterpart for the activation free energy change: $\Delta G^{\ddagger} = \Delta H^{\ddagger} - T\Delta S^{\ddagger}$. Thus the free energy of activation has contributions from both an enthalpy change and an entropy change. The enzyme must act to lower the reaction barrier either by lowering the enthalpy in the transition state or by increasing the entropy of that state, or possibly both at the same time. The transition state in many reactions involves straining bonds in the substrate. If the enzyme were to use its own functional groups to hold tightly to the strained substrate, the enzyme might decrease the activation enthalpy for the reaction. In other cases a favorable entropy change might be gained if the substrate (and the enzyme's active site) were to release waters of hydration on forming the transition state.

General Mechanisms for Catalysis

Enzymes use a variety of chemical mechanisms:

- *General acid–base catalysis*, using a moiety (usually an amino acid side chain) in the enzyme. The side chain must, of course, be capable of donating or accepting protons, and it should do so reversibly, to regenerate the original state of titration of the enzyme (that is the mark of a catalyst; it is regenerated after the reaction). The pH range over which a particular side chain can do this will strongly depend on the chemical nature of that side chain's ionizable group. Broadly speaking, acidic side chains, like those with carboxylic acids, function below pH 5; the imidazole group of histidine operates well in the pH range around 6; and side chain amino groups perform this sort of reversible titration around pH 10–11. **Table 6-2** summarizes the expected pH ranges for the titration of the common functional groups found in proteins.
- *Nucleophilic catalysis*, using covalent bonds between enzyme and substrate, with an amino acid side chain on the enzyme acting as a nucleophile. Nucleophiles are electron-rich moieties, and such groups on the enzyme tend to attack electron-poor regions on the substrate. Examples of potential nucleophiles in an enzyme include the hydroxyl groups on the side chains of serine, threonine, or tyrosine (especially if they are first ionized). The thiol group of cysteine also can act as a nucleophile, and the imidazole ring of histidine may function as a nucleophile, in reactions where it helps to transfer phosphate groups.
- *Electrophilic catalysis*, where the enzyme withdraws electron density from a reaction center. This might be done in a variety of ways—for example, using H^+ transfer to the substrate,

Titrable Group	Approximate pK_a	Titrable Group	Approximate pK_a
C-terminal α-carboxylic acid	3	β-Sulfhydryl	8
γ- and β-Carboxylic acid	4–5	Phenolic hydroxyl	9–10
Imidazole	6–7	ε-Amino	10–11
N-terminal α-amino	8	Guanidino	12–13

Table 6-2 Titrable Functional Groups of Enzymes and the pH Range Over Which They Are Titrated

or a metal ion (Zn^{2+} is commonly used by enzymes) or a positively charged amino acid side chain (e.g., the terminal amino group of lysine, or the side chain of arginine), or an "electron sink" nitrogen on a cofactor, to help in withdrawing electron density.

- *Proximity effects*, aligning and juxtaposing moieties on substrate and enzyme for rapid reaction. This can be important for enzymes acting on two substrate molecules or substrate and cofactor molecules simultaneously. For example, enzymes performing redox reactions on a substrate often use a cofactor to accept or donate electrons. To pass the electrons, the substrate and the cofactor must be positioned close together, with just the right mutual orientation.
- *Bond strain*. An enzyme may change its conformation to cause the substrate's bonds to approximate those of the transition state (a *transition state* is a transient state in which the molecule has partially undergone reaction, and is at the point of highest free energy along the reaction pathway). This generally weakens the bond and makes it more reactive.
- *Charge neutralization*. This can facilitate substrate binding or help to stabilize an intermediate.
- *Environmental effects*. Here the solvent or other molecules help to stabilize the transition state, thereby promoting reaction.

In many cases, an enzyme will use two or more of these mechanisms to catalyze a reaction. A later section in this chapter looks at a few selected enzymes in detail and focuses on their use of acid–base catalysis and nucleophilic catalysis, as these mechanisms are quite common.

Classes of Enzymes and Types of Reactions

A systematic classification of enzymes has been developed by the International Enzyme Commission, based on the types of reactions that are catalyzed. The six major enzyme classes are listed in **Table 6-3**. Each of these major classes has subclasses, sub-subclasses, and so on, to describe the huge number of different enzyme-catalyzed reactions and the differences among the proteins catalyzing them. Once thoroughly characterized, an enzyme may be assigned an "EC" (Enzyme Commission) number that reflects the precise category of reaction catalyzed and the particular protein involved. For example, ribonuclease A from bovine pancreas has the identifier EC 3.1.27.5.

Note the use of the suffix of *-ase* to indicate an enzyme. Older names may not reflect this convention, however. For example, we have names like "chymotrypsin" and "pepsin." Also, abbreviations are very common, such as using "RNase" for "ribonuclease."

Under modern conventions, the name of an enzyme is constructed to indicate both the type of reaction and the principal substrate or product of the reaction. For example, "dehydrogenase," "reductase," and "oxidase" all indicate participation in redox reactions, albeit in different ways and by different mechanisms.

Enzyme Class	Type of Reaction	Examples
Oxidoreductases	Reduction–oxidation (redox)	Lactate dehydrogenase, dihydrofolate reductase
Transferases	Move chemical group	Creatine kinase, hexokinase
Hydrolases	Hydrolysis; bond cleavage with transfer of functional group to water	Chymotrypsin, lysozyme, RNase A
Lyases	Non-hydrolytic bond cleavage	Fumarase
Isomerases	Intramolecular group transfer (isomerization)	Triose phosphate isomerase, methylmalonyl CoA mutase
Ligases	Synthesis of new covalent bond between substrates, using ATP hydrolysis	RNA polymerase, pyruvate carboxylase

Table 6-3 Six Principal Classes of Enzymes

Ribonuclease A: Acid–Base Catalysis

Background

RNase A is a digestive enzyme that hydrolyzes RNA. It is a very rugged enzyme, easily obtained in large quantities. Its crystal structure is known; this structure confirms notions about its mechanisms that were developed before the detailed structure was obtained. The origin of specificity here is basically that of a lock-and-key fit of substrate with enzyme, although some evidence indicates that the enzyme also changes conformation upon taking up substrate. There is a well-defined binding cleft for the substrate. The enzyme forms a 2′,3′ cyclic phosphate intermediate in a two-stage mechanism. There is a strong pH dependence, with a characteristic bell-shaped activity curve (**Figure 6-7**). These properties are related to the protonation and deprotonation of two key histidine residues in the active site.

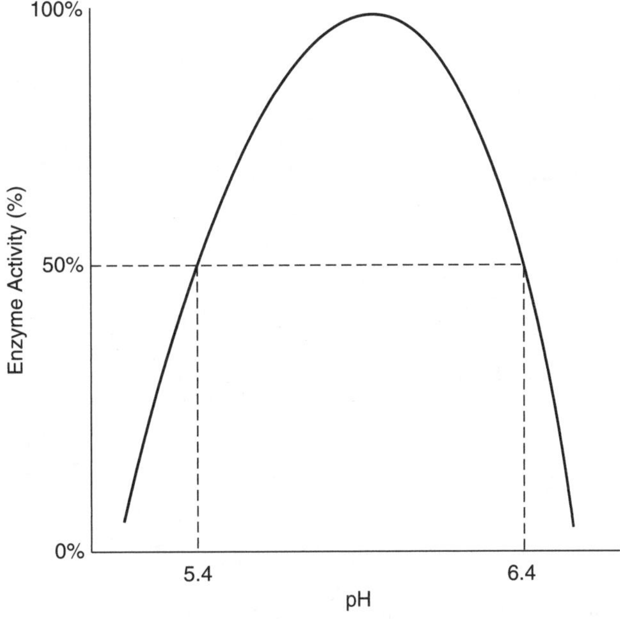

Figure 6-7 Ribonuclease A activity as a function of pH.

Substrate Binding: Key Points

- The binding site contains several proton acceptor/donor groups—His 12, His 119, Lys 7, Lys 41, and Lys 66—not all of which necessarily participate in catalysis but which may help to hold a negatively charged RNA chain onto the enzyme.
- There is high specificity for a pyrimidine ring on the 3′ side of the cleaved bond; purines are too large to fit (an example here of steric selectivity). Also, a network of hydrogen bonds attach the enzyme to the substrate to hold it moderately tightly in the active site.
- There is low specificity for any particular base on the 5′ side. Binding here is mainly through ionic attraction: The negatively charged phosphodiester backbone of RNA is held by the positively charged Lys and Arg side chains.

The enzyme will bind single-stranded DNA, too. It will not cleave it because DNA lacks the 2′-OH on the ribose sugar, so the sugar cannot form the 2′,3′ cyclic intermediate.

Mechanism

The reaction can be conveniently divided into two stages, each with its own transition state, going to and from a semi-stable intermediate. Both stages involve concerted general acid–base catalysis by His 12 and His 119, which produces the observed pH dependence (Figure 6-7).

First Stage (Figure 6-8)

Step 1: Unprotonated His 12 takes a proton from the 2′-OH, while protonated His 119 starts to donate a proton to the 5′-O. Simultaneously, the 2′-O starts to bond to phosphorus, forming a pentacovalent intermediate (this is the transition state, en route to the 2′,3′ cyclic intermediate). The negative charge on the intermediate is stabilized by the nearby positively charged Lys 41 side chain.

Step 2: The bond between P and the 5′-O breaks, a proton is finally transferred from His 119 to this oxygen, and the bond between P and the 2′-O is fully formed. This

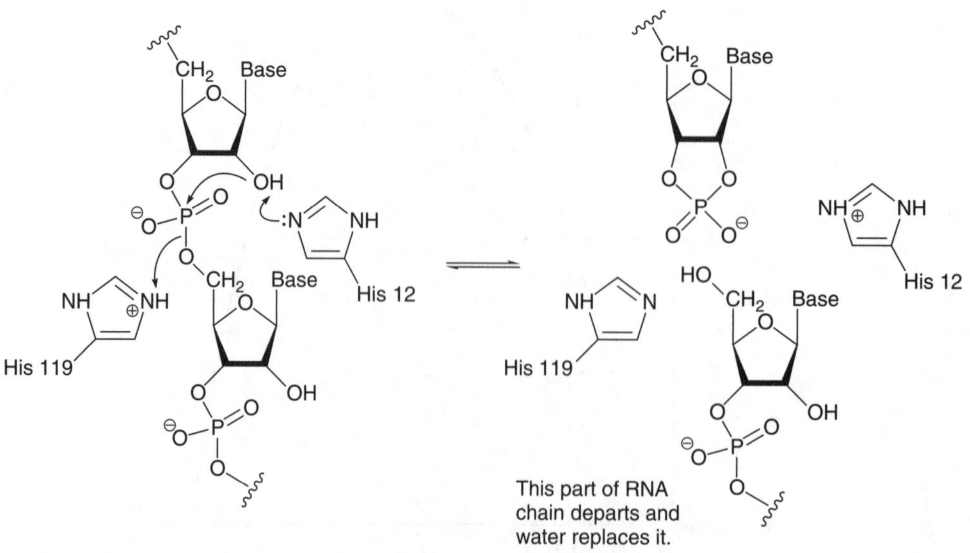

Figure 6-8 The first stage of RNA chain cleavage by ribonuclease A.

yields the 2′,3′ cyclic intermediate; this cyclic form is not a transition state, but rather a semi-stable reaction intermediate.

Notice that this first stage requires that His 12 be electrically neutral (unprotonated) and that His 119 already have a proton bound. This implies that the solution pH must be acidic enough to titrate His 119 and add a proton there, but not so extreme as to titrate His 12 also. At 25°C, the pK_a values of these histidines are approximately 5.4 and 6.4 (their local environments are different, so they have different acidities). If the pH is much more acidic than 5.4, or much more alkaline than 6.4, then the activity of the enzyme will drop sharply, because one or the other of the histidines has been mostly titrated to the wrong state.

Second Stage (Figure 6-9)

Step 3: The 5′-OH end leaves the site, and a molecule of water enters.

Step 4: Ionized His 12 donates a proton to 2′,3′ cyclic phosphate, as neutral His 119 takes a proton from H_2O, leaving OH^- next to the cyclic phosphate.

Step 5: OH^- attacks the cyclic phosphate, forming a pentacovalent intermediate. "In-line" nucleophilic displacement takes place on the phosphorus. (This is the second transition state, en route from the 2′,3′ cyclic intermediate to the final product.)

Step 6: The 2′-OH is reformed, with the 3′ carbon carrying the phosphate group.

Points to Note

- There is concerted catalysis by two residues.
- This is a case of general acid–base catalysis, by both of those residues.
- There is role reversal for these residues, from stage 1 to stage 2.
- Nucleophilic displacement has a trigonal bipyramidal transition state for the pentacovalent phosphorus.
- The 2′,3′ cyclic intermediate is *not* a transition state; it is a semi-stable intermediate.
- The pH-activity curve is explained by the roles and states of titration of His 12 and His 119.
- A proton from His 12 goes to the nearby neutral oxygen, not the anionic oxygen, on the phosphorus.

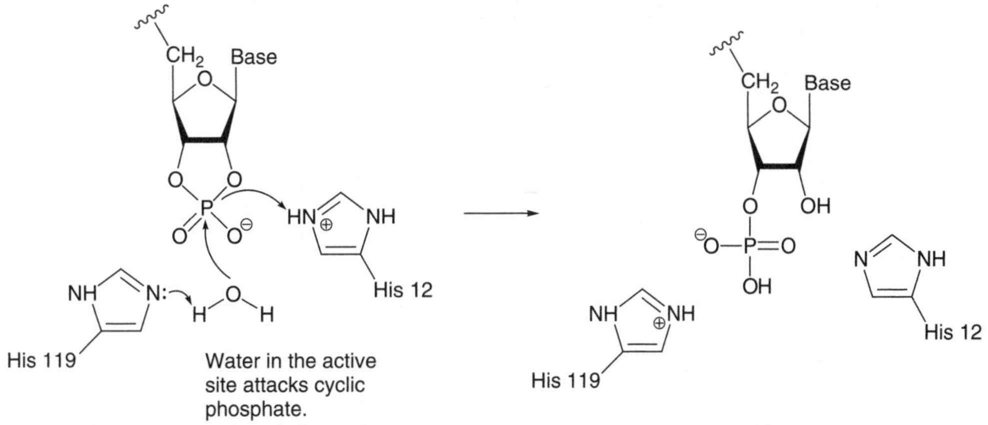

Figure 6-9 The second stage of RNA chain cleavage by ribonuclease A.

Chymotrypsin and Other Proteases: Covalent Catalysis and Nucleophiles

Background

The amide bonds in a protein are typically quite stable and resist hydrolysis. It requires special catalytic apparatus to cleave these bonds, which the class of enzymes known as proteases can provide. Chymotrypsin is one of these proteases. It is a digestive enzyme, secreted by the pancreas. It cuts the amide backbone of proteins and prepares them for further degradation to amino acids and peptides.

Chymotrypsin preferentially cleaves peptides on the carboxyl side of aromatic or large nonpolar residues. The side chain of such a residue is held in a hydrophobic pocket in the enzyme's active site; this pocket provides most of the specificity of the enzyme toward aromatic and nonpolar residues. The amide linkage of the substrate is placed close to three important residues of the enzyme: Asp 102, His 57, and Ser 195. The side chains of these three amino acids form a *catalytic triad* that facilitates the cleavage. The serine residue plays a key catalytic role; to emphasize its importance, chymotrypsin and its relatives that use the same reaction mechanism are known as *serine proteases.*

Origins of Substrate Specificity

The related enzymes trypsin and elastase (both serine proteases) show different substrate specificities than chymotrypsin; these enzymes have slightly different pockets for binding substrate (**Figure 6-10**). Trypsin has a carboxyl group buried at the bottom of its pocket, and it preferentially cleaves substrates with positively charged side chains. Elastase has two protruding hydrophobic groups in the pocket that block large side chains from entering the pocket. Accordingly, elastase has specificity toward small nonpolar side chains instead.

Similar principles govern the specificity of the carboxypeptidases. These enzymes cleave polypeptide chains specifically at the carboxyl-terminus (albeit by a different mechanism than that used by the serine proteases). Carboxypeptidase A has a large nonpolar pocket for binding substrate, and this enzyme preferentially cuts next to residues with aromatic or bulky aliphatic side chains like leucine or isoleucine (also tryptophan). Carboxypeptidase B has an ionized aspartic acid residue in the bottom of a similar pocket, so it shows a preference for substrates with positively charged groups like lysine that would fit well in its binding pocket.

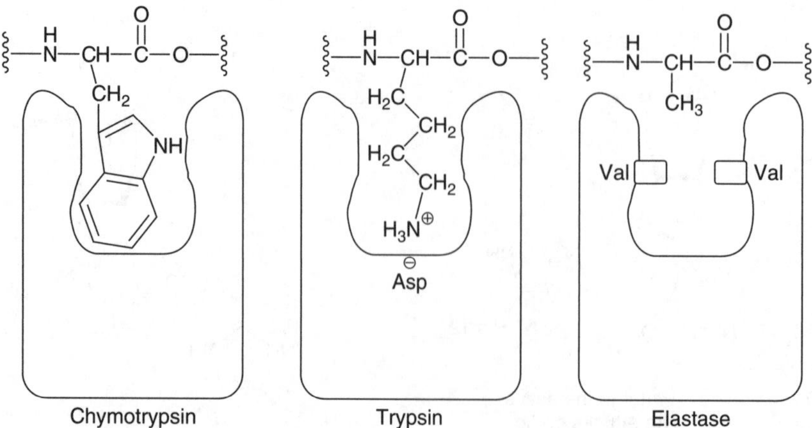

Figure 6-10 The differences in features of the active sites of three proteases explain their substrate selectivity.

Reaction Mechanism for Chymotrypsin

Hydrolysis of the amide linkages in proteins is a difficult reaction to perform in water without using a catalyst. Chymotrypsin speeds up the reaction by a factor of a billion ($10^9\times$) or more. The mechanism does not involve the direct attack of water on the amide bond because this attack has a high activation barrier and would produce very slow reaction kinetics. Instead, the enzyme forms a covalent linkage to an intermediate on the pathway to the product (which is a cleaved peptide bond), and then uses water to hydrolyze the bond holding this intermediate on the enzyme. This intermediate can actually be isolated, under special circumstances. Thus the reaction involves two stages, just as the mechanism for RNase A involves two distinct stages. Because the intermediate is an acyl group held via a covalent bond to the enzyme, we speak here of covalent catalysis and an *acyl-enzyme intermediate*.

First Stage (Figure 6-11)

Step 1: A substrate peptide chain enters the active site. Asp 102 is already ionized and forms a strong hydrogen bond to the ring of His 57. This increases the ability of His 57 to pull a proton from the —OH on the side chain of Ser 195; removal of this proton generates a strongly nucleophilic alkoxide anion on Ser 195. (Here we see a role for acid–base equilibria, although the base is not directly involved in acting on the substrate but instead is internal to the enzyme.)

Step 2: The Ser 195 anion attacks the peptide carbonyl (a nucleophilic attack), forming a tetrahedral transition state. The negative charge on the carbonyl (an "oxyanion") is stabilized by the "oxyanion hole" formed from amide nitrogens along the peptide chain backbone of the enzyme.

Step 3: The transition state quickly collapses and leaves the substrate carbonyl attached to the side chain of Ser 195. This is now a partially stable acyl-enzyme intermediate, held by a covalent bond in the active site.

Step 4: The remainder of the substrate chain (amino side) leaves the active site.

Second Stage

Step 5: Water enters the active site; it interacts strongly with His 57 and becomes polarized.

Step 6: The polarized water attacks the acyl-enzyme carbonyl (another nucleophilic attack), resulting in development of the negative charge again on the oxygen of the carbonyl group (stabilization again in the oxyanion hole) and formation of another tetrahedral transition state.

Step 7: The tetrahedral transition state collapses, with part of the water (—OH) attached to the carbonyl, and the other hydrogen going to His 57.

Step 8: The carboxylic acid so formed leaves the active site, which has now been regenerated and is ready to accept another substrate molecule.

Points to Note

- There is a "catalytic triad" of amino acid residues Asp 102, His 57, and Ser 195 in the active site.
- There are two discernible stages within this mechanism, with two transition states and one main semi-stable reaction intermediate.
- The semi-stable intermediate is covalently bound to the enzyme through Ser 195 (the "acyl-enzyme intermediate").

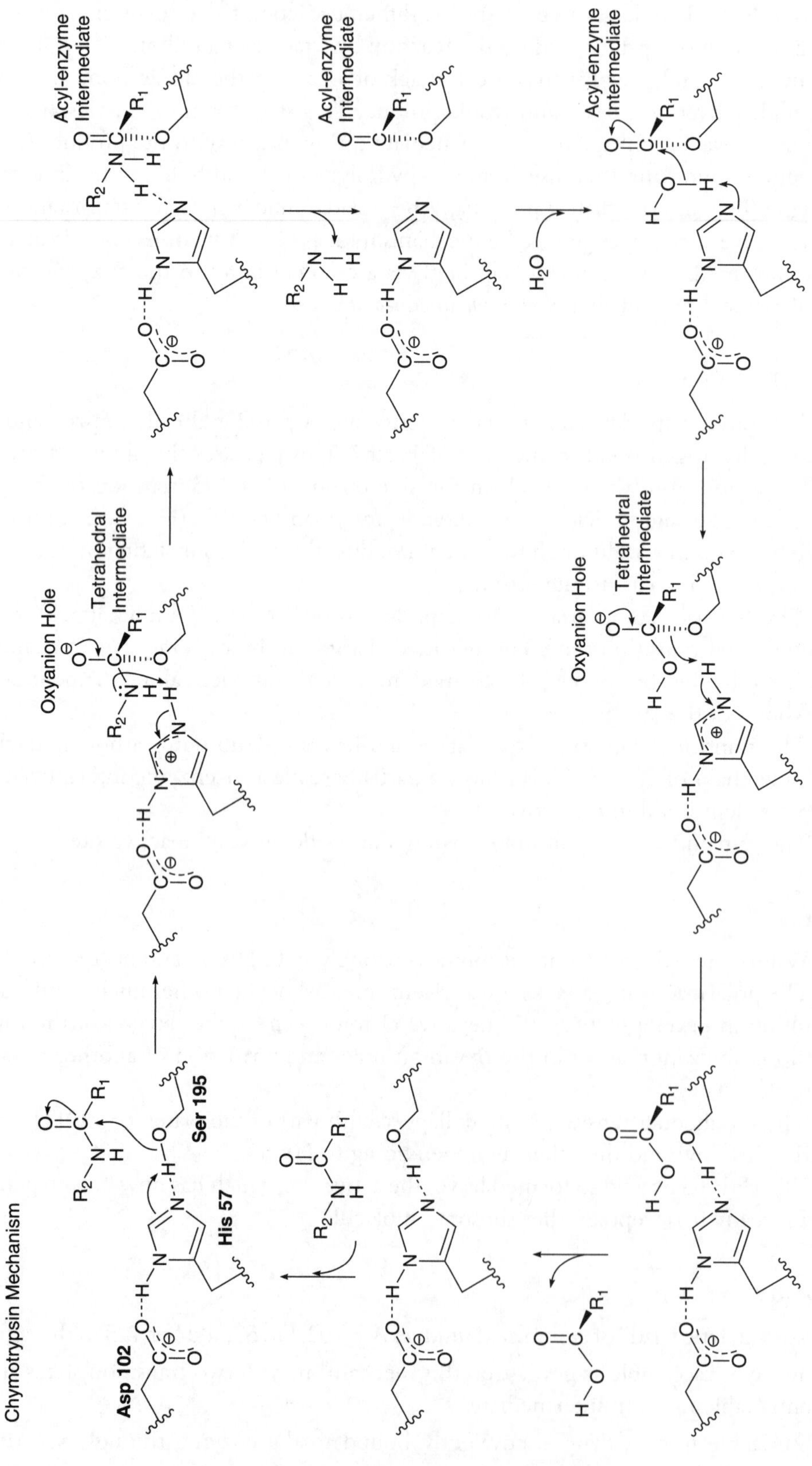

Figure 6-11 Peptide chain cleavage mechanism for chymotrypsin.

- General acid–base catalysis here involves hydrogen bonds and proton transfers across the three members of the catalytic triad.
- Highly polarized oxygen atoms, either from the Ser 195 side chain or from water, carry out nucleophilic attacks.

Other Proteases

Enzymologists have discovered three other major classes of proteases: the cysteine proteases, the aspartyl proteases, and the metalloproteases. All three classes activate the carbonyl of the substrate toward nucleophilic attack, albeit by different mechanisms. The cysteine proteases use a cysteine residue, with an S — H group on the side chain, in place of a serine in the active site. The enzyme papain, from papaya fruit, is an example of a cysteine protease.

The aspartyl proteases have a pair of aspartic acid groups in place of the serine of chymotrypsin. The ionized aspartates polarize a local water molecule, which then acts as the nucleophilic attacking agent. Two clinically important examples of this class are the HIV protease and the kidney enzyme renin (involved in the regulation of blood pressure).

The third class of proteases uses a metal ion cofactor to aid in catalysis. Enzymes that use metal ions in catalysis are called *metalloenzymes*. In particular, *metalloproteases* use a metal ion, usually Zn^{2+}, in the active site to help polarize the substrate and activate it for attack. The carboxypeptidases mentioned earlier are examples of this phenomenon.

Clinical Application

The human immunodeficiency virus (HIV) is responsible for the disease of acquired immune deficiency syndrome (AIDS), one of the great epidemics of our time. (There are, in fact, two closely related forms of the virus: HIV-1 and HIV-2. HIV-2 is less virulent and has a different DNA sequence than HIV-1.) The life cycle of the virus depends on the proteolytic processing of two major polypeptides encoded by the virus. This is accomplished by a viral protease; host cell enzymes cannot perform this processing. If the viral protease were specifically inhibited, it would disrupt the virus life cycle, thereby blocking multiplication and distribution of the virus. Thus a great deal of research has gone into finding and developing drugs that would specifically inhibit the viral protease without interfering with normal cellular processes.

The HIV protease is a homodimeric protein with a twofold rotationally symmetric structure; the substrate binding site extends across the dimer interface and has considerable symmetry itself. Each of the monomer subunits contributes a catalytic aspartate residue to the active site; each subunit also contributes a β-hairpin loop or "flap" that helps to bind substrate.

The twofold symmetry of the active site originally guided researchers to developing inhibitors that themselves would have this twofold symmetry (or at least approximate the symmetry), and that would also mimic the natural substrate or, even better, the transition state in the proteolytic reaction catalyzed by the enzyme. Subsequent studies, drawing on crystal structures of the enzyme with bound ligands, have indicated that perfect symmetry in an inhibitor is not necessary for good affinity or selectivity.

(Continued)

Figure 6-12 shows a selection of inhibitors of the HIV protease. These compounds resemble the natural polypeptide substrate to some degree; notice the presence of amide linkages and of projecting bulky nonpolar groups. A key feature in these compounds is the presence of a secondary alcohol —OH group near the center of the compound, replacing an amide linkage. This alcohol group mimics the tetrahedral transition state of the reaction, but, of course, is not hydrolyzable by the protease. Their resemblance to the transition state enables these inhibitors to bind tightly to the protease to inhibit it.

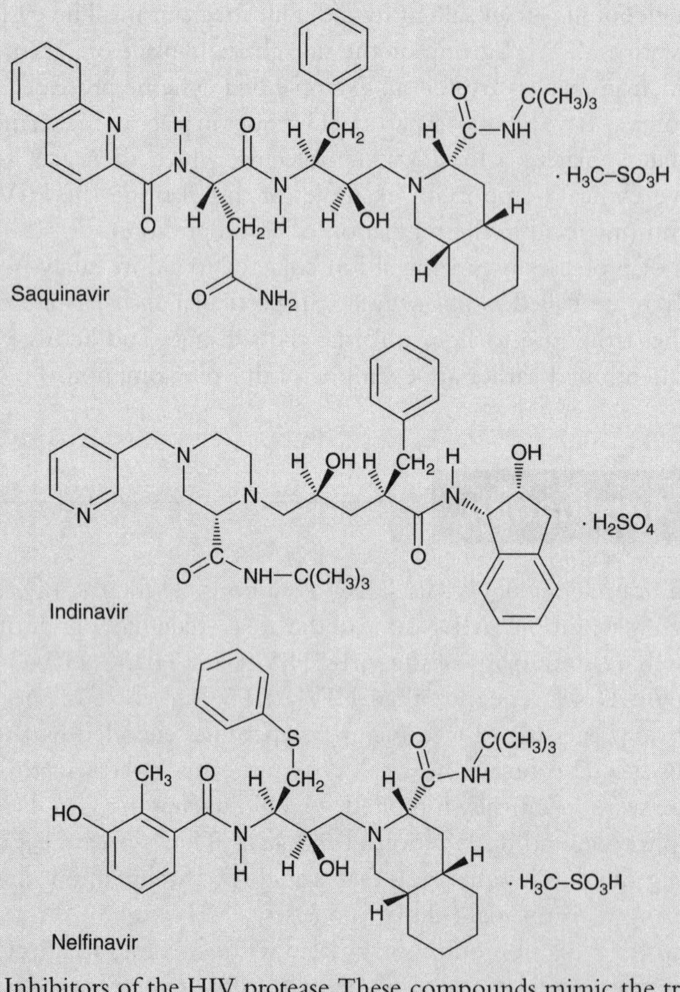

Saquinavir

Indinavir

Nelfinavir

Figure 6-12 Inhibitors of the HIV protease. These compounds mimic the transition state of the proteolytic reaction; they are tightly bound by the enzyme but cannot be hydrolyzed.

Carbonic Anhydrase: Metal Ions and Electronic Strain

Physiological Background

Carbon dioxide (CO_2) is produced by the cell in aerobic metabolism of carbohydrates, lipids, and amino acids. CO_2 rapidly and spontaneously reacts with water to produce the relatively strong acid, carbonic acid, which then spontaneously ionizes to release a proton and generate bicarbonate anion (**Figure 6-13**).

$$O{=}C{=}O + H_2O \underset{k_{-1}}{\overset{k_{+1}}{\rightleftharpoons}} HO{-}C({=}O){-}OH \underset{k_{-2}}{\overset{k_{+2}}{\rightleftharpoons}} HO{-}C({\cdots}O)^{\ominus}{\cdots}O + H^{\oplus}$$

Figure 6-13 Hydration of CO_2 forms carbonic acid, which then ionizes to give bicarbonate anion.

In humans, the CO_2 generated in actively respiring tissue is transported through the blood by red blood cells in the form of bicarbonate. Enzymes called carbonic anhydrases (CA) perform this conversion of CO_2 to bicarbonate in the red blood cells, speeding up the naturally occurring reaction. In the lung, the enzymes reverse the reaction to release CO_2 for exhalation.

CO_2 and bicarbonate, and the action of various carbonic anhydrases, come up in several other places in metabolism and physiology. For example, the proper intra-ocular pressure in the vitreous humor of the eye is maintained by a physiological mechanism that involves the conversion of CO_2 to bicarbonate, as catalyzed by one form of carbonic anhydrase. Pertinent to primary metabolism, bicarbonate is used in a carboxylation reaction at the start of gluconeogenesis; another bicarbonate-dependent carboxylation reaction helps to kick off fatty acid biosynthesis; and bicarbonate appears yet again in nitrogen excretion, in the formation of urea.

In humans, at least seven different forms of carbonic anhydrase are present. Some are membrane bound; others are found in the cytosol; and at least one type is found in mitochondria. **Table 6-4** summarizes selected features of various mammalian carbonic anhydrase enzymes.

Isoform	Distribution	Function
CA I (cytosolic)	Primarily in red blood cells, gastrointestinal epithelia, also eye, sweat glands, salivary glands, and elsewhere	Promotion of gas, fluid, and ion transfer; bicarbonate secretion, CO_2 excretion and transport. Five to six times as abundant as CA II, but only 15% as active.
CA II (cytosolic)	Widely distributed in secretory and absorbing epithelia, but found in virtually all tissues	Promotion of gas, fluid, and ion transfer; bicarbonate and acid secretion, CO_2 excretion and transport. High-activity isozyme.
CA III (cytosolic)	Mainly in red skeletal muscle, but also found in rat livers, salivary glands, prostate gland, brain, colon, mammary gland, and elsewhere	Facilitation of CO_2 diffusion. Possible role in muscle contraction. Acid–base homeostasis, in liver.
CA IV (membrane-bound glycoprotein in nonhumans)	Lung, kidney, perhaps elsewhere	Reabsorption of bicarbonate in proximal renal tubules. Transport of H^+ and bicarbonate in lung, and facilitation of CO_2 transfer.

Table 6-4 Activities and Distribution of Isoforms of Carbonic Anhydrase

Isoform	Distribution	Function
CAV (mitochondrial)	Kidney, liver, perhaps elsewhere	Provide bicarbonate for initial steps in gluconeogenesis and ureagenesis.
CAVI (secreted glycoprotein)	Salivary gland	pH regulation in saliva, protection of esophagus and stomach.

Table 6-4 Activities and Distribution of Isoforms of Carbonic Anhydrase (Continued)

Origins of Substrate Specificity

All forms of carbonic anhydrase have a common feature: They carry a zinc ion that is a key cofactor for catalysis (refer back to Figure 6-1). The zinc ion, Zn^{2+}, is bound or ligated to four moieties, typically three histidine residues and a water molecule or hydroxide anion, depending on pH. The zinc ion is characteristically buried at the bottom of a cone-shaped dimple or pit in the enzyme's surface; the pit is approximately 1.5 nm (15 Å) deep and 1.5 nm across. The conical depression that forms the active site has a hydrophobic face for binding substrate or ligands like cyanide, and a hydrophilic face that is thought to provide a route for shuttling protons in and out, to regenerate the active site after catalysis.

Reaction Mechanism

The zinc ion acts here as an electrophile in drawing electron density toward itself, but in so doing it promotes the ionization of the bound water molecule. The resulting hydroxide ion that is retained by the zinc ion then acts as a nucleophile in attacking a molecule of CO_2. This is the basis for the reaction mechanism by which carbonic anhydrase acts on CO_2 (**Figure 6-14**).

Steps in Reaction

Step 1: Zinc ion with a bound hydroxide anion sits at the bottom of the active site as a molecule of CO_2 enters and is held on the nonpolar face of the cavity.

Step 2: The CO_2 shifts toward the zinc ion, and the hydroxide ion attacks it, forming bicarbonate.

Step 3: Water enters the active site and displaces the bicarbonate ion toward the nonpolar face.

Step 4: The bicarbonate anion is released and a new molecule of water replaces it at the zinc. The bound water is acidic, with a (formal) positive charge.

Step 5: A proton is transferred from the zinc-bound water to a neighboring His 64, regenerating the zinc-bound hydroxide.

Step 6: The proton on His 64 is shuttled away from the active site through residues on the hydrophilic face of the active site.

Points to Note

- The zinc is strongly held by three histidine residues; it, in turn, holds a hydroxide ion formed from water.
- The zinc polarizes the bound water to enable hydroxide attack on the CO_2.
- Neighboring residues participate in a network of hydrogen bond that hold substrate molecules and transfer protons.

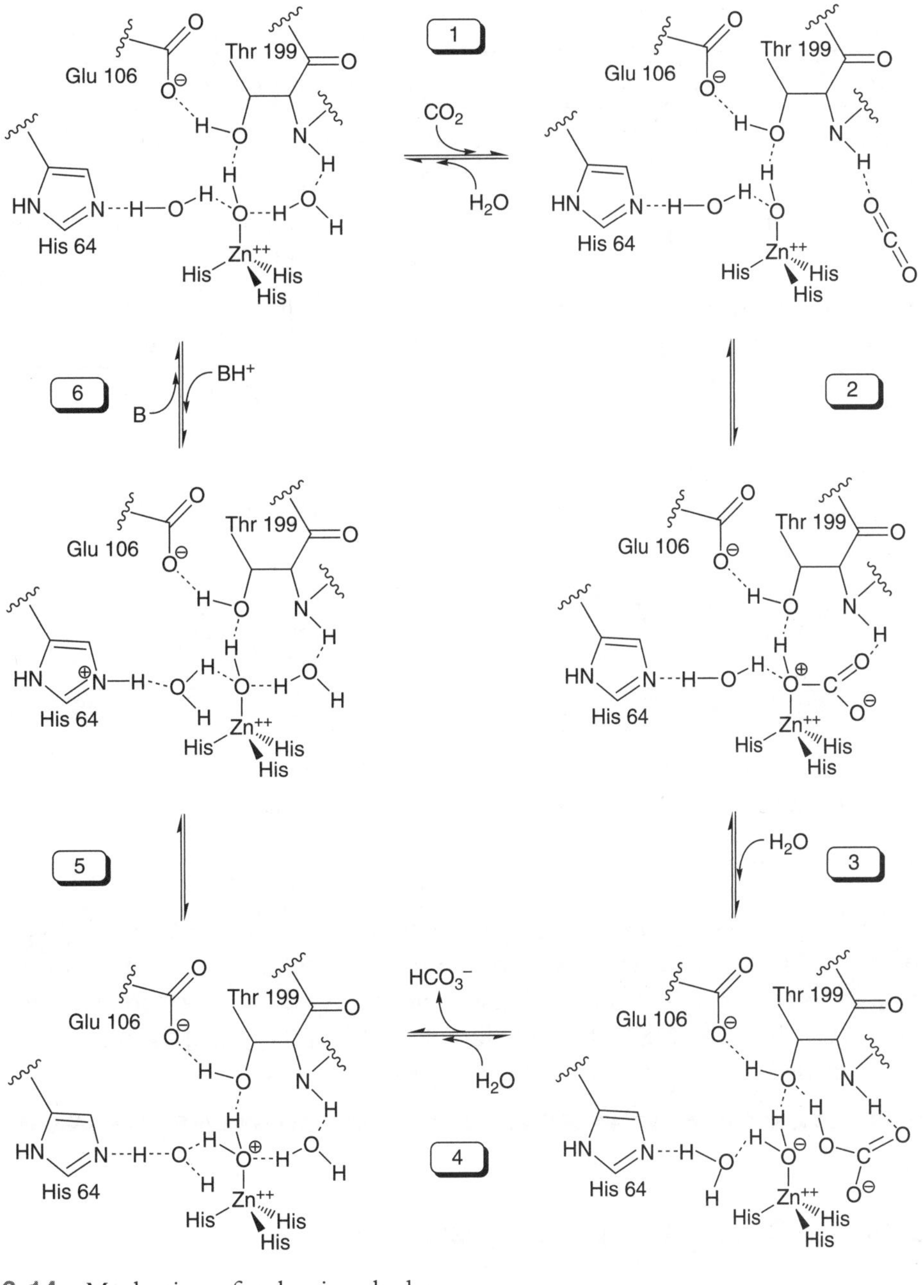

Figure 6-14 Mechanism of carbonic anhydrase.

Source: Adapted with permission from V.M. Krishnamurthy et al. (2008). Carbonic anhydrase as a model for biophysical and physical-organic studies of proteins and protein-ligand binding. *Chem. Rev.* 108:946–1051. Copyright 2008 American Chemical Society.

Clinical Application

Inhibitors of carbonic anhydrase are used in a variety of clinical settings, as shown in **Table 6-5**. Sulfonamides are highly effective inhibitors of carbonic anhydrase (**Figure 6-15**). These compounds bind to the zinc in the active site and block entry of

(Continued)

Disorder	Effect of Inhibition
Glaucoma	Reduction of aqueous humor formation
Acute mountain sickness	Decrease formation and lower pH of cerebrospinal fluid
Toxicity due to urinary excretion of acidic drugs or metabolites	Urinary alkalinization; solubilization of acidic drugs or metabolites

Table 6-5 Selected Clinical Applications of Inhibitors of Carbonic Anhydrase

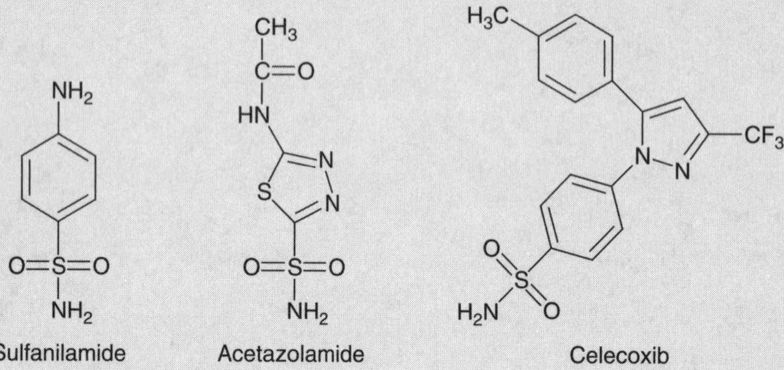

Figure 6-15 Sulfonamide drugs.

CO_2 or bicarbonate. Acetazolamide has been widely prescribed for glaucoma, to reduce intraocular pressure. Sulfanilamide, one of the original "sulfa" drugs, is an antibacterial agent (it helps block nucleotide synthesis), but it also inhibits carbonic anhydrase. Celecoxib (Celebrex), an NSAID used to inhibit cyclo-oxygenase 2, was recently shown to (unexpectedly) inhibit carbonic anhydrase quite effectively.

Introduction to Cooperativity and Allosterism

Allosterism

Proteins often have multiple binding sites on their surface, where substrate, cofactors, ions, and other small molecules may attach themselves. The binding of a small molecule (a ligand) at one site on a protein can affect the binding properties at another site on the same protein. Often this is done through a change in conformation at the second site, induced by the binding of the ligand at the first site. We then speak of the ligand as an *allosteric effector* and the protein as an *allosteric protein*. The term *allosteric* comes from the Greek words *allos* (meaning "other") and *steros* (meaning "shape"); allosteric means "other shape," implying a change in conformation.

The ligands that affect conformation and binding properties this way can be quite simple, like protons; they can be small organic molecules as well, from earlier or later reactions in a biochemical process. In some enzymes the ligand might even be the substrate, acting here in a noncatalytic role as an allosteric effector as well as in a reactive role of course.

Multisubunit proteins can transmit shape changes across the interface between subunits. A good example here is the way in which hemoglobin changes shape as it takes up oxygen molecules (see the discussion later in this chapter). Some enzymes have special regulatory subunits that bind allosteric effectors, as well as special catalytic subunits where the main chemical business takes place. Shape changes in the regulatory subunits can be propagated to the catalytic subunits across the interfaces between the two kinds of subunits.

Allosterism plays a major role in the regulation of activity of key enzymes. These enzymes tend to be large proteins that contain multiple subunits, multiple catalytic sites, and multiple sites for binding allosteric effectors. Some effectors serve to inhibit the enzyme, without binding in or near the active site; other effectors can actually increase the activity of the enzyme by driving a shape change that leads to more or better active sites.

Allosterism has been found in a number of membrane-bound proteins important for signal transduction. Several drugs are thought to produce their pharmacological effects through allosterism—that is, by binding at secondary sites that affect the conformation of the receptor and thus its activity.

Cooperativity

When the binding of one molecule of ligand facilitates the binding of a second molecule, the result is called positive *cooperativity*. In this scenario, the binding sites are not acting independently of each other, but instead are affecting each other's behavior, with uptake of the first ligand increasing the binding affinity for the second ligand. This pattern arises in many multisubunit enzymes, particularly those involved in catalyzing key steps in metabolic pathways. It is tied closely to allosteric effects, or changes in shape, in the subunits of those enzymes. Cooperativity also appears in other biochemical systems, most notably in the transport of oxygen by the protein hemoglobin. In fact, cooperativity is probably easier to understand with these transport proteins than it is with the more complicated kinetic behavior of multisubunit enzymes.

Mammalian hemoglobin is a tetramer, composed of two α subunits and two β subunits, with each subunit carrying a single heme group. The four subunits pack closely together, and the interfaces between subunits have many noncovalent interactions. With four heme groups, hemoglobin has the capacity to hold four O_2 molecules when fully saturated.

Hemoglobin is well known for its characteristic sigmoid curve for binding oxygen (**Figure 6-16**). This oxygenation curve has three phases: an initial flat portion at low $[O_2]$ and low degrees of oxygen binding; then a sharp rise in oxygen binding over a very limited range of $[O_2]$; and lastly a flattened portion (a "plateau"), leading to the saturation of available oxygen-binding sites. The result is a sort of flattened S-shape for the oxygenation curve (a sigmoid curve).

Hemoglobin does not avidly bind a first molecule of O_2; the initial affinity for oxygen is apparently low. If one is bound, however, then the uptake or binding of another O_2 becomes more likely—that is, the affinity for O_2 has increased. Similarly, binding of a second O_2 increases the affinity for a third O_2. This uptake of O_2 is reflected in the sharp rise in the oxygenation curve. Eventually, the hemoglobin's four heme groups may have all acquired a molecule of oxygen, which corresponds to the "plateau" in the oxygenation curve.

The sigmoid curve, with its apparent changes in oxygen affinity, can be explained in terms of conformational changes in the protein as it takes up O_2. Upon binding a molecule of O_2, the heme group flexes in such a way that neighboring amino acids must shift position, and in turn their neighbors must also shift. These changes in atomic position can propagate over quite

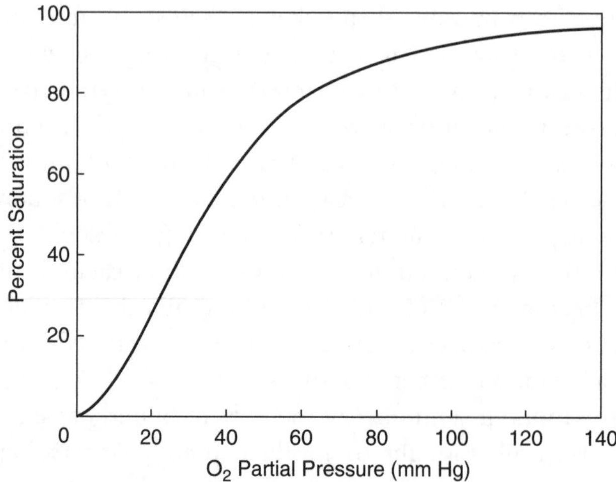

Figure 6-16 The oxygenation curve of hemoglobin shows a characteristic sigmoid shape, due to cooperative interactions among the subunits.

long distances within a subunit, up to and across the interface between neighboring subunits, and then over to the heme groups in those neighbors. The propagated conformational change enables the subunits to communicate and affect one another's affinity for O_2.

Before any oxygen is bound, the subunits in hemoglobin are all in a low-affinity state, denoted for historical reasons as the *T* (or *taut*) conformation. After the first O_2 is bound and the conformation around that heme group has changed, there will be a strong tendency for neighboring subunits (which do not yet have O_2 bound to their hemes) to switch conformation to the *R* (or *relaxed*) state. The subunits are interacting through the propagated changes in atomic positions; they are "cooperating." In the R state, these unoxygenated subunits have higher affinity for O_2. This characteristic explains the sudden increase in oxygen affinity over a very limited range of O_2 concentrations. The increase in oxygen affinity is an example of positive cooperativity, which here is closely tied to the allosteric or conformational changes in hemoglobin. (The actual process of switching all four subunits is rather complicated, involving differences in oxygen affinity and interfacial contacts between the α and β subunits.)

Two main models of allosterism are distinguished: the concerted model and the sequential model. Both can incorporate positive cooperativity to help explain the activity of multisubunit enzymes and proteins.

The Concerted or MWC Model of Enzyme Allosterism and Cooperativity

Monod, Wyman, and Changeux (MWC) were the authors of the paper that first described the concerted model. **Figure 6-17** is a sketch of how this model works; for simplicity, it presents only a dimeric enzyme.

Basic Assumptions in the MWC Model

- The enzyme has two or more identical subunits.
- Subunits can switch between two (or more) conformations—for example, R and T.
- Each subunit has one or more binding sites (for substrate or effector).
- The affinity of the site for the ligand depends on that subunit's conformation; the R conformation is usually chosen to indicate the one with higher affinity (or activity) for ligand.

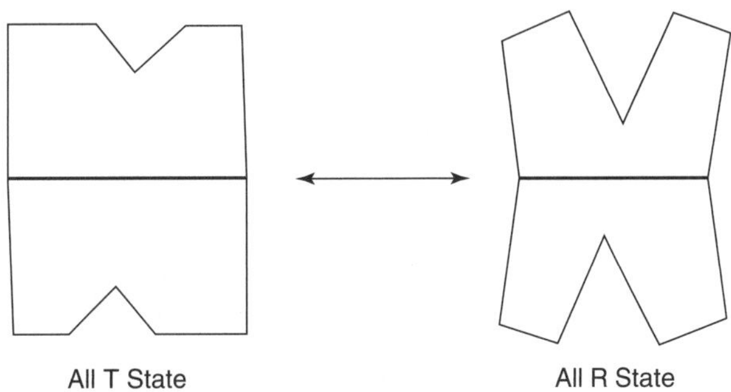

Figure 6-17 The concerted model of enzyme activation, for a dimeric enzyme.

- Conformational changes in subunits occur in a concerted manner—for example, all-R or all-T, but not mixed R and T in same enzyme. (Hence we use the terms "concerted," "two-state," and "all-or-none" when describing the model.)

Qualitative Behavior of the Model

Activators bind to the R form and increase its concentration at the expense of the T form, thereby raising the activity level. Inhibitors bind to the T form, causing any transition to the R state to be more difficult, and shifting the activity curve to the right (higher substrate concentrations are then required for the same level of activity).

The main problem with the MWC model is its requirement that all subunits in the enzyme change conformation simultaneously. Despite this drawback, it has been quite successful in explaining the behavior of hemoglobin in binding oxygen, and in explaining the concentration–activity relationships observed with enzymes such as aspartate transcarbamoylase and various dehydrogenases.

The Sequential or KNF Model

Koshland, Nemethy, and Filmer (KNF) were the authors of the paper that first proposed the sequential model. **Figure 6-18** is a sketch of how this model works. For simplicity, again we show only a dimeric enzyme, with two conformations available to its subunits.

Basic Assumptions in the KNF Model

Like the MWC model, the KNF model applies to multisubunit enzymes, whose subunits switch between two (or more) conformations. There are possibly several binding sites per subunit, whose affinity or activity depends on the conformation of the subunit. However, unlike those in the MWC model, the subunits in the KNF model can change conformation one at a time (hence the "sequential" description of the model).

Qualitative Behavior of the Model

Notice that for the dimeric enzyme there are now four—not two—states shown. This difference arises because the subunits can change shape, one at a time; the overall change in activity is sequential and more gradual than in the MWC model. This makes the KNF model a more realistic representation than the MWC model with its "all-or-none" shape change requirement. There can be mixed states in the KNF model, where some of the subunits have changed shape and others have not.

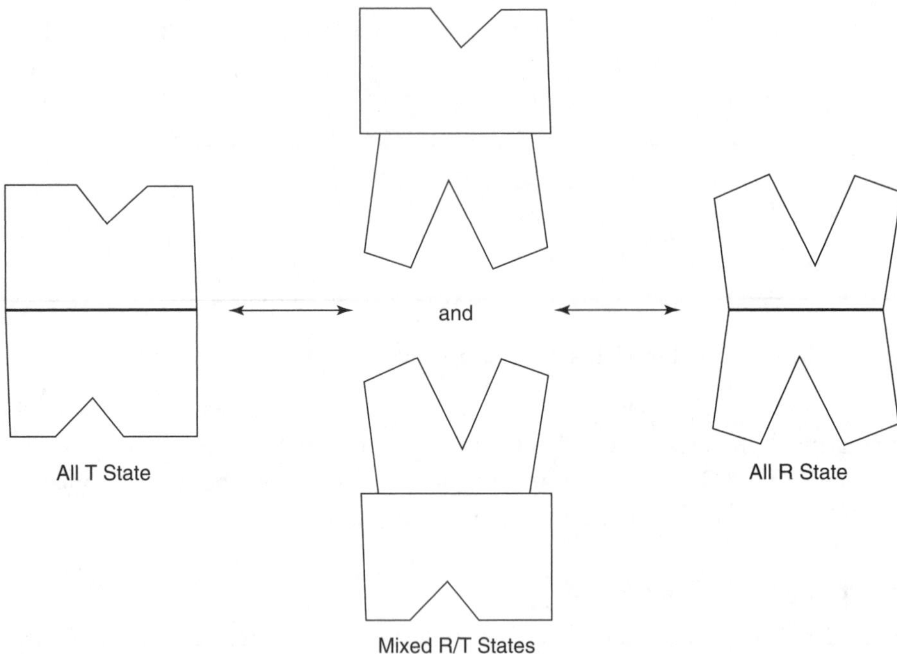

Figure 6-18 The sequential model of enzyme activation, for a dimeric enzyme.

As in the MWC model, allosteric effectors produce their effects by binding to either the R or T conformations preferentially. If they prefer the R conformation, then the enzyme overall becomes more active. If the effector prefers the T conformation, then the enzyme will be less active.

Aspartate Transcarbamoylase: An Allosteric Enzyme

Background

Aspartate transcarbamoylase (ATCase) is a key enzyme in pyrimidine biosynthesis. It catalyzes the first (committing) step in this pathway (**Figure 6-19**), so it is tightly regulated. Feedback inhibition is provided by cytidine triphosphate (CTP) and by uridine triphosphate, the end products of the pathway.

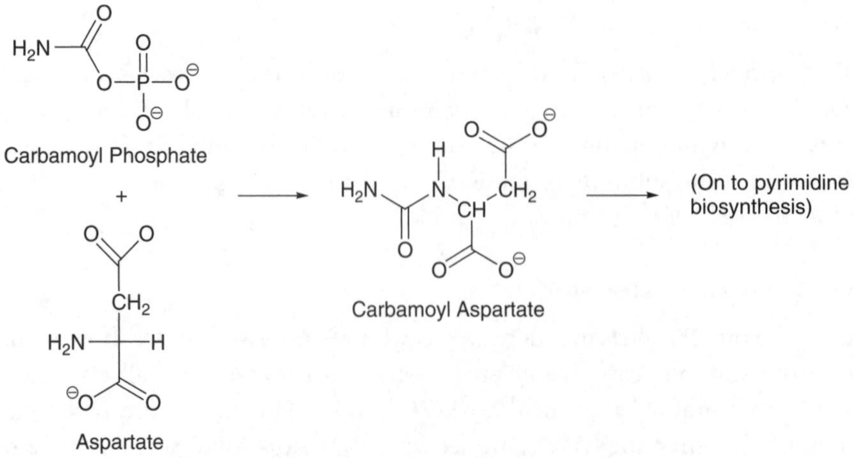

Carbamoyl Phosphate

+

Aspartate

⟶

Carbamoyl Aspartate

⟶

(On to pyrimidine biosynthesis)

Figure 6-19 Formation of carbamoyl aspartate, the reaction catalyzed by aspartate transcarbamoylase (ATCase), and the first step in the pathway leading to pyrimidine biosynthesis.

Structure and Conformational Changes

The bacterial enzyme is particularly well studied, so we discuss it here. The enzyme shows large conformational changes, and there is a high degree of cooperativity present, making this system a good example of allosterism and cooperativity.

The enzyme has multiple subunits of two different types. The first subunit type (denoted as type r) regulates the activity but does not catalyze the reaction; this subunit type binds nucleotides like ATP or CTP, then alters their conformation to affect the activity occurring at the second type of subunit. The second subunit type (denoted as type c) is, of course, where catalysis takes place; it binds the substrates of the enzyme, aspartate and carbamoyl phosphate. The intact enzyme has a subunit stoichiometry of $r_6\, c_6$; overall, there are 12 peptide chains in the intact enzyme. These chains are formed into two catalytic trimers and three regulatory dimers.

Upon binding substrate, large changes occur in the quaternary structure of the enzyme, involving substantial rotations and displacements of subunit chains (**Figure 6-20**). Note the large central cavity that opens up in the R form (this form is the more active) compared to the T form; notice how subunit contacts become modified during this transition.

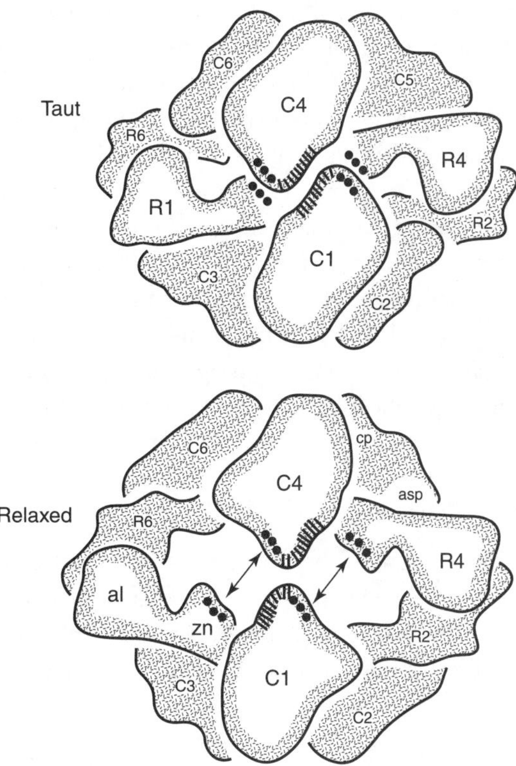

Figure 6-20 ATCase shows large quaternary structural changes upon activation from the compact T state to the open R state. ATCase has six catalytic subunits (denoted as C in the diagram) and six regulatory subunits (denoted as R). Note the change in subunit position and in contacts between subunits, along with more subtle changes in subunit shape, as the substrates aspartate (asp) and carbamoyl phosphate (cp) are bound.

Source: Adapted with permission from J.E. Gouaux and W.N. Lipscomb. (1990). Crystal structures of phosphonoacetamide ligated T and phosphonoacetamide and malonate ligated R states of asparate carbamoyltransferese at 2.8-A resolution and neutral pH. *Biochemistry* 29:389–402. Copyright 1990 American Chemical Society.

Shown in Figure 6-20 is a site for binding a zinc cofactor (zn) on a regulatory subunit, along with sites for substrate aspartate (asp) and carbamoyl phosphate (cp) on one of the catalytic subunits. Aluminum (al) was used in the crystal structure determination but is not really a substrate or effector.

Catalytic Mechanism

Two substrates are available to bind into the catalytic site: carbamoyl phosphate and aspartate. Which binds first—or does the order even matter?

In fact, there is a well-defined temporal order to binding: first carbamoyl phosphate (CP), then aspartate. Carbamoyl phosphate is relatively unstable in solution (it has a half-life of approximately 5 minutes at 37°C), so it makes sense to bind it and hold onto it to protect it from degradation in free solution. Later, when aspartate becomes available, carbamoyl phosphate is rapidly converted to product.

The active site has one positively charged pocket (not two, as might be expected for an enzyme binding two negatively charged substrates). This positively charged pocket can bind either aspartate or CP. Binding of CP alone will induce the enzyme to change its shape slightly in a way that enhances its affinity for CP in the pocket. The shape change also creates a binding site for aspartate, a site that was not present before. This change explains the required temporal ordering of the binding. Binding of CP also weakens the interactions that hold the enzyme in the T conformation, which will help in the transition to the more catalytically active R conformation.

When aspartate binds to an enzyme site holding a molecule of CP, the aspartate is oriented so that its α-amino group can make a nucleophilic attack on the carbonyl carbon of CP. Having the CP molecule already bound also makes the region more electropositive, which lowers the pK_a of the α-amino group of aspartate and helps promote catalysis. Binding of aspartate makes the site more electronegative and triggers the movement of positively charged residues in the rest of the enzyme, leading to the large conformational change observed for the T-to-R switch. In the R form, the substrates are forced closer together, which lowers the activation energy for the reaction.

The nucleophilic attack involves a tetrahedral intermediate for the transition state; this is a nucleophilic attack on the carbonyl of CP (**Figure 6-21**). There is a possible role for His 134 (with a positive charge) to stabilize the negative charge on the oxygen of the carbonyl; electronic strain may also play a role. The phosphate is also a good leaving group for a nucleophilic displacement reaction.

Activation and Inhibition Patterns

Figure 6-22 shows how the activity of the enzyme is sensitive to the concentration of several pertinent small molecules. These small molecules are allosteric effectors. ATP activates the enzyme, whereas pyrimidine nucleotides (CTP or UTP) inhibit it. Notice how the activity curve is shifted to higher substrate concentrations in the presence of UTP or CTP.

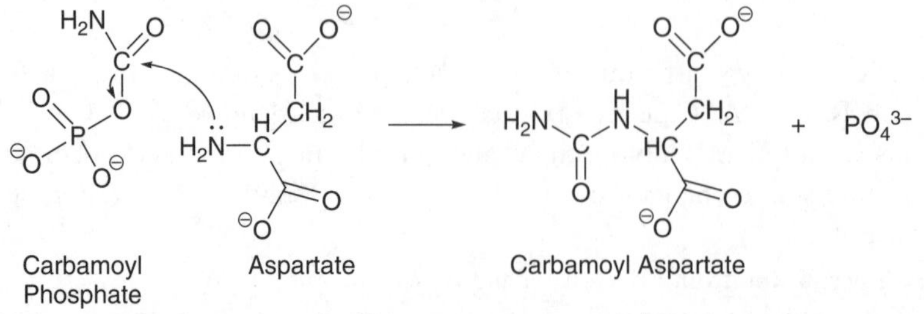

Carbamoyl Phosphate + Aspartate → Carbamoyl Aspartate + PO_4^{3-}

Figure 6-21 Formation of carbamoyl aspartate involves the nucleophilic attack of the amino group of aspartate on the carbonyl of carbamoyl phosphate, with displacement of the phosphate.

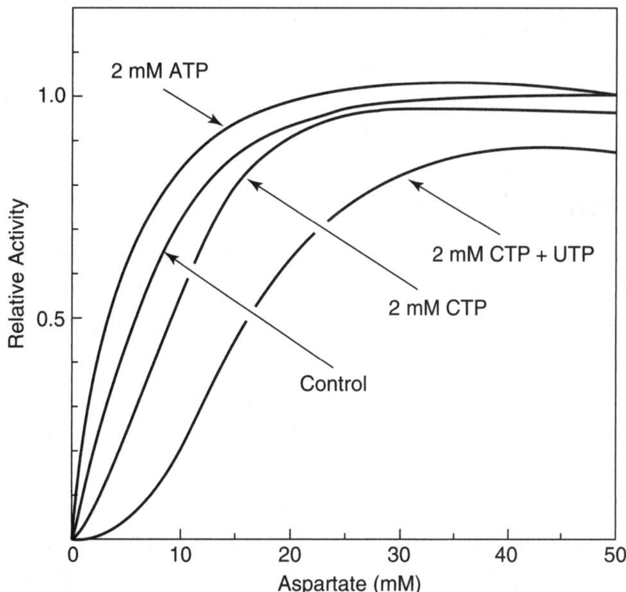

Figure 6-22 The effect on ATCase activity of some small-molecule allosteric effectors. Pyrimidine nucleotides (CTP or UTP) inhibit the enzyme, while ATP activates it.

Source: Adapted from J.R. Wild et al. (1989). In the presence of CTP, UTP becomes an allosteric inhibitor of aspartate transcarbamoylase. *Proc. Natl. Acad. Sci. USA* 86:46–50, with permission of Dr. J.R. Wild.

The activity curve has a characteristic sigmoid shape, rather like the letter "S." Activity is low at low concentrations of substrate. Then, at some intermediate concentration, a sharp rise in activity occurs, followed by a flattening of the curve as full activity is approached. Without substrate, the enzyme's subunits are in the T state, with low activity. As the concentration of substrate rises, a sudden change in activity occurs as the enzyme changes conformation to the more active R state. The change to the R state involves cooperative interactions among the subunits.

The sigmoid activity curves reflect cooperative interactions among the subunits. The origin of this cooperativity is the change in conformation promoted by the binding of aspartate in the active site of a c-type subunit. Having one catalytic site switch conformation will weaken the interactions at other sites on neighboring subunits that are holding them in the T state. This weakening makes it more probable that those other sites will now switch conformation to the more active R state. With two or more catalytic sites now in the high-activity conformation, the observed enzymatic activity rises sharply. Of course, when all the subunits have finally changed to the R state, then no further increase in activity is possible, and the activity curve flattens out.

Binding the first molecule of aspartate is not very likely: The affinity is low in the T state, and there is not much catalytic activity because the local conformation does not promote reactivity. If one aspartate is bound and causes that first subunit to switch to the R state, however, then it becomes much more likely that a neighboring site will switch and bind another CP and aspartate. Thus, for a very small increase in concentration of aspartate, the enzymatic activity rises steeply. In this way, the system resembles oxygen binding by hemoglobin.

Regulation by Covalent Modification

The binding of only one or a few hormone molecules to their receptors on a cell can lead to quite dramatic changes in the physiology of that cell, and can cause systemic or whole-body responses. Clearly, the original signal (hormone binding) has been amplified in such a case. This amplification is achieved by using signaling cascades that rely in part on a series of covalent modifications of a set of enzymes in the cell. The key here is that each activated (and modified) enzyme in the cascade can act on several—perhaps hundreds or thousands—substrate molecules so that one event (the binding of one hormone molecule) leads to many thousands of chemical changes inside the cell. Often, such cascades use covalent modifications such as phosphorylation or peptide cleavage to achieve this signal amplification.

Reversible Phosphorylation

The modification here is the attachment or removal of phosphoryl groups on the side chains of certain amino acids. Most often these are serine, threonine, or tyrosine residues, all of which have an —OH group on the side chain where a phosphoryl moiety can be attached. The cofactor ATP is typically the donor of the phosphoryl group. Attachment of a phosphoryl group is performed by enzymes called protein kinases; removal of the groups is performed by protein phosphatases. The use of ATP provides a link to the overall state of the cell in terms of its stores of energy.

As an application of the signal cascade regulatory mechanism, consider the chain of processes that stimulate glycogen breakdown and release of glucose into the bloodstream. In the "fight or flight" response, the hormone epinephrine binds to receptors on the surface of target cells. Its binding stimulates an internal enzyme that converts many molecules of ATP into a correspondingly large number of molecules of cyclic AMP (cAMP). The cAMP then binds to and activates (among other targets) protein kinase A. This kinase phosphorylates and activates another kinase (phosphorylase b kinase), which in turn phosphorylates and activates glycogen phosphorylase. Activated glycogen phosphorylase proceeds to break down glycogen chains and to release glucose (after some further processing). Perhaps 100 to 1000 molecules of glycogen phosphorylase become activated as the result of one molecule of epinephrine binding to a receptor on the cell, and perhaps 10,000 or more molecules of glucose are liberated.

Proteolysis

Quite apart from simple proteolytic digestion of dietary protein, cleavage of the peptide backbone in a polypeptide can lead to profound changes in its biological activity. For example, certain peptide hormones are synthesized as longer precursor polypeptide chains that must be cleaved in specific locations to create the active hormone; the processing of insulin is just one example. In regard to enzymes, specific proteolysis of precursor proteins may be needed to convert a catalytically inactive precursor (called a zymogen) into the catalytically proficient form (the enzyme proper). This is the process by which such digestive enzymes as trypsin and chymotrypsin are formed; proteolytic processing of their catalytically inert precursors, trypsinogen and chymotrypsinogen, is needed to generate the catalytically competent enzymes.

Other Major Types of Covalent Modification

Several other types of covalent modifications have been found. As with phosphorylation, these alterations involve attachment of groups to the side chains of certain amino acids. Some common changes are profiled here:

- Acylation, involving lipid attachment, for targeting the protein to membranes
- Glycosylation, with attachment of a sugar or carbohydrate, for targeting and molecular recognition (e.g., by the immune system—recall the A-B-AB-O types of blood)
- Methylation and acetylation (acetylation and de-acetylation of histone proteins is important, for example, in regulation of gene expression)

QUESTIONS FOR DISCUSSION

1. Monoamine oxidase has a pH activity profile with a maximum at approximately pH 9.5, a midpoint for the ascending branch at approximately pH 7.5, and a midpoint for the descending branch at approximately pH 10.3. Suggest possible active-site residues for this enzyme. Use Table 6-1 to justify your choices.
2. Lysozyme acts to cleave glycosidic bonds in polysaccharides. A proposed mechanism is shown in **Figure 6-23**, emphasizing the catalytic roles of two acidic residues in the active site. The rate of polysaccharide hydrolysis as a function of pH shows a maximum at approximately pH 5.2, with a midpoint for the ascending branch at approximately pH 3.9 and a midpoint for the descending branch at approximately pH 6.7. Describe the state of titration (ionized or not) of Asp 52 and Glu 35 at pH 3.0, on the ascending branch at pH 3.9, at the maximum at pH 5.2, on the descending branch at pH 6.7, and at pH 8.0.
3. For the following enzymes, decide whether the suggested amino acid could replace the indicated active-site residue, to maintain activity. Explain your choice in each case.
   a. Chymotrypsin: Replace serine 195 with (A) threonine; (B) cysteine; (C) alanine.
   b. Ribonuclease A: Replace histidine 12 with (A) lysine; (B) tyrosine; (C) cysteine.
   c. Carbonic anhydrase: Replace glutamate 106 with (A) lysine; (B) aspartate; (C) tyrosine.
4. The Zn(II) cofactor in human carbonic anhydrase isozymes I and II can be replaced by Co(II) with nearly complete restoration of enzymatic activity. Mg^{2+} and Ca^{2+} are both divalent cations present in biological systems at much higher concentrations than either zinc or cobalt. Why can't magnesium or calcium replace zinc (or cobalt) as a cofactor for carbonic anhydrase?
5. Interestingly, carbonic anhydrase can also act as an esterase, hydrolyzing *p*-nitrophenyl acetate, for example. Suggest a possible mechanism for this esterase action.
6. Figure 6-14 shows three inhibitors of carbonic anhydrase. Which structural features do they have in common?
7. A bacterial proline racemase interconverts the two stereoisomers of proline. It is strongly inhibited by pyrrole-2-carboxylic acid. However, tetrahydrofuran-2-carboxylic acid is not an inhibitor. Draw the structures of all four compounds. What does this suggest

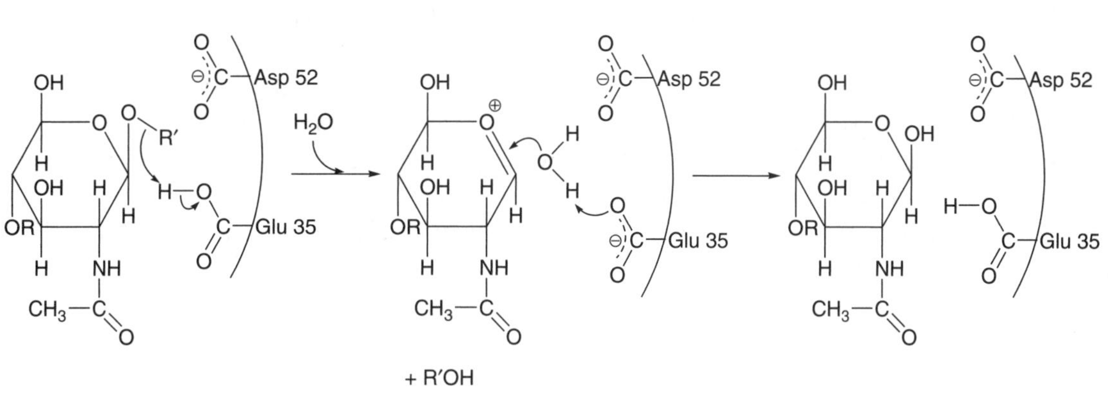

Figure 6-23 Mechanism for action of lysozyme, emphasizing acid–base catalysis by the side chains of Glu 36 and Asp 52.

about the configuration about the α-carbon of the substrate over the course of the isomerization reaction?

8. Chymotrypsin and some other proteases can hydrolyze ester bonds, albeit not nearly as well as they cleave peptide bonds. Review the peptidase action of chymotrypsin and propose a mechanism for its action as an esterase.
9. The L isomer of benzylsuccinate effectively inhibits carboxypeptidase A. Compare the structure of L-benzylsuccinate with the structures of the immediate products of peptide hydrolysis, and explain why L-benzylsuccinate is such an effective inhibitor.
10. How might alkyl phosphonates act as inhibitors of esterases? Compare the transition state for ester hydrolysis to the configuration about the tetrahedral phosphorus atom in the phosphonate.
11. Myoglobin is an oxygen-binding protein, very similar to hemoglobin except that myoglobin is a monomer of a single polypeptide chain with a single heme group, whereas hemoglobin is a tetramer. The oxygenation curve for myoglobin is in the shape of a hyperbola, unlike the sigmoid curve of hemoglobin. Is the oxygenation of myoglobin cooperative? Can you explain mathematically the origin of the hyperbolic shape of its oxygenation curve, using simple chemical equilibria principles?

REFERENCES

D. M. Blow. (1976). "Structure and mechanism of chymotrypsin," *Accts. Chem. Res.* 9:145–152.

W. A. Eaton et al. (1999). "Is cooperative oxygen binding by hemoglobin really understood?", *Nature Struct. Biol.* 6:351–357.

J. T. Edsall. (1980). "Hemoglobin and the origins of the concept of allosterism," *Fed. Proc.* 39:226–235.

D. E. Hansen and R. T. Raines. (1990). "Binding energy and enzymatic catalysis," *J. Chem. Educ.* 67:483–489.

D. E. Koshland. (1958). "Application of a theory of enzyme specificity to protein synthesis," *Proc. Natl. Acad. Sci. USA* 44:98–104.

V. J. Krishnamurthy et al. (2008). "Carbonic anhydrase as a model for biophysical and physical–organic studies of proteins and protein-ligand binding," *Chem. Rev.* 108:946–1051.

G. E. Lienhard. (1973). "Enzymatic catalysis and transition-state theory," *Science* 180:149–154.

W. N. Lipscomb. (1994). "Aspartate transcarbamylase from *Escherichia coli*: Activity and regulation," *Adv. Enzymol.* 68:67–151.

C. P. Macol et al. (2001). "Direct structural evidence for a concerted allosteric transition in *Escherichia coli* aspartate transcarbamoylase," *Nature Struct. Biol.* 8:423–426.

F. M. Richards and H. W. Wyckoff. (1971). "Bovine pancreatic ribonuclease," in *The Enzymes* Vol. IV, 3rd ed. (Ed. P. D. Boyer), Academic Press, New York.

A. G. Splittgerber. (1985). "The catalytic function of enzymes," *J. Chem. Educ.* 62:1008–1012.

CHAPTER 7

Models for Enzyme Kinetics

Learning Objectives

1. Define and use correctly the terms *turnover number*, K_M, *Michaelis constant*, V_{max}, *enzyme saturation, maximal velocity, "kinetically perfected" enzymes, competitive inhibitor, mixed inhibition, irreversible inhibition,* and *suicide substrate*.
2. Describe the general two-step reaction model for the Michaelis-Menten treatment of enzyme kinetics. State under which conditions the reaction is essentially bimolecular and overall second order, and under which conditions it is apparently unimolecular and first order.
3. Interpret various graphs (compute slopes, intercepts) of enzyme kinetic data, deducing from them numerical values for various enzyme parameters (k_{+2}, k_{cat}, V_{max}, K_M, K_I).
4. Draw a diagram showing kinetic relations among enzyme, substrate, and inhibitor, to illustrate the concept of competitive inhibition.
5. Give examples of competitive inhibition, naming both enzyme and inhibitor, that are relevant to pharmacy.
6. Explain the basis for the toxicity of heavy metals, in terms of enzyme action.
7. Describe the basis for active-site-directed irreversible inhibition. Give examples of this type of inhibition, naming both enzyme and inhibitor, that are relevant to pharmacy.
8. State the basic concept behind the interest in enzyme inhibitors as pharmaceutical agents.
9. Explain the rationale behind combination chemotherapy.
10. List the four basic strategies for the design of enzyme inhibitors. Give practical examples or applications of each strategy.

Why Study Enzyme Kinetics?

The study of enzyme kinetics is a powerful way to investigate an enzyme's mechanism, leading to a better understanding of general cell metabolism as well as an understanding of drug action and the design of medicinal agents.

Kinetic assays with enzymes are widely used in drug discovery and development. Generally, these tests involve inhibition of a specific enzyme that has been chosen as a drug target. For example, the drug acetazolamide for treating glaucoma was developed by studying how well different kinds of sulfonamides would inhibit carbonic anhydrase, an enzyme involved in maintaining electrolyte and fluid balance (among many other activities) in cells. The anticancer drug methotrexate, which targets the enzyme dihydrofolate reductase, was developed by studying how different compounds (resembling the natural substrates of the enzyme) could produce changes in the enzyme's reaction kinetics. This enzyme catalyzes a key reaction in the biosynthesis of precursor nucleotides for DNA and RNA, so its inhibition could block cell growth and replication, thereby producing an antibiotic or anticancer action.

Tests for the presence or absence of specific enzymes, employing kinetics, are used clinically in diagnosing various pathologies. Serum levels of lactate dehydrogenase are often used in diagnosing the extent of a myocardial infarction; poisoning by organophosphorus insecticides can be diagnosed by examining levels of circulating cholinesterase; and other enzyme tests are used to check the functioning of the heart, liver, skeletal muscle, and other organs.

The Michaelis-Menten model is widely used as a first-order or approximate description of how enzymes work. It can be applied to many different types of enzymes. It also serves as a starting point for describing the action of inhibitors of enzyme action. Because many drugs act by inhibiting certain key enzymes, this is an especially important application. Much of the same mathematical apparatus can also be used to describe the action of drugs or hormones at receptors, the interaction of gene-regulatory proteins with nucleic acids, and the functioning of membrane-bound transport proteins and ion channels. Thus a study of this model and its equations can be applied not only to enzyme kinetics but also to areas in pharmacology and molecular biology.

As noted earlier, many drugs function as inhibitors of enzymes to produce a therapeutic effect. Several different general types of inhibition are possible, which can be exploited by medicinal chemists in developing new drugs. Also, combinations of inhibitors can sometimes be more effective than using a single inhibitor, in blocking a biochemical pathway and producing the desired overall effect. This chapter briefly introduces the general strategies used to design and develop these valuable drugs.

The Michaelis-Menten Model

To present the Michaelis-Menten model, we first review the basic reaction scheme. This discussion sets up some of the mathematical treatment, leading to a rate law for the model. Depending on the concentration of substrate relative to a compound parameter called the Michaelis constant, the rate law can show some unusual behavior, unlike rate laws in simpler chemical kinetic systems. This outcome calls for some detailed explanation, and we give examples of parameter values and their interpretation. Along the way, we also introduce some specialized enzymological terminology and concepts.

A Single Substrate in a Two-Step Reaction Mechanism

We return to the scheme presented in Chapter 6 for enzyme catalysis, in which the enzyme acts on a single substrate. To recapitulate, we first put the enzyme (E) in contact with the substrate (S), then have the chemical reaction take place and the enzyme release the product (P).

$$E + S \rightleftharpoons E \cdot S \rightarrow E + P \tag{7-1}$$

The enzyme makes contact with the substrate by diffusion; this interaction leads to a reaction intermediate, a complex denoted as E · S, that has some persistence. The E · S complex is not the same as an activated complex or transition state; in fact, the E · S complex may be quite stable. The E · S complex then passes over some sort of activation barrier, through a transition state (not shown in Equation 7-1; see **Figure 7-1**), for a chemical reaction that yields the product (P). Alternatively, the complex (E · S) could fall apart and the enzyme and substrate diffuse away from each other.

Notice that the second step is written with an arrow that points only "forward," implying that the reaction is irreversible. The model ignores any back-reaction that reconverts product (P) back into the complex E · S. This convenient mathematical simplification gives a good approximate account of enzyme behavior for many systems, particularly when a substantial energetic barrier exists to transforming product plus enzyme back into the reaction intermediate (E · S).

Of course, many enzyme-catalyzed reactions are, in fact, reversible. Generally, in the case of a fully reversible reaction, the height of the barrier separating the intermediate E · S from the product (E + P) is relatively low. Unfortunately, accounting for the back-reaction leads to more complicated mathematics than are found in the simple, irreversible reaction model, so these complications are better left to more specialized texts on enzyme kinetics.

A Simple Rate Law for this Mechanism

First, we introduce some rate constants into the two-step model:

$$\mathrm{E} + \mathrm{S} \underset{k_{-1}}{\overset{k_{+1}}{\rightleftharpoons}} \mathrm{E}\cdot\mathrm{S} \xrightarrow{k_{+2}} \mathrm{E} + \mathrm{P} \tag{7-2}$$

Here k_{+1} is the forward rate constant for the meeting of E with S to form the complex E · S. This is a bimolecular reaction step. For the reaction in the reverse direction, k_{-1} is the rate constant

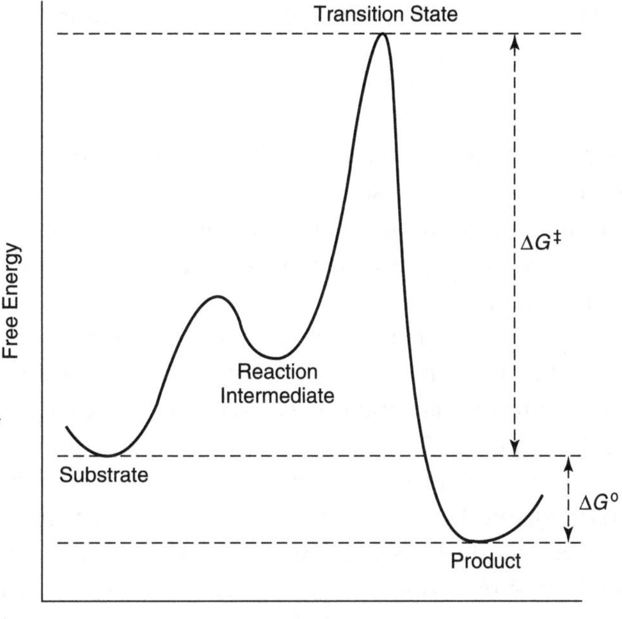

Figure 7-1 Reaction progress diagram, showing the thermodynamic favorability of the reaction (free energy of the product is lower than that of the substrate) and the high kinetic barrier to the reaction.

for the dissociation of this complex. This is a unimolecular reaction step. Lastly, k_{+2} is the rate constant for the breakdown of E · S to form E + P; it is also a unimolecular reaction step.

Unimolecular rate parameters (such as k_{-1} and k_{+2} in the Michaelis-Menten scheme) have units of reciprocal time—that is, sec^{-1} or "per second" (sometimes "per minute" or "per hour," but the time unit of seconds is preferred when using SI units). Bimolecular rate parameters (such as k_{+1} in the Michaelis-Menten scheme) have dimensions of reciprocal concentration–reciprocal time—for example, units of L/mol-sec ($molarity^{-1}$ sec^{-1} or M^{-1}-sec^{-1}) or "per molar per second."

In chemical kinetics, the rate of reaction is conventionally symbolized by v (italic lowercase vee). For this model, the reaction rate is regarded either as the rate of appearance of product (so that $v = d[P]/dt$) or as the rate of disappearance of substrate (so that $v = -d[S]/dt$). Notice the difference in sign between these two expressions. The minus sign in the second expression serves as a reminder that the amount of substance being monitored (here, the substrate) is decreasing.

Appendix 7-1 shows how to obtain an expression for the rate law for this system. The fundamental result is that, for this model, the rate of reaction is

$$v = \frac{[E_0][S]k_{+2}}{[S] + \left(\dfrac{k_{+2} + k_{-1}}{k_{+1}}\right)} = \frac{[E_0][S]k_{+2}}{[S] + K_M} \tag{7-3}$$

Here, the quantity $[E_0]$ is the total enzyme concentration. Notice the quantity in the denominator within the brackets. This is the Michaelis constant, symbolized by K_M. A careful check of the units of this expression reveals that all the units of time cancel out, leaving K_M with units of concentration.

Overall, the dimensions on the right side of the last equality in Equation 7-3 will be found to be concentration over time, or in terms of common units, molarity per second (M-sec^{-1}). This, of course, matches the units of v, on the left side of the equation.

Terminology

The quantity $(k_{+2} + k_{-1})/k_{+1}$ is defined as K_M, the *Michaelis constant.* It can be related to a dissociation constant for the enzyme–substrate complex, under special circumstances. Indeed, it has the correct units to be a dissociation constant (commonly described in units of molarity). In other circumstances, however, it includes certain kinetic effects; in this situation, it cannot be treated as a dissociation constant.

The *turnover number,* k_{cat}, is the maximum number of substrate molecules converted, or turned over, to product per unit time per active site. The qualification "per active site" is important because many enzymes are multimeric, with several catalytic sites. When there is only the one intermediate species, E · S, and when both formation and dissociation of this complex are fast, k_{cat} is simply equal to k_{+2}. However, with more complicated kinetic schemes that involve more intermediates than just E · S, then the rate constants from these added steps contribute to k_{cat}. Mathematically, k_{cat} sets a lower bound to the rate constant for these steps. With these more complicated reactions, the rate law should now be amended to read

$$v = \frac{[E_0][S]k_{cat}}{[S] + K_M} \tag{7-4}$$

Notice the replacement of k_{+2} by k_{cat}. In these more complicated kinetic cases, k_{cat} may not refer to just a single step in the reaction but instead may contain contributions from several kinetic steps. Also, it may not be a "constant" but instead may include some dependence on concentrations. However, it still provides a measure of the rate "per site" for multisite enzymes.

The reaction rate will be maximized when all of the active sites on all of the enzyme molecules are filled and are ready to carry out a chemical or catalytic step. We describe this scenario as *saturating* the enzyme with substrate and note that it requires generally that $[S] \gg K_M$. Now the only limiting factor is in forming product P from the complex. Then we have a *maximum velocity* of reaction V_{max}:

$$V_{max} = k_{cat}[E_0] \tag{7-5}$$

All of these enzyme parameters depend on the specific reaction being catalyzed. If the substrate, temperature, pH, salt, or buffer concentration is changed, then the numerical values of these parameters may change as well.

Molecularity and Reaction Order of Enzyme Kinetics

Enzyme kinetics has an unusual feature in that, as the concentration of substrate increases, we seem to have second-order kinetics that gradually switches over to first-order kinetics. Why does this happen? The molecularity of the individual steps has not changed: E joins with S to form E · S in a bimolecular reaction, and the E · S complex falls apart, one way or another, in a unimolecular step. Nevertheless, the overall reaction order seems to change, depending on whether we have mostly free enzyme or mostly saturated enzyme present in solution.

When [S] is low by comparison to K_M, we have mostly free enzyme in the system; there is not a high enough concentration of substrate to drive it into forming a complex with the enzyme. For low values of [S] by comparison to K_M, we can (approximately) ignore the factor of [S] that appears in the denominator of the general rate law expression because it is so small in comparison to K_M. However, we still have a factor of [S] in the numerator, and we cannot neglect it because it is multiplying everything else in the numerator; it is not adding to anything there. The result is an *approximate* rate law:

$$\text{Rate} = v = \frac{k_{+2}[E_0][S]}{K_M} \tag{7-6}$$

Notice that this approximate expression is second order; it is used when we have mostly free enzyme in the system (with no substrate yet bound). This factor explains why the kinetics start by showing second-order behavior.

The combination k_{+2}/K_M (or more generally k_{cat}/K_M) has the units of a second-order rate constant. Indeed, k_{cat}/K_M appears to be an *effective* second-order rate constant. It can be shown mathematically that the quantity k_{cat}/K_M actually sets a lower bound to the true rate constant for enzyme–substrate association.

Now consider the other situation: When [S] is much greater than K_M, and the enzyme active sites are filled with substrate, then the rate v approaches V_{max}. Because [S] is much greater than K_M, in the general expression for the rate we can (approximately) neglect the factor K_M in the denominator compared to the factor [S]. We can then cancel factors of [S], top and bottom, in the expression and arrive at the approximate relation

$$\text{Rate} = k_{+2}[E_0] = V_{max} \tag{7-7}$$

This is a first-order rate law, with only one concentration—that of the enzyme—because we cancelled out the factors of [S]. Because we have saturated all the enzyme molecules with substrate, we have the maximal rate V_{max}.

Units of Enzyme Activity

The traditional unit (symbol U) of enzyme activity is the amount of enzyme that can convert one *micromole* of substrate into products in one minute. Note the time unit and amount of matter here. The SI unit of activity is the katal (symbol kat), which is the amount of activity that converts one mole of substrate into products in one second. This unit is not widely used, given that most assays use quite small amounts of material, not an entire mole. However, the unit of the microkat sometimes shows up in the literature; this unit is based on the conversion of one *micromole* of substrate per second, which is much closer to the amounts of material actually used in assays. A useful conversion is that 1 microkat equals 60 (traditional) units of activity.

Numerical Values of Kinetic Parameters

Table 7-1 presents numerical values for kinetic parameters for some common enzymes. Carbonic anhydrase is one of the fastest-acting enzymes known. Its turnover number is extremely high. Indeed, with adequate substrate present, this enzyme operates essentially under "diffusion control": As fast as substrate enters the active site, it is converted. However, carbonic anhydrase has only a weak affinity for its substrate; its K_M value of 8000 micromolar would require a substrate concentration of 8 millimolar to reach half its maximal velocity (see the discussion of Eq. 7-14 later in this chapter for details on the connection between half-maximal velocity and the K_M parameter).

Lactate dehydrogenase is somewhat slower acting but has higher affinity for its substrate (it would reach half-maximal velocity with a substrate concentration a bit greater than 0.1 millimolar). Elastase is very slow kinetically (fewer than 10 molecules turned over per active site per second), and it binds the (artificial) substrate weakly. Fumarase has a high turnover number and fairly good affinity for its substrate.

Interpretation of the Michaelis Parameter

If we think of the enzyme merely taking up substrate, without any catalysis, we would have the binding equilibrium $E + S \rightleftharpoons E \cdot S$, with an equilibrium constant for dissociation of

$$K_S = \frac{[E][S]}{[E \cdot S]} = \frac{k_{-1}}{k_{+1}} \qquad \text{(dissociation)} \qquad (7\text{-}8)$$

Enzyme–Substrate	K_M (micromolar)	k_{cat} (per second)
Carbonic anhydrase–CO_2	8000	6×10^5
Lactate dehydrogenase–pyruvate	140	1×10^3
Elastase–Ac-Pro-Ala-Pro-Ala-NH_2	3900	8.5
Fumarase–fumarate	27	2.7×10^3

Table 7-1 Selected Enzymes and Their Kinetic Parameters

We can separate the Michaelis parameter into this "equilibrium" constant, plus a correction:

$$K_M = K_S + \frac{k_{+2}}{k_{+1}} \tag{7-9}$$

Thus the Michaelis parameter can be approximated by the dissociation constant K_S for the E · S complex, but only if the quantity k_{+2}/k_{+1} is much smaller than K_S—that is, if the rate of catalysis is much slower than the rate at which the E · S complex falls apart back to E + S.

Meaning of k_{cat}/K_M

For saturating concentrations of substrate, the maximal rate of reaction is given by $V_{max} = k_{cat}[E_0]$. To saturate the active sites, we must have $[S] \gg K_M$. But what happens under the opposite condition, when most of the active sites are vacant? What limits the rate then, and can we find an expression to describe the rate under these conditions?

Most of the active sites are vacant when the substrate concentration is low, such that $[S] \ll K_M$. If we neglect [S] by comparison to K_M in the denominator of Equation 7-4, then the rate equation becomes

$$v = \left(\frac{k_{cat}}{K_M}\right)[E_0][S] \tag{7-10}$$

This equation has the form of a second-order rate law, so the quantity (k_{cat}/K_M) appears to be a second-order rate constant: It has the proper units, and it multiplies two concentration quantities. Strictly speaking, however, it is not a true second-order rate constant because this is only an approximate rate law.

If we substitute for K_M in the quantity k_{cat}/K_M, we get the relation

$$\frac{k_{cat}}{K_M} = \frac{k_{cat}\,k_{+1}}{k_{-1} + k_{cat}} \tag{7-11}$$

If the rate of product formation (the chemical step, governed by k_{cat}) is much faster than the dissociation rate of the enzyme–substrate complex (that is, if $k_{cat} \gg k_{-1}$), then the quantity (k_{cat}/K_M) approaches k_{+1}. We can interpret this to mean that the overall rate of reaction is approaching that for the rate of encounter of free enzyme with free substrate. In free solution, this rate cannot be faster than the rate at which E and S diffuse together; that is, the upper limit for (k_{cat}/K_M) is set by diffusion. Numerically this puts the upper limit on (k_{cat}/K_M) between 10^8 and $10^9\ M^{-1}\ sec^{-1}$. Enzymes with numerical values of (k_{cat}/K_M) in this range are said to be *kinetically perfected*; the rate of catalysis cannot be further improved without somehow reducing the time for E to reach S. For example, some multisubunit enzymes, in catalyzing multistep reactions, are organized so that they do not depend on diffusion after the first step, but instead transfer the products of intermediate reactions directly from one active site to the next. This processive style of action allows for great efficiency in catalysis.

The specificity of an enzyme for one substrate over another can be quantitatively measured using k_{cat}/K_M. Suppose that an enzyme can act on two different substrates, A and B, to form products P and Q, respectively. We set up the reactions so that the initial concentrations of A and B are the same; we also set up the scenario so that [A] is much lower than the Michaelis constant for than substrate, and [B] is likewise much lower than its corresponding Michaelis constant. We can then ask about the rate of consumption of A versus B, using a ratio of the two rates (actually, we use the approximate rate laws that are good when substrate is limiting):

$$\frac{v_A}{v_B} = \frac{k_{cat}^A / K_M^A}{k_{cat}^B / K_M^B} \tag{7-12}$$

Equation 7-12 shows that the specificity, in terms of overall rate of reaction, of the enzyme for A versus B depends on both K_M and k_{cat} together, not on just K_M alone or k_{cat} alone. The catalytic step alone does not guarantee specificity for A over B, because binding before reaction is important; conversely, strong binding of a substrate does not lead to a preference without considering how fast the bound substrate is converted into product.

Graphical Representations of the Michaelis-Menten Model

It is possible to determine numerical values for k_{cat} and K_M by graphing enzyme kinetic data. These graphical schemes are widely used in presenting and interpreting enzyme kinetic data, in both publications and public presentations, so it is useful to have a good grasp of how they are related mathematically to the underlying data. They also have their weaknesses, which must be guarded against, to avoid over-interpreting or misinterpreting data.

Determining the Initial Rate of Reaction

The initial rate of reaction, v, is determined by setting up the enzymatic reaction with a certain measured amount of enzyme and a measured amount of substrate. The progress of the reaction is followed by measuring (usually) the appearance of product P (although sometimes the disappearance of substrate is measured instead).

Next, we plot the concentration of product as a function of time. This plot (**Figure 7-2**) generally shows a high slope initially, then "falls over" to give lower slope values at longer

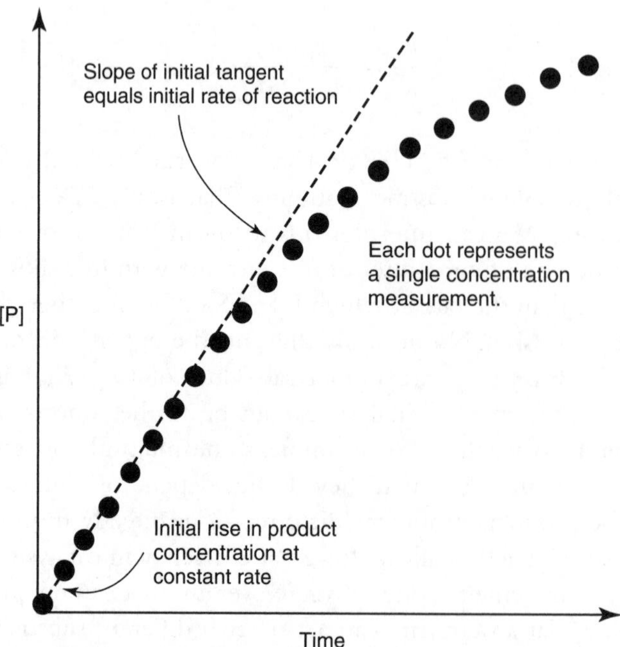

Figure 7-2 The accumulation of product with time for an enzyme-catalyzed reaction. The initial rate or velocity of the reaction is the initial slope of the plot of [P] versus time.

times. The slope at any particular time point equals $d[\mathrm{P}]/dt$, so it is the rate of reaction at that time point. By carefully measuring the slope at several time points close to the beginning of the reaction, we can determine the initial rate of reaction (initial velocity). We can then use these initial velocity values in a second plot, the "direct plot," to help determine the Michaelis parameter K_M and the maximal velocity V_{max}.

Direct Plot

In a direct plot, we plot the initial velocity on the y-axis, as a function of initial substrate concentrations [S] on the x-axis, from the basic equation

$$v = \frac{[\mathrm{E}_0][\mathrm{S}]k_{cat}}{[\mathrm{S}] + K_\mathrm{M}} \tag{7-13}$$

In this format, the basic Michaelis-Menten equation yields a hyperbola. One asymptote is the horizontal line where the velocity has reached its maximum: $v = V_{max}$. The plot gradually rises toward this asymptote, where the enzyme is saturated with substrate (**Figure 7-3**). The initial slope of this plot equals V_{max}/K_M.

A useful feature of the direct plot is that, at the point on the graph where the reaction rate is half the maximum velocity, the corresponding substrate concentration equals the numerical value of K_M. To see this relationship, note that the basic rate law equation can be written as follows:

$$v = \frac{[\mathrm{E}_0][\mathrm{S}]k_{cat}}{[\mathrm{S}] + K_\mathrm{M}} = V_{max}\left(\frac{[\mathrm{S}]}{[\mathrm{S}] + K_\mathrm{M}}\right)$$
$$= \frac{1}{2} V_{max} \qquad \text{when } [\mathrm{S}] = K_\mathrm{M} \tag{7-14}$$

Thus, when [S] numerically equals K_M, the initial rate is at half its maximum value. This provides a way to estimate K_M: Plot the initial rate of reaction as a function of [S], find the maximum (plateau) for the initial rate, then drop back along the plot to where v is half this value, and find the corresponding concentration of S. This numerical value for [S] equals the numerical value of K_M.

In a strict mathematical sense, the initial velocity never actually reaches its maximum value but merely approaches it as [S] becomes very large. Due to uncertainties in the amount of product formed, vertical scatter (noise) may exist within the data used in a direct plot. The

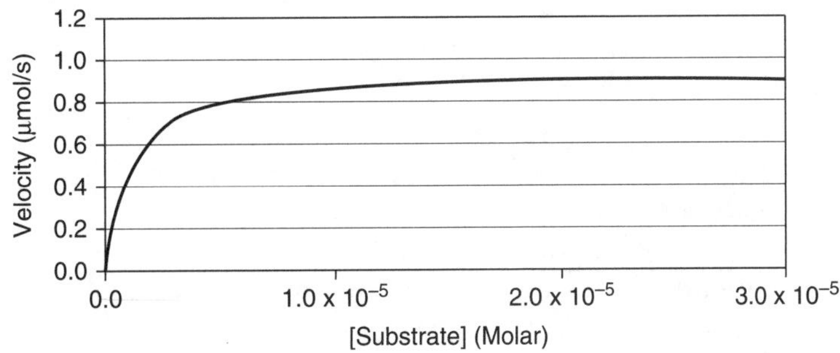

Figure 7-3 The direct plot representation of enzyme kinetic data. Initial rates for a constant enzyme concentration, from experiments done with initial substrate concentrations [S], are plotted as a function of [S].

scatter can obscure the approach to saturation, suggesting that saturation has been achieved, when it actually has not. This issue can lead to errors in estimating the half-maximal velocity, and thus in estimating the numerical value of K_M. For accurate determination of the Michaelis constant (and k_{cat}, too), we should instead use nonlinear statistical curve-fitting of Equation 7-13 to the data.

Double-Reciprocal (Lineweaver-Burk) Plot

Instead of using nonlinear curve-fitting to derive parameter values, it is possible to transform the data to produce a linear plot, which is perhaps easier to interpret. The Michaelis-Menten equation can be rearranged into the form

$$\frac{1}{v} = \frac{K_M}{V_{max}} \cdot \frac{1}{[S]} + \frac{1}{V_{max}} \tag{7-15}$$

This equation suggests a plot of $(1/v)$ as a function of $1/[S]$. The plot should be a straight line, with a slope of K_M/V_{max}. The x-axis intercept will be at $-1/K_M$, and the y-axis intercept will be at $1/V_{max}$ (**Figure 7-4**).

This linearized plot is not without its difficulties. For instance, because reciprocals are used, the largest initial velocities and largest substrate concentrations will be plotted near the crossing of the x- and y-axes. Small concentrations and velocities will lie far out along the axes. Small absolute errors in determining concentration and velocity values can, however, produce large relative errors when either [S] or v is small. Thus this plot tends to misweight the data, in a statistical sense.

A very useful qualitative feature of this plot is its utility in judging whether an enzyme system is following the Michaelis-Menten model. Curvature in such a plot indicates a failure of the system to follow the strict Michaelis-Menten model. One common reason for the existence of curvature is the presence of multiple catalytic sites per enzyme, which may interact to augment or hinder activity beyond what would happen if the catalytic sites acted independently

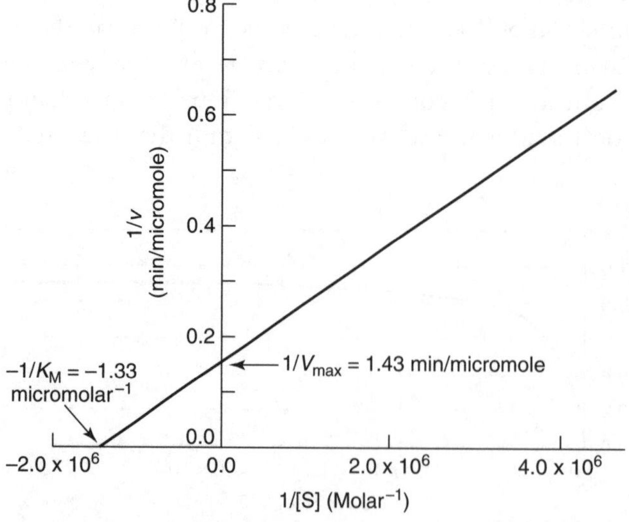

Figure 7-4 A double-reciprocal (Lineweaver-Burk) plot of enzyme kinetic data. According to the Michaelis-Menten model, such a plot should yield a straight line whose intercept on the vertical axis will equal $1/V_{max}$, and whose intercept on the horizontal axis will equal $-1/K_M$.

of one another. With the activity altered, the plot becomes curved, and it is fairly easy to detect this curvature by eye.

Other linearized plots of enzyme kinetic data are the Eadie-Hofstee plot of v against $v/[S]$, from the equation

$$v = -K_M \cdot \frac{v}{[S]} + V_{max} \tag{7-16}$$

and the Hanes-Woolf plot of $[S]/v$ against [S], from the equation

$$\frac{[S]}{v} = \frac{K_M}{V_{max}} + \frac{[S]}{V_{max}} \tag{7-17}$$

Although these linear plots are visually appealing, if there is scatter in the data the plots can hide serious deviations of the actual system from the idealized Michaelis-Menten model. Nevertheless, they are useful for quick determinations (which may have substantial error) of the parameters. However, it quickly becomes a rather tedious chore to prepare graph after graph. For accurate determinations of the parameters, and for testing whether a system is adequately described by the Michaelis-Menten model, one should use proper computer software and analyze the data carefully, using nonlinear curve-fitting methods. Widely available programs that run on personal computers can easily handle this task.

Reversible Competitive Inhibition

General Concepts

Most inhibitors produce their effects in reducing the overall rate of reaction by forming a complex with the enzyme. *Competitive inhibitors* compete with substrate for binding to the enzyme; formation of the E · S complex is reduced while a new type of complex, E · I, is formed. Once bound, the inhibitor I has little or no tendency to react (**Figure 7-5**). A competitive inhibitor has no effect on the catalytic step; k_{cat} and k_{+2} are the same (although other inhibitor types might change k_{+2}). Formation of the E · I complex reduces the free enzyme concentration, and hence the tendency of the E · S complex to form. The net effect is to reduce the rate of reaction.

In the simplest picture of competitive inhibition, the inhibitor I binds directly in the active site and so blocks S from binding. However, the binding mode of I may not be exactly the same

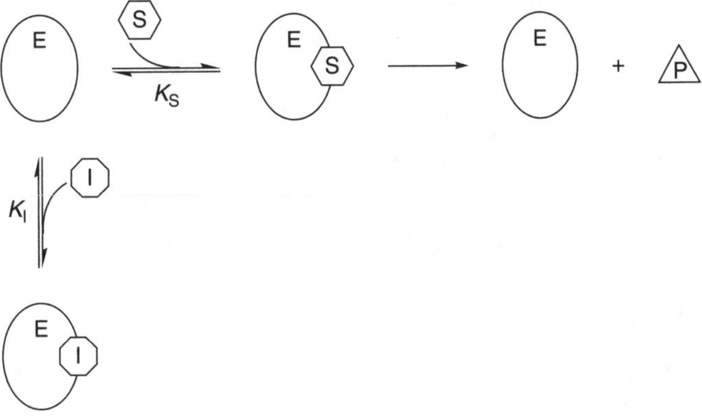

Figure 7-5 Schematic for competitive inhibition.

as for S. For example, different points of contact with the surface of the enzyme may be used by the inhibitor, which still binds in such a way as to block binding by the substrate.

Mathematics of Competitive Inhibition

To describe competitive inhibition, the kinetic scheme must be augmented to include inhibitor binding:

$$\mathrm{E \cdot I} \underset{k_{+i}}{\overset{k_{-i}}{\rightleftharpoons}} \mathrm{I + E + S} \underset{k_{-1}}{\overset{k_{+1}}{\rightleftharpoons}} \mathrm{E \cdot S} \underset{k_{-2}}{\overset{k_{+2}}{\rightleftharpoons}} \mathrm{E + P} \tag{7-18}$$

Conservation of mass of enzyme gives the relation $[\mathrm{E_0}] = [\mathrm{E \cdot S}] + [\mathrm{E \cdot I}] + [\mathrm{E}]$; the total amount of enzyme present must be in complex with substrate or with inhibitor, or else free in solution. Substituting this condition on $[\mathrm{E_0}]$ into the basic equation gives

$$v = \frac{[\mathrm{E_0}][\mathrm{S}]k_{cat}}{[\mathrm{S}] + K_{\mathrm{M,\,apparent}}} = V_{max}\left(\frac{[\mathrm{S}]}{[\mathrm{S}] + K_{\mathrm{M}}\left(1 + \frac{[\mathrm{I}]}{K_{\mathrm{I}}}\right)}\right) = \frac{V_{max}}{1 + \frac{K_{\mathrm{M}}}{[\mathrm{S}]}\left(1 + \frac{[\mathrm{I}]}{K_{\mathrm{I}}}\right)} \tag{7-19}$$

where the inhibitory constant K_{I} is

$$K_{\mathrm{I}} = \frac{k_{-i}}{k_{+i}} = \frac{[\mathrm{E}][\mathrm{I}]}{[\mathrm{E \cdot I}]} \tag{7-20}$$

From Equation 7-19, it appears as though K_{M} has increased by a factor of $1 + ([\mathrm{I}]/K_{\mathrm{I}})$; equivalently, in the rate law we have a modified or apparent Michaelis constant, $K_{\mathrm{M,\,apparent}}$:

$$K_{\mathrm{M,\,apparent}} = K_{\mathrm{M}}\left(1 + \frac{[\mathrm{I}]}{K_{\mathrm{I}}}\right) \tag{7-21}$$

Notice that K_{I}, like K_{M}, has the dimensions of a dissociation constant. Unlike K_{M}, however, the inhibitory constant (as defined in Equation 7-20) really is an equilibrium dissociation constant.

In competitive inhibition, a higher concentration of substrate can restore the original rate of reaction. This higher [S] corresponds to an effective increase in K_{M}. Physically what happens is that as the concentration of S increases, the equilibrium of E with E · S and E · I shifts away from E · I and toward E · S, which then permits the catalytic reaction step to occur and so form product. The maximum velocity is still the same, however; V_{max} does not change.

Graphical Representation for Competitive Inhibition

For competitive inhibition, the double-reciprocal plot is still linear. The intercept on the vertical axis is the same, so V_{max} has not changed. However, the slope of the plot increases as [I] increases, reflecting the change in the apparent Michaelis constant (**Figure 7-6**).

Uncompetitive Inhibition

Uncompetitive type of inhibition is relatively uncommon in enzymology. The underlying principle is that the inhibitor preferentially binds to the E · S complex, not to the free enzyme, and forms an E · S · I complex. No E · I complex is formed. The E · S · I complex is catalytically

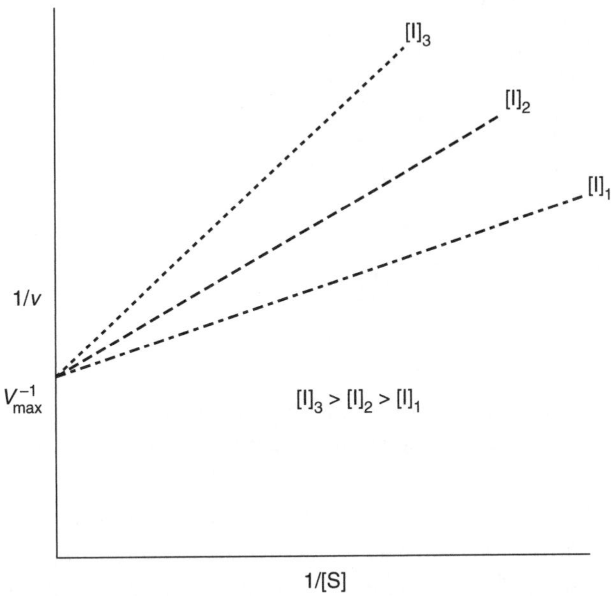

Figure 7-6 A double-reciprocal plot showing the effects of different concentrations of a competitive inhibitor. Competitive inhibition alters the slope of the plot and the intercept on the horizontal axis, but does not affect the intercept on the vertical axis; V_{max} is unchanged in competitive inhibition, but K_M becomes larger.

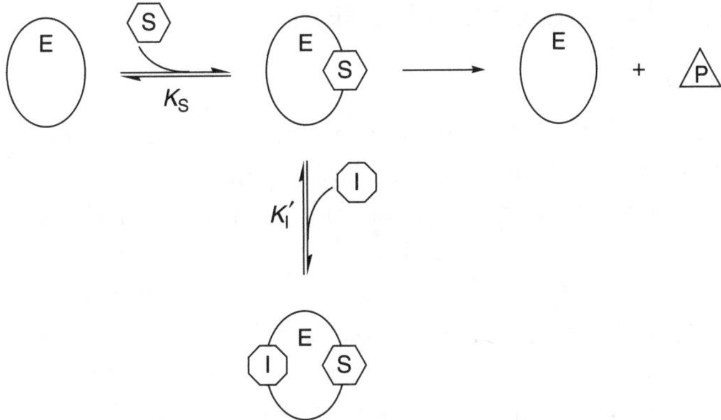

Figure 7-7 Schematic of uncompetitive inhibition.

inert (**Figure 7-7**). It can be shown mathematically that, for uncompetitive inhibition, K_M is decreased in magnitude, and V_{max} is reduced as well; by comparison, in competitive inhibition, only K_M is affected. For uncompetitive inhibition, it is not possible to overcome the inhibition and so reach V_{max} by adding more and more substrate. Adding more substrate in the presence of an uncompetitive inhibitor simply gives the inhibitor more E · S complexes to bind to, and more opportunities to inhibit the enzyme.

"Mixed" and Noncompetitive Inhibition

In mixed inhibition, the inhibitor I can form a complex both with free enzyme E and with the enzyme–substrate complex E · S. The E · I and E · S · I complexes are both catalytically inactive. Notice how this model includes both competitive and uncompetitive inhibition—hence the name "mixed" inhibition (**Figure 7-8**).

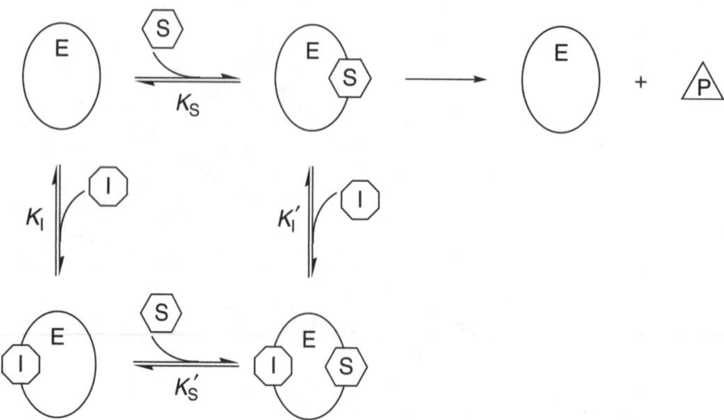

Figure 7-8 Schematic of mixed inhibition. Noncompetitive inhibition is a special case of mixed inhibition, where the inhibitor binds with equal affinity to either E alone or the E·S complex.

Because I will bind to the E · S complex, it is not possible to overcome inhibition by adding more substrate. The maximum velocity achievable now is something less than that achieved when no inhibitor is present. This is unlike the case of competitive inhibition, where adding S can overcome inhibition, but it does resemble the case of uncompetitive inhibition.

Noncompetitive inhibition is a special case of mixed inhibition. For noncompetitive inhibition, the inhibitor has the same affinity for either E or the E · S complex; that is, K_I is numerically equal to K_I'. For mixed inhibition the quantities K_I and K_I' are allowed to be different.

Active-Site-Directed Irreversible Inhibition

Irreversible Inhibition

Generally the irreversible inhibition of an enzyme entails covalent attachment of the inhibitor to the enzyme or some covalent modification, involving key residues of the enzyme, by the inhibitor. The catalytic activity of the enzyme is completely lost, and it can be restored only by synthesizing new enzyme molecules. Many drugs that target enzymes are irreversible inhibitors of those enzymes.

To gain specificity and affinity, and to avoid side effects from unwanted reactions with other enzymes, inhibitors can be designed to bind in or near the enzyme's active site. A typical drug-design strategy in these circumstances is to synthesize a compound that resembles the natural substrate of the enzyme. Once bound, the compound forms a covalent attachment to the enzyme. The covalent attachment prevents the inhibitor from dissociating from the enzyme—hence the inhibition is considered irreversible.

Clinical Application

A famous example of irreversible inhibition involves aspirin, which targets and covalently modifies a key enzyme involved in inflammation. Aspirin (acetylsalicylic acid) contains a reactive acetyl group, and the active site of the target enzyme (prostaglandin H synthase, also called cyclo-oxygenase; see Chapter 13) contains a serine residue. The acetyl group from aspirin can react with this serine's side chain, specifically with the —OH group, to acetylate it (**Figure 7-9**). This modification introduces a bulky group into the enzyme's active site that blocks the entry of the enzyme's regular substrate, arachidonic acid.

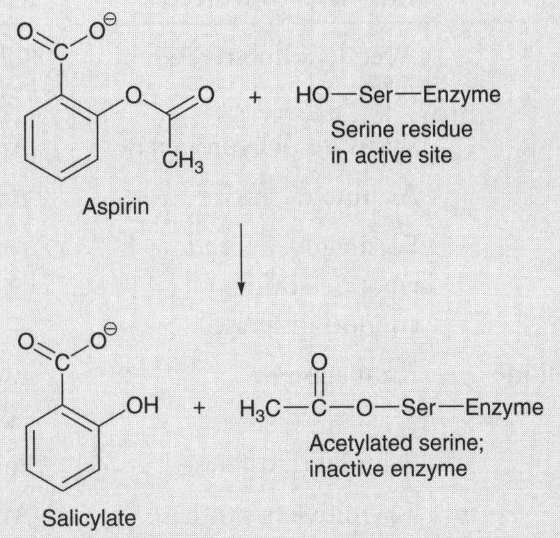

Aspirin + HO—Ser—Enzyme (Serine residue in active site) → Salicylate + $H_3C—C(=O)—O—Ser—Enzyme$ (Acetylated serine; inactive enzyme)

Figure 7-9 Acetylsalicylic acid (aspirin) irreversibly inhibits cyclo-oxygenase by acetylating a key serine residue in the enzyme's active site.

The enzyme would normally convert the arachidonic acid into chemical messengers involved in inducing the symptoms of inflammation (among other things). When the substrate is unable to enter the chemically modified active site, however, the enzyme is inhibited and these chemical messengers are not made, so inflammation is reduced. Because the acetyl group is covalently attached, the inhibition is irreversible. Eventually, the body synthesizes new enzyme molecules, which restores the body's normal ability to produce those chemical messengers and produce inflammation.

"Suicide Substrates"

Sometimes an inhibitor is unreactive until the enzyme attempts to use it as a substrate. At that point, the compound binds covalently to the active site and inhibits the enzyme permanently. The enzyme "kills itself" by this sort of reaction; thus the inhibitor is described as a "suicide inhibitor." This situation is slightly different from the irreversible inhibition strategy where the inhibitor needs no activation by the enzyme to become covalently attached.

Clinical Application

Penicillin is a good example of a suicide inhibitor; it is unreactive until the bacterial transpeptidase "accepts" it as a substrate; it then becomes covalently linked, irreversibly, in the enzyme's active site.

Another example is physostigmine. This toxic compound is a natural product, derived from calabar beans. It reacts with acetylcholinesterase, forming an acyl derivative in the enzyme's active site and blocking the degradation of acetylcholine in nerve cell junctions. Although quite toxic in its own right, physostigmine is used in small doses to treat the effects of anticholinergic agents.

Drug	Enzyme Inhibited	Clinical Use
Neostigmine	Acetylcholinesterase	Glaucoma, myasthenia gravis
Organo-arsenicals	Pyruvate dehydrogenase	Antiprotozoal
D-Cycloserine	Alanine racemase	Antibiotic
Azaserine	Formylglycinamide ribonucleotide aminotransferase	Anticancer
4-Hydroxy-androstenedione	Aromatase	Estrogen-mediated breast cancer
Chloramphenicol	Peptidyl transferase	Antibiotic
5-Fluorouracil	Thymidylate synthase	Anticancer
Disulfiram	Aldehyde dehydrogenase	Alcoholism

Table 7-2 Examples of Active-Site-Directed Irreversible Inhibitors

Table 7-2 lists several examples of active-site-directed irreversible inhibitors.

Heavy Metal Toxicity

Many enzymes have sulfhydryl groups that are needed either for catalytic activity or for structural reasons. These groups can form tight bonds with heavy metals such as mercury, lead, silver, and even iron and copper. Once the heavy metal atom is bound, the sulfhydryl cannot function in catalysis. Also, the presence of the metal atom can distort the structure of the enzyme and affect its catalytic ability. One treatment for syphilis, no longer in use in the United States, exploited just such a sensitivity of enzymes in the spirochete *Treponema pallidum* to mercury and bismuth.

Nerve Agents

Many chemical warfare agents react with enzymes to inhibit them. Certain organic phosphates (e.g., sarin) are extremely toxic, targeting acetylcholinesterase. Derivatives are used agriculturally to kill insects (e.g., parathion, Dursban; see **Figure 7-10**).

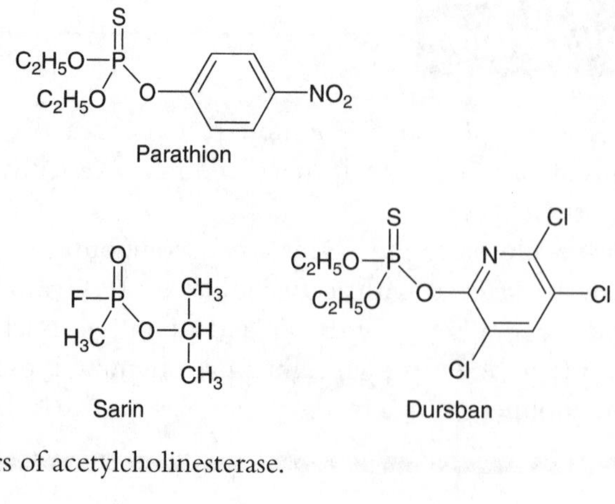

Parathion

Sarin

Dursban

Figure 7-10 Inhibitors of acetylcholinesterase.

Introduction to Design of Enzyme Inhibitors

Enzymes as Drug Targets

A key principle in drug design and development is that of identifying a target for drug action. By picking a key enzyme and inhibiting it, one can reduce the concentration of the metabolites and/or build up the concentration of substrate(s), thereby obtaining a clinically useful response. Some examples of such inhibitors currently in use include the following:

- Statins inhibit HMG CoA reductase, leading to lower cholesterol levels.
- Gleevec inhibits a protein kinase and blocks proliferation of cancer cells.
- Aspirin inhibits a cyclo-oxygenase and reduces inflammation.

Combination Chemotherapy

In combination chemotherapy, the main idea is to combine two inhibitors that target the same (or a related) pathway to achieve an enhanced response, greater than might be achieved with either inhibitor alone.

As an example, one very effective antibacterial combination is trimethoprim and sulfamethoxazole; the combination is called co-trimoxazole. Sulfamethoxazole targets dihydropteroate synthetase and reduces folate synthesis. Trimethoprim then targets dihydrofolate reductase (the next step in the folate pathway) and blocks synthesis of tetrahydrofolic acid. Tetrahydrofolic acid is required in purine synthesis, pyrimidine synthesis, and the synthesis of certain amino acids, so this drug combination is very effective in halting bacterial growth (**Figure 7-11**).

A variation on this idea is to use one compound to protect the other from metabolic degradation. For example, in treating bacterial infections clavulanic acid sulbactam may be combined with penicillin (**Figure 7-12**); the clavulanic acid blocks bacterial β-lactamase, which would otherwise degrade the penicillin. This drug combination keeps the penicillin free to block the key enzyme involved in cell wall synthesis by bacteria.

Examples of Inhibitor Design

Four basic strategies can be used in inhibitor design: mimic the substrate; mimic the transition state; irreversibly react with a key residue; or change the enzyme's conformation or state of assembly.

Substrate Mimics

Substrate mimics are usually competitive inhibitors. The strategy here is to use compounds that have much—but not all—of the chemical features of the substrate, so that they fit into the active site and are held relatively tightly, but do not themselves react and do not let substrate react.

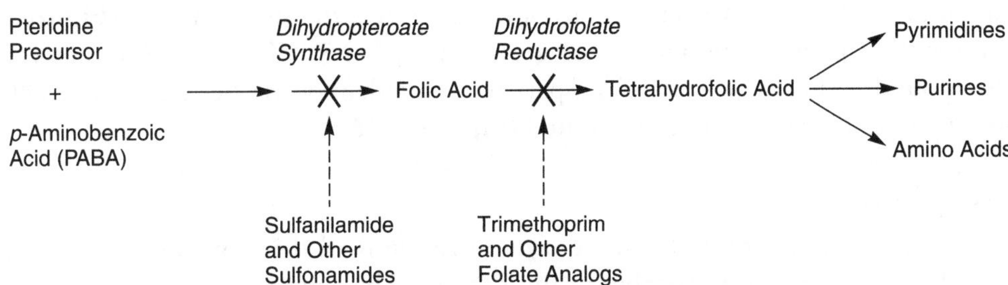

Figure 7-11 Combination chemotherapy to inhibit bacterial growth by blocking folic acid biosynthesis.

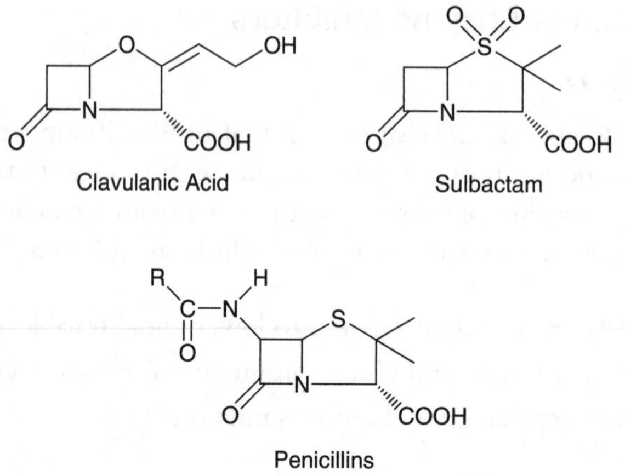

Figure 7-12 Agents for combination chemotherapy to inhibit bacterial growth by blocking cell-wall biosynthesis. Here the clavulanic acid and sulbactam serve to extend the action of penicillin.

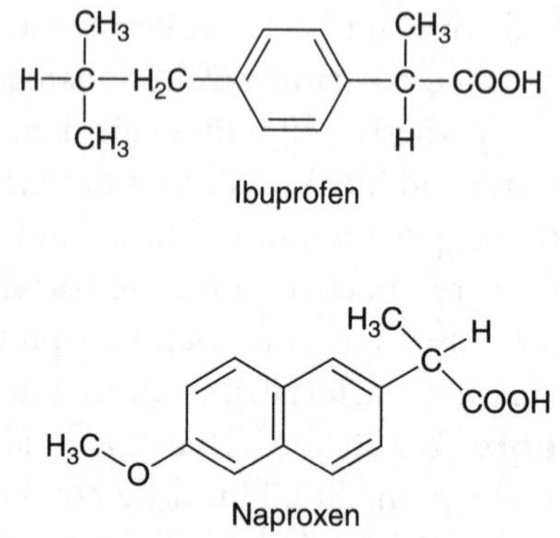

Figure 7-13 Ibuprofen and naproxen are competitive inhibitors of cyclo-oxygenase (also known as prostaglandin H_2 synthase), acting as anti-inflammatory drugs.

For example, ibuprofen and related compounds occupy the active site to inhibit prostaglandin synthetase, thereby acting as anti-inflammatory drugs (**Figure 7-13**).

Transition State Mimics

Compounds can be made that resemble the transition state (the high-energy intermediate in the reaction diagram) but that cannot go on to complete the reaction. These compounds should bind more tightly to the enzyme than does the natural substrate, given that one way in which enzymes function is to stabilize the transition state by binding tightly to it. An example here is the compound 2′-deoxycoformycin, a diazepine ring with a ribose substituent (**Figure 7-14**). It very potently inhibits adenosine deaminase, with $K_I = 2.5 \times 10^{-12}$ M. Another example is the compound PALA, which inhibits aspartate transcarbamoylase because it resembles the transition state as the two substrates are joined (**Figure 7-15**).

Irreversible Inhibition

A compound with good affinity for the enzyme may be used that contains a reactive group that can link covalently and irreversibly to the enzyme. The action of aspirin, in acetylating a key serine residue in the active site of cyclo-oxygenase (Figure 7-9), is perhaps the best-known example of this sort of inhibition.

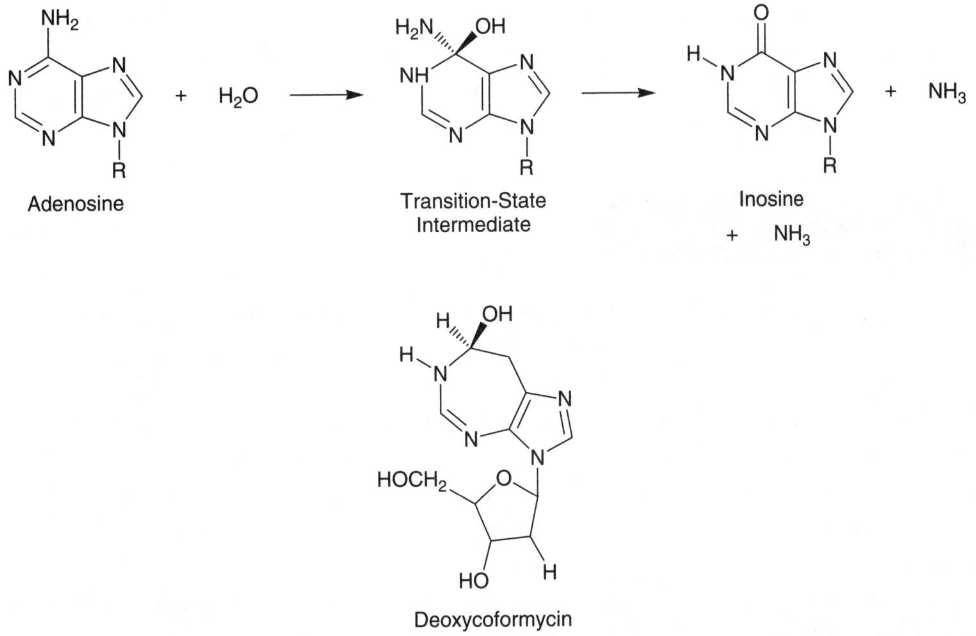

Figure 7-14 Adenosine deaminase is potently inhibited by the transition state analog deoxycoformycin.

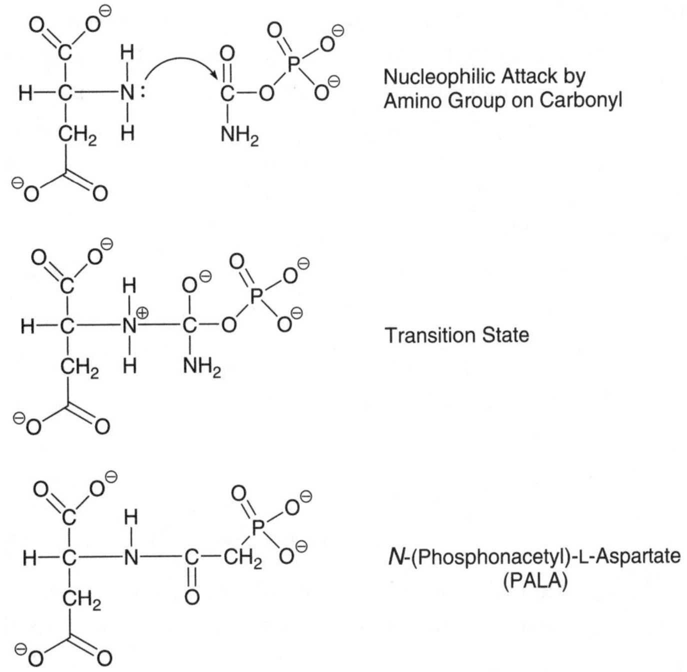

Figure 7-15 *N*-(Phosphonacetyl)-L-aspartate (PALA) resembles the transition state for combining aspartate with carbamoyl phosphate. PALA is a potent inhibitor of the enzyme aspartate transcarbamoylase.

Uncompetitive Inhibitors

A classical uncompetitive inhibitor forms a ternary complex with the enzyme and the substrate, and blocks turnover of the substrate into product; at the same time, the inhibitor forms negligible amounts of complex with the free enzyme. To do so, presumably the inhibitor would not compete with substrate in forming complexes with the enzyme. Instead, it might bind to a different site on the enzyme or protein, away from the active site, or it might combine with groups on both the substrate and the enzyme. The inhibitor might then somehow interfere with binding of substrate in the correct conformation or with catalysis in some way; another possibility is that the inhibitor could block the proper association of enzyme subunits. Such inhibitors are much more challenging to discover and develop, and are not very common.

Clinical Application

One example of an uncompetitive inhibitor arises in the search for drugs to treat cases of poisoning by methanol or ethylene glycol. Liver alcohol dehydrogenase is the major enzyme responsible for the metabolism of ethanol, using NAD^+ as a cofactor in the reaction. This enzyme has relatively broad specificity and not only acts on ethanol but also oxidizes methanol to formaldehyde (a toxic metabolite that reacts with proteins); it will also oxidize ethylene glycol to glycoaldehyde (which then leads eventually to oxalic acid, another quite toxic metabolite). Accidental ingestion of either methanol or ethylene glycol causes many cases of poisoning each year.

Tetramethylene sulfoxide and 3-butylthiolane 1-oxide (**Figure 7-16**) are uncompetitive inhibitors of the dehydrogenase, with respect to ethanol as the substrate. These sulfoxides form strong ternary complexes with the enzyme and the NAD^+ coenzyme, and they block turnover of substrate into the oxidized product. Their structure resembles the presumed intermediate between the alcohol substrate and the aldehyde product, although it does not appear that they are truly transition state analogs. An advantage of using these uncompetitive inhibitors to treat poisoning cases is that the inhibition is not reversed by increasing levels of substrate, unlike with competitive inhibitors; the inhibitors remain effective even with high levels of the dangerous substrate, methanol or ethylene glycol.

Tetramethylene Sulfoxide

3-Butylthiolane 1-Oxide

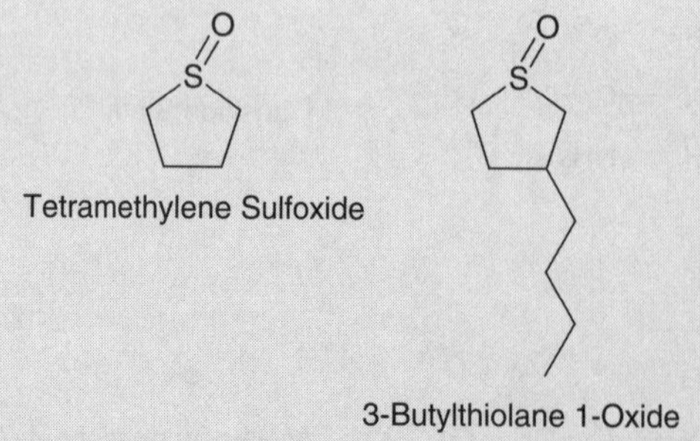

Figure 7-16 Tetramethylene sulfoxide and 3-butylthiolane 1-oxide are potent uncompetitive inhibitors of liver alcohol dehydrogenase. (Note the possibility of several stereoisomers of the latter compound.)

QUESTIONS FOR DISCUSSION

1. **Figure 7-17** is a plot of the absorbance changes, due to product formation, observed in a 1-cm path length cuvet as the enzyme papain acts on an artificial substrate. Initial substrate concentrations (s_i) are shown. Assume that the product has an optical extinction

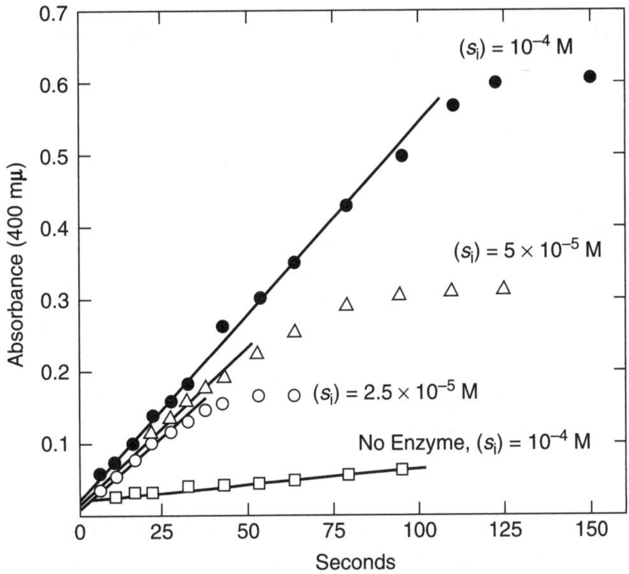

Figure 7-17 Activity of papain on an artificial substrate.

Source: Adapted with permission from J.F. Kirsch and M. Igelström. The kinetics of the papain-catalyzed hydrolysis of esters of carbobenzoxyglycine. Evidence for an acyl-enzyme intermediate. (1966). *Biochemistry* 5:783–791. Copyright 1966 American Chemical Society.

coefficient of $6.4 \times 10^3\ M^{-1}\ cm^{-1}$ at 400 nm, and that Beer's law applies. What is the initial rate of reaction for an initial substrate concentration of 100 micromolar?

2. **Figure 7-18** is a double-reciprocal plot of the activity of the enzyme papain on an artificial substrate; $1/v_i$ is the reciprocal of the initial velocity of the reaction. What is V_{max} for this enzyme with this substrate? If the enzyme concentration is 3.3×10^{-7} molar, what is k_{cat} for this enzyme with this substrate? Can you estimate a K_M value for this reaction?

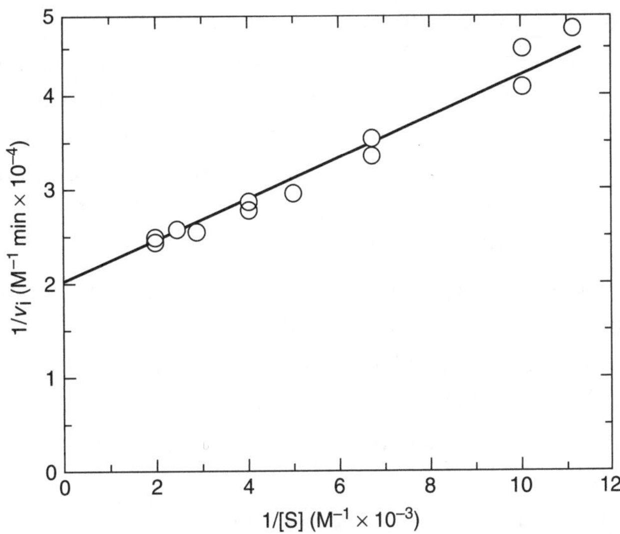

Figure 7-18 Double-reciprocal plot of papain activity on an artificial substrate.

Source: Adapted with permission from J.F. Kirsch and M. Igelström. The kinetics of the papain-catalyzed hydrolysis of esters of carbobenzoxyglycine. Evidence for an acyl-enzyme intermediate. (1966). *Biochemistry* 5:783–791. Copyright 1966 American Chemical Society.

[S] (micromolar)	V_I (micromol/min)
1.0×10^{-1}	8.24×10^{-1}
2.0×10^{-1}	1.47
5.0×10^{-1}	2.80
1.0	4.00
2.0	5.09
5.0	6.09
10.0	6.51

Table 7-3 Enzyme Kinetic Data for Question 3

3. Use the data in **Table 7-3** to deduce V_{max} and K_M values for an enzyme-catalyzed reaction that obeys Michaelis-Menten kinetics.
4. Suppose that an inhibitor binds to an enzyme at a site far removed from the active site. As the inhibitor binds, it drives a shape change in the enzyme that warps the active site such that substrate can no longer fit into, and be acted upon by, the active site. Which type of inhibition is this: competitive, noncompetitive, uncompetitive, or perhaps something else? Explain your choice.
5. Now suppose that instead of driving a shape change, the bound inhibitor in Question 4 has an arm that extends over the cleft of the active site, so that it blocks the entry of substrate into that site. Which kind of inhibition is this? Explain your choice.
6. Qualitatively distinguish (in words) between competitive and noncompetitive inhibition. How could you distinguish between the two types of inhibition by using graphs of kinetic data? Which data would you need? Which patterns would you see?
7. Irreversible inhibitors are often quite toxic. Why? Can you name some well-known irreversible (and highly toxic) enzyme inhibitors?
8. A patient with a bacterial infection is taking folate supplements while you treat the infection with co-trimoxazole. The infection persists. Review the action of co-trimoxazole, and propose an explanation for the persistence of the infection.
9. Subtilisin is a bacterial serine protease. Mutation of the serine residue to alanine, in the active site of subtilisin, reduces k_{cat} by a factor of 1 million, with little change in K_M. Propose an explanation of this fact.
10. Methotrexate binds to dihydrofolate reductase with a free energy change of -56.9 kJ/mol. What is the inhibitory constant K_I for methotrexate?
11. What would be the kinetic consequences if a substrate had exactly the same affinity for both the R and T forms of an allosteric enzyme?
12. What is the ratio of [S] to K_M when the velocity of an enzyme-catalyzed reaction is 20% of V_{max}?
13. A problem in algebra: Derive a suitable equation that would lead to a straight-line plot of enzymatic inhibition data (observed rate as a function of inhibitor concentration, for a fixed substrate concentration), to get the inhibitory constant K_I from the slope or intercept in that plot.

REFERENCES

V. K. Chadha, K. G. Leida, and B.V. Plapp. (1983). "Inhibition by carboxamides and sulfoxides of liver alcohol dehydrogenase and ethanol metabolism," *J. Med. Chem.* 26:916–922.

A. Cornish-Bowden. (1995). *Fundamentals of Enzyme Kinetics*, Portland Press, London.

A. R. Fersht. (1974). "Catalysis, binding and enzyme–substrate complementarity," *Proc. R. Soc. Lond. B* 187:397–407.

H. Lineweaver and D. Burk. (1934). "The determination of enzyme dissociation constants," *J. Am. Chem. Soc.* 56:658–666.

I. H. Segel. (1975). *Enzyme Kinetics*, Wiley-Interscience, New York.

R. Wolfenden and M. J. Snider. (2001). "The depth of chemical time and the power of enzymes as catalysts," *Acc. Chem. Res.* 35:938–945.

APPENDIX 7-1 DERIVATION OF THE MICHAELIS-MENTEN EQUATION

First Version: Equilibrium Approximation

In 1913, Michaelis and Menten proposed a kinetic scheme for simple enzyme kinetics:

$$E + S \underset{k_{-1}}{\overset{k_{+1}}{\rightleftharpoons}} E \cdot S \xrightarrow{k_{+2}} E + P \tag{7-22}$$

Michaelis and Menten supposed that the first step was rapid and reversible, and that an equilibrium constant for this step could be written as follows: $K_S = [E][S]/[E \cdot S]$. The second step was taken as the chemical transformation step, with a first-order rate constant k_{cat}.

$$v = k_{+2}\,[E \cdot S] \tag{7-23}$$

The total enzyme concentration $[E_0]$ and the free enzyme concentration $[E]$ are connected by mass conservation:

$$[E] = [E_0] - [E \cdot S] \tag{7-24}$$

With a bit of algebra, this gives

$$[E \cdot S] = \frac{[E_0][S]}{K_S + [S]} \tag{7-25}$$

Now we substitute this expression into the equation for v:

$$v = \frac{[E_0][S]\,k_{+2}}{K_S + [S]} \tag{7-26}$$

Notice that this equation is based on the assumption that the enzyme–substrate complex is in a rapid equilibrium with the free enzyme and free substrate. This is an approximation, however, which is good only when the rate of chemical transformation is slow by comparison to the rate of dissociation of the enzyme–substrate complex.

Second Version: Steady-State Approximation

In 1925, Briggs and Haldane assumed a kinetic scheme very much like that of Michaelis and Menten, and they analyzed the case when the forward rates of both steps were comparable. They assumed that the concentration of the enzyme–substrate complex was constant or in a "steady state"—that is, that they could write a rate equation for this intermediate when it did not change in concentration:

$$\frac{d[\mathrm{E}\cdot\mathrm{S}]}{dt} = 0 = k_{+1}[E][S] - k_{+2}[\mathrm{E}\cdot\mathrm{S}] - k_{-1}[\mathrm{E}\cdot\mathrm{S}] \tag{7-27}$$

Once again, using conservation of mass, the quantity $[\mathrm{E}\cdot\mathrm{S}]$ can be replaced:

$$[\mathrm{E}\cdot\mathrm{S}] = \frac{[\mathrm{E}_0][\mathrm{S}]}{[\mathrm{S}] + \left(\dfrac{k_{+2} + k_{-1}}{k_{+1}}\right)} \tag{7-28}$$

Then the rate of reaction is

$$v = \frac{[\mathrm{E}_0][\mathrm{S}]\ k_{+2}}{[\mathrm{S}] + \left(\dfrac{k_{+2} + k_{-1}}{k_{+1}}\right)} = \frac{[\mathrm{E}_0][\mathrm{S}]\ k_{+2}}{[\mathrm{S}] + K_{\mathrm{M}}} \tag{7-29}$$

The quantity $(k_{+2} + k_{-1})/k_{+1}$ is defined as K_{M}, the Michaelis constant. It is related to the equilibrium constant K_{S} of the original Michaelis-Menten equation by

$$K_{\mathrm{M}} = K_{\mathrm{S}} + (k_{+2}/k_{+1}) \tag{7-30}$$

When $k_{-1} \gg k_{+2}$, this equation simplifies to $K_{\mathrm{M}} = K_{\mathrm{S}}$ and we have the original Michaelis-Menten expression for the rate of reaction.

CHAPTER 8

Basic Concepts in Metabolism

Learning Objectives

1. Define and use correctly the terms *intermediary/primary metabolism, catabolism, anabolism, pathway, feedback, committed step, Crossover Theorem, compartmentalization, reciprocal regulation, vitamin, activated group carrier, ATP, phosphoanhydride, phosphoester, energy charge, adenylate charge, coenzyme A, thioester, pantothenic acid, thioester, nicotinamide, niacin, NADH, NADPH, pellagra, flavin,* $FADH_2$*,* $FMNH_2$*, riboflavin,* and *flavoprotein*.
2. List major food components, and compare their relative energy values.
3. Distinguish between vitamins and minerals, and between fat-soluble vitamins and water-soluble vitamins. List the main biochemical functions for these vitamins and minerals. Explain the concept of turnover in metabolism, and describe how it relates to a proper daily diet.
4. List the three main stages in catabolism. Summarize in a diagram the main pathways for the digestion of foodstuffs.
5. Describe the concept of feedback, as applied to metabolic pathways. Distinguish between positive and negative feedback. Identify important common features of metabolic regulation involving key steps and end products.
6. List and describe four major mechanisms for control of metabolism.
7. Recognize the structure of ATP and identify phosphoester and phosphoanhydride bonds in the structure. Explain how ATP functions as a "carrier" of free energy in metabolism, and describe the cycling of ATP with ADP. Explain why ATP serves as a "good" donor of phosphoryl groups, giving the structural and electronic basis for this behavior.
8. Recognize the structure of coenzyme A. Identify functionally important chemical groups on this molecule and relate them to coenzyme A's function as a carrier of activated acyl groups. Relate the structure of coenzyme A to that of the precursors, adenosine, pantothenic acid, and β-mercaptoethylamine.
9. Recognize the structures of NAD^+, NADH, $NADP^+$, NADPH, FAD, and $FADH_2$. For each, explain its role in metabolism. Identify functionally important chemical groups on these molecules. Relate their structures to those of their respective precursor vitamins.
10. Explain the role of kinetic stability in the metabolic functioning of ATP, NADH, and $FADH_2$.

Regulation of Metabolism

Intermediary or *primary metabolism* is the collection of reactions responsible for the generation of energy for the cell, and the use of this energy and simple organic precursor molecules to make more complicated molecules for the cell. *Anabolism* is the subset of these reactions that leads to the synthesis of new or more complicated molecules from simpler precursors, while *catabolism* is the collection of reactions responsible for the breakdown of energy-yielding molecules.

In these reactions, there is usually an orderly progression of chemical transformations leading from some precursor to some final product. The set of linked reactions from precursor to final product, together with the catalyzing enzymes, cofactors, and regulatory factors, is often referred to as a *pathway* for that product. Pathways may be branched, and they can interlink with one another. There are also examples of "cyclic" pathways that apparently close back on themselves (as in the urea cycle or the Krebs/citric acid cycle). **Figure 8-1** gives some examples of these different types of pathways.

Most pathways are tightly regulated and coordinated with other pathways, as part of the overall physiology of the cell. This interaction allows the cell to conserve resources and avoid wasteful expenditures of materials, energy, or time. Irregularities or loss of regulation in pathways can easily lead to pathologies; we will see many examples of disease states due to defects in metabolic regulation of one pathway or another.

Feedback in Metabolic Regulation

The concept of *feedback* comes from systems engineering. Consider a very abstract representation of a system as composed of some sort of input (e.g., an aural signal like a voice, or precursor chemicals in a biochemical pathway), some sort of amplifying and transforming processor (e.g., a microphone and an electronic amplifier, or a set of biochemical reactions), and finally output of some kind (e.g., the sound from an electronic speaker, or the biochemical product of a pathway). Feedback returns a portion of the output of a system as input. Positive feedback results in amplification of the original input—that is, there is more output. In contrast, negative feedback results in less output. An example of positive feedback is the screech or howl sometimes experienced with an electronic amplifier/microphone system. Examples of negative feedback include a thermostat, where a rise in temperature shuts off the furnace generating the heat, or the pupil of the eye, where a brighter light causes the pupil to contract and reduce the influx of light onto the retina.

Enzymes and Metabolic Pathways

The input here is the first substrate in the pathway (plus any small-molecule effectors that might be acting on enzymes of the pathway); the output is the last product of the path; the amplifier is the (set of) enzymes involved. **Figure 8-2** depicts the general pattern. Note that two or more enzymes may be involved in a pathway, and that one or more of them may be regulated, to control metabolic flow through the pathway.

Negative Feedback in Metabolism

Inhibition of enzymes is often used to control metabolic pathways, thereby providing for greater metabolic efficiency. Often there is also allosterism in such systems; the product molecule binds to a regulatory site (different from the catalytic site) on the key enzyme(s) and inhibits that enzyme by causing a change in its conformation. In Figure 8-2, the product C may bind to enzyme E_1 and slow down conversion of precursor to intermediate A.

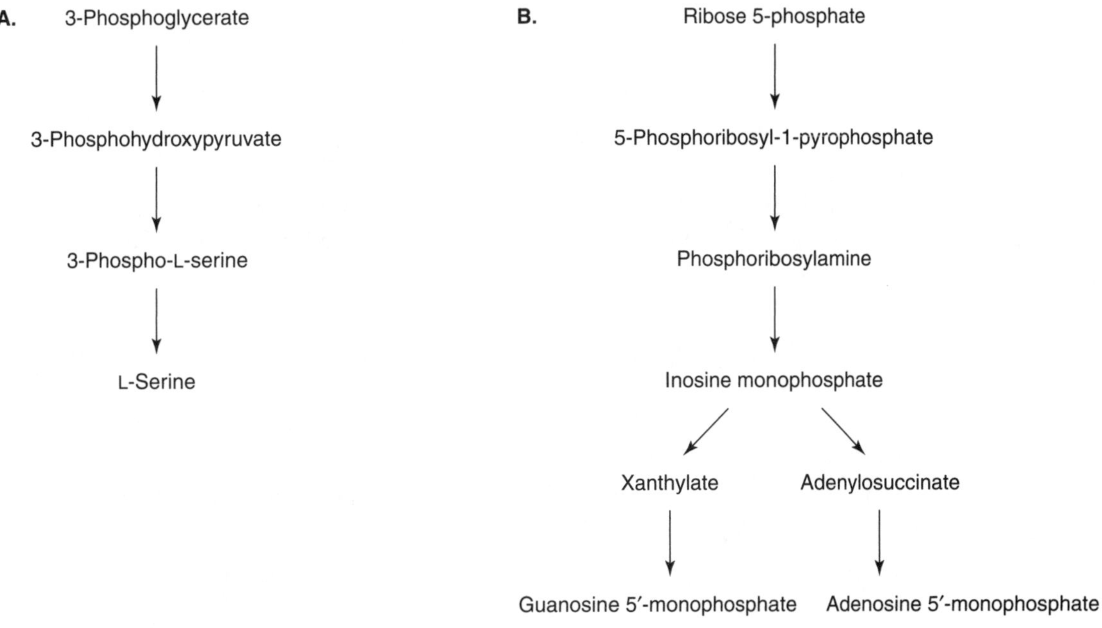

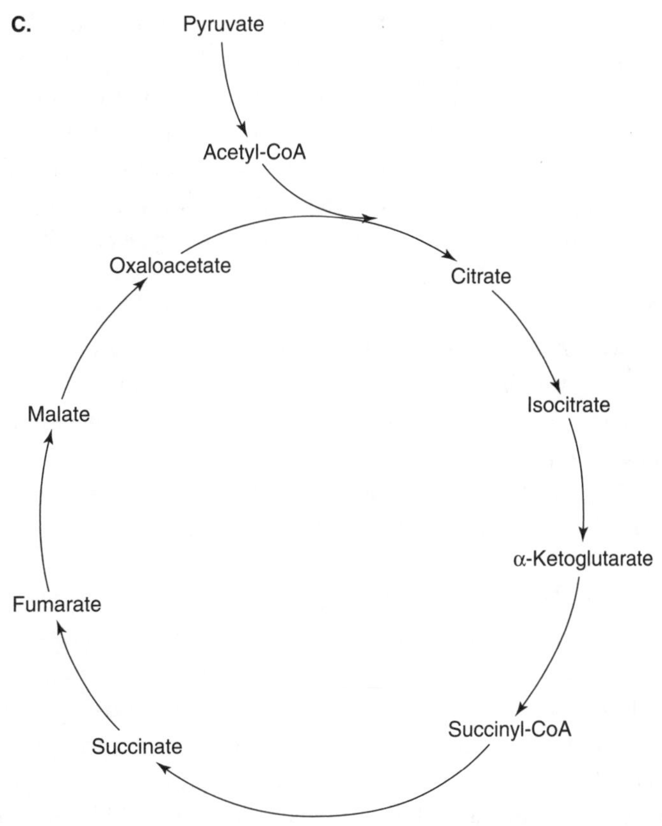

Figure 8-1 Different types of biochemical pathways. **A.** The biosynthesis of the amino acid serine is a typical linear pathway. **B.** Purine biosynthesis shows a branch at the point where inosine 5′-monophosphate is made. **C.** The citric acid cycle is a famous example of cyclical pathway.

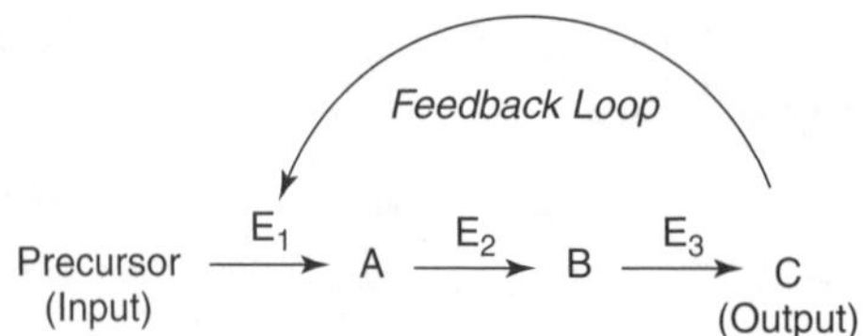

Figure 8-2 The concept of feedback in a biochemical pathway. The end product C acts on the first enzyme of the pathway. In negative feedback, product C inhibits enzyme E_1; in positive feedback, product C stimulates the enzyme.

Important features of negative feedback in metabolic pathways include the following:

- Generally the first unique step of a pathway (also called the *committed step*) is regulated; there may be other points for regulation as well.
- The end product C is an inhibitor, and in complicated pathways feedback may also be exerted by intermediates along the pathway.
- The end product C may or may not resemble the precursor or substrate at the committed step.

Examples of negative feedback are quite common in biochemistry, and later chapters will present several instances of this type. One example of negative feedback has already been given, in Chapter 7. That chapter included a discussion of the allosteric control of the activity of the enzyme aspartate transcarbamoylase (ATCase) by nucleotides. The pyrimidine nucleotides CTP and UTP are products of the pyrimidine biosynthetic pathway. They reduce the amount of their own synthesis by allosterically inhibiting the upstream enzyme ATCase, binding to regulatory subunits and causing a conformational change in the multisubunit enzyme. Notice that these structurally complicated pyrimidine nucleotide end products do not resemble the regular substrates for ATCase (a simple amino acid and a simple phosphorylated organic compound).

Positive Feedback

In positive feedback, there is activation—not inhibition—by a product of the pathway. Binding of product molecules to regulatory sites on key enzymes may stimulate or activate those enzymes (by changing their shape; e.g., by allosterism) to produce greater conversion of the precursor to the ultimate product of the pathway.

In feed-forward (not "feedback," but closely related to it), a precursor—not a product—serves to activate a key enzyme (perhaps to "prepare" for more throughput). Allosterism is possible here as well.

Positive feedback and feed-forward mechanisms appear much less frequently than negative feedback mechanisms in biochemistry. One system that incorporates feed-forward is found in the path for the synthesis of glycogen, a storage carbohydrate polymer. Here the key enzyme glycogen synthase is allosterically activated by glucose-6-phosphate, a phospho-sugar produced at an earlier step in the path. Interestingly, an example of positive feedback is found in the related path for the breakdown of glycogen. In this other system, AMP allosterically activates glycogen phosphorylase to start the breakdown of glycogen and the synthesis of ATP. As ATP levels rise, so do AMP levels, which leads to even more glycogen breakdown, and even more ATP. (Other controls at work here damp out a possible runaway breakdown of the body's entire supply of glycogen.)

The Crossover Theorem

Perturbing a metabolic pathway by adding an activator or an inhibitor of one of the enzymes in the pathway results in changes in metabolite concentrations before and after a control enzyme's step, with the changes occurring in opposite directions. For example, adding an inhibitor will typically result in an increase in the concentration of the control enzyme's substrate(s) and a decrease in the concentration of its product(s). The appearance of such opposite changes in concentration, or a "crossover" in concentrations relative to the normal values, has been dubbed the *Crossover Theorem* by biochemists. (Of course, this isn't a theorem in the mathematical sense, but rather a convenient label for the phenomenon.)

The Crossover Theorem can be applied to rationalize some aspects of certain metabolic diseases. Diseases such as phenylketonuria (PKU), galactosemia, and many others are due to a deficiency in enzyme activity in a normal metabolic pathway. The blockage at one point interrupts the flow from precursor to final metabolite; metabolites from the steps before the point of blockage accumulate, whereas normally they exist at low concentrations. As their concentrations increase, minor reactions of these metabolites start to occur, and the concentration of unusual metabolic by-products rises. Also, a characteristic decrease in the concentration of metabolites that are downstream from the point of blockage often occurs. The appearance in the body of the unusual metabolites can be useful in deducing the exact defect causing the disease. This effect is used, for example, in diagnosing such diseases as phenylketonuria or maple syrup urine disease (see Chapter 14 for more details on these diseases).

Insights from the Crossover Theorem can lead to strategies to treat disease states. For example, one could try to reduce serum cholesterol levels by blocking the synthesis of cholesterol with a drug that will inhibit a key enzyme in the cholesterol biosynthetic pathway. Exploitation of this mechanism has, in fact, has led to several drugs that successfully reduce high cholesterol levels. The drug lovastatin is a good example: It inhibits the enzyme HMG-CoA reductase, which catalyzes a key step in this pathway (**Figure 8-3**), and this inhibition reduces overall cholesterol levels in the patient.

Major Metabolic Control Mechanisms

There are several mechanisms by which the cell or organism can regulate metabolism.

Concentration

Concentration mechanisms include control of the level of enzyme(s), substrates, cofactors, and other substances. With more enzyme present, more substrate can be converted to product per unit time. Thus more "throughput" occurs with more catalyst present. Conversely, with less enzyme present, there is less throughput and less product made. The level of enzyme is usually under genetic control, involving regulation of gene expression. Recall that proteins (enzymes) are subject to degradation (turnover) by proteolytic enzymes, so concentration changes represent another route to reduce the amount of catalyst and, therefore, to reduce the throughput. Similarly, regulation of cofactor abundance can help or hinder the throughput. Of course, supplying more substrate is necessary if greater throughput is to be achieved.

Compartmentalization

Major opposing pathways are often located in different intracellular membrane-bound organelles or compartments (*compartmentalization*). These pathways are separated by membrane barriers, with specialized transport systems to carry material across the membranes. The transport system itself may be regulated as well. This allows control of concentrations (as discussed in the preceding subsection), separation of competing processes, and so on. Some examples of compartments and compartmentalized processes would include (1) the nucleus, with replication of DNA, or synthesis of mRNA; (2) mitochondria, with the citric acid cycle and fatty acid oxidation; and (3) the cytosol, with glycolysis and fatty acid synthesis.

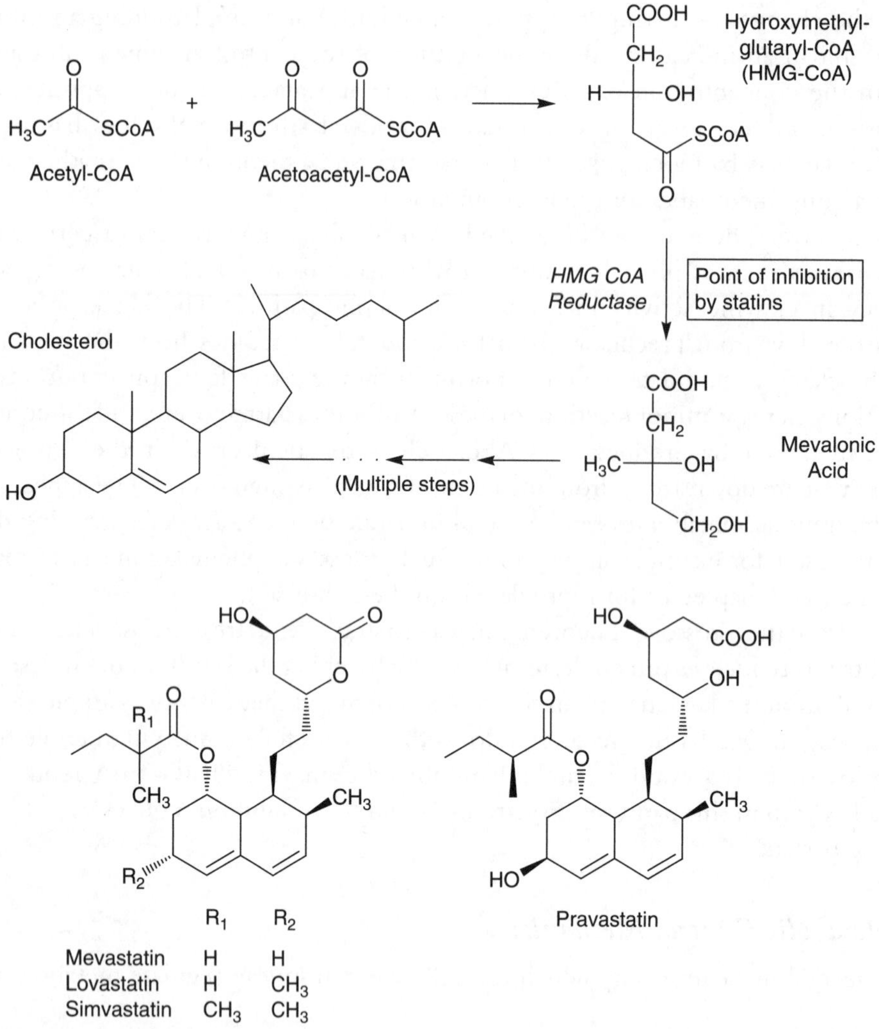

	R_1	R_2
Mevastatin	H	H
Lovastatin	H	CH_3
Simvastatin	CH_3	CH_3

Figure 8-3 The biosynthesis of cholesterol can be interrupted at a key reaction where statins inhibit the enzyme HMG-CoA reductase.

Enzyme Activation or Deactivation

With enzyme activation/deactivation mechanisms, control is exerted at the level of the degree of catalytic activity (as opposed to amount of catalyst, as discussed earlier). Two main mechanisms exist: covalent modification and ligand binding.

Covalent modifications that alter enzymatic activity include phosphorylation, glycosylation, adenylation, ADP ribosylation, proteolytic processing, and more. These changes are often used in signaling cascades. The covalent modifications may or may not be reversible. For example, phosphorylation is often reversible, with one kind of enzyme (a kinase) catalyzing attachment of a phosphoryl group, and another kind of enzyme (a phosphatase) removing the group. Balancing the relative activities of these kinases and phosphatases is an important process for the cell. Chapter 9 gives more details as to how this is accomplished in the metabolism of carbohydrates; Chapter 13 considers it further in the context of lipid metabolism.

Reversible, noncovalent binding by allosteric effectors can raise or lower enzyme activity. Often the concentrations of these effectors are connected to the overall metabolic state of the cell. See the example of the inhibition of the enzyme ATCase, in Figure 6-22, which is inhibited by pyrimidine nucleotides, the end product of the pyrimidine biosynthetic pathway. Here the rise in pyrimidine nucleotide concentration in the cell automatically reduces biosynthesis of exactly those same compounds.

Hormones

Hormones serve as chemical messengers for communication between cells and tissues. They are bound to specific receptors on membranes, and either carried inside the cell and released for further action, or stimulate the receptor in some fashion to generate a continuation of the "signal" inside the cell. This latter mechanism involves intracellular "second messengers" for signaling pathways (e.g., Ca^{2+} ions, certain nucleotides, special sugar derivatives). Hormones can play a role in any of the three previously discussed control mechanisms.

Reciprocal Regulation of Competing Pathways

Generally speaking, a competent cell contains enzymes for both synthesizing and breaking down the same set of biochemical compounds—for example, for synthesizing and degrading complex carbohydrates. This could lead to problems if the activities of the two sets of enzymes were not well controlled: one set would be using valuable cellular resources (e.g., energy, reducing power) to make "expensive" biochemicals, while the other set of enzymes would be tearing these compounds apart as fast as it could. These opposing behaviors would clearly not be to the cell's advantage, if not closely controlled.

One way to avoid this conflict, as noted earlier, is to segregate the enzymes by compartmentalization, separating them by one or more biomembranes. Nevertheless, in many cases, for proper biochemical functioning, the enzymes must coexist in the same cellular compartment (for example, a membrane will slow down cellular responses, but if the enzymes are in the same compartment, responses can be much faster). Then, depending on the immediate physiological state, one set of enzymes or the other must be shut off while the other set is active. This idea is termed *reciprocal regulation.*

Reciprocal regulation can be achieved by using either or both of two of the control mechanisms just discussed: the covalent modification of enzymes to alter their activity and the noncovalent binding of small effector molecules to alter enzymatic activity. Both mechanisms can be employed at the same time, to regulate a pair of competing pathways.

For example, in carbohydrate metabolism, glycolysis breaks down sugars; in contrast, gluconeogenesis generates sugars from simple precursors. These two opposing pathways operate in the same cellular compartment, so their relative rates can be quickly adjusted in response to the abundance of carbohydrates in the environment, the need for new sugar molecules to supply other tissues, and so on. The two pathways are regulated primarily by allosteric effector binding to key enzymes.

Another example of reciprocal regulation, this time involving covalent modification for enzyme regulation, comprises glycogen synthesis and its breakdown by glycogenolysis (not to be confused with glycolysis). Again, the two opposing processes are located in the same cellular compartment (the cytosol) and there is a need to be able to switch the two processes on and off relatively rapidly, without the delays associated with gene expression for synthesis of the enzymes of the pathways, or with proteolysis of cellular proteins. For both synthesis and breakdown of glycogen, the processes are regulated principally by reversible phosphorylation, with interlocking chains of protein kinases and phosphatases. These mechanisms will be laid out in more detail in the next chapter.

Diet and Nutrition

A proper diet should supply energy for daily functions, building blocks for growth, and replacements as needed to maintain homeostasis. The energy will come from the oxidation of foodstuffs such as carbohydrates and lipids. While the body possesses the capacity to make a very large number of the necessary building blocks for proteins, nucleic acids, and biomembranes, there are some particular constituents it cannot make—notably, a number of amino acids and certain species of fatty acids. These substances are termed "essential" to a proper diet, and a deficiency in their supply will lead to pathologies. In addition, the body needs to acquire from the diet small amounts of vitamins and inorganic compounds or elements, for use as cofactors for enzymes or for transport proteins (such as the iron in hemoglobin), and for structural purposes (e.g., calcium and phosphate for bones). Finally, the body must dissolve and transport all these substances, so it requires an ample supply of water.

Water

The body needs to dissolve a wide variety of substances—nonpolar, polar, and ionic. The remarkable capacity of water to dissolve such a wide range of chemicals is exploited throughout biology. Truly, water can be termed the "matrix of life."

The human body consists of 65% to 70% water. Water is regularly lost through respiration (breathing), sweating, and excretion (through urinary and fecal routes). Extra fluid loss can occur through prolonged sweating, vomiting, diarrhea, or extensive burn injuries. Conversely, fluid retention can occur with certain diseases, particularly those affecting water or sodium excretion.

Major Food Components

Most foods are complex mixtures of carbohydrates, lipids, and protein, plus small amounts of vitamins and minerals. The carbohydrates, lipids, and protein can all supply energy to the body as well as provide building blocks for growth and replacement.

Carbohydrates in the diet include both simple (monomeric and dimeric) and complex (polymeric) sugars. Common dietary carbohydrates include glucose and fructose (monomeric sugars), sucrose and lactose (disaccharides), and starch and cellulose (both polymeric; cellulose is not digestible by humans). Digestion of carbohydrates starts with hydrolysis of the complex polymeric forms down to monomeric and dimeric sugars. Some of the monomeric sugar is used directly for biosynthesis and some is stored as glycogen, but most is oxidized to release energy in the process called glycolysis.

Dietary lipids ("fats") are also complex, and the various classes of lipid can serve quite different purposes—for example, as a source of energy, as membrane building blocks, for communication between cells, and so on (see Chapter 5). Triglycerides are the form of dietary lipid that is mostly used for energy. As with carbohydrates, digestion starts with hydrolysis to release the constituent fatty acids and glycerol. The fatty acids are then oxidized in a very orderly process to release the energy stored in the C—H and C—C bonds. The glycerol may also be oxidized, or used in biosynthesis.

Proteins are the dietary source of amino acids; again, digestion hydrolyzes dietary protein to release the constituent monomeric amino acids. These monomers can be used directly for biosynthesis of new protein in the body, as building blocks for other compounds (e.g., glycine in the synthesis of nucleic acid bases), or as a source of energy for the body.

Carbohydrates, lipid, and protein differ in their energy content. Note that the densest dietary source of energy is fat or lipid, due to the highly reduced state of the hydrocarbon

Nutrient	Approximate Energy Value (kJ/g)	Recommended Percentage of Energy Intake for Adults
Carbohydrate	17	45–65
Fat	38	20–35
Protein	17	10–35

Table 8-1 Three Main Classes of Food Components and Their Energy Content

Source: J. J. Otten, J. P. Hellwig, and L. D. Meyers (eds.). (2006). *Dietary Reference Intakes: The Essential Guide to Nutrient Requirements*, Institute of Medicine, National Academies Press, Washington, DC, p. 70.

chains in the lipids compared to the more oxidized carbon chains in amino acids (protein) or carbohydrates. Furthermore, due to the need to excrete the nitrogen associated with protein, the useful energy content of protein is considerably reduced from what might be expected on the basis of calorimetry. **Table 8-1** compares the energy value to the body of these three different fuels and gives the current recommended intake of each for the average adult.

Main Pathways for Digestion of Foodstuffs

In terms of digestion, we are concerned here with catabolism in primary metabolism—that is, how foodstuffs are digested and used by the body. The digestive system breaks down complex polymers such as proteins and polysaccharides into simple monomeric or oligomeric units. Thus the compounds of concern to primary metabolism generally are small organic molecules with molecular weights less than 1000 g/mol, not polymers such as DNA and proteins.

Catabolism proceeds through three stages:

- Stage I is essentially the breakdown of polymeric foodstuffs to monomeric constituents. Proteins are broken down to amino acids, carbohydrates to simple sugars, and lipids to fatty acids and glycerol. Relatively little energy is generated at this stage. In humans, stage I processes occur mostly in the gastrointestinal tract and are catalyzed by enzymes secreted into the mouth and gut. The breakdown is further aided by secreted acid (in the stomach) and by solubilizing agents such as bile salts; the latter compounds are especially important for breakdown and absorption of the less-soluble lipid components of the diet.
- Stage II is the conversion of monomeric constituents (generated in stage I) to simple metabolic intermediates. These reactions take place inside cells, after delivery by the circulatory system of the monomeric constituents from the digestive tract. There is typically little release of useful free energy in these reactions; energy may actually be consumed in some of them. Two key examples of the simple compounds generated in stage II are (1) the simple organic acid pyruvate and (2) acetyl groups linked to a carrier compound, coenzyme A (commonly abbreviated as CoA). Both pyruvate and acetyl-CoA will appear repeatedly in later chapters of this book. Two examples of major metabolic pathways involved in stage II of catabolism are glycolysis (for the breakdown of glucose) and β-oxidation of fatty acids.
- Stage III is the ultimate degradation of simple intermediates to CO_2, H_2O, NH_3, and urea, followed by excretion of these end products (e.g., by the urea cycle). These processes are catalyzed by intracellular enzymes. Generation of useful energy and reducing power for the cell occurs mostly at this stage. The citric acid cycle links stages II and III, operating on acetyl groups generated primarily from the breakdown of sugars and fatty acids. The

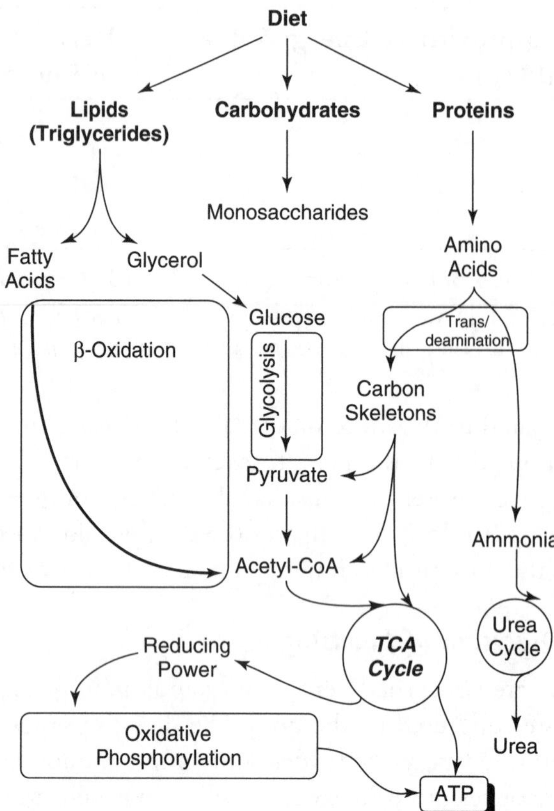

Figure 8-4 Summary diagram of catabolism, showing how the breakdown of foodstuffs leads to energy generation for the cell.

energy from oxidation of these acetyl groups is stored temporarily in the form of reduced cofactors. The oxidation of these cofactors by complicated membrane-bound enzymes called respiratory complexes is strongly coupled to the action of the ATP synthase, which captures much of the energy released in this stage.

Figure 8-4 shows the main pathways for the breakdown of polymeric foodstuffs into simple organic compounds, and finally the release (and capture) of energy from these processes. Note the convergence onto the TCA cycle. The reducing power generated by the TCA cycle will be used by mitochondrial respiratory complexes to make more ATP.

Vitamins and Minerals

Vitamins are small organic molecules that can perform chemical functions (often in enzyme catalysis) not allowed by the chemistry of ordinary amino acids, sugars, or lipids. Minerals are inorganic elements—often ions—needed for structural, catalytic, osmotic, electrochemical, or binding functions in the body. The vitamins cannot be made by the body and, therefore, must be obtained from the diet; likewise, minerals must be taken in as a regular part of the diet. **Table 8-2** and **Table 8-3** summarize the minerals and vitamins needed in the human diet.

Vitamins and minerals are excreted daily; that is, they are subject to turnover. They do not persist in the body indefinitely, and they must be replaced if the body is to continue with normal metabolic activities. Thus the diet must include sufficient amounts of minerals and vitamins to allow for replacement of the lost (degraded, excreted) factors. Generally, minerals and vitamins

Mineral	Main Function
Calcium	Bone and teeth; signal transduction and conduction; blood coagulation
Chloride	Main anion in body fluids
Fluoride	Bone and teeth
Iodine	Thyroid hormones
Iron	Oxygen transport and storage; redox; electron transport
Magnesium	Cofactor for enzymes
Phosphorus	Bone; phosphate esters
Potassium	Main intracellular cation
Sodium	Main extracellular cation
Sulfur	Bile acid conjugation; connective tissue biopolymers

Table 8-2 Major Minerals Required in Human Nutrition

Vitamin	Function	Disease Associated with Deficiency
Fat Soluble		
A	Vision, cellular differentiation	Night blindness
D	Calcium metabolism	Rickets, osteomalacia
E	Lipid antioxidant	Lipid peroxidation
K	Blood coagulation enzymes	Inability to clot blood
Water Soluble		
Cobalamin (B_{12})	Isomerization of methylmalonyl CoA to succinyl CoA; conversion of homocysteine to methionine	Pernicious anemia; megaloblastic anemia; homocysteinuria; central nervous system degeneration
Biotin	Carboxylation reactions	Deficiency rarely occurs; dermatitis, alopecia
C (ascorbic acid)	Hydroxylation reactions; biosynthesis of collagen	Scurvy
Folic acid	Wide variety of reactions involving H- and C-transfers	Megaloblastic anemia
Niacin (B_3)	Redox reactions	Pellagra
Pantothenic acid (B_5)	Acyl carrier in fatty acid metabolism; acetyl carrier in many reactions	Deficiency rarely occurs
Pyridoxine (B_6)	Transaminations	Anemia
Riboflavin (B_2)	Redox reactions	Deficiency rarely occurs
Thiamine (B_1)	Oxidative decarboxylation reactions	Beri-beri

Table 8-3 Vitamins and Their Functions

are needed only in small amounts. The U.S. Department of Health and Human Services and the U.S. Department of Agriculture jointly publish dietary guidelines that lay out the expected average amounts of vitamins, minerals, and macronutrients such as fat, carbohydrate, and protein needed to maintain health.

Vitamins can be grouped according to their solubility in water (see Table 8-3). The water-soluble vitamins include ascorbic acid (vitamin C) and the B vitamins. Fat-soluble vitamins include vitamins A, D, E, and K. Table 8-3 also compares the roles of vitamins and notes pathologies associated with vitamin deficiencies.

Fat-Soluble Vitamins

Vitamin A is really three separate but chemically related compounds: retinol, retinal, and retinoic acid (**Figure 8-5**). When converted to the retinal form, these compounds serve as an essential cofactor for the protein rhodopsin, responsible for vision in rod cells. Vitamin A also plays a role in the growth and remodeling of various tissues, especially epithelial tissue. It is mainly stored in the liver, but must be transported to other tissues via the bloodstream, and then inside the cell, by carrier proteins. A natural dietary source rich in vitamin A is, of course, liver; vitamin A can also be derived from the provitamin, β-carotene, found in plants.

Vitamin D is generated by the action of sunlight on 7-dehydrocholesterol; the photo-oxidative reaction leads to vitamin D_3 (cholecalciferol; **Figure 8-6**). This compound is further oxidized in liver and kidney to the final, active compound, known as 1,25-dihydroxycholecalciferol. Vitamin D is responsible for maintaining proper bone mineralization, through regulation of the metabolism of calcium and phosphate. Strictly speaking, it functions more as a hormone and not as a cofactor for an enzyme or transporter protein. It binds to a receptor protein in the cytoplasm and is carried to the cell nucleus, where the protein–vitamin complex regulates the expression of certain genes. In this respect, the function of vitamin D resembles the action of steroid hormones, which also operate through receptor proteins to regulate gene expression. In the modern diet in industrialized and developed countries, fortified milk and dairy products serve as the major dietary source of vitamin D; fish oil and egg yolks are food sources that are naturally rich in this vitamin.

Vitamin E is quite nonpolar and dissolves well in the nonpolar interior of lipid bilayers (**Figure 8-7**). It serves primarily as an antioxidant in biomembranes, protecting the membranes and the embedded proteins against oxidative attack of free radicals and peroxides. Like vitamins A and D, vitamin E is actually a mixture of compounds, called tocopherols. Nuts and vegetable oils are especially rich in vitamin E.

Vitamin K is a collection of related compounds, based on the core structure of menadione (**Figure 8-8**). It is required for the clotting of blood; this vitamin is a cofactor in enzyme-catalyzed reactions that carboxylate particular glutamate residues in proteins involved in the blood-clotting cascade. Vitamin K is found in green leafy vegetables; it is also synthesized by bacteria in the gut, typically in quantities that satisfy normal adult needs without dietary supplementation.

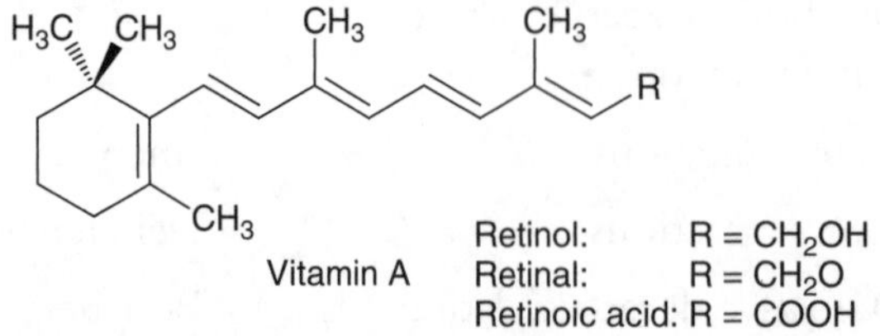

H_3C CH_3 CH_3 CH_3 R CH_3

Vitamin A

Retinol: R = CH_2OH
Retinal: R = CH_2O
Retinoic acid: R = COOH

Figure 8-5 Vitamin A includes three related compounds: retinol, retinal, and retinoic acid.

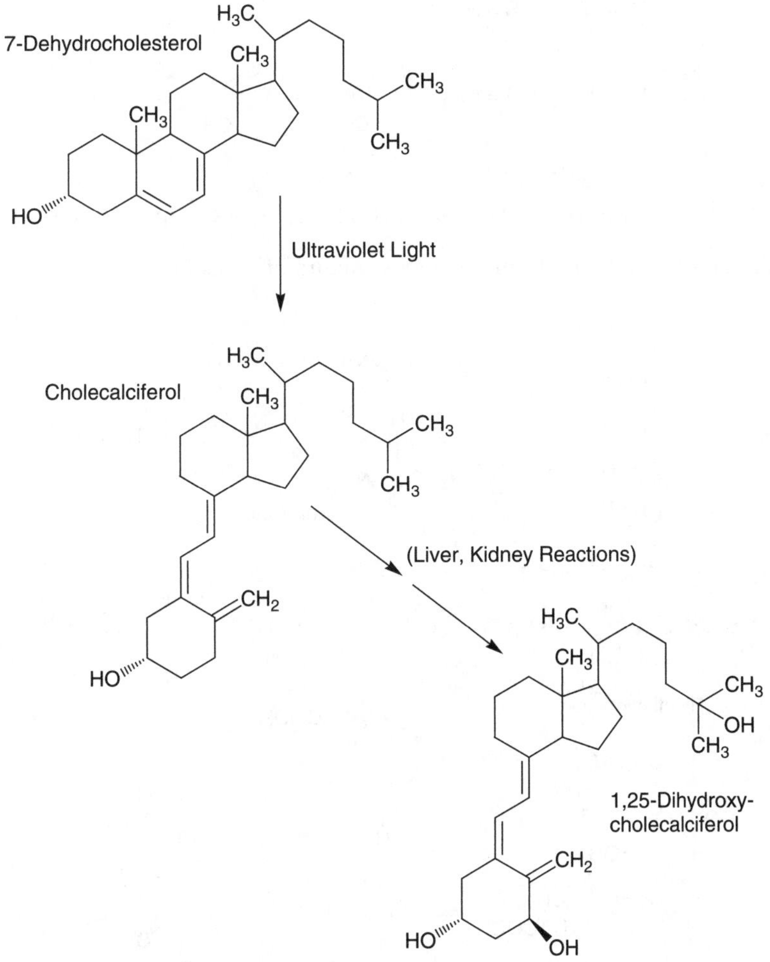

7-Dehydrocholesterol

Ultraviolet Light

Cholecalciferol

(Liver, Kidney Reactions)

1,25-Dihydroxy-cholecalciferol

Figure 8-6 Vitamin D is formed by the action of ultraviolet light on a precursor (7-dehydrocholesterol), with processing of the product by the liver and kidney, to yield 1,25-dihydroxycholecalciferol.

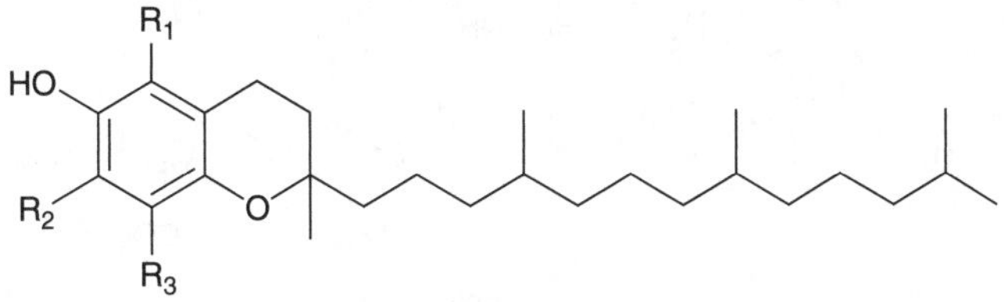

Tocopherol	R_1	R_2	R_3
α-	CH_3	CH_3	CH_3
β-	CH_3	H	CH_3
γ-	H	CH_3	CH_3
δ-	H	H	CH_3

Figure 8-7 Vitamin E includes several different species of tocopherols.

Water-Soluble Vitamins

The collection of vitamins shown in **Figure 8-9** is known as the vitamin B complex. This complex includes thiamine (vitamin B_1), riboflavin (vitamin B_2), niacin (vitamin B_3), pantothenic acid (vitamin B_5), pyridoxine (vitamin B_6), cobalamin (vitamin B_{12}), folic acid, and biotin. All of these vitamins are processed by the body into cofactors for enzymes involved in metabolism.

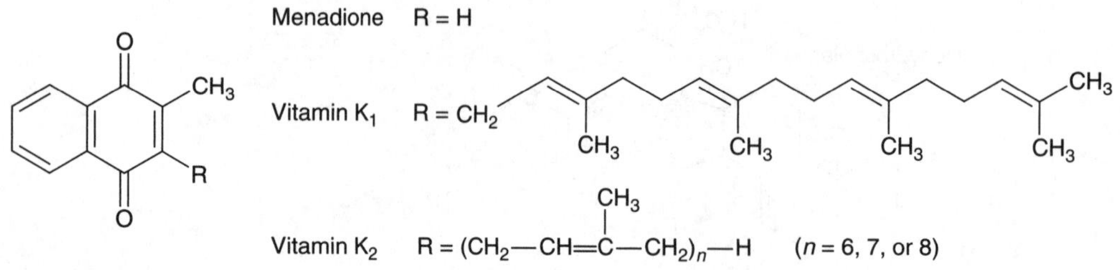

Menadione R = H

Vitamin K_1 R = CH_2

Vitamin K_2 R = $(CH_2—CH{=}C(CH_3)—CH_2)_n—H$ (n = 6, 7, or 8)

Figure 8-8 Vitamin K is built up from the core structure of menadione.

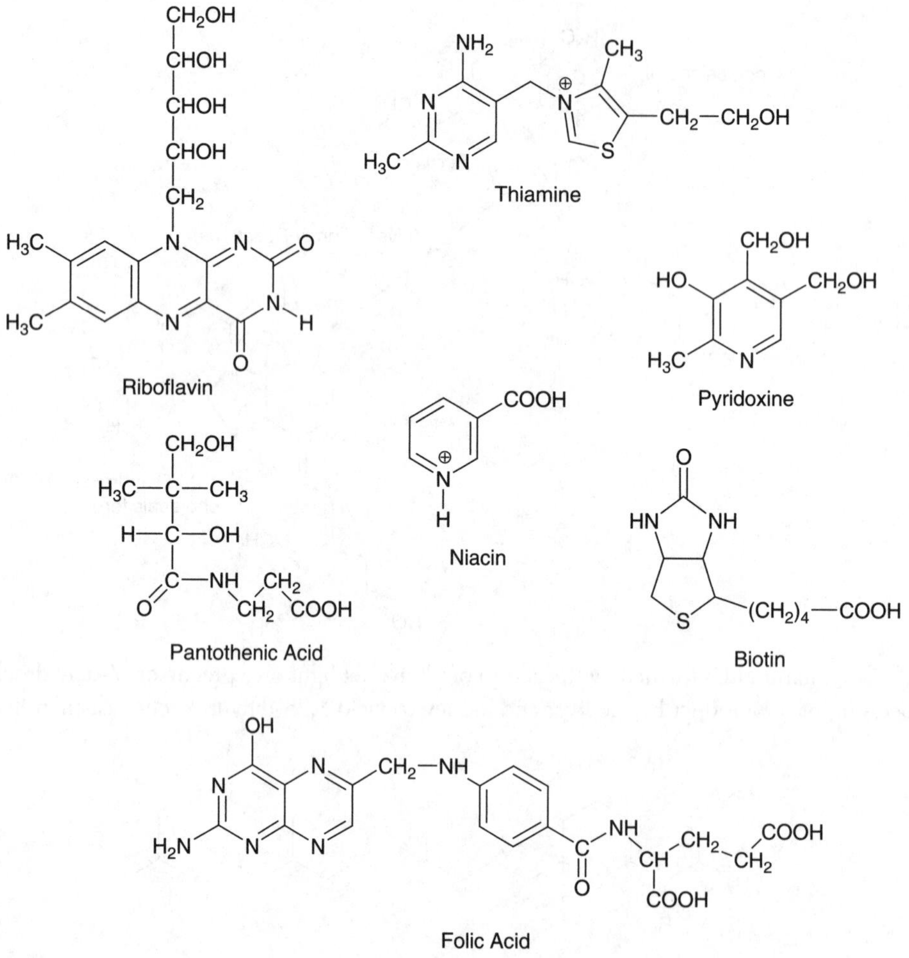

Thiamine

Riboflavin

Pyridoxine

Niacin

Pantothenic Acid

Biotin

Folic Acid

Figure 8-9 Structures of several of the B-complex vitamins (see Figure 13-9 for the more complicated structure of vitamin B_{12}).

Thiamine is found in meat, yeast, whole grains, and nuts. It is involved in decarboxylation reactions and the transfer of acyl groups. Thiamine pyrophosphate (TPP) is the corresponding activated cofactor.

Riboflavin serves as a cofactor in numerous biochemical redox reactions, where its ability to accept and donate electrons one at a time is quite valuable. Dietary sources of riboflavin include meat, nuts, and legumes. The chemistry of riboflavin is discussed later in this chapter.

Niacin is processed by the body into nicotinamide adenine dinucleotide; its role in biochemical redox is also discussed later. As with riboflavin, dietary sources of niacin include meat, nuts and legumes.

Pantothenic acid is found in yeast, grains, egg yolk, and liver. It is an important part of coenzyme A, discussed later in this chapter, and it helps in the transfer of acyl groups.

Pyridoxine, found especially in liver, yeast, nuts, and beans, is activated by attachment of a phosphate group; the basic chemistry of the corresponding enzyme cofactor, pyridoxal phosphate, is discussed in Chapter 14. It plays a major role in the interconversion of amino acids and keto acids, and in the biosynthesis of neurotransmitters (serotonin and dopamine) and sphingolipids.

Cobalamin is synthesized by bacteria; plants and animals are not able to make it. Dietary sources include liver, kidney, eggs, and cheese. Because plants do not make this vitamin, it is especially important for those following a vegetarian diet to supplement their diet with cobalamin. This vitamin is needed for key reactions in the catabolism of certain fatty acids, in the biosynthesis of nucleotides, and in the metabolism of amino acids. Chapters 13 and 14 have more information on the role of cobalamin in biochemistry.

Folic acid (folate) is found in liver, yeast, and leafy vegetables. In particular, it is needed for the synthesis of nucleotides, but it plays a role in many other biochemical reactions as well. It is discussed in Chapter 13 and 14 alongside cobalamin.

Biotin is available from a wide variety of foods. It is also made by gut bacteria; in fact, this bacterial source can supply most or all of the needs of a normal healthy adult. Biotin serves as a cofactor in carboxylation reactions.

Vitamin C (ascorbic acid) is found in fresh fruits and vegetables, and is the vitamin whose deficiency is famously associated with scurvy (pathologic changes in connective tissue, especially the gums, and a weakening of the walls of blood vessels leading to a tendency to hemorrhage). Vitamin C acts as a reducing agent and is a source of electrons in certain biochemical reactions, particularly in helping to maintain metal ion cofactors in a more reduced state (e.g., iron in the ferrous Fe^{2+} state as opposed to the ferric Fe^{3+} state).

Minerals

Table 8-2 identifies the major inorganic species found in the body and relates them to their respective biochemical roles. Additionally, trace amounts of other elements are needed to maintain good health—for example, molybdenum, cobalt, chromium, selenium, and copper. Copper atoms are cofactors in certain respiratory complexes performing redox reactions in mitochondria, and molybdenum is a cofactor in enzymes responsible for purine degradation. However, in many cases the functions of these trace elements are incompletely known.

Adenosine 5′-Triphosphate

To speed up many reactions, a common biochemical solution is to use *activated group carriers*. The idea here is to reduce the energetic barrier to the reaction of interest by preparing one or more of the reactants to react especially readily (under the right circumstances, of course, generally in the active site of a particular enzyme). If not in the proper active site environment, however, the activated group carrier should not react much on its own; that is, it ought to be kinetically stable, if not thermodynamically stable. **Table 8-4** lists some common carriers of activated groups in biochemistry. These carriers are very often derived from vitamins. Refer back to the list of vitamins and see if you can match entries in Table 8-4 with their respective vitamin precursors.

A key carrier in biochemistry of an activated chemical group is the molecule ATP (adenosine 5′-triphosphate). The activated group here is the chain of phosphoanhydride linkages of the triphosphate moiety. As discussed in Chapter 4, ATP is a nucleotide, composed of an organic

Carrier Molecule	Group Carried in Activated Form
ATP	Phosphoryl
Coenzyme A and lipoamide	Acyl (from a carboxylic acid, e.g., acetic acid)
Thiamine pyrophosphate	Aldehydic
Biotin	CO_2
Tetrahydrofolate	One-carbon units (e.g., methylene, formyl)
S-Adenosylmethionine	Methyl

Table 8-4 Examples of Activated Group Carriers

base (adenine), a sugar (ribose), and a triphosphate group. Our interest here is not in its role in RNA and DNA synthesis and degradation, but instead in the energetic consequences of hydrolyzing the phosphoanhydride linkages in the triphosphate group.

ATP Structure

Figure 8-10 shows the structure of ATP. The sugar is linked to the base through a glycosidic bond to the N9 position of the adenine, while the triphosphate moiety is linked to the sugar at the C5′ position. The triphosphate group is normally ionized under physiological conditions.

Note the presence of two *phosphoanhydride* linkages in the triphosphate group. Anhydrides are formed by the condensation of two acids; here the acid is phosphoric acid. From your previous course work, you may be familiar with acetic anhydride (formed by condensing two molecules of acetic acid). It is also possible to have a mixed anhydride, formed by condensing two different species of acid, such as acetic acid with phosphoric acid.

Hydrolysis of Phosphoanhydride Bonds

ATP has two phosphoanhydride bonds. When hydrolyzed, each can yield a large amount of free energy. The bonds are thus sometimes described as "high energy." What is really meant, however, is that hydrolysis of the bond leads to the release of a large amount of free energy, not that the electrons in the bonds are somehow in an excited state.

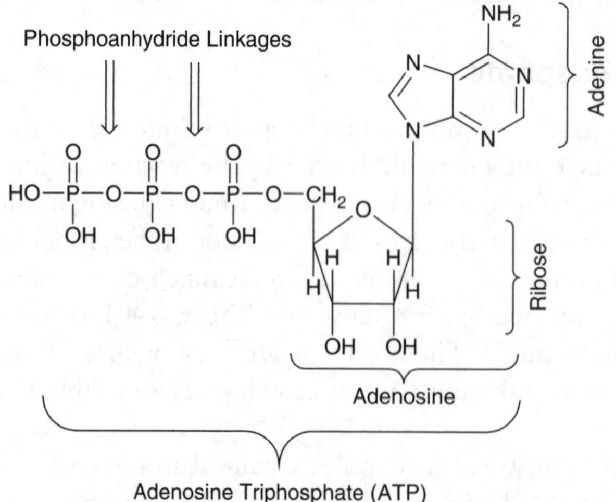

Figure 8-10 Structure of adenosine triphosphate.

The products of hydrolysis are ADP, AMP, inorganic phosphate (PO_4^{3-} or HPO_4^{2-}, abbreviated as P_i), and possibly pyrophosphate (abbreviated as PP_i). The two main modes of hydrolysis and the corresponding standard state free energy changes are given in Equations 8-1 and 8-2:

$$ATP + H_2O \rightleftharpoons ADP + P_i \quad \Delta G'^{\circ} = -30.5 \text{ kJ/mol} \quad (8\text{-}1)$$

$$ATP + H_2O \rightleftharpoons AMP + PP_i \quad \Delta G'^{\circ} = -45.6 \text{ kJ/mol} \quad (8\text{-}2)$$

(Note that we do not usually write the charges of ATP, P_i, and other reactants and products, even though the phosphates are generally ionized under physiological conditions.)

These hydrolysis reactions are highly favorable due to three factors:

- Resonance stabilization of the hydrolysis products versus ATP
- Acid dissociation at pH 7 of the acid products (giving the ionized phosphate groups)
- Greater electrostatic repulsion of charges in ATP versus hydrolysis products

Driving an Unfavorable Reaction by Coupling to ATP Hydrolysis

The (net) hydrolysis of ATP in the cell can provide a source of negative free energy change, and this process can be coupled to other biochemical reactions that may be distinctly unfavorable (going "uphill" in terms of free energy). However, because of the coupling, and because the free energy released by ATP hydrolysis is so negative, the overall (coupled) reaction can run "downhill." The release of free energy from hydrolysis of the ATP can shift equilibrium constants in coupled reactions by a large factor, as much as 10^8. The shift in the equilibrium constant can drastically change the equilibrium ratio of products over reactants, such that products become overwhelmingly predominant; that is, the ATP hydrolysis drives the reaction toward the formation of products that otherwise would be formed in vanishingly small amounts.

Anhydride linkages are generally thermodynamically unstable in aqueous solution. The hydrolysis reaction, however, may take a long time to occur. Thus ATP is kinetically stable, but thermodynamically unstable. It has a large negative free energy for hydrolysis of its phosphoanhydride linkages but the rate of attack on the phosphoanhydride bonds by water is very slow in the absence of any catalyst; at pH 7, the half-life of ATP in water is several hours. This kinetic stability allows the cell to transport ATP to sites where it can be degraded by particular enzyme systems, to do useful work for the cell at a rapid rate.

Coupling of ATP hydrolysis to reactions that are thermodynamically unfavorable does not generally occur through the direct hydrolysis of ATP itself. More often than not, ATP provides the driving free energy more indirectly, through a series of group transfers. This involves covalent bond formation and breakage, and is generally a two-step process:

- Step 1: Attach part of the ATP molecule (e.g., a phosphate, PP_i, or AMP) covalently to the substrate or to an amino acid in the enzyme. This raises the overall free energy, an "investment."
- Step 2: Detach the adduct (typically via a displacement reaction) and release P_i, PP_i, AMP, or another product. This is now equivalent to ATP hydrolysis and is usually *very* favorable in terms of free energy, so it lowers the overall free energy of the reaction; here is our "return on investment."

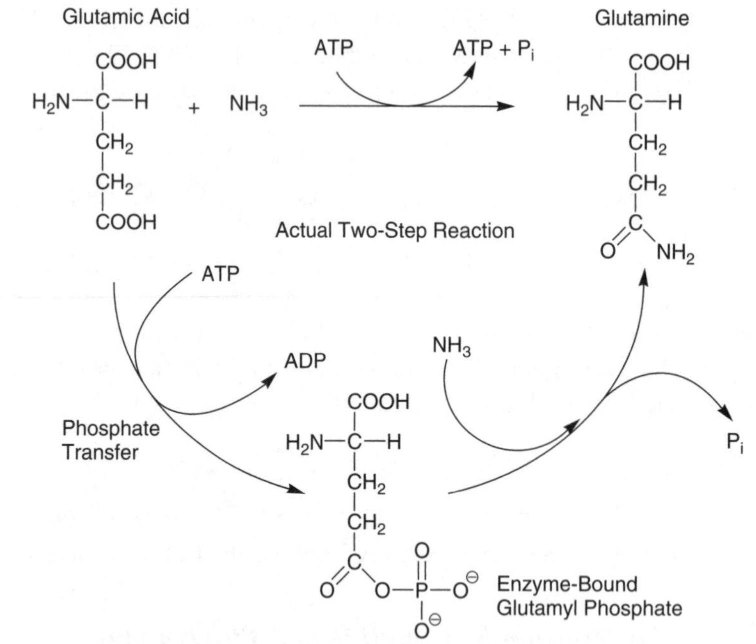

Figure 8-11 Example of how ATP can help drive an otherwise unfavorable biochemical reaction. Although such reactions are often shown schematically as occurring in only one step, in reality two or more intermediate steps may be involved.

Many—if not most—of these coupling reactions involving ATP hydrolysis actually take two steps, although they are often written as simple one-step reactions. An example is shown in **Figure 8-11**. The point here is that the phosphate group is first transferred to activate the otherwise kinetically inert molecule of glutamic acid; it is then displaced from the glutamyl moiety, serving as a good leaving group. This process is *not* a simple hydrolysis.

ATP is formed from the diphosphate precursor, ADP, during primary metabolism of fuels such as sugars. It can then be used in a multitude of cellular tasks that call for a source of free energy to drive an otherwise unfavorable process. **Figure 8-12** summarizes the formation of ATP in the cell and its use in energy-demanding processes. Note the "recycling" of ATP.

ATP serves as a carrier of activated phosphoryl groups, transferring the terminal phosphate onto proteins, sugars, nucleosides, and many other biochemicals. Recall that reversible phosphorylation is an important mechanism for regulating enzyme activity.

The Energy Charge

The concept of an *energy charge* (sometimes referred to as the *adenylate charge*) is a convenient way to keep track in the cell of the potential for performing work in general (e.g., biosynthesis, mechanical work). It is a method of counting the available phosphoanhydride linkages, allowing for their interconvertibility. It emphasizes ATP, ADP, and AMP (the adenylate nucleotides), as they are present in much higher concentrations than other nucleotides such as GTP. Here is the mathematical definition of this quantity:

$$\text{Energy charge} = \frac{[\text{ATP}] + \frac{1}{2}[\text{ADP}]}{[\text{ATP}] + [\text{ADP}] + [\text{AMP}]} \tag{8-3}$$

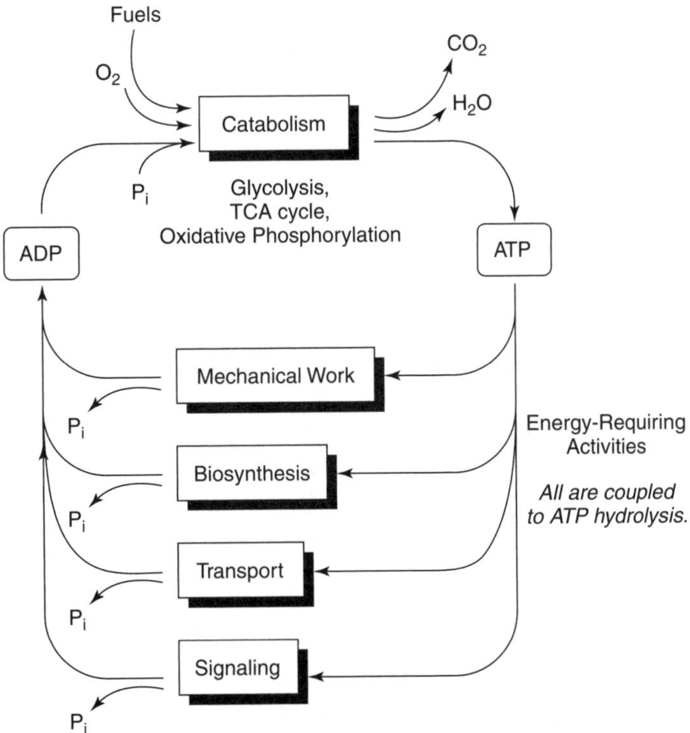

Figure 8-12 ATP is generated by catabolic reactions, and its hydrolysis is used to help drive a variety of energy-demanding processes; the ADP from hydrolysis can be readily recycled back to ATP.

The energy charge is a ratio of available phosphoanhydride linkages to the entire pool of adenine nucleotides. Note how ADP is counted in the numerator, but at only half the value for an equal concentration of ATP, because ATP has twice the number of phosphoanhydride linkages. The relation is defined this way so that the energy charge conveniently varies from zero (no ATP or ADP available; all adenylates are in the form of AMP) up to 1 (all adenylates are now in the form of ATP; no AMP or ADP).

In general, pathways that generate energy (ATP) are inhibited by a high energy charge; conversely, pathways that consume energy are stimulated by a high energy charge. The rates of reaction in these pathways reflect the degree of stimulation or inhibition. The pathways are controlled to maintain homeostasis—that is, to keep the energy charge at a relatively high level (approximately 0.80 to 0.95 for most cells). This can also be thought of as "buffering" the cell's energy level, by analogy to the action of buffers in acid–base systems; the system resists change.

Figure 8-13 compares schematically the rate of energy generation in the cell to the rate of energy consumption, as the energy charge varies from low to high. Notice how the steepest parts of the two curves appear in the region of the "desired" energy charge (from 0.8 to 0.95). This allows large changes of rate for small changes in energy charge so that the cell rapidly restores its energy balance.

Other "High-Energy" Compounds

Table 8-5 lists a number of other biochemicals whose hydrolysis to release phosphate gives up a large amount of free energy. Note that the values in Table 8-5 apply to standard-state concentrations of all reaction participants, at pH 7; conditions in vivo will be quite different, so the driving force for these reactions in vivo will likely also be quite different.

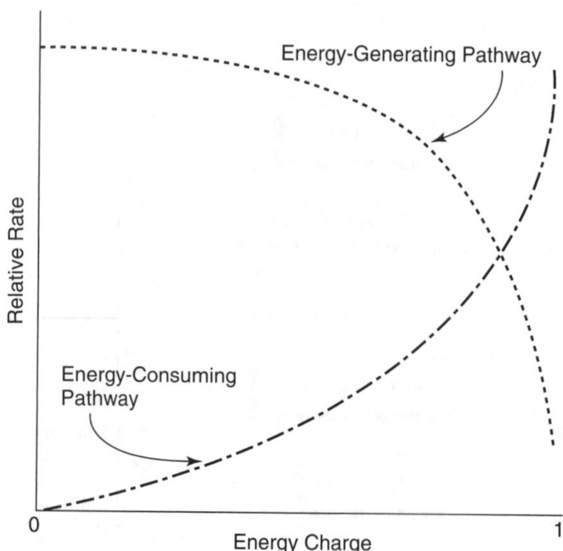

Figure 8-13 The rates of energy-generating and energy-consuming reactions in the cell are balanced against each other to maintain cellular homeostasis.

"High-Energy" Compound That Reacts with Water	Hydrolysis Product	Standard-State Free Energy Change $\Delta G'^{\circ}$(kJ/mol)
Phospho*enol*pyruvate (PEP)	Pyruvate + P_i	−61.9
1,3-bisphosphoglycerate	3-Phosphoglycerate + P_i	−49.4
Creatine phosphate (phosphocreatine)	Creatine + P_i	−43.1
Acetyl-CoA	Acetate + CoASH	−31.4
ATP	ADP + P_i	−30.5
Glucose-1-phosphate	Glucose + P_i	−20.9
Glycerol-1-phosphate	Glycerol + P_i	−9.2

Table 8-5 Energetics of Hydrolysis of "Energy-Rich" Biochemicals

Source: Compilation by W. P. Jencks. (1976). *Handbook of Biochemistry and Molecular Biology*, 3rd ed., Vol. I (ed., G. D. Fasman), CRC Press, Cleveland, OH, pp. 296–304.

ATP is found approximately in the middle of the list. In vivo, the free energy change available from ATP hydrolysis is probably near −50 kJ/mol, due to in vivo concentrations that are considerably different (e.g., millimolar and not molar) from the standard-state concentrations assumed in Table 8-5. Depending on the local concentrations of reactants and products, ATP hydrolysis may help to drive some unfavorable reactions (e.g., muscle contraction, biosynthetic reactions) or ATP may be synthesized (from ADP, by phosphoryl group transfer) by coupling this reaction to one of the more "energetic" hydrolysis reactions described earlier. For example, in muscular contraction the initial depletion of muscle cell stores of ATP can be partially restored very quickly by using creatine phosphate to re-phosphorylate the ADP that is building up.

Basis for High Free Energy of Hydrolysis

Phosphate ester hydrolysis releases much less free energy than ATP phosphoanhydride hydrolysis. Why? A typical phosphate ester hydrolysis would proceed as follows:

$$\text{Glycerol-1-phosphate} + H_2O \rightleftharpoons \text{Glycerol} + P_i \quad \Delta G'^{\circ} = -9.2 \text{ kJ/mol} \qquad (8\text{-}4)$$

The difference is due to the resonance stabilization of ADP and P_i (products of hydrolysis) versus ATP, and the greater electrostatic repulsion of charges in ATP versus products ADP and P_i. These factors do not apply to hydrolysis of standard phosphoesters.

Other biochemicals also have a high free energy of hydrolysis or of phosphoryl group transfer—namely, phosphocreatine phosphate (important in muscles) and phosphoenolpyruvate. Their reaction can also help drive coupled reactions toward the formation of (otherwise unlikely amounts of) product.

In ATP and these other compounds, the phosphoanhydride bonds are normal chemical bonds, not bonds where the electrons are excited. They simply have a large free energy release when hydrolyzed. Don't be misled by terminology like "high-energy bonds."

Coenzyme A: Carrier of Activated Acyl Groups

The name coenzyme A is often abbreviated to CoA; the "A" comes from the adenosine nucleotide part of the structure. To emphasize the role of the reactive thiol group, we shall occasionally use the abbreviation CoASH instead of CoA.

Structure of Coenzyme A

Figure 8-14 shows the detailed structure of *coenzyme A*. There are three major parts here: the adenine nucleotide, the *pantothenic acid* moiety (vitamin B_5), and the *mercaptoethylamine*. This last group carries the main reactive site, a thiol group. Note the use of the nucleotide "handle" for holding the coenzyme on the enzyme. Many enzymes have a special pattern of folding of the polypeptide chain to form a site on the protein surface that will specifically hold or bind the adenosine moiety.

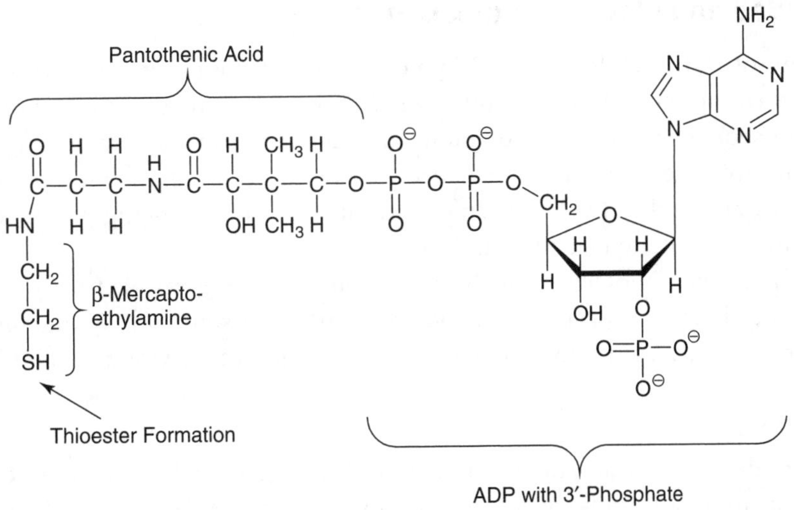

Pantothenic Acid

β-Mercapto-ethylamine

Thioester Formation

ADP with 3′-Phosphate

Figure 8-14 Structure of coenzyme A.

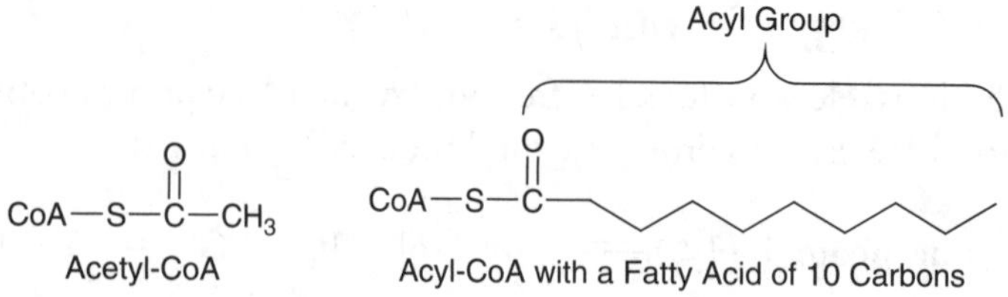

$$\text{CoA—S—}\overset{\text{O}}{\overset{\|}{\text{C}}}\text{—CH}_3$$

Acetyl-CoA

Acyl Group

CoA—S—C(=O)— (10-carbon chain)

Acyl-CoA with a Fatty Acid of 10 Carbons

Figure 8-15 Coenzyme A in its role as a carrier of acyl groups.

Coenzyme A in its role as a carrier of acyl groups is shown in **Figure 8-15**. Note the *thioester* linkage, formed from the acid carboxylate of the acetic acid or fatty acid and the thiol group of the coenzyme. The linkage is similar to, though not as stable as, the more familiar oxyesters of organic chemistry.

Function

Coenzyme A is a good example of a reactive group joined to an adenine nucleotide. The reactive group is the thiol moiety, which forms a thioester linkage with fatty acids. The carbon chain of the acid (the acyl group) may be as small as 2 carbons, as in acetic acid, which joins with CoA to form acetyl-CoA. Alternatively, it may be a much longer chain of 16 carbons, as in palmitic acid, which joins with CoA to form palmitoyl-CoA.

Coenzyme A serves as a carrier of acyl groups in two major ways:

- Transferring two-carbon acetyl groups in fuel oxidation
- Carrying longer alkyl chain building blocks in the synthesis of fatty acids

Acylated CoA is a reactive intermediate, ubiquitous in biochemistry. The thioester here is less stable than the corresponding oxyester, because the sulfur atom is less effective in delocalizing electrons. Thus there is less resonance stabilization of the acyl CoA thioester compared to the oxyester (less C-to-S double-bond character). When the bond is broken, more free energy is liberated from the thioester. This outcome favors transfer of the acyl group; that is, it activates the acyl group. As a consequence, we regard CoA as a carrier of an activated acyl group. Compare this perspective to the notion of ATP as a carrier of activated phosphoryl groups.

Nicotinamides and Flavins: Redox Cofactors

The side chains of amino acids are especially poor at performing reversible electron transfers—that is, at performing reductions or oxidations. Much of intermediary metabolism, however, consists of the sequential oxidation of molecules derived from foodstuffs. Hence there is a need for small molecules that can act reversibly in redox reactions, helping to perform those oxidations in degrading the "fuel" molecules and capturing the reducing power for later use in making ATP, in biosynthetic reactions, and in other processes.

Some of these helper molecules involve metal ions and the reversible transfer of electrons to and from the metal center. In this section, we look instead at some purely organic compounds that are very commonly used in biochemical redox systems, the flavins and the nicotinamides.

Nicotinamides

The nicotinamides contain an adenine nucleotide as part of their structure (**Figure 8-16**). The *nicotinamide* moiety is itself "basic," and is joined to a sugar, so the complete compound is regarded as a sort of dinucleotide: nicotinamide adenine dinucleotide (*NADH*) and nicotinamide

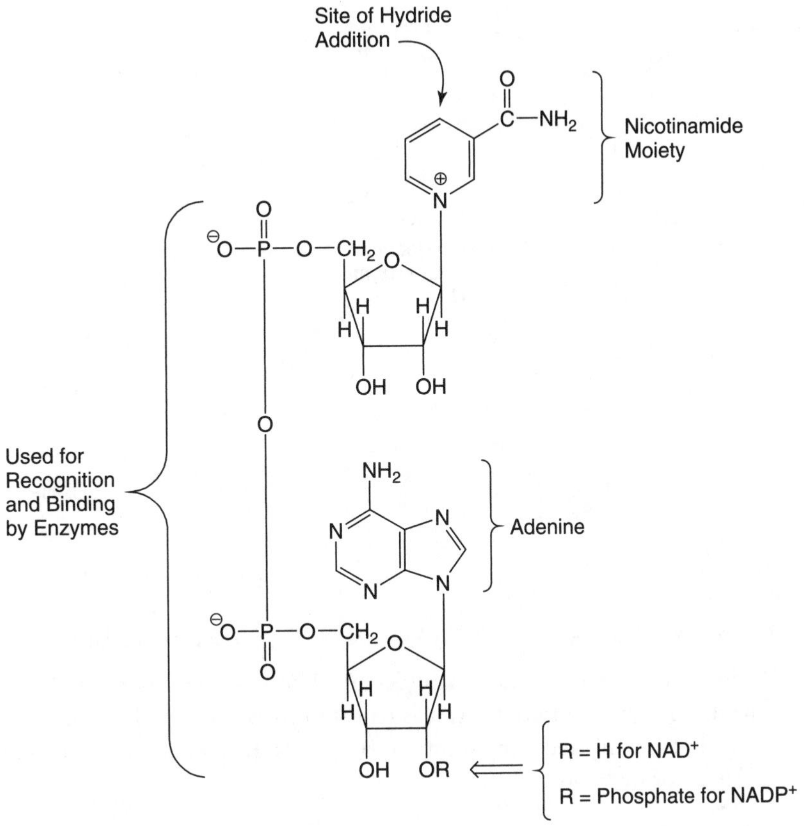

Figure 8-16 Structure of the nicotinamide coenzymes.

adenine dinucleotide phosphate (*NADPH*). *Niacin* is the common name for nicotinic acid, the precursor to nicotinamide. The two nicotinamides have distinct roles: NADH is used mainly in the oxidation of fuel molecules, while NADPH is used mainly in biosynthesis where reductions are performed.

Nicotinamides are fairly stable kinetically when free in solution; they are only slowly oxidized by dissolved O_2. This property makes them useful for transferring electrons from one site in the cell to another. Although NADH and NADPH may be kinetically stable, however, they are still thermodynamically unstable and will react—slowly!—with dissolved oxygen.

The reactive site for reduction is the 4 position on the pyridine ring. The positively charged ring nitrogen in the pyridine moiety of NAD^+ or $NADP^+$ (see **Figure 8-16**) acts as an electron sink, helping the ring system accept a hydride anion (a hydrogen nucleus with two electrons). These coenzymes can either accept or donate electrons, depending on their redox state. Both nicotinamides are two electron carriers; both electrons are transferred in a concerted mechanism. The reaction can be readily reversed and the nicotinamides recycled for many rounds of electron transfer, so it is proper to regard these compounds as coenzymes.

The nucleotide "handle" for binding to enzymes has many moieties for noncovalent interactions with the enzyme. The binding may be either tight or relatively loose. Nicotinamides can be released into solution from the enzyme because they are not covalently bound. This characteristic technically makes them a co-substrate in the reaction, rather than a prosthetic group (prosthetic groups are held tightly and are not released into solution).

Fundamental redox chemistry for the nicotinamides is shown in **Figure 8-17**, which emphasizes the cycling between states of oxidation. Generally, different enzymes are involved

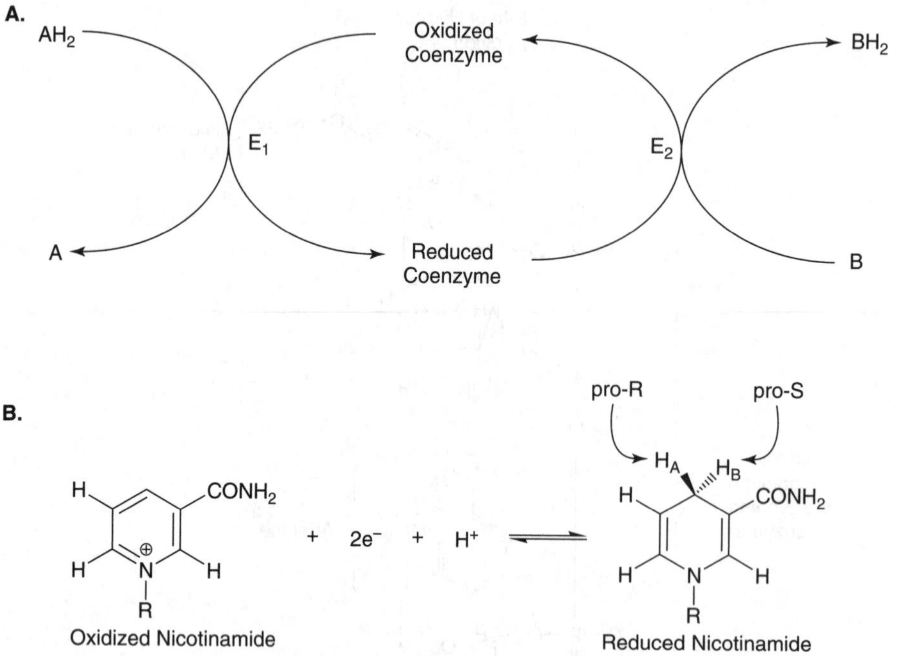

Figure 8-17 Redox cycling for the nicotinamides. **A.** The oxidized coenzyme is converted to its reduced form by enzyme E_1, while substrate AH_2 is oxidized to product A; then the reduced coenzyme is re-oxidized by enzyme E_2, while reducing substrate B to BH_2. **B.** Reduction of the oxidized nicotinamide by two equivalents of hydrogen.

in the oxidation reactions versus the reduction reactions for the coenzyme. Note the difference between oxidized and reduced forms of the nicotinamide ring. Also note the possibility, after reduction, of distinguishing one hydrogen at the N4 position from the other, as the two faces of the pyridine ring are not identical. This distinction can play a role in the detailed stereochemistry of hydride transfer by the reduced cofactor.

When working with redox reactions involving nicotinamides and flavins, you must be very careful to distinguish between hydrogen ions (H^+, which does not carry an electron), hydride ions (H^-, which carries two electrons), and hydrogen atoms (H, which carries a single electron). You should convince yourself that the reaction described previously does, indeed, involve the transfer of two electrons onto the nicotinamide. This reaction can also be thought of as the addition of a hydride ion, equivalent to a hydrogen nucleus plus two electrons, onto the ring system. It is easy to lose track of the electrons in these reactions; note that diagrams in this and other texts may not depict balanced chemical reactions, and that electrons or protons may not be explicitly represented.

Pellagra and Dietary Deficiency of Niacin

Tryptophan is the biosynthetic precursor to niacin in those organisms that can make niacin. **Figure 8-18** compares the vitamin niacin (nicotinic acid) to its precursor tryptophan and to the biologically relevant nicotinamide used to make NADH and NADPH. For reference, the structure of the poisonous vegetable alkaloid nicotine is shown as well.

Humans lack the capacity to synthesize adequate amounts of niacin from tryptophan. This problem can be exacerbated if tryptophan is lacking in the diet. Because nicotinamides are

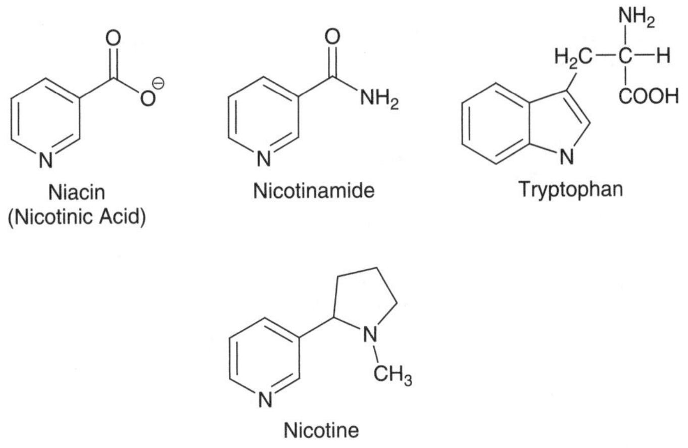

Niacin (Nicotinic Acid)

Nicotinamide

Tryptophan

Nicotine

Figure 8-18 The nicotinamides are derived from dietary niacin, not from nicotine.

so widely used in cellular chemistry, a deficiency in their supply is a very serious matter, and symptoms will spread throughout the body.

In the southern rural United States, the diet is traditionally rich in corn, but unfortunately corn lacks tryptophan. Poor people, in relying on a corn-rich diet, might therefore suffer from *pellagra*. This disease manifests itself first with a characteristic roughness of the skin and diarrhea. In extreme cases, dementia and even death can result. Fortunately the cure is cheap—dietary supplementation with niacin. Unfortunately, pellagra still appears occasionally in alcoholics, who often have an imbalanced diet.

Do not confuse niacin and nicotinamide with the addictive natural product, nicotine. Niacin and nicotinamide will cure pellagra, but nicotine will not.

Roles of Nicotinamides in the Cell

Figure 8-19 summarizes the differences between NADH and NADPH in terms of their biochemistry in the body. Note that NADH is involved primarily in catabolism leading to energy production (oxidative phosphorylation) in the form of ATP, while NADPH is generated by catabolic reactions and then used in biosynthetic reactions.

Flavins: $FADH_2$, $FMNH_2$

Riboflavin, or vitamin B_2, is the precursor to $FADH_2$ and $FMNH_2$. Like the nicotinamides, the *flavins* participate in electron transfer reactions. Usually these flavins are very tightly bound to the enzyme; they qualify as prosthetic groups. Enzymes carrying these compounds are called *flavoproteins*.

As with the nicotinamides, the nomenclature of these cofactors is unusual. Flavin mononucleotide (FMN in the oxidized form, $FMNH_2$ in the reduced form) and flavin adenine dinucleotide (FAD in the oxidized form, $FADH_2$ in the reduced form) both contain the basic isoalloxazine ring with a linked sugar–phosphate complex (the sugar here is ribitol). The combination of the sugar–phosphate complex with a basic ring qualifies this compound to be called a "nucleotide," although, of course, it does not appear in RNA or DNA. In FAD or $FADH_2$, an adenosine is combined with this "nucleotide"; thus biochemists have referred to the compound as a "dinucleotide."

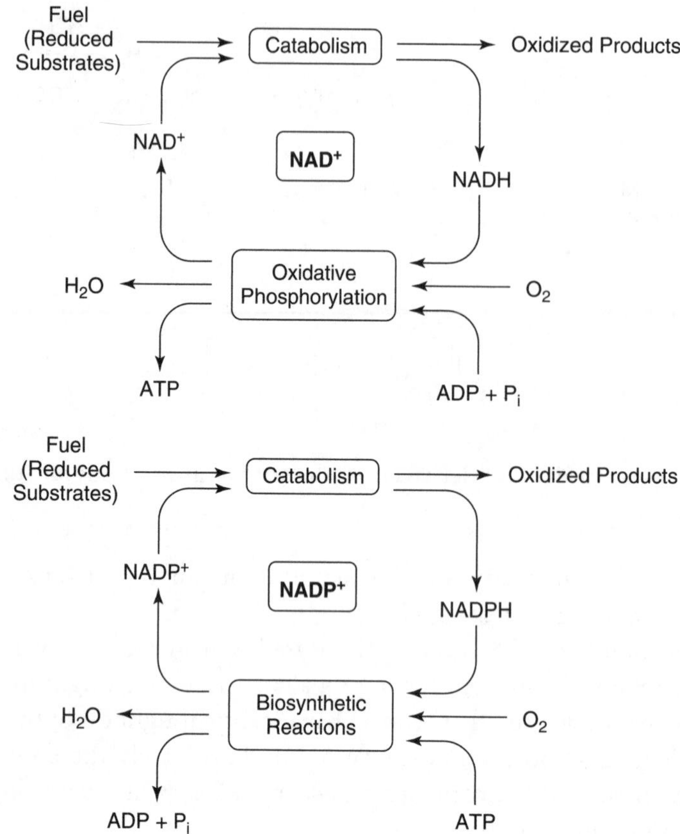

Figure 8-19 Comparison of the biochemical roles of NAD^+/NADH and $NADP^+$/NADPH in the cell. NADH is important in energy generation for the cell through oxidative phosphorylation; NADPH is important for biosynthetic reactions.

Another point of similarity to the nicotinamides is that again we have an adenine nucleotide joined to a reactive group, the isoalloxazine ring (**Figure 8-20**). Also like the nicotinamides, the flavin molecules can carry two electrons (along with two protons; note that there is no change in electrical charge on the molecule).

Unlike the nicotinamides, flavin cofactors can transfer electrons one at a time; the nicotinamides always donate or receive them two at a time. Also unlike the nicotinamides, the flavins are not kinetically or thermodynamically stable against oxidation. Flavins will readily react with dissolved oxygen and other oxidants, so these prosthetic groups are generally buried, away from casual contact with the solvent, at the enzyme's active site.

Fundamental redox chemistry for flavins is shown in **Figure 8-21** (the reactive isoalloxazine ring's behavior is emphasized, as it is the same for both FAD and FMN). Note the reactive sites and scheme for one-electron transfer reactions involving a *semiquinone* intermediate.

The free energy change or redox potential for these reductions depends on the local environment around the flavin group. Interactions with surrounding protein moieties will (slightly) distort electron orbitals on the flavin, thereby affecting their tendency to gain or lose electrons. This remarkable sensitivity results in considerable variation in the relative stability of the various forms, depending on which protein holds the flavin; binding of the flavin to one species can strongly favor the oxidized form, while binding to a different enzyme species will favor (perhaps only slightly) the reduced form.

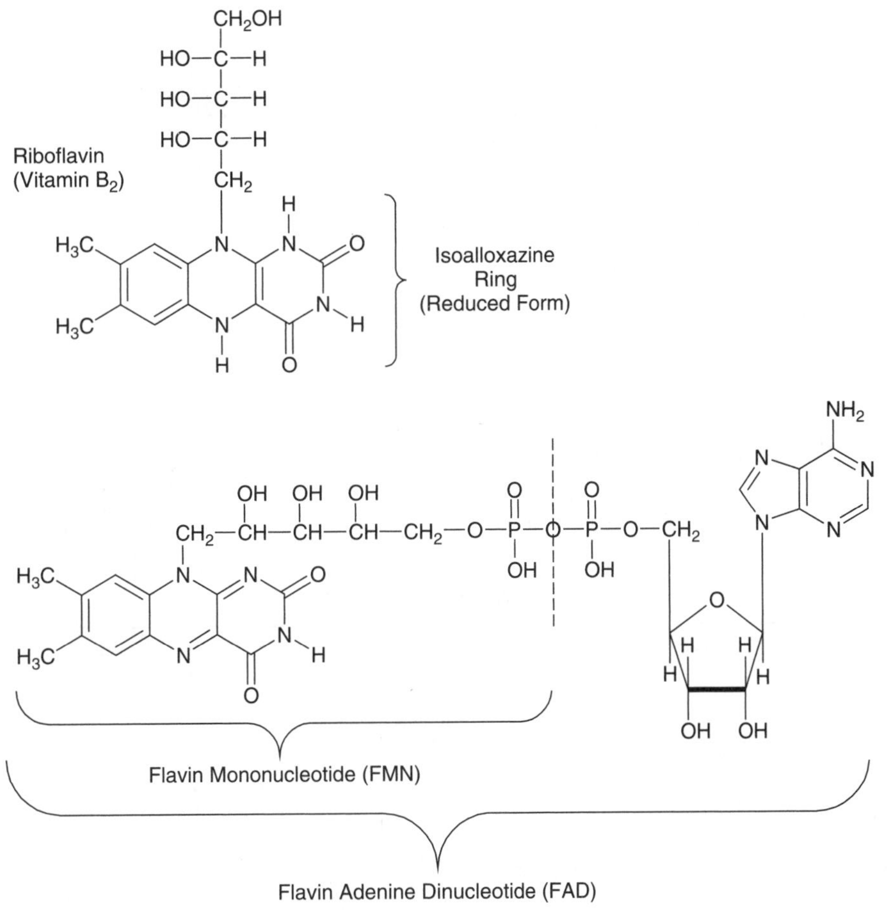

Figure 8-20 Structures of riboflavin and the derived cofactors, flavin mononucleotide (FMN) and flavin adenine dinucleotide (FAD).

QUESTIONS FOR DISCUSSION

1. If the concentrations of ATP and ADP were both 4 mM in a cell, would it be possible to have an energy charge of 0.85? Why or why not?
2. What would be some of the likely biochemical consequences if an individual suffered from an inability to absorb adequate amounts of phosphate from food? Consider regulation of enzymatic activity in biochemical pathways along with the synthesis and reuse of enzymatic cofactors.
3. Acetyl phosphate is a mixed anhydride of acetic acid and phosphoric acid.
   a. Hydrolysis of acetyl phosphate has $\Delta G'^{\circ} = -46.9$ kJ/mol. What is the chemical basis for this favorable hydrolysis?
   b. Under biochemical standard state conditions, could this reaction drive the phosphorylation of ADP to ATP? What about the phosphorylation of 3-phosphoglycerate to 1,3-bisphosphoglycerate?
4. In vivo, creatine phosphate is used to drive the phosphorylation of ADP to ATP.
   a. The hydrolysis of creatine phosphate has $\Delta G'^{\circ} = -43.1$ kJ/mol. What is the chemical basis for this favorable hydrolysis?

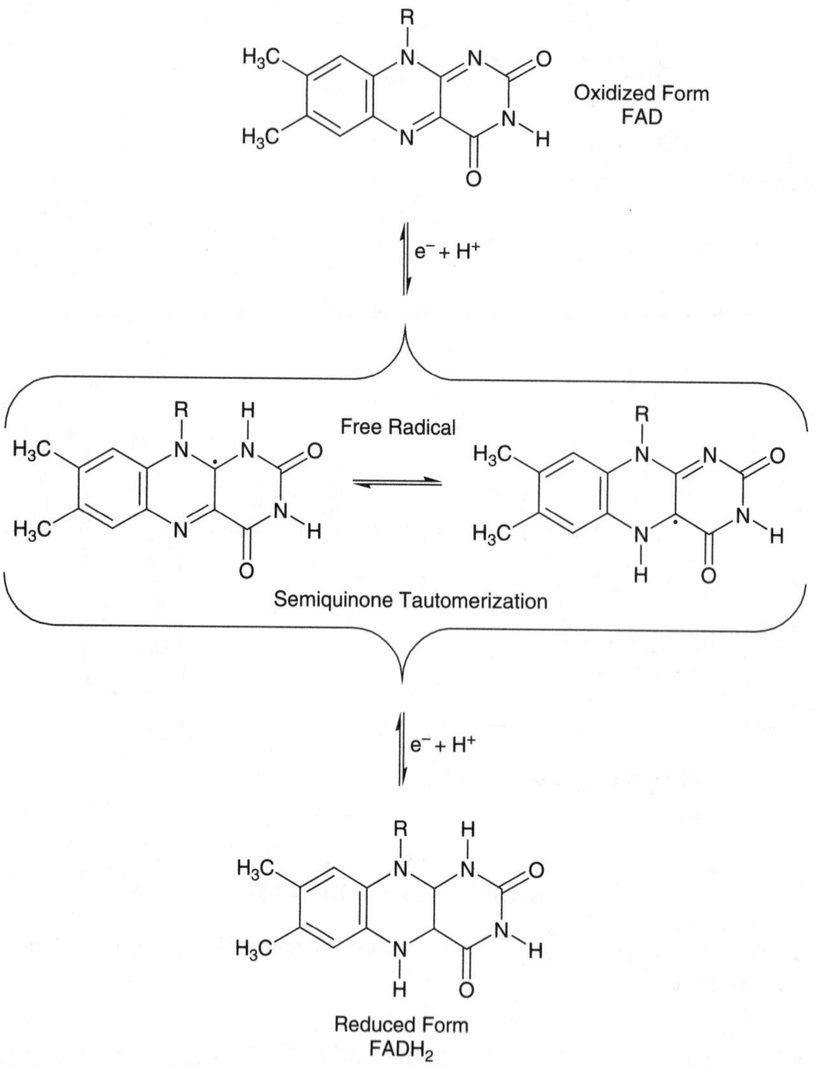

Oxidized Form FAD

$e^- + H^+$

Free Radical

Semiquinone Tautomerization

$e^- + H^+$

Reduced Form $FADH_2$

Figure 8-21 Sequential one-electron reductions of flavins, showing the intermediate semiquinone free radical and its possible tautomerization.

b. What is $\Delta G'^\circ$ for coupling creatine phosphate hydrolysis to ADP phosphorylation?

c. In resting vertebrate muscle, typical concentrations of creatine phosphate are approximately 25 mM, while creatine concentrations are approximately 13 mM. Typical adenine nucleotide concentrations here would be [ATP] = 4 mM and [ADP] = 0.013 mM. Calculate $\Delta G'$ for rephosphorylation of ADP by creatine phosphate under these conditions.

5. Patients undergoing renal dialysis may suffer from vitamin deficiencies. Why?
6. Bile is needed for emulsification of dietary lipids and lipid-like molecules, as a part of their digestion and absorption. Patients suffering from biliary obstruction may show an unusual sensitivity to bruising, and their blood clotting time is unusually extended. Propose an explanation for these effects.
7. Patients suffering from Wilson's disease absorb excessive amounts of copper from the diet; furthermore, these patients tend to excrete too little copper. Why might physicians treat such patients with increased amounts of dietary cysteine or with drugs such a D-penicillamine or dimercaptopropanol? Why might dietary supplementation with zinc also help?

REFERENCES

P. Belenky, K. L. Bogan, and C. Brenner. (2006). "NAD^+ metabolism in health and disease," *Trends Biochem. Sci.* 32:12–19.

G. F. Combs, Jr. (2008). *The Vitamins: Fundamental Aspects in Nutrition and Health*, Elsevier/ Academic Press, Amsterdam.

D. Fell. (1997). *Understanding the Control of Metabolism*, Portland Press, London.

F. Franks. (2000). *Water: A Matrix of Life*, 2nd ed., Royal Society of Chemistry, Cambridge, UK.

P. J. Roach. (1991). "Multisite and hierarchal protein phosphorylation," *J. Biol. Chem.* 266:14139–14142.

J. N. Spencer. (1985). "Heat, work, and metabolism," *J. Chem. Educ.* 62:571–574.

S. S. Zimmerman. (1984). "Using concepts of exercise and weight control to illustrate biochemical principles," *J. Chem. Educ.* 61:882–885.

CHAPTER 9

Major Pathways of Carbohydrate Metabolism

Learning Objectives

1. Define and use correctly the terms *glycolysis, GLUT protein, nicotinamide pool, aerobic* versus *anaerobic metabolism, lactate fermentation, thermodynamic inefficiency, hexokinase, phosphofructokinase (PFK), gluconeogenesis, glucose 6-phosphatase, pyruvate carboxylase, lactate dehydrogenase, Cori cycle, isoenzyme (isozyme), glycogen, glycogenin, glycogenolysis, glycogen synthase, phosphorolysis, second messenger, cyclic AMP, glycogen phosphorylase, McArdle's disease,* and *galactosemia*.
2. Explain how glycolysis produces metabolic energy as well as intermediates for further metabolic reactions.
3. Diagram the glycolytic pathway. Describe how glycolysis can be divided into three stages.
4. List and describe the reactions in glycolysis, in correct metabolic order. List the intermediates (the compounds) in the glycolytic pathway. Note where ATP is consumed and where it is produced. Note the role of nicotinamide cofactors.
5. Describe how sucrose can enter the glycolytic pathway; note the two points of entry. Describe how galactose can enter the glycolytic pathway; relate defects in this process to the disease of galactosemia.
6. Explain how glycolysis is regulated. Describe how allosterism is important for regulating phosphofructokinase. List and describe other enzymes important in regulating glycolysis.
7. Explain how pyruvate may be converted to acetyl-CoA, to ethanol, or to lactate. Relate the latter two reactions to the regeneration of NAD^+ for continued glycolytic functioning.
8. Describe the major physiological functions of gluconeogenesis, glycogen synthesis, and glycogenolysis. Note important precursors for each of these pathways. List important organs or tissues, and intracellular locations, for each of these pathways.
9. Describe the regulation of gluconeogenesis, glycogen synthesis, and glycogenolysis. Note key enzymes, activators, and inhibitors. Connect the regulation of these pathways to physiological states and functions.
10. Describe the linkages among gluconeogenesis, glycogen synthesis, and glycogenolysis, as well as their connections to glycolysis and the TCA cycle. Relate these linkages to the regulation of these pathways.

11. Compare glycolysis to gluconeogenesis, noting points in common and points of disparity.
12. Compare glycogen synthesis to glycogen breakdown, noting points in common and points of disparity.
13. Compare and contrast insulin versus glucagon in terms of their effects on glycolysis and gluconeogenesis. Do the same for insulin versus glucagon or epinephrine in terms of their effects on glycogen metabolism.
14. Describe the Cori cycle and relate it to the glycolytic pathway, tissue-specific pools of reduced and oxidized nicotinamides, gluconeogenesis, and the functioning of the H and M isozymes of lactate dehydrogenase.
15. Describe the structure of glycogen, and relate it to the biological advantages of glycogen as an energy-storage polymer. Explain why this structure is efficient.
16. Describe the function of glucose 6-phosphatase in the liver, and compare it to what happens in brain and muscle.
17. Explain the role of UDP-glucose in glycogen synthesis and in the interconversions of monosaccharides (e.g., galactose and glucose).
18. List several examples of different glycogen storage diseases. Relate each to the underlying biochemical defect, and explain the connection to clinical symptoms.
19. Recognize the structures of glucose, glucose-1-phosphate, glucose-6-phosphate, UDP-glucose, pyruvate, and cyclic AMP.

Glycolysis

Glucose is the major form of carbohydrate presented to cells after absorption from the gut (**Figure 9-1**). It is the major fuel used by the brain; several other specialized tissues are also highly dependent on glucose as fuel.

Glycolysis is the primary pathway for the metabolism of glucose and other sugars (carbohydrates). Another name for this pathway is the Embden-Meyerhof pathway. Glycolysis comprises the cell's set of reactions for the breakdown of sugars so that energy can be recovered. It is performed by all cells of the body and takes place in the cytosol. The net reaction is conversion of glucose to pyruvate: A six-carbon molecule (glucose) is broken into two three-carbon molecules (pyruvate).

Carbohydrate Digestion and Glucose Uptake by Cells

Salivary amylase acts on ingested carbohydrates (oligomers and polymers containing sugars such as glucose, mannose, lactose, and fructose) to cleave $\alpha(1 \rightarrow 4)$ glycosidic bonds, randomly,

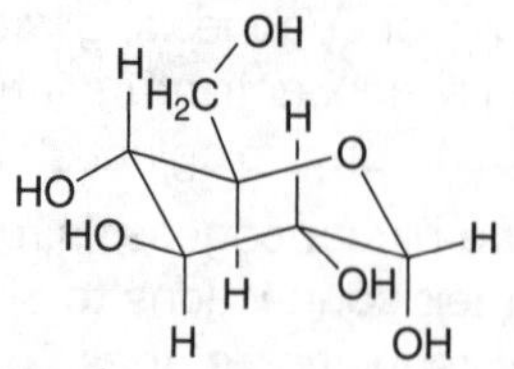

OH
H
H_2C
H
O
HO
HO
H
H
OH
H
OH

Figure 9-1 Structure of β-D-glucose.

to produce smaller units of eight or fewer sugar units. In the stomach, the very acidic pH stops the action of amylase; little further enzymatic hydrolysis occurs in the stomach. Upon passage into the small intestine, secretions from the pancreas neutralize the acid, and various digestive enzymes are released; these then cleave the oligosaccharides to form monosaccharides and disaccharides. The disaccharides are further hydrolyzed to monosaccharides at the brush border. Some sugars are absorbed by simple passive diffusion (notably pentoses), but others are taken up by facilitated diffusion or by active transport via specific carrier proteins. The sugars then pass into the portal blood system for metabolism in the liver; they may also be stored there as glycogen. Sugars (from glycogen or from gluconeogenesis; see the discussion later in this chapter) can also be released by the liver into the bloodstream.

How does glucose enter the cell? Glucose from the bloodstream enters through the action of glucose transporters, transmembrane proteins that specifically bind glucose. The binding region changes conformation and expels the bound glucose on the other side of the membrane. Both the conformational change and the transport reaction are reversible.

These transporter proteins share many features with enzymes. Notably, they are specific for particular substrates, they have a characteristic rate of action (how fast they pass the substrate across the membrane), and they can be inhibited, especially by analogs of the substrate. Their enzymatic characteristics (e.g., K_M values) reflect their physiological role. A high K_M value means the transporter works only when lots of glucose is present. Conversely, a low K_M value means that the transporter has high affinity for glucose and will bind and transport it even when glucose concentrations are very low.

Humans have a number of different glucose transporters (*GLUT proteins*); at least 14 members have been identified, with each type having a different role. GLUT1 and GLUT3 are found in almost all cell types, have a K_M value of approximately 1 mM, and are responsible for basal glucose transport (they transport glucose even when blood glucose levels are low). GLUT1 is especially important for sugar transport into brain cells.

GLUT2 is found mainly in liver and pancreatic cells. This particular transporter has a high K_M for glucose (15–20 mM); the high K_M value means that this transporter works only when blood glucose levels are very high. Thus the pancreas, which secretes insulin, senses the blood glucose level and adjusts its rate of secretion accordingly. Also, the liver takes up glucose only when blood glucose levels are high; when blood glucose levels drop, this constraint "spares" the blood glucose for its uptake by brain and muscle (and the liver may actually release glucose into the bloodstream then).

GLUT4 has a K_M of approximately 5 mM and is found in muscle and adipose tissue. In fat cells, many of these transporter proteins are found in the interior of the cell. Insulin acts on fat cells to cause a translocation of these "interior" transporters to the cell surface, where they increase the uptake of glucose dramatically (up to a threefold change in glucose transport).

GLUT5 appears to be a transporter that is specific for fructose; it is expressed in several different types of tissue. GLUT7 transports both glucose and fructose; it works in the small intestine and colon to absorb these sugars from the gut.

Three Stages of the Glycolytic Pathway

Figure 9-2 lays out the glycolytic pathway. Three main sections of the pathway can be distinguished. The first part works on the six-carbon molecule (glucose), readying it for oxidation. The second part splits the six-carbon molecule into two three-carbon fragments (dihydroxyacetone phosphate or DHAP, and glyceraldehyde 3-phosphate) and then interconverts them. The third part operates on one of these three-carbon molecules (glyceraldehyde

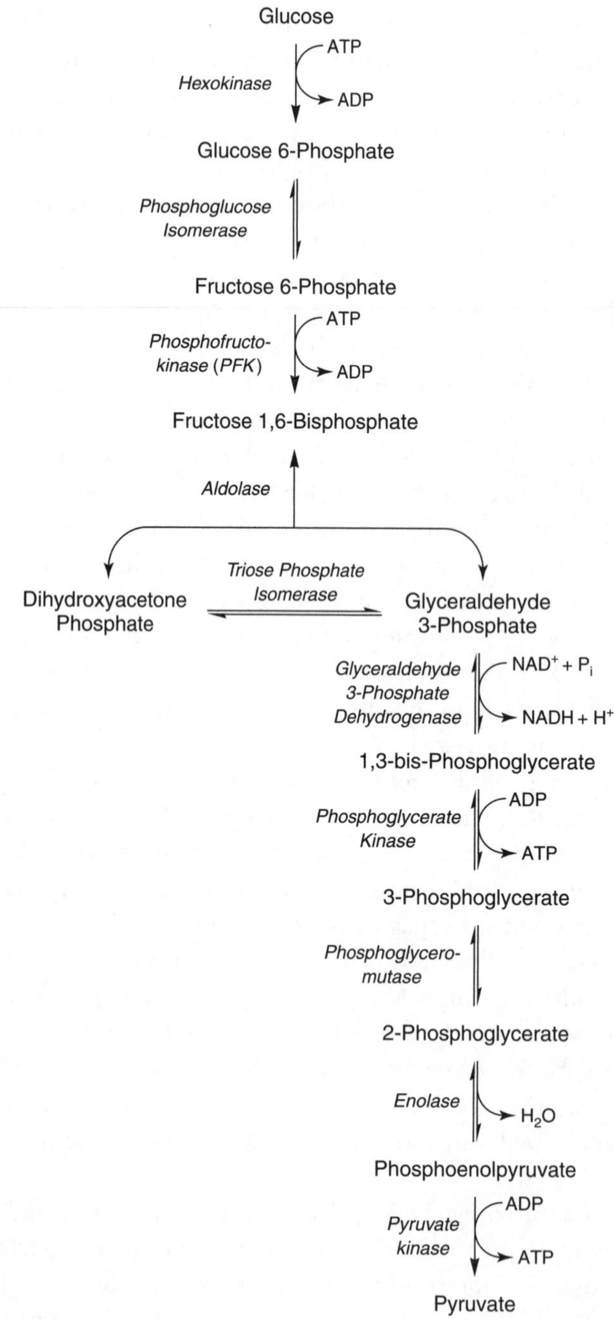

Figure 9-2 The pathway of glycolysis.

3-phosphate), oxidizing it to yield energy. The three-stage model can be summarized as follows: prepare, split, and oxidize glucose.

Notice that one glucose molecule will generate two molecules of pyruvate, thanks to the interconversion of dihydroxyacetone phosphate with glyceraldehyde 3-phosphate by the triose phosphate isomerase enzyme.

Energetics of Glycolysis

The overall process leads to the generation of energy-rich phosphoanhydride bonds, in ATP, from the breakdown of energy-rich compounds bearing phosphate groups. This transformation is referred to as substrate-level phosphorylation. Later, we will consider oxidative phosphorylation, where electron transport drives the formation of ATP; this latter process is quite different from glycolysis and substrate-level phosphorylation. (Photosynthetic organisms can also employ a third process to make ATP, known as photophosphorylation.)

The thermodynamics of glycolysis has several important features:

- There is net ATP production. The pathway consumes 2 units in stage I, but produces $2 \times 2 = 4$ units in stage III. Thus there is net production of 2 units of ATP per 1 molecule of glucose entering the path. It costs energy to make ATP, but its production is possible because overall there is release of free energy, from top to bottom, in the pathway.
- Glycolysis is a "downhill" process. Overall the process runs "downhill" in free energy: Both ΔG and $\Delta G'^\circ$ are less than or equal to zero for the entire process (**Table 9-1**). There are, however, some "uphill" steps with ΔG and $\Delta G'^\circ \geq 0$. The numbers for the individual steps vary a bit with the source: Authorities differ somewhat, depending on which tissues were analyzed (e.g., muscle cells versus red blood cells). The reaction interconverting DHAP with glyceraldehyde 3-phosphate is the only one with any significant discrepancy. Some data sources or interpretations also neglect to account for running two molecules of glyceraldehyde 3-phosphate through the lower part of the pathway.
- The sign and value of $\Delta G'^\circ$ are helpful, but do not tell the whole (thermodynamic) story. Recall that in the living cell, reactions are *not* at equilibrium, so $\Delta G'^\circ$ is indicative but not a true measure of free energy changes in vivo. However, from knowledge of the concentrations of metabolites in vivo, estimates can be made of ΔG values for conditions in vivo. These values, which are often quite a bit different from those calculated under standard-state conditions, tend to indicate that glycolysis is, indeed, a favorable process in vivo.
- Not all the free energy is captured in making ATP. Glycolysis does not "harness" all the free energy to use in making ATP. If we calculate the free energy change needed for the net synthesis of two phosphoanhydride bonds (there is a net gain of two ATP molecules), and compare it to the free energy change resulting from converting glucose into two molecules of pyruvate, we find that the two numbers do not match. In fact, it seems that more free energy is released by the glucose-to-pyruvate conversion than is absorbed by the phosphoanhydride formation.
- The apparent *thermodynamic inefficiency* of glycolysis is deceptive. It appears that glycolysis is an inefficient process that "wastes" free energy that could otherwise be put to use in making more ATP. Where does the "excess" free energy go? Into heat. This outcome, in fact, may be useful for maintaining body heat in animals. Insects such as bees may take advantage of this process to "warm up" before flight. Also, note that the reactions in the glycolytic pathway are potentially reversible: if they were run backward, they could consume ATP, not produce it. The cell will "sacrifice" some free energy to drive reactions in the required direction and ensure a sufficient ATP level for the cell. See the first reaction in the glycolytic pathway as an example.

Glycolysis is Anaerobic

No Direct Oxygen Use in Glycolysis

There is no direct consumption of oxygen in the glycolytic pathway. Glycolysis produces ATP for the cell *anaerobically*, without direct consumption of oxygen. This is *not* the major route to ATP production, however. Oxidative phosphorylation will do this, in an *aerobic* (oxygen-requiring)

Reaction	Enzyme	ΔG′° (kJ/mol)	ΔG (kJ/mol)*	ATP Formed
Glucose → glucose-6-P	Hexokinase	−16.7	−33.4	−1
Glucose-6-P → fructose-6-P	Phosphogluco-isomerase	+1.7	0 to +25	
Fructose-6-P → fructose-1,6-bis-P	Phosphofructo-kinase-1	−14.2	−22.2	−1
Fructose-1,6-bis-P → DHAP + G3P	Aldolase	+23.8	−6 to 0	
DHAP → G3P	Triose-phosphate isomerase	+7.5	0 to +4	
G3P → 1,3-BPG	Glyceraldehyde-3-phosphate dehydrogenase	+6.3	−2 to +2	
1,3-BPG → 3-PG	Phosphoglycerate kinase	−18.8	0 to +2	+2
3-PG → 2-PG	Phosphoglycero-mutase	+4.4	0 to +0.8	
2-PG → PEP	Enolase	+7.5	0 to +3.3	
PEP → Pyruvate	Pyruvate kinase	−31.4	−16.7	+2
Net		**−29.9**	**−35.2 to −80.3**	**+2**

Table 9-1 Correlation of Free Energy Changes and ATP Synthesis in Glycolysis

*For erythrocytes, at pH 7.

Source: Adapted with permission from D. L. Nelson and M. M. Cox. (2008). *Lehninger Principles of Biochemistry*, 5th ed., W. H. Freeman, New York.

set of reactions. Later chapters on the citric acid cycle and on oxidative phosphorylation discuss this topic in more detail.

Under anaerobic conditions (such as blockage of oxygen transport to the cells), glycolysis can continue and energy generation is possible, but only for a short time. This occurs because, as glycolysis proceeds, the *nicotinamide pool* (the collection of free and bound molecules of NAD^+ and NADH) in the cell is becoming mostly reduced (to NADH). Eventually, glycolytic energy production stops when the cell has too little NAD^+ left.

Aerobic Metabolism and Nicotinamides: An Indirect Dependence on Oxygen

Glycolysis does not depend directly on oxygen; there are no reactions in glycolysis that involve molecular oxygen. However, certain of the reactions do depend on the availability of oxidized nicotinamide (NAD^+); the enzymes catalyzing these steps are performing redox reactions, and they need the nicotinamide to act as an electron acceptor (the electron donor here is the sugar molecule that is being slowly oxidized, piece by piece). How does the body (re)generate the necessary NAD^+ for the cell to continue with glycolysis?

Under aerobic conditions, the pool of oxidized nicotinamide is regenerated as the NADH is used in conjunction with oxidative phosphorylation. Exactly how this feat is accomplished is covered elsewhere (see Chapter 11). This other set of reactions does, indeed, require adequate supplies of molecular oxygen, so there is indirectly a coupling of continued glycolysis and the consumption of oxygen by the cell.

As an aside, even if molecular oxygen were supplied to the cell, recall that nicotinamides do not react directly with oxygen, and the cell cannot directly oxidize them with molecular oxygen. Thus this pathway is not a route to regenerate NAD^+ for continued glycolytic action.

Other Substrates for Glycolysis

Many other oxidizable "fuel" molecules can be fed into the glycolytic pathway. Some may require some preprocessing before entering the pathway. **Figure 9-3** summarizes how a number of common sugars can enter glycolysis. Notice that not all the sugars enter at the top of the pathway as glucose; instead, they may enter at some later stage. Notice also that the breakdown of lipids can provide glycerol, which can be converted to an intermediate in the glycolytic pathway.

These interconversions among sugars often use a uridine diphosphate (UDP) moiety as an activating group. For UDP-glucose, the attachment occurs through the C1 carbon on glucose (**Figure 9-4**).

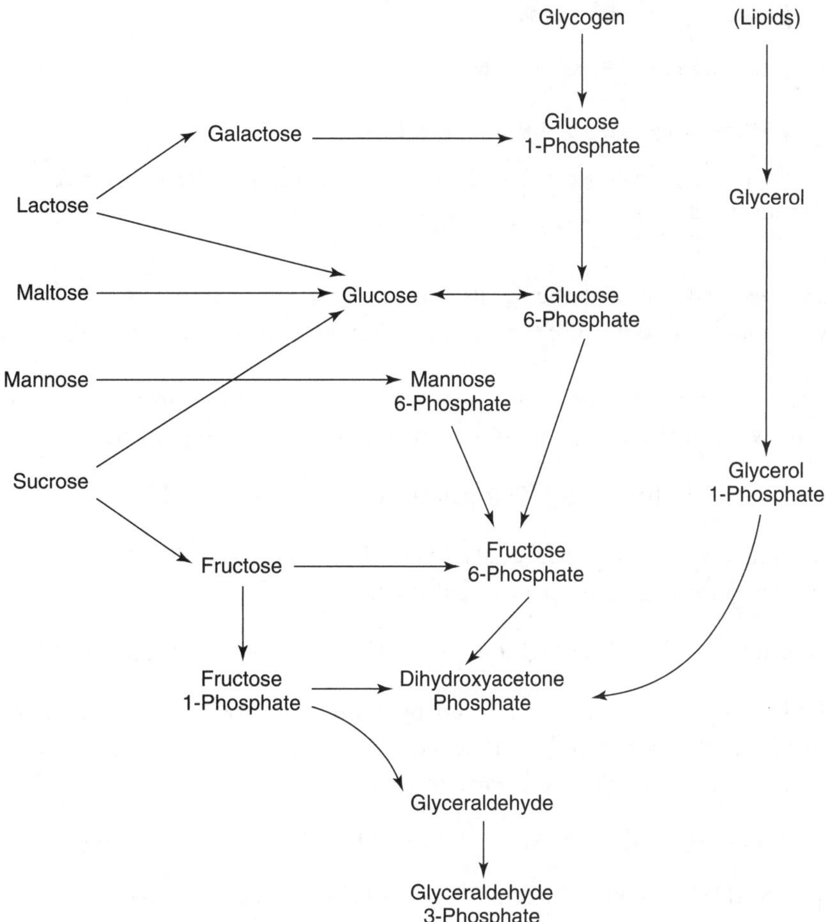

Figure 9-3 Several different sugars, as well as the glycerol from the breakdown of certain lipids, can be used in glycolysis.

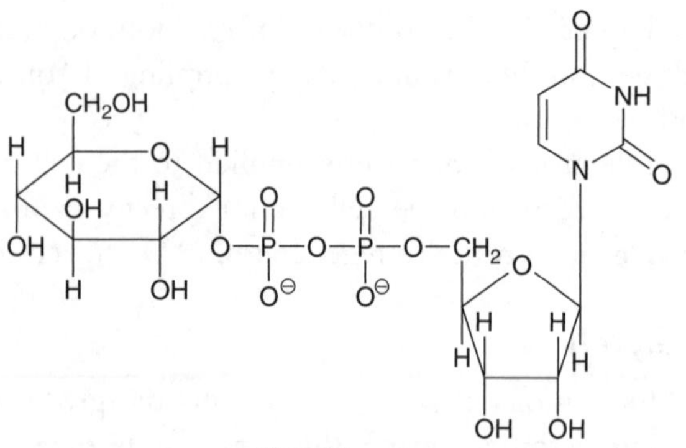

UDP-Glucose

Figure 9-4 Structure of uridine diphosphate glucose (UDP-glucose).

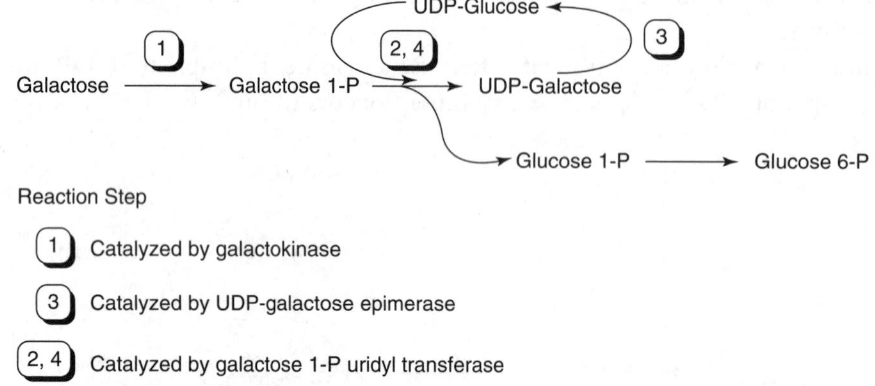

Figure 9-5 Galactose can be converted to glucose 6-phosphate, thereby entering the glycolytic pathway. See the text for details.

As an example of the use of the UDP moiety in sugar interconversions, we look at how galactose may be converted to glucose 6-phosphate. This process involves several steps (**Figure 9-5**).

Step 1: This reaction is catalyzed by galactokinase. Note the consumption of ATP in the phosphorylation reaction; energy is consumed to start the conversion.

$$\text{Galactose} + \text{ATP} \rightarrow \text{galactose 1-P} + \text{ADP} + \text{H}^+ \tag{9-1}$$

Step 2: This reaction is catalyzed by galactose 1-P uridyl transferase. Here the uridyl moiety is transferred from glucose over to galactose.

$$\text{Galactose 1-P} + \text{UDP-glucose} \rightarrow \text{UDP-galactose} + \text{glucose 1-P} \tag{9-2}$$

Step 3: This *two-step* reaction is catalyzed by UDP-galactose 4-epimerase. Note how the (tightly bound) nicotinamide is first reduced in forming the 4-keto intermediate, then re-oxidized when the glucose is formed.

$$\text{UDP-galactose} + \text{NAD}^+ \rightarrow \text{NADH} + \text{4-keto intermediate}$$

$$\text{NADH} + \text{4-keto intermediate} \rightarrow \text{UDP-glucose} + \text{NAD}^+ \tag{9-3}$$

Step 4: The "new" UDP-glucose is used in a repetition of step 2 (Equation 9-2) to get glucose 1-P by transferring its UDP moiety onto a phosphorylated galactose. Note the "recycling" here of the UDP-sugars.

Clinical Application

Galactosemia is a genetic disease that is most commonly due to the absence of galactose 1-P uridyl transferase activity; a less-common form is due to deficiency in galactokinase (see Figure 9-5). Loss of galactose 1-P uridyl transferase activity blocks step 2 in the reaction scheme for the interconversion of glucose and galactose. (What would happen if galactokinase activity were absent?) An accumulation of galactose in the blood results. The deficiency is due to an autosomal recessive gene. Heterozygotes usually express enough enzyme to accommodate ordinary dietary intake of galactose, but their systems may be overwhelmed if challenged with a large amount of galactose. In the case of a homozygous recessive individual, the buildup of unmetabolized galactose eventually causes liver damage, mental retardation, and cataracts.

The treatment is relatively simple in concept: Exclude galactose from the diet! In practice, this is not so simple. Recall that lactose is a disaccharide of glucose and galactose. Milk is a major dietary source of lactose (and hence of galactose), so people with a deficiency in the ability to metabolize galactose should definitely avoid dairy products.

Do not confuse galactosemia with common lactose intolerance. The latter condition has to do with the breakdown of lactose in the gut. Normally, the disaccharide lactose is cleaved into monosaccharides by the digestive enzyme lactase. In the absence of lactase activity, the uncleaved disaccharide is taken up by gut bacteria and metabolized by them to produce gas (CO_2) as well as acidic metabolic end products that tend to draw water into the intestines. This process produces bloating, flatulence, cramping, and diarrhea. Simple lactose intolerance is treatable with an enzymatic preparation taken with the meal. The enzyme will hydrolyze the lactose into galactose and glucose, which can then be absorbed and metabolized by the body.

Fructose is one of the most common simple sugars in the diet. Normally it is absorbed from the gut through the action of GLUT5 and GLUT7, passing through the intestinal enterocytes, and then into the bloodstream via GLUT2. It is eventually delivered to the liver for further metabolism. Fructose can be phosphorylated to fructose 6-phosphate by hexokinase. At this point, the fructose 6-phosphate is ready to enter the glycolytic pathway (see Figure 9-2). In the liver, however, this is not the main pathway for the breakdown of fructose. Instead, in the liver the enzyme fructokinase phosphorylates the sugar to form fructose 1-phosphate, which undergoes a different but related set of reactions to produce the same triose phosphates as fructose 6-phosphate.

These triose phosphates are produced through the action of the enzyme aldolase on the phosphorylated sugar. Three enzymatic forms of aldolase exist: Aldolase A is expressed in most body tissues; aldolase B is expressed predominantly in the liver, and aldolase C is found primarily in the brain. The liver form, aldolase B, has the unusual ability to cleave both fructose 1,6-bisphosphate and fructose 1-phosphate with nearly equal facility; the other two forms of aldolase do not have this ability. This behavior is quite important for liver metabolism of fructose, because (thanks to the activity of liver fructokinase) most of the fructose will be converted to fructose 1-phosphate, not fructose 6-phosphate.

Aldolase B cleaves fructose 1-phosphate to DHAP and glyceraldehyde. Note that the second product here is not glyceraldehyde 3-phosphate, as we start with only a mono-phosphorylated sugar. (Glyceraldehyde can also arise in the liver through the metabolism of glycerol, as a by-product of the breakdown of triglycerides.) The glyceraldehyde can be phosphorylated (by a triose kinase) to give glyceraldehyde 3-phosphate, which brings us back to the two triose phosphates at the center of the glycolytic pathway.

Clinical Application

A deficiency in aldolase B leads to the disease known as hereditary fructose intolerance. The incidence of this disease is low, affecting approximately 1 in every 20,000 to 30,000 newborns. Hereditary fructose intolerance is a recessive inherited genetic disease, and a number of genetic variants have been characterized. Symptoms of the disease characteristically become apparent early in life, when young infants are first exposed to foods containing fructose. These symptoms include bloating, nausea, and vomiting. If the disease is left untreated, severe damage to the liver and kidney can occur.

If aldolase B activity is deficient, then the liver cannot accommodate all of the fructose 1-phosphate generated by the action of fructokinase; thus fructose 1-phosphate will tend to build up and not be further metabolized. This buildup will deplete the local pool of ATP as well as the local pool of inorganic phosphate because the phosphates will be trapped in the unmetabolized fructose 1-phosphate. This will have widespread effects throughout the cell, as many other cellular processes depend on adequate supplies of ATP and phosphate. Phosphate is especially necessary for the breakdown of glycogen (discussed later in this chapter) to release glucose to the bloodstream when blood sugar levels drop. A deficiency in aldolase B activity can lead to severe hypoglycemia following ingestion of fructose, as the incoming fructose will sequester a major fraction of the available phosphate, thereby blocking glycogen breakdown and glucose release. Fructose 1-phosphate will eventually build up to the point where it inhibits fructokinase, which will decrease liver uptake of fructose and raise blood levels of this sugar; thus a high serum level of fructose is a characteristic feature of the disease.

Hereditary fructose intolerance can be relatively benign if diagnosed early. Patients are treated by managing the diet to avoid fructose and sucrose. Sorbitol should also be avoided, because it can be metabolized to fructose. There is, unfortunately, no cure for the disease, and adherence to the strict diet must be maintained throughout the whole lifetime.

Points of Chemical Interest

Ten distinct chemical reactions occur within the glycolytic pathway, involving six different types of reactions. **Figure 9-6** gives a pictorial representation of the six types of reactions. More details on the types of reactions and the enzymes catalyzing them are found in **Table 9-2**.

Glycolysis consumes ATP in stage I, in the phosphorylation of glucose and of fructose 6-phosphate, so it appears that this pathway consumes cellular energy stores. ATP is later generated in stage III, however, so this process actually results in a net gain in the amount of ATP for the cell instead of a loss.

Glycolysis uses NAD^+ as a coenzyme in redox reactions, generating NADH. Glycolysis does not directly use molecular oxygen, but adequate oxygenation is needed for glycolysis to continue.

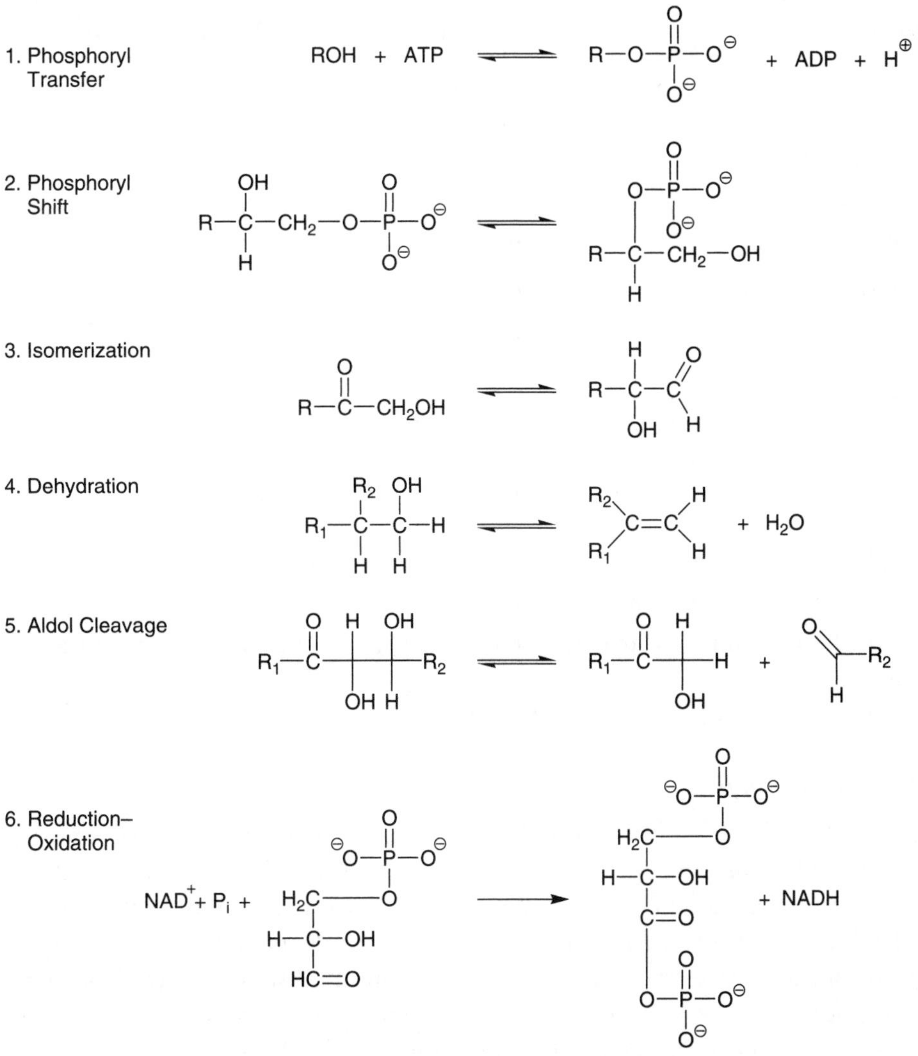

1. Phosphoryl Transfer
2. Phosphoryl Shift
3. Isomerization
4. Dehydration
5. Aldol Cleavage
6. Reduction–Oxidation

Figure 9-6 The six types of chemical reactions occurring in glycolysis.

Reaction	Type of Reaction	Enzyme Involved
Glucose → Glc 6-P (ATP consumed)	Phosphoryl group transfer	Hexokinase
Glc 6-P → Fructose 6-P	Isomerization	Glucose 6-P isomerase
Fructose 6-P → fructose 1,6-bis-P (ATP consumed)	Phosphoryl group transfer	Phosphofructokinase-1
Fructose 1,6-bis-P → DHAP + glyceraldehyde 3-P	Aldol cleavage	Aldolase
DHAP → glyceraldehyde 3-P	Isomerization	Triose phosphate isomerase
Glyceraldehyde 3-P → 1,3-bis-phosphoglycerate	Oxidation/ reduction, phosphorylation	Glyceraldehyde 3-P dehydrogenase

Table 9-2 Classification of Glycolytic Reactions by Type

Reaction	Type of Reaction	Enzyme Involved
1,3-bis-Phosphoglycerate → 3-phosphoglycerate (ATP generated)	Phosphoryl group transfer	Phosphoglycerate kinase
3-Phosphoglycerate → 2-phosphoglycerate	Phosphoryl group shift	Phosphoglycerate mutase
2-Phosphoglycerate → PEP	Dehydration	Enolase
PEP → Pyruvate (ATP generated)	Phosphoryl group transfer	Pyruvate kinase

Table 9-2 Classification of Glycolytic Reactions by Type (Continued)

There are multiple points of interconnection to other pathways:

- Through DHAP to lipid metabolism
- Through the use of sugars other than glucose
- Through the generation of pyruvate and its linkage to the metabolism of the amino acid alanine
- Through pyruvate's entry to the TCA cycle

Regulation of Glycolysis

Regulation of metabolic pathways can be complicated. The original analysis of glycolytic regulation focused on one enzyme, *phosphofructose kinase* (PFK). This enzyme catalyzes the first unique step in this pathway, the so-called committed step. If the activity of this enzyme limited the rate of entry to the pathway, then the overall activity of the pathway can be easily controlled. The concept of such "pacemaker" enzymes and "committed steps" controlling metabolism is simple and appealing, but is very often an over-simplification of the true regulatory system.

Various experiments have cast doubt on the theory of PFK as the main controlling entity for glycolysis. For example, cloning and over-expression of PFK in host cells result in little or no effect on the flux through the pathway. There are also strong theoretical grounds for suspecting that individual steps in glycolysis do not exert decisive control. Instead, to achieve a relatively large change in flux through the pathway, the cell could change the activities of several enzymes simultaneously (including *hexokinase* and *pyruvate kinase*); this mechanism is favored by the evidence and by theory.

Glycolysis appears to be controlled primarily at three sites. For simplicity, we start with the main site of regulation.

Regulation at Phosphofructokinase-1

Several different *isozymes* of PFK exist (isozymes are products of different genes, with different catalytic and regulatory behaviors, but catalyzing the same overall reaction), and phosphofructokinase-1 (PFK-1) is the most important form. This tetrameric enzyme can change its shape, yielding a concomitant change in activity (allosterism). Feedback from products is a key factor in altering the enzyme's activity.

PFK-1 is inhibited by ATP and citrate but is activated by ADP or AMP or cAMP or fructose 2,6-bisphosphate (formed by action of PFK-2, an enzyme not in the glycolytic pathway). (See **Figure 9-7**.) Overall, this permits activation of glycolysis when ATP (i.e., cellular energy) is low, whereas glycolysis will be inhibited when ATP is high.

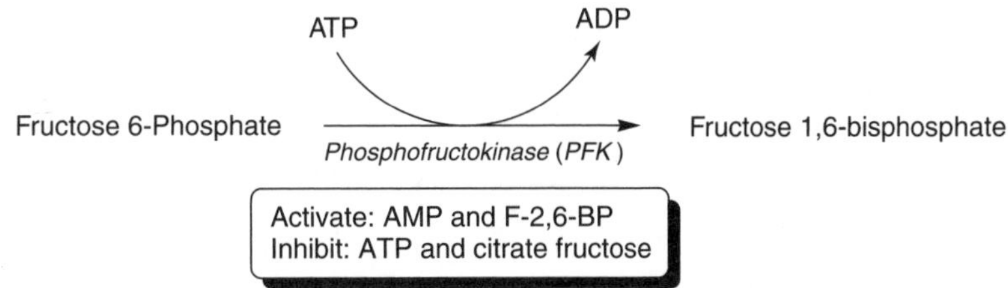

Figure 9-7 The activity of phosphofructokinase is sensitive to the energy charge of the cell and is closely regulated.

Hexokinase

Why not regulate the pathway exclusively through hexokinase? After all, it looks like it catalyzes the "committing step." Hexokinase is not involved in the first unique step of glycolysis. Also, its product (glucose 6-phosphate) is used for other metabolic purposes, such as the interconversion of hexoses and the generation of reducing power in the phosphogluconate pathway (see Chapter 12).

Hexokinase is inhibited by glucose 6-phosphate. This compound is also used in other pathways, so exerting control via this compound's concentration allows fine-tuning of glycolysis in concert with other pathways. Actually, in humans, several different forms of this enzyme are present, differing in their activity and sensitivity to regulation.

Pyruvate Kinase

Pyruvate kinase catalyzes the last reaction in the path, where the phosphorylation of ADP to ATP is coupled to the conversion of phosphoenolpyruvate to pyruvate. This enzyme controls outflow from the glycolytic path, in connection with a somewhat complicated "feed-forward stimulation" mechanism that will not be described here. This enzyme is allosterically inhibited by ATP; thus a product of glycolysis acts to inhibit its own formation. Feedback is negative in this case. Also, ATP inhibition produces overall sensitivity of the glycolytic pathway to the energy charge in the cell. A high energy charge leads to a slowing down of the path producing ATP.

Why Does Alanine Inhibit Pyruvate Kinase?

In addition to its sensitivity to ATP levels, pyruvate kinase is inhibited by the amino acid alanine. If the function of the glycolytic pathway is to produce energy for the cell, what does alanine have to do with energy metabolism? In a reversible reaction, alanine can be converted to pyruvate (see Chapter 14 for details of this transamination reaction), the end product of glycolysis. As we will see, pyruvate will be further oxidized in the TCA cycle; that is, pyruvate itself is used as fuel for the cell. Thus high levels of alanine are a signal that fuel for the cell is (at least potentially) abundant and that glycolytic activity may be reduced. This relationship is another example of linkage between metabolic paths—in this case, that for carbohydrates and that for amino acids.

Linkage of Glycolysis to Pyruvate Metabolism

Pyruvate is the end product of the glycolytic pathway (see the structure in **Figure 9-8**) and a key precursor for the TCA cycle and for the synthesis of fatty acids and amino acids. Several different reactions are possible for pyruvate:

- *Lactate fermentation*: conversion to lactic acid, by lactate dehydrogenase. Reduction of pyruvate to lactate will regenerate NAD^+, necessary for continued glycolytic function.
- *Alcoholic fermentation*: conversion to ethanol, via acetaldehyde. Pyruvate decarboxylase catalyzes the first reaction, alcohol dehydrogenase the second. Reduction of acetaldehyde

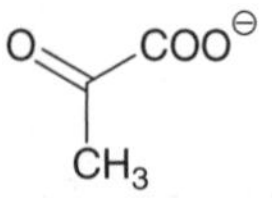

Figure 9-8 Structure of pyruvate.

regenerates NAD^+. Alcoholic fermentation is an important pathway for yeast, as exploited by brewers and winemakers, but not for higher organisms.

- Oxidative decarboxylation to form acetyl CoA, for entry into the TCA cycle. This process involves reduction of NAD^+ to NADH, which is catalyzed by pyruvate dehydrogenase. It is a very important metabolic path for pyruvate.
- (Trans)Amination to form alanine. Chapter 14, on amino acid metabolism, has more details on this process.
- Carboxylation to form oxaloacetate. This process can be important for proper turnover rates in the TCA cycle (see material on the citric acid or TCA cycle in Chapter 10).

Lactate fermentation is especially important for muscle tissue. When muscles perform sustained exertion, they use ATP for muscular contraction. The local stores of ATP (and other useful sources of phosphoanhydrides) may not be enough to sustain the exertion, so the ADP must be re-phosphorylated to ATP. This phosphorylation will deplete local stores of molecular oxygen; also the transport of oxygen to these tissues may not be adequate to sustain the exertion. In such cases, glycolysis will be called upon to produce ATP anaerobically. As glycolysis proceeds, the local pool of NAD^+ is converted to NADH through this mechanism. Without re-oxidation of the NADH (as by oxidative phosphorylation, the oxygen-consuming process that also makes ATP), glycolysis would eventually stop. Lactate fermentation provides an alternative way to regenerate locally the pool of NAD^+, by allowing glycolysis to make ATP, so that muscular exertion can continue.

Central Metabolic Role of Glucose 6-Phosphate

Glucose 6-phosphate is a phosphorylated sugar (**Figure 9-9**) that is used in glycogen synthesis, offering a way for the cell to store sugar locally. It is also used in the pentose phosphate pathway to produce NADPH (for reductive biosyntheses). Furthermore, it is a precursor for ribose, the important sugar that is needed for nucleotide synthesis. **Figure 9-10** shows how glucose 6-phosphate connects these paths.

Glycolysis is linked physiologically to the breakdown of glycogen (*glycogenolysis*) and the generation of sugar molecules de novo (*gluconeogenesis*). These three pathways are intricately intertwined, and their concerted regulation requires a delicate balancing act on the part of the cell.

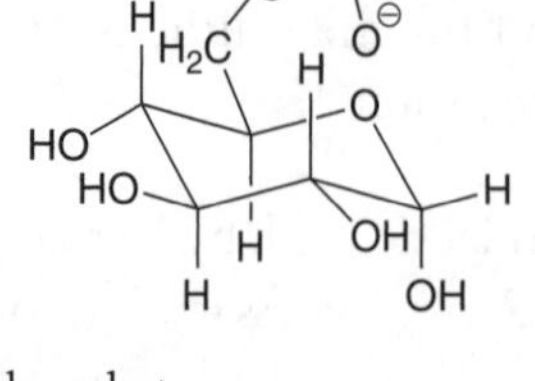

Figure 9-9 Structure of glucose 6-phosphate.

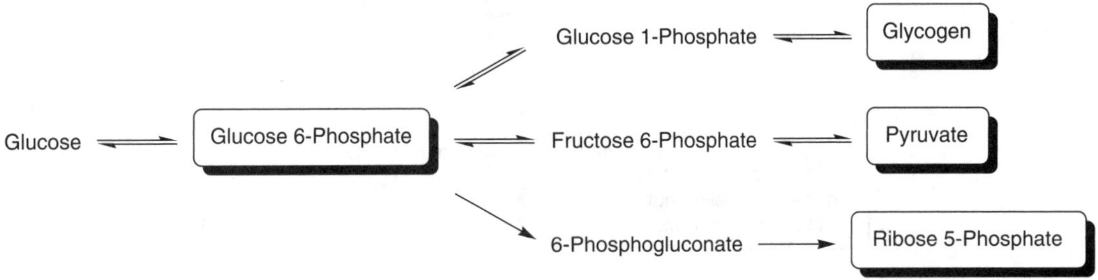

Figure 9-10 Glucose 6-phosphate is central to glycolysis, glycogen formation, and the synthesis of ribose 5-phosphate (as well as the generation of NADPH).

Gluconeogenesis

Gluconeogenesis is the pathway leading from simple noncarbohydrate precursors to the sugar glucose. These precursors include glycerol (from the breakdown of triglycerides) and some species of amino acids, as well as lactic acid that may have been derived through glycolysis. The body converts these precursors into pyruvate, oxaloacetate, or dihydroxyacetone phosphate, which can then enter the biosynthetic pathway to glucose.

In mammals, gluconeogenesis occurs mostly in the liver, with some glucose made in the kidneys as well. Glucose is not made in muscle, nerve cells, or other locations. During conditions of starvation, liver gluconeogenesis becomes the major source of glucose for muscle and brain cells. Glucose made in the liver by gluconeogenesis must be transported by the bloodstream to other tissues where it will be used.

The combination of glucose transport to actively working tissues combined with the reverse transport of lactate from those tissues back to the liver is called the Cori cycle. The Cori cycle is the mechanism by which the body maintains adequate supplies of glucose for tissues that do not themselves perform gluconeogenesis. It is important for maintaining those tissues when glucose is not available by absorption from the gut (e.g., during overnight fasting or under conditions of starvation).

The Biosynthetic Pathway to Glucose

The enzymes for gluconeogenesis are located mostly in the cytosol. However, as shown in **Figure 9-11**, the process can be thought of as starting in the mitochondria, with pyruvate going to oxaloacetate, then to malate, and then eventually to 2-phosphoenolpyruvate out in the cytosol. Transport across the mitochondrial membrane is involved in the early steps of the pathway.

Four special enzymes are used to avoid three glycolytic reactions that are especially unfavorable to synthesis of glucose. The gluconeogenic reactions involved in these special steps, indicated by stars in Figure 9-11, are (1) the conversion of pyruvate to PEP, in multiple steps; (2) the conversion of fructose 1,6-bisphosphate to fructose 6-phosphate; and (3) the conversion of glucose 6-phosphate to glucose. It is important to realize that gluconeogenesis is not glycolysis in reverse!

Glucose 6-phosphatase plays a special role here. This enzyme is found in the liver and kidneys, where gluconeogenesis and glycogenolysis occur. It catalyzes removal of the phosphate group from glucose 6-phosphate. Glucose 6-phosphate is the immediate product of gluconeogenesis and (less directly) of glycogenolysis, so the removal of the phosphate group enables the prompt release of glucose to the bloodstream and its transport to other tissues where it is needed. Tissues such as muscle lack this enzyme, so these tissues tend to retain glucose after it has been phosphorylated.

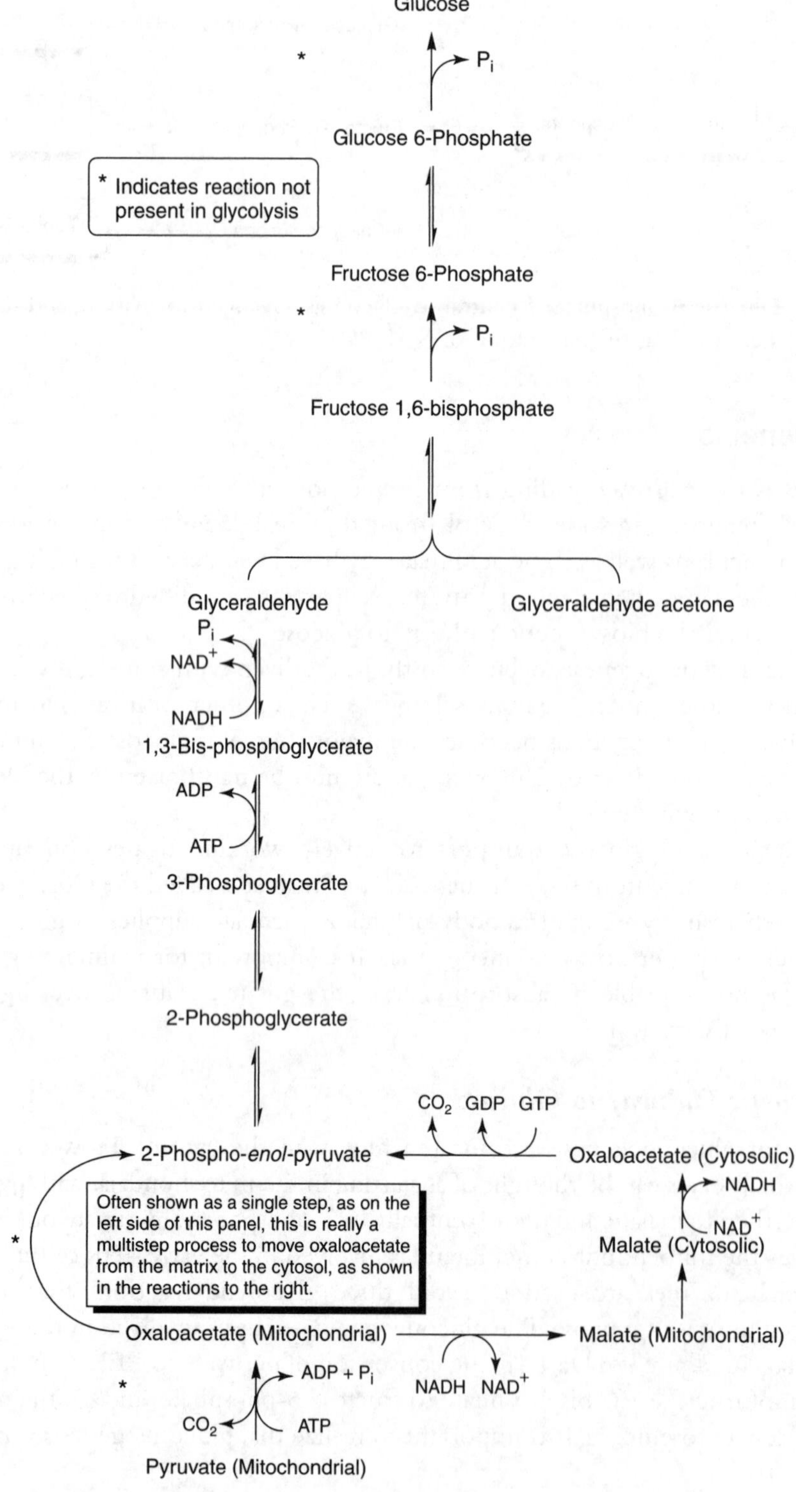

Figure 9-11 The pathway for gluconeogenesis.

Note the use of carbon dioxide in carboxylating pyruvate to form oxaloacetate. This mitochondrial reaction is driven at the expense of ATP hydrolysis. The CO_2 is then released in the cytosol, as oxaloacetate is decarboxylated to give 2-phosphoenolpyruvate. Note also the unusual use of GTP in this latter reaction.

Redox reactions, involving nicotinamides, occur in the mitochondria and in the cytosol. Partial cancellation of NADH generation (in the malate to oxaloacetate reaction) occurs as a result of the subsequent conversion of 1,3-bisphosphoglycerate to glyceraldehyde 3-phosphate. Overall there is net consumption of NADH by gluconeogenesis.

Net Reaction in Gluconeogenesis

The joining of two pyruvate molecules, with the input of energy and reducing power, leads to a single molecule of glucose:

$$2 \text{ pyruvate} + 4 \text{ ATP} + 2 \text{ GTP} + 2 \text{ NADH} + 2 \text{ H}^+ + 6 \text{ H}_2\text{O}$$
$$\rightarrow \text{glucose} + 6 \text{ P}_i + 4 \text{ ADP} + 2 \text{ GDP} + 2 \text{ NAD}^+ \qquad (9\text{-}4)$$

with $\Delta G'^\circ = -37.7$ kJ/mol (-9 kcal/mol).

Gluconeogenesis consumes four ATP, two GTP, and two NADH molecules, while glycolysis produces two ATP and two NADH molecules. The extra free energy is needed in gluconeogenesis to drive an otherwise unfavorable process. The net cost of a round trip through glycolysis and gluconeogenesis is four phosphoanhydride bonds (recall that GTP and ATP are energetically equivalent).

Regulation of Gluconeogenesis

Like glycolysis, gluconeogenesis is regulated at several points. First there is the entry point, where pyruvate is converted to oxaloacetate by *pyruvate carboxylase*. Pyruvate has another major metabolic pathway that it can enter, the TCA cycle via the pyruvate dehydrogenase complex (see Chapter 10), so it is important to balance these two paths at the outset. The two enzymes' activities are regulated by levels of acetyl-CoA. Acetyl-CoA is a product of oxidation of pyruvate by pyruvate dehydrogenase; it is also derived from the breakdown of fatty acids and certain amino acids.

$$\text{Pyruvate} + \text{NAD}^+ + \text{CoASH} \rightarrow \text{Acetyl-S-CoA} + \text{NADH} + \text{H}^+ + \text{CO}_2$$
$$\Delta G'^\circ = -8.0 \text{ kcal/mol} \qquad (9\text{-}5)$$

Thus high levels of acetyl-CoA generally signal that the cell has enough fuel and does not need to oxidize pyruvate. It is then a good time to store up fuel for future use or for transport to tissues that need energy. Thus, when its levels increase, acetyl-CoA will inhibit its own production. At the same time, acetyl-CoA binds to pyruvate carboxylase and stimulates it. In this way, pyruvate is diverted away from energy production and toward energy storage.

A second point of regulation is at the reaction catalyzed by fructose bisphosphatase-1 (FBPase-1). The reaction catalyzed by FBPase-1 is just the reverse of the one in glycolysis catalyzed by PFK-1. While PFK-1 is activated by AMP, it is just the opposite for FBPase-1; this enzyme is strongly inhibited by AMP. Because both glycolysis and gluconeogenesis take place in the same cellular compartment, this pattern of activation/inhibition provides a very tidy way of reciprocally controlling the two opposing pathways and making them sensitive to the energy charge in the cell. (See also the effects of AMP on glycogen breakdown.)

Feedstocks for Gluconeogenesis

For animals, the carbons involved in gluconeogenesis come from three principal sources:

- Lactate and pyruvate (which are easily interconverted; see the later discussion of the Cori cycle and the role of lactate dehydrogenase)

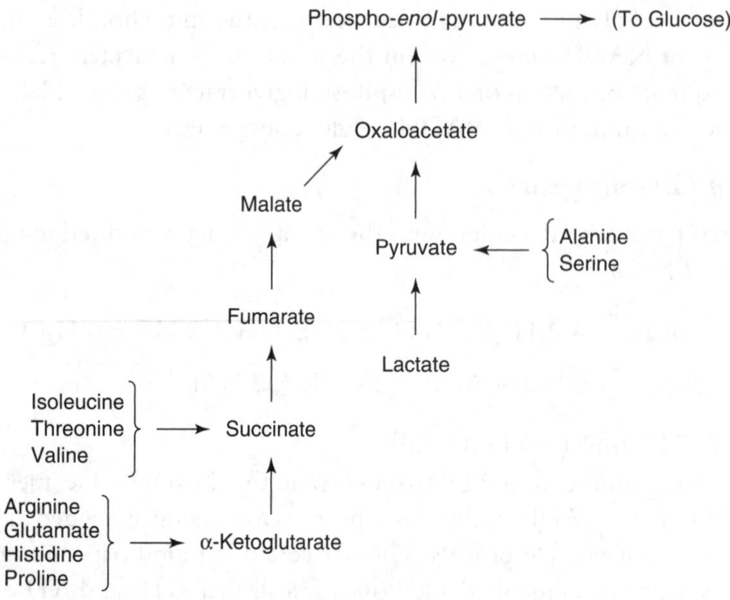

Figure 9-12 Sources of carbon atoms for gluconeogenesis.

- Glycerol, mainly from triglycerides (fat)
- Glucogenic amino acids (from protein)

(Plants can perform photosynthesis, which is a fourth source for them.) **Figure 9-12** summarizes these sources. Keep these sources in mind as we study the metabolism of lipids and amino acids in later units.

The Cori Cycle and Lactate Dehydrogenase

The *Cori cycle* connects anaerobic glycolysis with gluconeogenesis, using separate tissues in the body to compartmentalize the two opposing processes. This cycle allows muscle to work anaerobically, generating lactate, while using the liver's capacity to absorb lactate and convert it into glucose.

Connecting Glycolysis to Gluconeogenesis: The Cori Cycle

Figure 9-13 shows how blood transports glucose from liver to muscle, and lactate from muscle to liver. As muscle cells work anaerobically, they generate lactate from pyruvate, which in turn regenerates the pool of NAD^+ necessary for continued glycolysis. The muscle tissue is unable to further oxidize lactate, however; lactate is a metabolic "dead end" in this sense. Somehow the lactate must be converted to a different form if it is to be further metabolized.

As lactate accumulates in the working muscle cells, it diffuses into the bloodstream and is transported to the liver. Inside liver cells, the lactate is then converted back into pyruvate (the reverse of the reaction that created the lactate in muscle). Now, however, the liver cells can use the pyruvate to make glucose, in the pathway of gluconeogenesis; in contrast, muscle cells cannot do so. The glucose made in this way can then be released from the liver into the bloodstream and returned to the actively working muscle, to sustain its action.

Role of Lactate Dehydrogenase

A key enzyme here is *lactate dehydrogenase* (LDH), a tetrameric enzyme that catalyzes the conversion of lactate to pyruvate, and vice versa. Lactate dehydrogenase is present in multiple

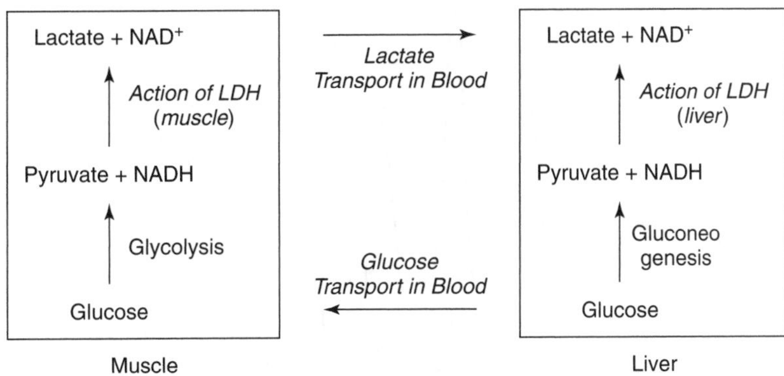

Figure 9-13 The Cori cycle. Glycolysis in active muscle tissue generates lactate, which is then released into the bloodstream. The lactate is used by the liver in gluconeogenesis to make fresh glucose, which is returned via the bloodstream to the muscle tissue.

forms in humans, called *isoenzymes*, or *isozymes* for short. As noted earlier, isoenzymes are enzymes that have different (maybe only slightly different!) amino acid sequences or covalent structures, but that catalyze the same reaction.

Different genes in the cell code for (nearly) the same type of enzyme subunit here. The different gene products do have somewhat different enzymatic characteristics; that is, they differ in their K_M values for lactate and pyruvate. Thus one type will preferentially bind pyruvate, while the other will preferentially bind and act on lactate. In some tissues, one type of subunit predominates, while in another tissue the other type of subunit is the most abundant.

The two types of LDH subunit are known as M (for muscle) and H (for heart). A tetramer of all H-type subunits would be designated as H_4-LDH; similarly, a tetramer of all M-type subunits would be designated as M_4-LDH. It is possible to find mixed forms as well—for example, with two M and two H subunits (H_2M_2), or one H and three M subunits (H_1M_3), or one M and three H subunits (H_3M_1). The proportions of these subunits of LDH differ from tissue to tissue; the H type predominates in cardiac muscle, while the M type is the major form in skeletal muscle and (curiously) in liver cells.

Figure 9-14 presents electropherograms for LDH, showing the five possible forms separated after electrophoresis. Panel A shows the "normal" pattern found in serum; panel B shows the aberrant pattern found after a myocardial infarction ("heart attack"). Notice how form 1 is elevated and form 3 reduced in this case. Heart muscle is rich in form 1 but low in form 3; the damage to heart tissue releases the form 1 LDH into the bloodstream, which then "swamps out" the normal pattern.

Aside on Multiple Forms of Enzymes

Multiple forms of a given enzyme might exist for many different reasons:

- Different, distinct gene products may be present simultaneously, possibly with differences in their expression. An example is malate dehydrogenase, in mitochondria versus the cytosol.
- Genetic variants (alleles) may exist. An example is glucose 6-phosphate dehydrogenase (to be discussed in detail in Chapter 12).
- Polymers of a single type of subunit may exist, with different numbers of subunits so associated. An example is glutamate dehydrogenase, which can vary from 250 kD to 1000 kD in mass, depending on how many subunits are joined (noncovalently) together.

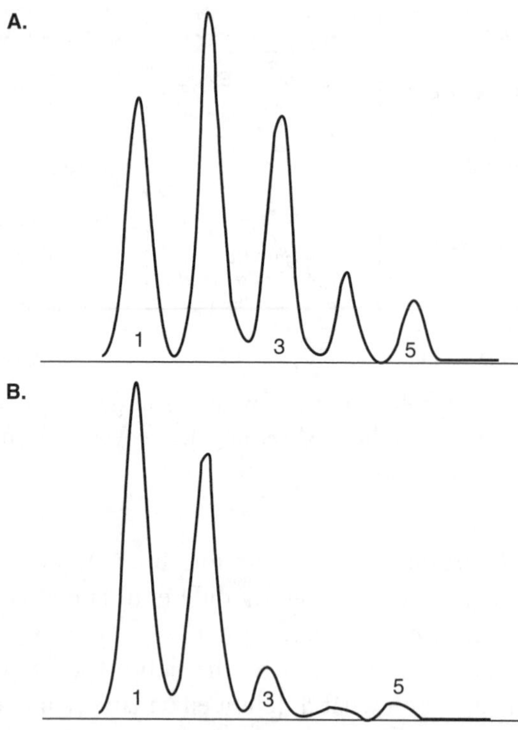

Figure 9-14 Electropherogram of isoforms of lactate dehydrogenase. **A.** The normal relative abundance in serum of the different forms of the enzyme. **B.** Alteration of the pattern when a myocardial infarction releases an abundance of the cardiac muscle form of the enzyme into the bloodstream.

- Hetero-polymers or hetero-oligomers are possible, composed of two or more different types of subunits. An example we have just discussed is lactate dehydrogenase, a tetramer with five different isozyme forms.
- Proteins can be covalently modified (e.g., by phosphorylation, glycosylation, or proteolytic processing), resulting in different forms of the same enzyme. Examples here include glycogen phosphorylase and certain lipases (in lipid metabolism; see Chapter 13).

The tissue specificity of various isozymes can be used diagnostically, as an indicator of local tissue damage. When tissues are damaged (e.g., in heart attack, cirrhosis of the liver, or bruising), they tend to leak enzymes into the bloodstream. The serum levels of these enzymes (particularly tracking of their rise and fall) are often assayed in clinical labs to diagnose and follow the course of a particular pathology. For example, the difference in isozyme forms of lactate dehydrogenase between cardiac muscle, liver, and skeletal muscle can enable healthcare providers to deduce whether a heart attack has occurred, whether there is liver damage, or whether there is just a lot of bruising of muscle tissue.

Tissue-specific expression of one isoform over another can be a part of metabolic regulation. For example, brain hexokinase has a K_M value of approximately 0.05 mM for glucose, while liver glucokinase has a K_M of approximately 10 mM for glucose. With its high affinity for glucose, brain hexokinase will "scavenge" available glucose down to low concentrations, to ensure energy production in the very active neural tissue. Conversely, with its low affinity for glucose, the liver glucokinase will function only when there is excess glucose circulating (normal [glucose] is approximately 5.5 mM), but then it will help the liver to remove the excess glucose from circulation and to store it as glycogen.

Clinical Application

Parasitic trypanosomes are responsible for several debilitating and devastating diseases, including leishmaniasis, Chagas' disease, and malaria. Interestingly, the bloodstream form of these parasites depends quite heavily on substrate-level phosphorylation of ADP to ATP, through glycolysis. Because the trypanosomal enzymes differ in sequence and structure from the corresponding human enzymes, selective targeting of the trypanosomal enzyme with an inhibitor, might be used to block replication of the parasite, while leaving the human host unaffected. In particular, trypanosomal glyceraldehyde-3-phosphate dehydrogenase (GAPDH) is under scrutiny for this purpose. The crystal structures of the enzyme from several different trypanosomes have now been determined, and there are appreciable differences in structure between human and trypanosomal enzyme around the site that binds the adenosyl moiety of the NAD^+ cofactor. Accordingly, adenosine analogs have been synthesized that selectively inhibit these enzymes. These inhibitors (one is shown in **Figure 9-15**) bind to and strongly inhibit the trypanosomal enzyme but do not interfere with human GAPDH function.

Because the trypanosomes depend so heavily on glycolysis, they have a corresponding requirement for high levels of NAD^+ to be regenerated from the NADH produced by glycolysis. This relationship suggests that targeting the parasitic form of the enzyme lactate dehydrogenase might be a viable approach. The crystal structures of the human LDH and the LDH from *Plasmodium falciparum* (which causes malaria) show differences in how the NADH cofactor is placed in the active site, and in the sequence and secondary structure of a loop region that folds down over the active site during catalysis. Compounds are being investigated that would exploit these differences, as part of the effort to produce selective and potent antimalarial agents. Figure 9-15 shows some heterocyclic, azole-based compounds that act as competitive inhibitors of the plasmodial LDH, competing with lactate to bind next to the NAD^+ cofactor in the active site.

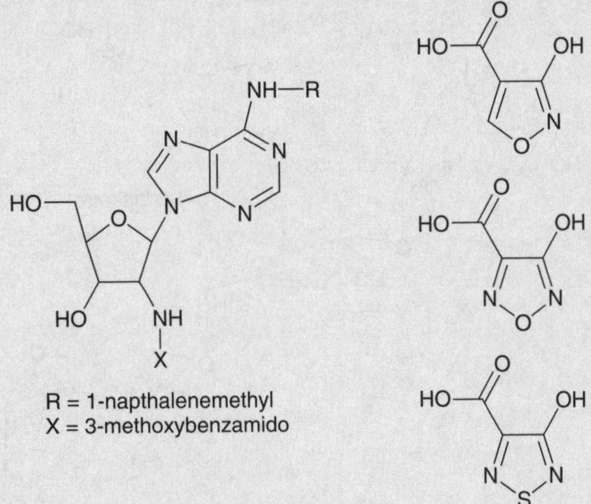

Figure 9-15 Inhibitors of trypanosomal enzymes. On the left is an inhibitor of trypanosomal glyceraldehyde 3-phosphate dehydrogenase; on the right are three inhibitors of trypanosomal lactate dehydrogenase.

Glycogenolysis and Glycogenesis

Glycogen is a cytosolic storage polymer for glucose; its formula is $(\text{glucose})_n$. A typical adult has approximately 200 grams of glycogen stored, mainly in the liver and muscle (roughly one day's worth of energy). Glycogen is broken down when ATP is needed by the cell or by distant tissues (hormonal communication of this need in distant tissues is discussed later in this section). The glucose is then fed into the glycolytic pathway for energy production purposes.

Structure of Glycogen

Glycogen is a highly branched polymer, thanks to two types of linkages between glucose residues. The majority of the residues are bonded through an $\alpha(1 \rightarrow 4)$ link, which leads to a straight chain of glucose residues. Occasionally, however, there is a second type of linkage, an $\alpha(1 \rightarrow 6)$ link, which leads to branches in the main chain (**Figure 9-16**). These branches help keep the polymer soluble by blocking close packing of the chains into a crystalline form. In addition, they provide many ends for chemical reactions—enzyme attack and rapid release of sugar, but they also ready resynthesis of the glycogen. Moreover, forming a polymer of glucose units reduces the osmotic stress on the cell. Recall that osmotic activity is proportional to the number of individual particles in solution. If the cell were to try to store all of these glucose molecules as individual units, rather than as a polymer, there would be a strong tendency for water to flood into the cell in response to the osmotic gradient, which could lead to rupture of the cell membranes.

Glycogen is built up from a small proteinaceous core particle (*glycogenin*). **Figure 9-17** schematically represents the glycogenin core and the high degree of branching of the glucose polymer chains, which blocks crystallization. Compare this branching to the structure of

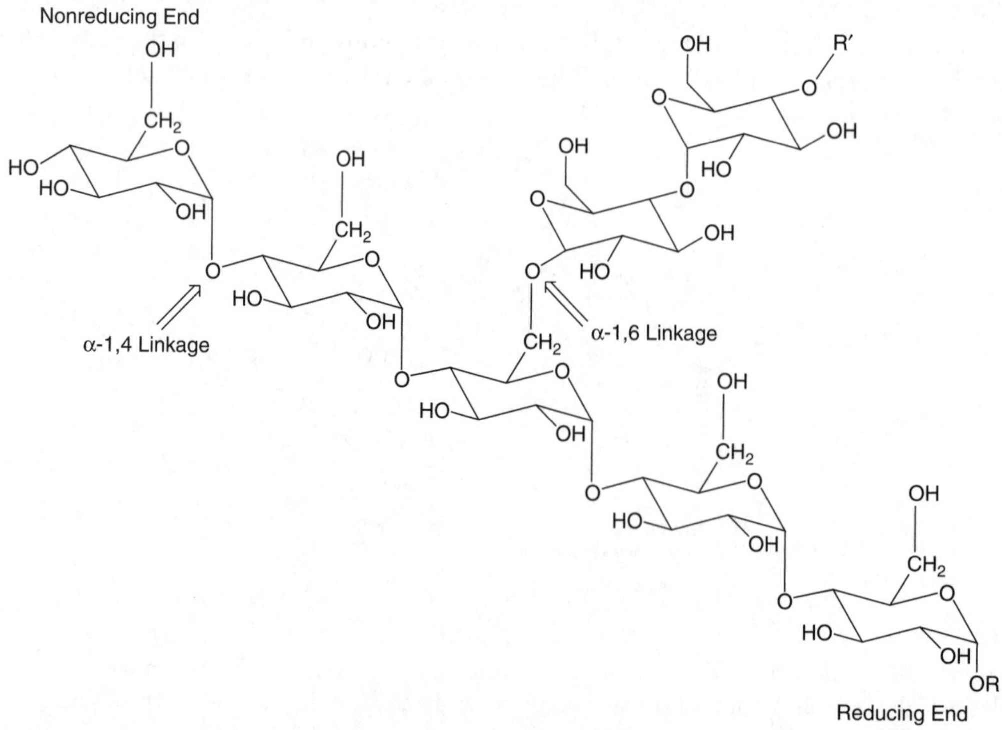

Nonreducing End

α-1,4 Linkage

α-1,6 Linkage

Reducing End

Figure 9-16 Structure of glycogen, showing both $\alpha(1 \rightarrow 6)$ and $\alpha(1 \rightarrow 4)$ linkages between glucose residues.

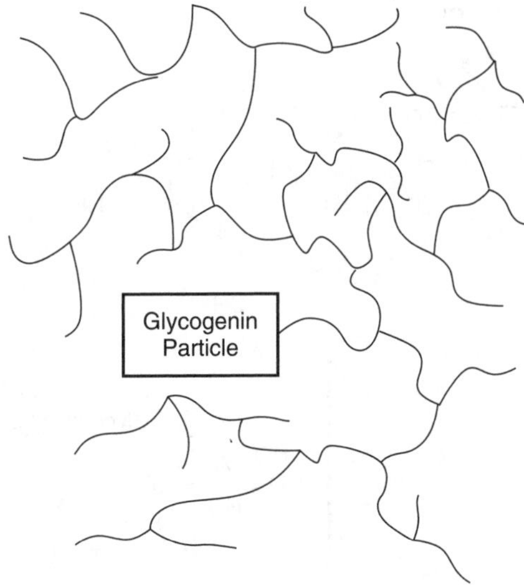

Figure 9-17 Schematic of a glycogen particle, showing the glycogenin core protein and the extensive branching of the attached glycogen chain.

cellulose, another glucose polymer; cellulose does not have branches and packs readily into semicrystalline arrays—an important factor in determining the mechanical strength of plant tissues. Notice also that the exposed ends in glycogen chains are the "nonreducing" ends; there is only one "reducing" end in a glycogen molecule, which is attached to the glycogenin particle. The exposure of the nonreducing ends permits ready breakdown as well as resynthesis of the chains. Special enzymes are needed for synthesizing and breaking down the branchpoints of the carbohydrate chains.

The carbohydrate chains are linked to the glycogenin protein through the phenolic hydroxyl group on a tyrosine residue. A short run of eight glucose residues must be attached to the protein before the synthase enzyme can start to make longer chains off this primer. It is thought that the glycogenin protein itself catalyzes the formation of this primer.

Glycogen Synthesis

Role of Uridine Diphosphate-Glucose

Synthesis and breakdown of glycogen occur by different paths. The synthetic pathway uses an activated intermediate, UDP-glucose (see Figure 9-4). By comparison, the breakdown pathway instead generates glucose 1-phosphate directly.

UDP-glucose is made by UDP-glucose pyrophosphorylase:

$$\text{Glucose 1-phosphate} + \text{UTP} \rightarrow \text{UDP-glucose} + \text{PP}_i \qquad (9\text{-}6)$$

This is a readily reversible reaction. However, the following hydrolysis of pyrophosphate to two phosphates—a very favorable hydrolysis of a phosphoanhydride bond—will drive the first reaction well toward the product side, as the pyrophosphate is depleted through hydrolysis.

Why use UDP, and not some other group, to activate the sugar for reaction?

- "Commitment": The reaction forming UDP-glucose is essentially irreversible due to hydrolysis of the pyrophosphate that is released.

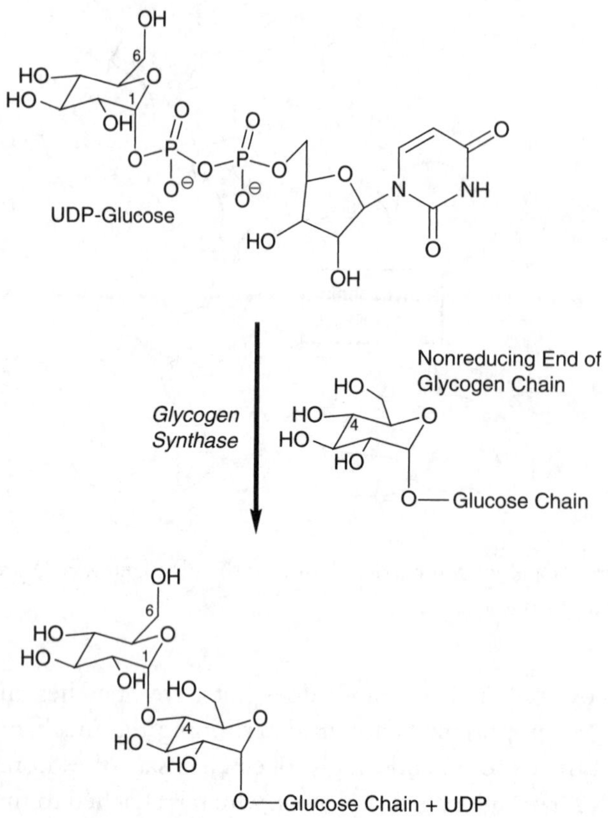

Figure 9-18 Action of glycogen synthase in using UDP-glucose to extend a glycogen chain.

- "Recognition": The UDP moiety forms a distinctive "handle" for other enzymes and proteins to recognize and bind to.
- "Displacement": The UDP group is a good leaving group in nucleophilic displacement reactions, lowering the energetic barrier to the reaction.

Action of Glycogen Synthase

Glycogen synthase uses the UDP-glucose to add glucose to the nonreducing end of a glycogen chain, forming an $\alpha(1 \rightarrow 4)$ link (**Figure 9-18**). This step actually requires a "primer" of at least four sugars on the end of a preexisting glycogen chain; the primer is made by another enzyme system. Subsequent branching of the glycogen chain is catalyzed by a special enzyme ("branching enzyme") that specifically forms $\alpha(1 \rightarrow 6)$ links. Defects in glycogen metabolism due to deficiencies in these enzymes are discussed later in this chapter.

Glycogen Breakdown

Action of Glycogen Phosphorylase

Glycogen phosphorylase a attacks the nonreducing end of a glycogen chain, releasing glucose 1-phosphate and shortening the chain by one residue. The enzyme acts repeatedly to degrade the chain back to a branch point. Degradation past branch points requires the action of a separate enzyme, the "debranching enzyme."

Glycogen phosphorylase removes a single sugar monomer by *phosphorolysis*, using inorganic phosphate (**Figure 9-19**). Notice that the product carries the phosphate group. This enzyme

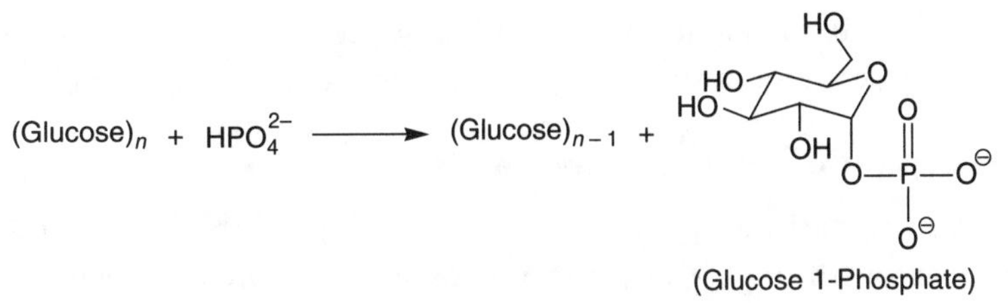

(Glucose)$_n$ + HPO_4^{2-} ⟶ (Glucose)$_{n-1}$ + (Glucose 1-Phosphate)

Figure 9-19 Action of glycogen phosphorylase in releasing glucose 1-phosphate from glycogen.

uses the cofactor pyridoxal phosphate (more on this cofactor later) in connection with amino acid metabolism. In this case, the cofactor probably helps the enzyme to maintain an active conformation but is not itself catalytically active.

Action of Phosphoglucomutase

The glucose 1-phosphate is isomerized by phosphoglucomutase to make glucose 6-phosphate (via the intermediate 1,6-bisphosphorylated sugar; **Figure 9-20**). Glucose 6-phosphate can then enter the glycolytic pathway, or be de-phosphorylated and released into the bloodstream.

Regulation of Glycogen Metabolism

Glycogen metabolism is subject to a complex control system; the uptake or release of glucose must mesh with several other systems. A pattern of interlocking cycles of activation/deactivation of enzymes catalyze successive steps in the process, with cycling of enzymes between two states. Regulation here depends on enzyme phosphorylation and dephosphorylation.

The synthesis and the breakdown of glycogen are under hormonal control. *Epinephrine* and *glucagon* are signaling agents (hormones) that will shut down glycogen synthesis; however, these same hormones also stimulate the breakdown of glycogen. The hormones are released at distant points in the body and travel through the circulation to the liver, where they signal a need for quick liberation of glucose (metabolic energy) to supply working cells (e.g., a need for glucose in muscle tissue). Under these circumstances, glycogen should not be synthesized, but instead should be broken down to release the glucose; hence, inhibition of glycogen synthesis and stimulation of glycogen phosphorolysis occur simultaneously. The effects of these hormones on two opposing enzyme systems in the same cellular compartment are a good example of reciprocal control in metabolic pathways.

In the overall physiology of the body, the hormone insulin generally opposes the effects of epinephrine or glucagon. All of these hormones are intimately connected to the control of energy metabolism in the body, and they all have strong effects on the metabolism of sugars

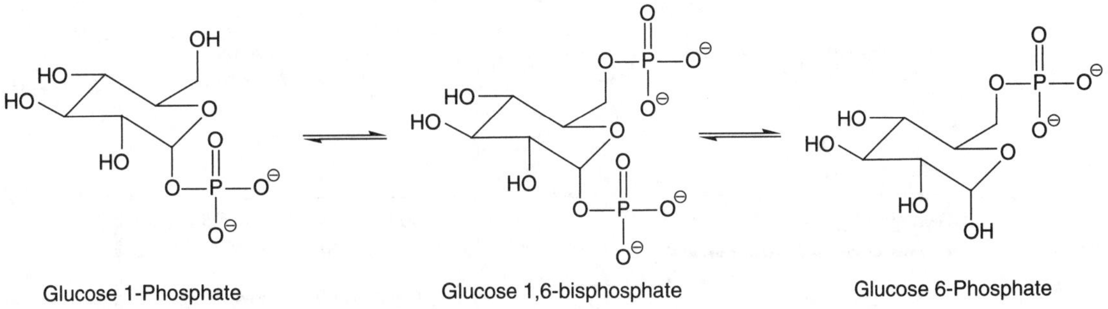

Glucose 1-Phosphate ⇌ Glucose 1,6-bisphosphate ⇌ Glucose 6-Phosphate

Figure 9-20 Reaction pathway for the conversion of glucose 1-phosphate to glucose 6-phosphate, via the bisphosphate intermediate.

(and of lipids as well). Here, insulin will stimulate glycogen synthesis and inhibit glycogen breakdown, which is just the opposite of what epinephrine or glucagon will do.

Hormonal Stimulation of Glycogen Synthesis

Figure 9-21 traces the pathway from hormonal binding to the extracellular domain of a transmembrane receptor, through the activation of various cytosolic enzymes, down to the ultimate effects on glycogen synthase and glycogen phosphorylase. Insulin binds to a receptor and activates a tyrosine kinase inside the cell. This kinase phosphorylates a protein kinase (the "insulin-sensitive" kinase), which in turn phosphorylates a particular phosphatase (phosphatase 1). (The action of a phosphatase is to remove phosphoryl groups—just the opposite reaction of phosphorylation.) Phosphatase-1 has two different targets. First, it acts on glycogen synthase and activates it. Second, it acts on phosphorylase kinase (not the phosphorylase, but the preceding enzyme in the path) and inactivates it. This permits coordinated regulation of glycogen synthesis and breakdown.

Hormonal Stimulation of Glycogen Breakdown

Glycogen breakdown is stimulated by epinephrine or glucagon. Two main actions can be seen here: The first is to stop the synthesis of glycogen, and the second is to stimulate breakdown of glycogen.

Glycogen synthase is inactivated by phosphorylation of a specific Ser residue. The *a* form (which is dephosphorylated) is the active one; the *b* form is the inactive phosphorylated form. The pattern of activation/inhibition is just the opposite for the phosphorylase (**Figure 9-22**).

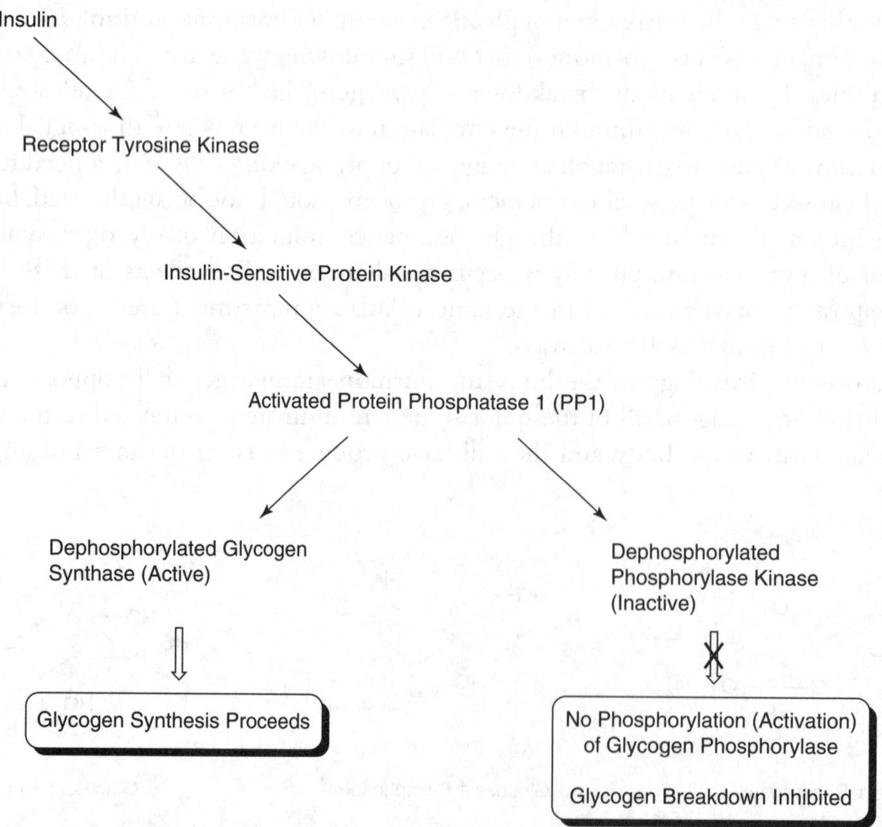

Figure 9-21 Hormonal stimulation of glycogen synthesis and blockage of glycogen breakdown.

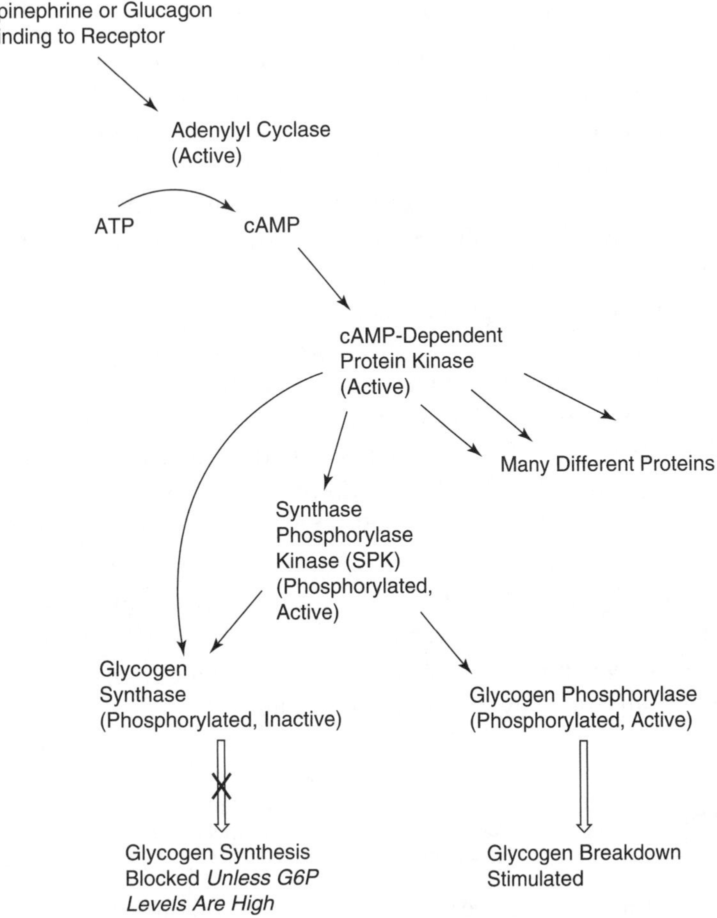

Figure 9-22 Hormonal blockage of glycogen synthesis and stimulation of glycogen breakdown.

Notice the key role of the *second messenger*, cyclic AMP (*cAMP*; **Figure 9-23**). The hormones are the chemical messengers outside the cell, whereas cAMP is the chemical messenger inside the cell. Its synthesis is stimulated by the binding of the hormones to a membrane-bound receptor, which in turn activates the cAMP–synthetic enzyme activity.

Calcium ion is also a general signaling agent, used here and in many other pathways inside the cell. Like cAMP, Ca^{2+} can serve as a second messenger, carrying a signal from outside the cell to pathways inside.

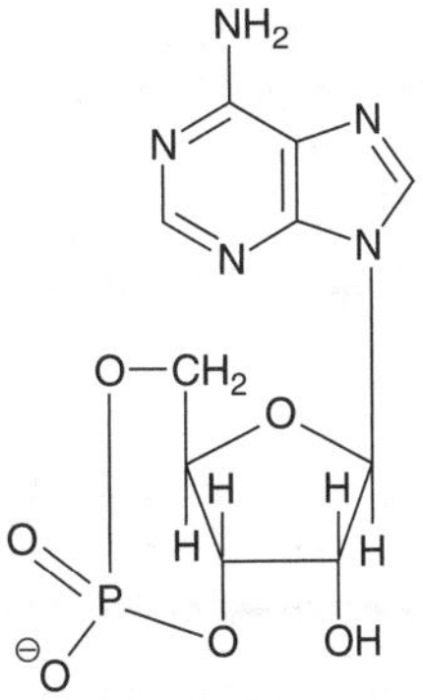

Figure 9-23 Structure of the "second messenger," cyclic adenosine monophosphate (cAMP).

Signaling Cascade and Amplification

The quick release of relatively large amounts of glucose from the liver occurs in response to hormonal signals, involving very dilute hormones. Here only a very small amount of the initiating hormone is needed to produce a very large cellular response: At several steps in the process, enzymes repeatedly generate molecules of product, which are then used in the next step of the process to stimulate the next enzyme, which then generates even more of its product, and so on. The combination of a multistep process with signal amplification at successive steps is termed a *signaling cascade*.

For example, suppose that a single molecule of epinephrine is sufficient to activate a single adenylyl cyclase enzyme. This enzyme is quite capable of turning over several dozen to a few hundred molecules of substrate, generating several dozen to a few hundred molecules of cAMP. Each of these cAMP molecules then can activate one molecule of protein kinase, so now we have perhaps several dozen to a few hundred activated protein kinases. Each of these protein kinases can then activate many molecules of phosphorylase kinase; in turn, the phosphorylase kinases each activate many molecules of phosphorylase. The end result is that it would be quite possible to have millions of molecules of glucose released for every molecule of hormone bound to its receptor (**Figure 9-24**). The various steps in the pathway can occur fairly quickly because they are enzyme-catalyzed reactions; there is no need to synthesize new enzymes, which is otherwise a slow cellular process. In this way, the cell can rapidly mobilize its glycogen stores with a signal from just a few hormone molecules.

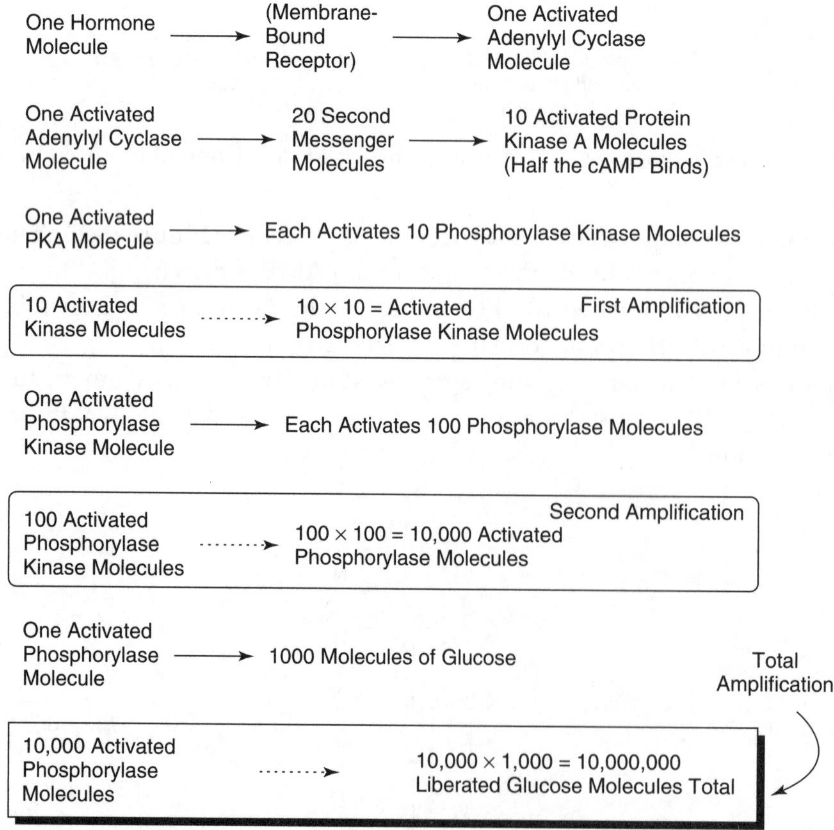

Figure 9-24 An estimate of the serial amplification of the signal due to the binding of a single hormone molecule, in causing the release of glucose from glycogen.

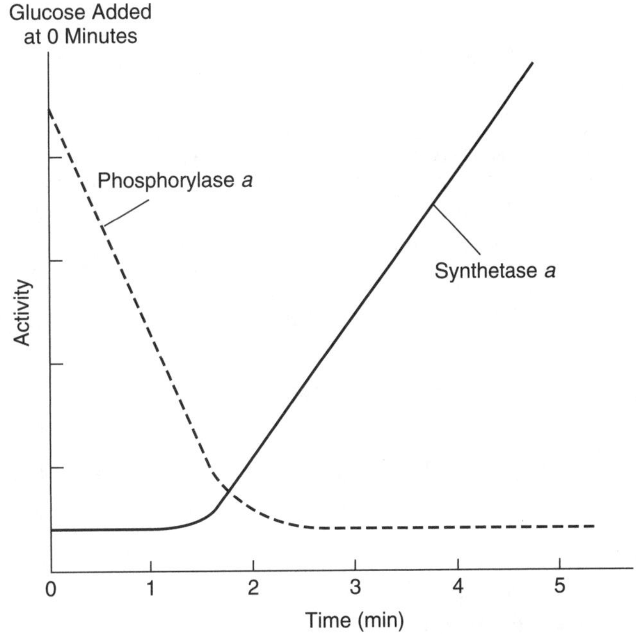

Figure 9-25 Concerted regulation of the activities of glycogen synthase and glycogen phosphorylase. Addition of glucose stimulates the synthase while leading to inhibition of the phosphorylase.

The cascade scheme—that of amplifying a weak initial signal into a massive amount of enzymatic activity—shows up elsewhere in biochemistry. For example, the same pattern of interlocking amplification cycles is seen in fatty acid breakdown and in the clotting of blood.

Coordination of Breakdown with Synthesis

The synthesis and breakdown of glycogen is coordinated: When one process is active, the other is shut off. **Figure 9-25** sketches the relative activities of the two key enzymes as a function of time after glucose is added to the growth medium.

The same hormone signaling system that activates one process inhibits the other. Thus we see the stimulation of synthesis and the inhibition of glycogen breakdown when levels of glucose rise. The signal hormone in this case would be insulin. The opposite pattern might be expected if glucose were low and a surge in epinephrine levels occurred. The rising epinephrine concentration would block glycogen synthesis and stimulate glycogen breakdown. This outcome can be traced back to the opposite effects of phosphorylation on the activities of glycogen synthase (inactive when phosphorylated) and glycogen phosphorylase (active when phosphorylated).

Clinical Application

Nine general types of glycogen storage disease have been identified (**Table 9-3**), all of which are due to defects in one or another enzymatic activity in glycogen synthesis or breakdown. The symptoms can usually be related in a straightforward way to the biochemical consequences of a deficiency in a particular enzyme. Here are a few examples.

(Continued)

Name	Type	Enzyme Deficiency	Tissues Chiefly Affected	Clinical Consequences
Von Gierke's disease	I	Glucose 6-phosphatase, or in transport system in endoplasmic reticulum	Liver, kidney	Severely enlarged liver, severe hypoglycemia, lactic acidosis, ketosis, hyperuricemia, hyperlipidemia
Pompe's disease	II	1,4-D-Glucosidase (lysosomal)	Liver, heart, muscle	Cardiac failure in infancy
Cori's disease	III	Amylo-1,6-glucosidase ("Debranching" enzyme)	Liver, muscle	Similar to type I, but milder
Andersen's disease	IV	"Branching" enzyme	Liver	Liver cirrhosis, death usually before age 24 months
McArdle's disease	V	Phosphorylase	Muscle	Muscle cramps, easily fatigued
Hers' disease	VI	Phosphorylase	Liver	Similar to type I, but milder
Tarui's disease	VII	Phosphofructokinase	Muscle	Similar to type V
	VIII	Phosphorylase kinase	Liver	Enlarged liver, hypoglycemia
	IX	Glycogen synthase	Liver	

Table 9-3 Glycogen Storage Diseases

Pompe's disease is due to a deficiency in a lysosomal glucosidase, also known as "acid maltase." The normal function of lysosomes is to break down proteins and nucleic acids, but they can also take up and digest glycogen. If the lysosomal glucosidase is missing or inactive, a buildup of undigested glycogen will occur inside the lysosomes, which will interfere with their proper digestive functioning. As a result, the whole cell is sickened; worse yet, because lysosomes are found in all types of tissue, all major organ systems can be affected. Pompe's disease appears early after birth, and generally proves fatal by 24 months.

McArdle's disease is caused by a deficiency in glycogen phosphorylase, principally in skeletal muscle. This phosphorylase is responsible for breaking down polymeric glycogen into monomeric glucose (actually, glucose 1-phosphate). If the glycogen phosphorylase activity is missing or inactive, the body will demonstrate a general inability to break down glycogen quickly. As a result, muscle tissue cannot use glycogen as a rapid energy source, and the muscle will depend on other sources of glucose when called upon for a sudden exertion (for example, lifting weights or running a short distance). This results in a buildup of lactic acid, which the affected individual experiences as painful cramps and muscular weakness.

QUESTIONS FOR DISCUSSION

1. Fructose can enter the glycolytic pathway after its conversion to fructose 1-phosphate by the enzyme fructokinase. Suppose you have just drunk a soda flavored with "high fructose corn syrup." What would be the metabolic consequences for serum levels of fructose if there were a deficiency in the activity of fructokinase?
2. Fructokinase in the liver is approximately 10 times faster in phosphorylating fructose than hexokinase is in phosphorylating glucose. Thus, to restore energy quickly to cells, it would seem that fructose would be preferred over glucose. Yet glucose is the preferred sugar for intravenous feeding. Why not use fructose in place of glucose in intravenous feeding?
3. Suppose that the enzyme PFK-1 is fully catalytically active, but does not respond allosterically to levels of ATP or AMP. What would be the metabolic consequences?
4. Explain why a mutation that leads to the complete loss of phosphofructokinase activity would be lethal.
5. Suppose that you were able to construct a bacterial cell line with a modified triose phosphate isomerase that could be allosterically stimulated by AMP and allosterically inhibited by ATP. Discuss how glycolysis and gluconeogenesis could be reciprocally regulated by such an enzyme. Also explain why such a new mutant is unlikely to arise in the wild. (*Hint:* Consider the fluctuating environment experienced by bacteria, especially the levels of oxygen.)
6. Why would a mutation leading to loss of triose phosphate isomerase activity lead to impaired ability to obtain energy from carbohydrates, but not be a lethal mutation?
7. The enzyme fructose-1,6-bisphosphatase-1 (FBPase-1) plays a key role in gluconeogenesis, generating fructose 6-phosphate from fructose 1,6-bisphosphate. What would be the metabolic consequences of a deficiency in the activity of this enzyme?
8. A deficiency in the glycogen debranching enzyme (Cori's disease) is associated with the characteristic symptoms of an enlarged liver, muscular weakness, and hypoglycemia. Explain why these symptoms arise.
9. Suppose that protein phosphatase-1 were mutated so that it no longer recognized and acted on the enzyme glycogen synthase. What would be the consequences?
10. In the synthesis of glycogen, the glycogen synthase uses UDP-glucose, rather than glucose. Explain why.

11. Suppose that a newborn infant is found to be unable to synthesize liver pyruvate kinase. Four clinicians gather around you and suggest the following predominant consequences:

    Clinician A: The infant will not be able to make GTP.

    Clinician B: The infant will not be able to make aspartate from oxaloacetate.

    Clinician C: The infant will produce excessively branched glycogen.

    Clinician D: The infant will have a greatly reduced capacity for glycolysis.

    Who is correct? Briefly explain the reasons for your choice.
12. Explain why lactate fermentation (the reduction of pyruvate to lactate) is especially important for muscle tissue in sustained exertion (e.g., running or swimming long distances). Why would liver cirrhosis compromise an athlete's ability to sustain such activity?
13. Suppose that a tumor of the pancreas resulted in the overproduction of insulin. How might this effect resemble a deficiency in the activity of glucose 6-phosphatase (von Gierke's disease)? What if the tumor resulted in lack of production of glucagon? How might you distinguish among these three cases? Which laboratory tests can you suggest?

REFERENCES

W. S. Bennett, Jr., and T. A. Steitz. (1978). "Glucose-induced conformational change in yeast hexokinase," *Proc. Natl. Acad. Sci. USA* 75:4848–4852.

A. Cornish-Bowden and M. L. Cárdenas. (1991). "Hexokinase and 'glucokinase' in liver metabolism," *Trends Biochem. Sci.* 16:281–282.

D. Fell. (1997). *Understanding the Control of Metabolism*, Portland Press, London.

T. T. Gleeson. (1996). "Post-exercise lactate metabolism: A comparative review of sites, pathways, and regulation," *Annu. Rev. Physiol.* 58:565–581.

H. G. Hers and L. Hue. (1983). "Gluconeogenesis and related aspects of glycolysis," *Annu. Rev. Biochem.* 52:617–653.

H. M. Holden, I. Rayment, and R. B. Thoden. (2003). "Structure and function of enzymes of the Leloir pathway for galactose metabolism," *J. Biol. Chem.* 278:43885–43888.

J. R. Knowles. (1980). "Enzyme-catalyzed phosphoryl transfer reactions," *Annu. Rev. Biochem.* 49:877–919.

R. C. Nordlie, J. D. Foster, and A. J. Lange. (1999). "Regulation of glucose production by the liver," *Annu. Rev. Nutr.* 19:379–406.

S. J. Pilkis and D. K. Granner. (1992). "Molecular physiology of the regulation of hepatic gluconeogenesis and glycolysis," *Annu Rev. Physiol.* 54:885–909.

W. S. Pray. (2000). "Lactose intolerance: The norm among the world's peoples," *Am. J. Pharm. Educ.* 64:205–207.

G. I. Shulman and B. R. Landau. (1992). "Pathways of glycogen repletion," *Physiol. Rev.* 72:1019–1035.

B. Thorens and M. Mueckler. (2990). "Glucose transporters in the 21st century," *Am. J. Physiol. Endocrinol. Metab.* 298:E141–E145.

E. van Schaftingen and I. Gerin. (2002). "The glucose-6-phosphatase system," *Biochem. J.* 362:413–532.

CHAPTER 10

Mitochondria and the Citric Acid Cycle

Learning Objectives

1. Define and use correctly the following terms: *mitochondrial matrix, cristae, mitochondrial porin, VDAC, adenine nucleotide carrier, tricarboxylate carrier, pyruvate dehydrogenase complex, thiamine pyrophosphate (TPP), lipoate, lipoamide, beri-beri, TCA cycle, anaplerosis/anaplerotic cycle, citrate synthase, isocitrate dehydrogenase,* α*-ketoglutarate dehydrogenase, pyruvate carboxylase, biotin, succinate dehydrogenase, three-point attachment model, glycerol phosphate shuttle,* and *malate–aspartate shuttle*.
2. Describe the organization of a typical mitochondrion, listing and locating membranes, enzymes, and important transporter proteins.
3. Describe the adenine nucleotide carrier or ATP-ADP translocase, and explain how it functions. List several other substrate transport systems important for mitochondria.
4. Describe the structure and composition of the pyruvate dehydrogenase complex. Write a scheme for the reactions it catalyzes. Relate the scheme to the structure and composition of the complex.
5. Describe how the pyruvate dehydrogenase complex is regulated. Describe the actions and effects of kinases and phosphatases involved in the regulation. Note other activators and inhibitors involved.
6. State the cellular locations of the enzymes of the TCA cycle. List several of the most important of these enzymes and describe the reactions they catalyze.
7. Diagram the TCA cycle. Name the metabolic intermediates, in correct order, of the TCA cycle. List the TCA cycle intermediates that participate in anaplerotic reactions, as biosynthetic precursors or as derived from compounds other than glucose. Describe how pyruvate can be used to make oxaloacetate; identify the role of biotin in the action of pyruvate carboxylase; and explain the pattern of regulation of this enzyme.
8. Describe generally the regulation of the TCA cycle, noting important activators and inhibitors, and their points of action.
9. Describe the overall function of the TCA cycle in metabolism, and explain its strict requirement for aerobic function. Relate TCA cycle regulation, along with its aerobic requirements, to physiological states.

10. Explain the consequences of a dietary deficiency in thiamine, and relate them to the disease known as beri-beri.
11. Explain how reducing equivalents are transported across the mitochondrial membrane. Diagram the glycerol phosphate shuttle. Relate it to the proper aerobic functioning of the TCA cycle and to aerobic glycolysis.
12. Recognize the structures of thiamine pyrophosphate and lipoic acid. State the metabolic functions of each.

Mitochondria

Mitochondria are the major site for aerobic (requiring molecular oxygen) energy generation in most eukaryotic cells. Muscle tissue and liver cells are generously supplied with mitochondria, because of the demand for energy. However, some cells (e.g., erythrocytes) do not have mitochondria and, therefore, do not use aerobic means for energy generation. Such cells may rely instead on glycolysis for their energy supply.

Mitochondrial Structure

Mitochondria have two lipid bilayer membranes, denoted as outer and inner membranes. The outer membrane is relatively permeable, thanks to the presence many copies of the *mitochondrial porin* protein. This protein forms pores across the outer membrane. Passage of material—specifically, anions such as phosphate as well as carboxylic acids—through the pore is controlled by a transmembrane voltage difference. An alternative name for the porin protein is *voltage-dependent anion channel* (*VDAC*). Such channels are open when the transmembrane voltage is low, but they close at higher voltages and reduce the flux of small ions, ATP, and other solutes.

The inner mitochondrial membrane is not so permeable as the outer membrane; most polar or ionic compounds cannot diffuse across it. Instead, the inner membrane is studded with numerous transmembrane proteins that import or export metabolites, phosphate, protons, and so on. These transporter proteins are specific for the particular molecules they carry across the membrane, as will be discussed later in this chapter. Neutral molecules, such as water, carbon dioxide, and oxygen, can pass through either membrane relatively freely.

Inside the inner membrane is the *mitochondrial matrix*, a cellular compartment containing many of the most important metabolic enzymes for the cell. This matrix contains enzymes of the tricarboxylic acid (TCA) cycle, fatty acid oxidation enzymes, and enzymes responsible for reactions appearing in the urea cycle and in gluconeogenesis (others are located in the cytosol; see **Figure 10-1**). Electron-transport chain proteins are bound to the inner membrane (see Chapter 11 for more details on these proteins). The matrix also contains genetic material (DNA) coding for certain key mitochondrial proteins; this material is complementary to the much greater genetic material found in the cell nucleus.

To increase the surface area available (so that more proteins can be embedded), the inner membrane is tightly folded or pleated, forming structures called *cristae*. The folding also allows close proximity of proteins and substrates to one another, providing greater efficiency in metabolism.

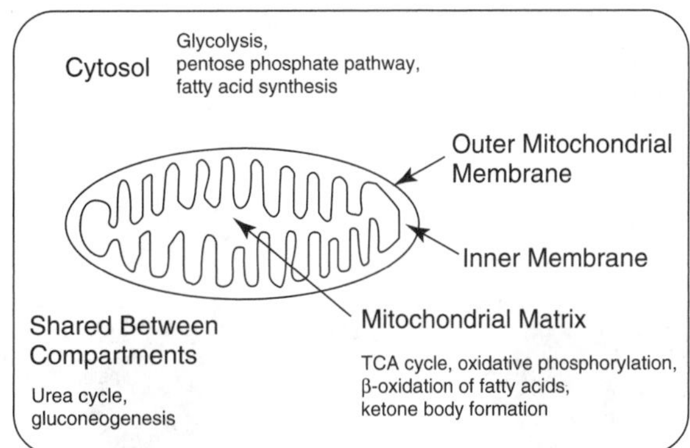

Figure 10-1 Schematized cell with mitochondrion, showing subcellular locations of major metabolic processes.

Substrate Transport Systems

Because the inner membrane is tightly sealed, passage across it is mediated by a number of transmembrane proteins that carry specific metabolites. Among the most important of these substrate transport systems are the following mechanisms:

- A translocase for ATP and ADP (the adenine nucleotide carrier)
- A dicarboxylate carrier, for malate, P_i, succinate, and so on
- A tricarboxylate carrier, primarily for citrate
- A pyruvate carrier
- A glutamate carrier
- The carnitine:acylcarnitine antitransporter
- The phosphate:hydroxide antitransporter

Of special interest are the adenine nucleotide carrier and the tricarboxylate carrier.

Adenine Nucleotide Carrier

ATP is made inside the matrix from ADP and inorganic phosphate (P_i); the phosphate enters through the action of its own distinct transporter system, with exchange of P_i for hydroxide anions (**Figure 10-2**). Transport of ATP and ADP across the inner mitochondrial membrane is the responsibility of the *adenine nucleotide carrier*. The functioning of this carrier (which is also called the translocase) is, of course, important in supplying ATP for the cytosol, from the phosphorylation of ADP inside the matrix. The entrance of ADP into the mitochondrial matrix requires the exit of ATP, which occurs by an antiport mechanism. It is driven by a favorable transmembrane electric potential, featuring movement of a negative charge outward.

Figure 10-3 describes schematically the transport action by the ATP translocase. The diphosphate nucleotide ADP is on the cytosolic side of the membrane, where it was generated when ATP was used up by one or another of the cellular processes (e.g., mechanical work, phosphorylation of proteins). ADP binds to the translocase, and the translocase undergoes a major shape change, "shoving" the ADP through its middle, in a process called eversion. (An umbrella everts, or goes inside-out, in a strong wind; so, too, with the translocase, in a fanciful sense.) The change in shape also reduces the affinity of the translocase for ADP. As a consequence, it releases the ADP to the matrix and will then bind ATP more strongly. Next,

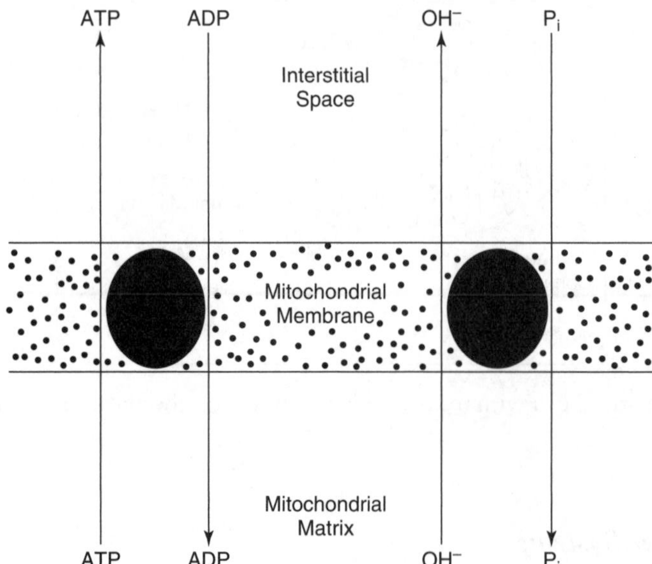

Figure 10-2 Entry of ADP and inorganic phosphate, and export of ATP, across the inner mitochondrial membrane.

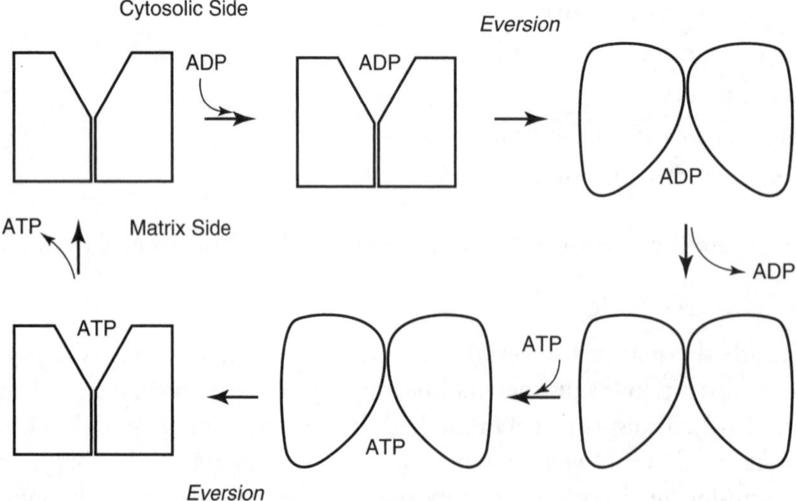

Figure 10-3 The ATP translocase and its eversion mechanism for antiport of ADP and ATP.

the everted translocase picks up a molecule of ATP from the matrix of the mitochondrion. The translocase now reverses its shape change, ejecting the ATP to the cytosolic side of the membrane. It is now ready to repeat the cycle.

The adenine nucleotide carrier is inhibited by the plant natural product atractyloside and by the bacterial toxin bongkrekic acid. Atractyloside binds to the translocase and stabilizes the conformation that binds ADP in preference to ATP; bongkrekic acid stabilizes the other conformation preferentially. In either case, the translocase is inhibited from changing conformation, so it cannot perform its usual duty of antiport of ADP and ATP.

Tricarboxylate Carrier

Reactions inside the matrix generate acetyl-CoA, which can then be used in the cytosol to synthesize fatty acids or sterols. Acetyl-CoA cannot itself cross the inner mitochondrial membrane. Instead, it is converted to citrate (by a reaction in the TCA cycle), and the citrate is exported to the cytosol, where it is cleaved to acetyl-CoA and oxaloacetate. The *tricarboxylate carrier* is responsible for exporting the citrate, in exchange for a dicarboxylate anion such as malate.

Citrate in the cytosol can also serve as an indirect measure of the energy state of the cell. In this role, it can act on certain cytosolic enzymes as an allosteric effector. For example, see the later material on the regulation of acetyl-CoA carboxylase, which affects the biosynthesis of fatty acids.

Pyruvate Dehydrogenase

Overview

Pyruvate is formed in the cytosol during glycolysis. It then enters the mitochondrial matrix, crossing the inner mitochondrial membrane by action of a special transmembrane protein, the pyruvate transporter protein. This process involves symport with protons. Once inside the matrix, under aerobic conditions the pyruvate is oxidized to acetyl-CoA in an oxidative decarboxylation:

$$\text{Pyruvate} + \text{NAD}^+ + \text{CoASH} \rightarrow \text{Acetyl-S-CoA} + \text{NADH} + \text{H}^+ + \text{CO}_2$$

$$\Delta G'^{\circ} = -33.4 \text{ kJ/mol} \qquad (10\text{-}1)$$

This central reaction of catabolism is catalyzed by the enzyme pyruvate dehydrogenase, an enzyme that is highly regulated. The large negative free energy change here shows that the product side of this reaction is highly favored. Note the generation of carbon dioxide and the role of the nicotinamide. The reduced nicotinamide generated here will later be oxidized, and the free energy released through this process will be captured for ATP synthesis; see Chapter 11.

The Pyruvate Dehydrogenase Complex

The *pyruvate dehydrogenase complex* is a very complex enzyme, with multiple subunits, a number of sequential reactions, and complex regulation. Much of what we know about it comes from studies of bacterial forms of the enzyme, but the human enzyme performs the same reactions and is regulated in a similar way.

In both prokaryotic and eukaryotic forms, the enzyme has the cofactors thiamine pyrophosphate (TPP), lipoic acid, and FAD bound quite tightly. It also acts on coenzyme A and NAD^+ (which are more loosely associated with the enzyme). There are three distinguishable types of subunits and three types of enzymatic activities, each associated with a different subunit.

For the enzyme from *E. coli*, the intact bacterial enzyme complex is extremely large, with a molecular weight of 5×10^6 daltons. The bacterial enzyme has 60 polypeptide chains, of three different types. There are 24 copies of the E_1 subunit type, 24 copies of the E_2 subunit type, and 12 copies of the E_3 subunit type. The human enzyme is somewhat different and a bit more complicated than the bacterial form. For example, in humans the E_1 subunit is actually composed of two types of polypeptide chains, α and β. Further, associated protein kinases and phosphatases help to regulate the activity of the enzyme by reversible phosphorylation. The entire complex is located inside the inner mitochondrial membrane. Depending on the source, the number of each type of subunit can vary, but there are certainly many copies of each subunit in the complex; total molecular weights of the whole eukaryotic enzyme assembly can be in the range of 7 million to 8.5 million.

The many subunits have close contacts with one another—a factor that is thought to help coordinate the action of the enzyme's different chemical actions by passing substrate from one subunit to the next and to help with allosteric regulation transmitted across interfaces between subunits. **Figure 10-4** illustrates the arrangement of the subunits in the bacterial form of the complex.

The general reaction catalyzed by this enzyme, an oxidative decarboxylation, is also seen with two other important enzymes: α-ketoglutarate dehydrogenase and branched-chain α-keto acid dehydrogenase (BCADH). The three enzymes are evolutionarily related, use the same cofactors, and employ the same general mechanism. α-Ketoglutarate dehydrogenase appears in the TCA cycle, and BCADH is important in amino acid metabolism.

Regulation of the Complex

The pyruvate dehydrogenase complex, its substrate pyruvate, and the product acetyl-CoA occur at the junction of several important metabolic pathways (**Figure 10-5**):

- Glycolysis, which produces pyruvate
- The tricarboxylic acid cycle, which consumes the product, acetyl-CoA, of the pyruvate dehydrogenase enzyme
- The transamination of pyruvate to alanine, and the reverse reaction, giving a link to amino acid metabolism
- The carboxylation of pyruvate to form oxaloacetate, a key intermediate in the tricarboxylic acid cycle

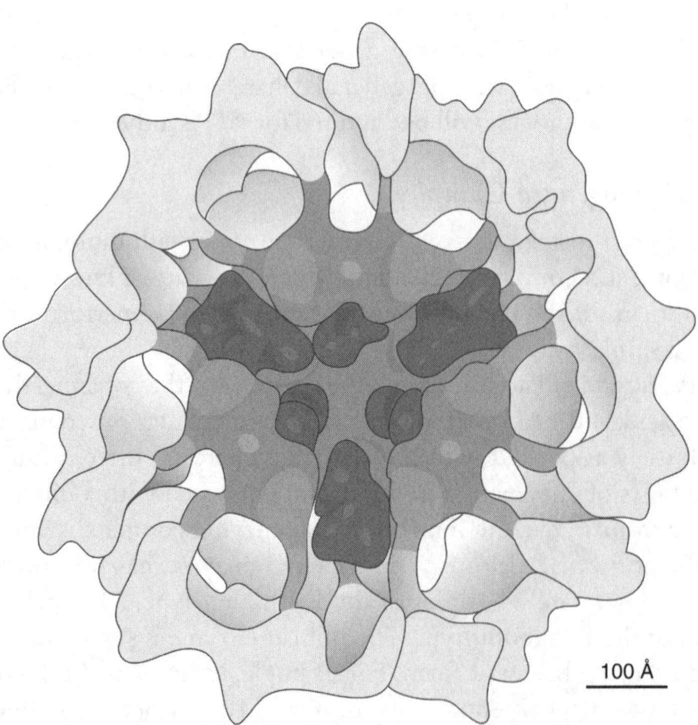

Figure 10-4 Cutaway view of the pyruvate dehydrogenase complex from *Azotobacter vinelandii*; the mammalian form of the complex is similar in structure. E_1 subunits are light gray, E_2 subunits are intermediate gray, and E_3 subunits are dark gray.

Source: Adapted with permission from Z. H. Zhou et al. (2001). "The remarkable structural and functional organization of the eukaryotic pyruvate dehydrogenase complexes," *Proc. Natl. Acad. Sci. USA* 98:14802–14807. Copyright 2001 National Academy of Sciences, U.S.A.

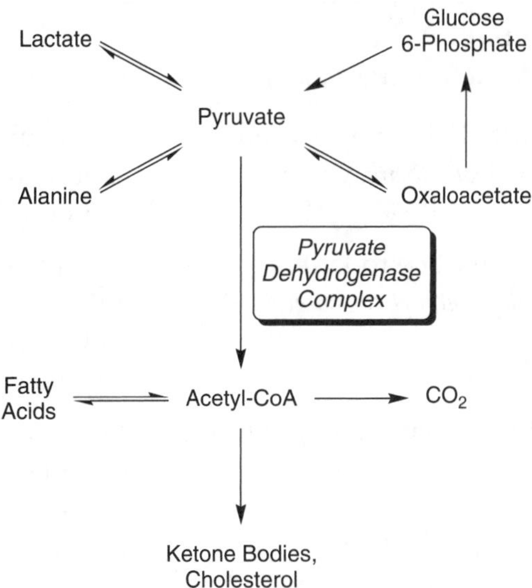

Figure 10-5 The central role in metabolism of the pyruvate dehydrogenase complex in converting pyruvate to acetyl-CoA.

It is very important for the cell to control the activity of the complex to coordinate all of these paths properly. Control of this enzyme complex is exerted in several ways:

- The AMP/ATP ratio allosterically regulates E_1 activity, producing sensitivity to the energy charge of the cell.
- The CoASH/acetyl-CoA ratio regulates E_2, so the enzyme is sensitive to demands for CoA or acetyl-CoA in other pathways.
- The NAD^+/NADH ratio regulates E_3, making the enzyme sensitive to the cell's redox balance.
- Cooperative, allosteric interactions from one type of subunit to another help to coordinate the overall activity of the complex and permit exact "fine-tuning" of its activity.
- Calcium ions stimulate the activity of the complex; Ca^{2+} is a common second messenger used to stimulate the general energy-producing pathways inside the cell.
- Phosphorylation (at high ATP levels) by specific kinases will inhibit the enzyme reversibly; dephosphorylation by specific phosphatases will activate the enzyme. Overall, this makes it sensitive to the energy charge.

Thus the enzyme is sensitive to both the energy charge of the cell and the oxidation–reduction state of the cell, while balancing its activity against demands for acetyl-CoA elsewhere in the cell.

Coenzymes and Prosthetic Groups of the Complex

Table 10-1 summarizes the various coenzymes or prosthetic groups used by the pyruvate dehydrogenase complex, noting which subunits are responsible for which catalytic activity. Two of these cofactors have not previously been introduced: thiamine and lipoic acid.

Thiamine

Thiamine from the diet is converted to *thiamine pyrophosphate* (*TPP*; **Figure 10-6**), then bound tightly as a prosthetic group in several enzymes (e.g., pyruvate dehydrogenase, α-ketoglutarate

Coenzyme or Prosthetic Group	Subunit (Attachment/*Name*)	Function of Subunit/ Coenzyme/Group
TPP	E_1 (tight but noncovalent) (*pyruvate decarboxylase*)	Nucleophilic attack on pyruvate, expulsion of CO_2, formation of hydroxyethyl group
Lipoic acid	E_2 (attached to Lys) (*dihydrolipoyl transacetylase*)	Accept acetyl group from TPP, pass it on to CoA and regenerate TPP (act as intermediate electron carrier)
Coenzyme A	Free in solution (binds to E_2)	Accept acetyl group from lipoamide, generate reduced lipoamide (act as intermediate electron carrier)
FAD	E_3 (tight but noncovalent) (*dihydrolipoyl dehydrogenase*)	Accept electrons from reduced lipoamide, transfer them to NAD^+
NAD^+	Free in solution (binds to E_3)	Accept electrons from $FADH_2$ and regenerate FAD

Table 10-1 Cofactors and Subunits of the Pyruvate Dehydrogenase Complex

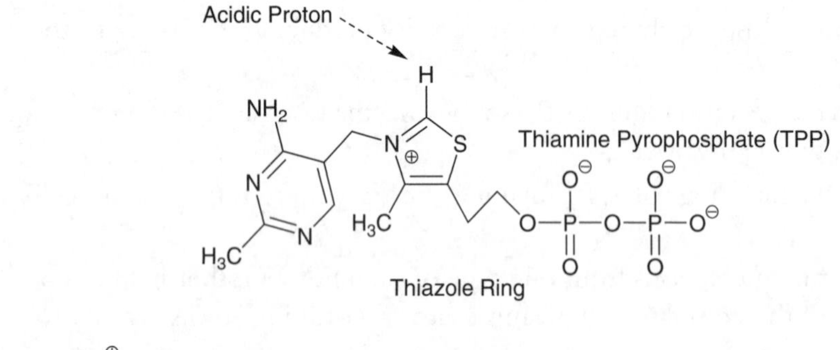

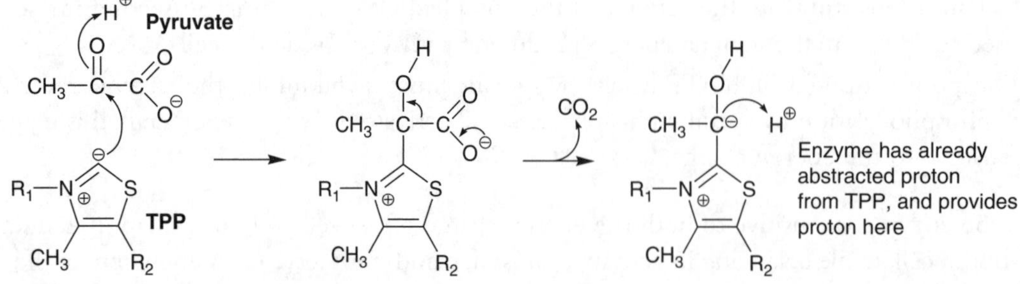

Figure 10-6 Structure of thiamine pyrophosphate (TPP), showing the acidic carbon of the thiazole ring, with details of the thiazole carbanion attack on pyruvate.

dehydrogenase, and transketolase). It helps in many different reactions. Broadly speaking, it plays two major roles, in the following processes:

- Degradation of α-keto acids, as with the enzymes pyruvate dehydrogenase and α-ketoglutarate dehydrogenase, via either non-oxidative decarboxylation or oxidative decarboxylation
- Transketolization (in connection with reactions of carbohydrates; see Chapter 12)

Enzyme	Function or Pathway
Transketolase	Pentose phosphate path; make ribose and generate NADPH
Pyruvate dehydrogenase complex	Prepare carbohydrates for entry to TCA cycle
α-Ketoglutarate dehydrogenase	TCA cycle; energy extraction
Branched-chain amino acid dehydrogenase	Amino acid catabolism

Table 10-2 Enzymes Using Thiamine Pyrophosphate as a Cofactor

TPP carries what are effectively activated aldehyde groups (α-hydroxylated alkyl groups) and participates in their transfer. The thiazole ring has an easily removed proton, whose departure leaves behind a very nucleophilic carbanion. This carbanion can readily attack carbonyl groups, such as those in aldehydes or ketones.

In the pyruvate dehydrogenase complex, the TPP acts on pyruvate. Figure 10-6 shows the attack on pyruvate's α-keto group. This action leads to a facile decarboxylation and a remaining carbanion that extracts a proton from a neighboring acidic group on the protein, giving hydroxyethyl TPP, an activated form of acetaldehyde.

Table 10-2 lists some enzymes that use TPP as a cofactor and describes its uses.

Lipoic Acid

Lipoic acid serves as an acyl carrier and as a two-electron carrier in the oxidative decarboxylation of α-keto acids (**Figure 10-7**). It accepts the aldehyde intermediate from TPP and oxidizes

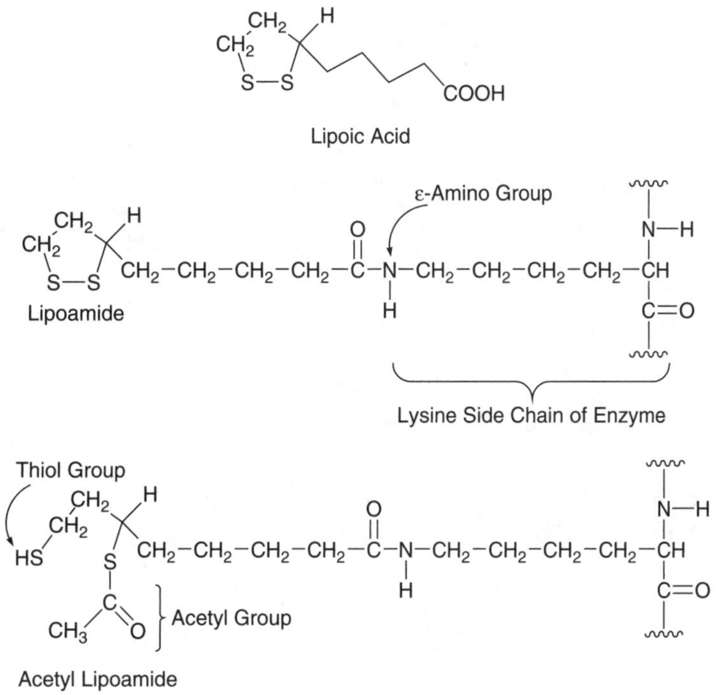

Lipoic Acid

ε-Amino Group

Lipoamide

Lysine Side Chain of Enzyme

Thiol Group

Acetyl Group

Acetyl Lipoamide

Figure 10-7 Structure of lipoic acid, the enzyme-bound lipoamide, and acetyl lipoamide.

it to what is effectively a carboxylic acid. In the case of the pyruvate dehydrogenase complex, this acyl group has only two carbons (making it an acetyl group). Lipoic acid also is important in fatty acid metabolism, in which it carries longer carbon chains. Lipoic acid is held on these enzymes by a covalent link—that is, an amide bond formed from the carboxyl group of lipoic acid and the ϵ-amino group of a particular lysine residue on the enzyme. Because it is held so tightly by the enzyme, it is considered to be a prosthetic group.

Lipoic acid or *lipoate* is the oxidized form of the free compound. Note the disulfide linkage here. When the compound is linked to an enzyme, it is referred to as *lipoamide*. When the enzyme-bound form is reduced and two thiol groups are formed from the disulfide group, it is called dihydrolipoamide. When an acyl group is attached, it becomes an acyl lipoamide (e.g., acetyl lipoamide).

Reaction Scheme for the Pyruvate Dehydrogenase Complex

Figure 10-8 summarizes schematically the reactions catalyzed by the pyruvate dehydrogenase complex. Subunit E_1 uses TPP to bind and activate pyruvate, in an oxidative decarboxylation. CO_2 leaves, but the remaining two carbons are bound to the TPP. Subunit E_2 contains a flexible lipoic acid group, covalently attached in the lipoamide form, that can make contact with multiple points within the complex. It swings the lipoamide group over to the site on E_1 where the TPP is holding the activated two-carbon fragment. The fragment is transferred to the lipoamide, and the TPP cofactor is regenerated, ready for another catalytic round. Next, the acyl lipoamide swings over to an adjacent site on E_2 where the two-carbon fragment is transferred to a waiting molecule of coenzyme A; the acyl-CoA is released and the reduced lipoamide chain swings over to a site on subunit E_3. On E_3, a redox reaction occurs using a bound flavin (FAD), which regenerates the oxidized form of lipoamide and readies it for another round of catalysis. The resulting $FADH_2$ is reoxidized on the E_3 subunit at the expense of a molecule of NAD^+, and the reduced nicotinamide is released to the mitochondrial matrix.

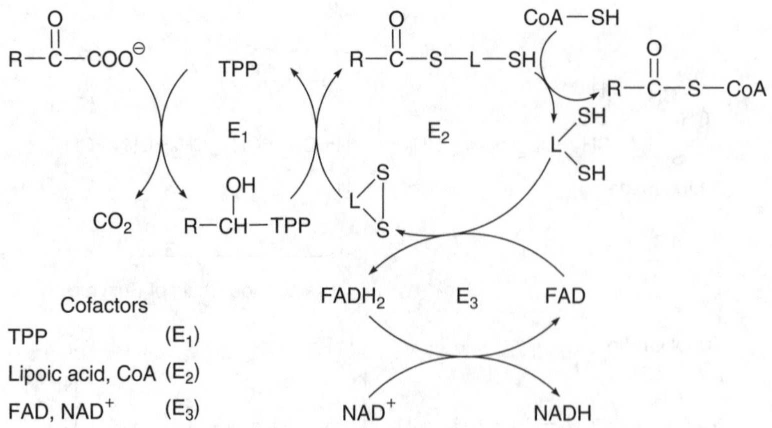

$R{-}C({=}O){-}COO^{\ominus}$ → (TPP, E_1) → CO_2 + $R{-}CH(OH){-}TPP$

$R{-}CH(OH){-}TPP$ + $L(S{-}S)$ → (E_2) → $R{-}C({=}O){-}S{-}L{-}SH$ + TPP

$R{-}C({=}O){-}S{-}L{-}SH$ + $CoA{-}SH$ → $R{-}C({=}O){-}S{-}CoA$ + $L(SH)_2$

$L(SH)_2$ + FAD → (E_3) → $L(S{-}S)$ + $FADH_2$

$FADH_2$ + NAD^+ → (E_3) → FAD + NADH

Cofactors

TPP	(E_1)
Lipoic acid, CoA	(E_2)
FAD, NAD^+	(E_3)

Figure 10-8 Reaction scheme for the pyruvate dehydrogenase complex.

Clinical Application

Beri-Beri

The disease known as *beri-beri* is due to a deficiency of thiamine (vitamin B_1) in the diet. This deficiency causes both neurologic and cardiovascular symptoms, including edema and heart enlargement. Beri-beri is still a health problem in some parts of Asia, and with malnourished populations in the Western world (especially with alcoholics). TPP is a prosthetic group in PDH, α-ketoglutarate dehydrogenase, and transketolase; these are key enzymes in carbohydrate metabolism. TPP is also found in BCADH, where it plays a role in amino acid metabolism. In beri-beri, we find high serum levels of pyruvate and α-ketoglutarate. Note how the Crossover Theorem can be applied here: Because the reactions that consume these compounds are blocked (by the absence of the necessary TPP), the body accumulates the reactants. The condition can be diagnosed by the low activity of transketolase (which requires TPP) in red blood cells.

Deficiencies in Activity of the PDH Complex

If the enzymatic activity of this enzyme is blocked or reduced, what will happen? The Crossover Theorem can be used here to make some qualitative predictions. For example, because pyruvate is not being acted on by the PDH complex, higher pyruvate levels should be found in serum. Also, higher alanine levels should be observed (because of the interconversion of this amino acid and its corresponding α-keto acid, pyruvate). There will likely be a general upset in energy production. The brain is especially sensitive to cellular energy levels; glycolysis by itself does not generate enough ATP to supply brain cells, and these cells depend on the further metabolism of pyruvate for adequate energy. Thus mental retardation and neurological upsets are very possible if this enzyme's activity is inhibited.

The Citric Acid or Tricarboxylic Acid Cycle

General Remarks

The *TCA cycle* lies between glycolysis (hence the appearance of pyruvate entering the cycle) and the electron transport system used in oxidative phosphorylation (discussed in the next chapter). It is connected to several other metabolic pathways as well. The TCA cycle is a central feature of living cells.

Figure 10-9 is a canonical representation of the TCA cycle, including the entry reaction catalyzed by the pyruvate dehydrogenase complex and the carboxylation reaction that connects pyruvate to the TCA cycle intermediate, oxaloacetate. **Table 10-3** lists the key enzymes by number and name, and notes the corresponding reaction.

Overall, two carbon atoms enter as an acetyl unit; two different carbon atoms leave as CO_2 (CO_2 can readily diffuse across membranes, and so exit from mitochondria). A total of eight electrons are extracted by redox reactions, in the form of three reduced nicotinamides and a reduced flavin. Also, a phosphoanhydride bond is generated for each turn of the cycle. Don't

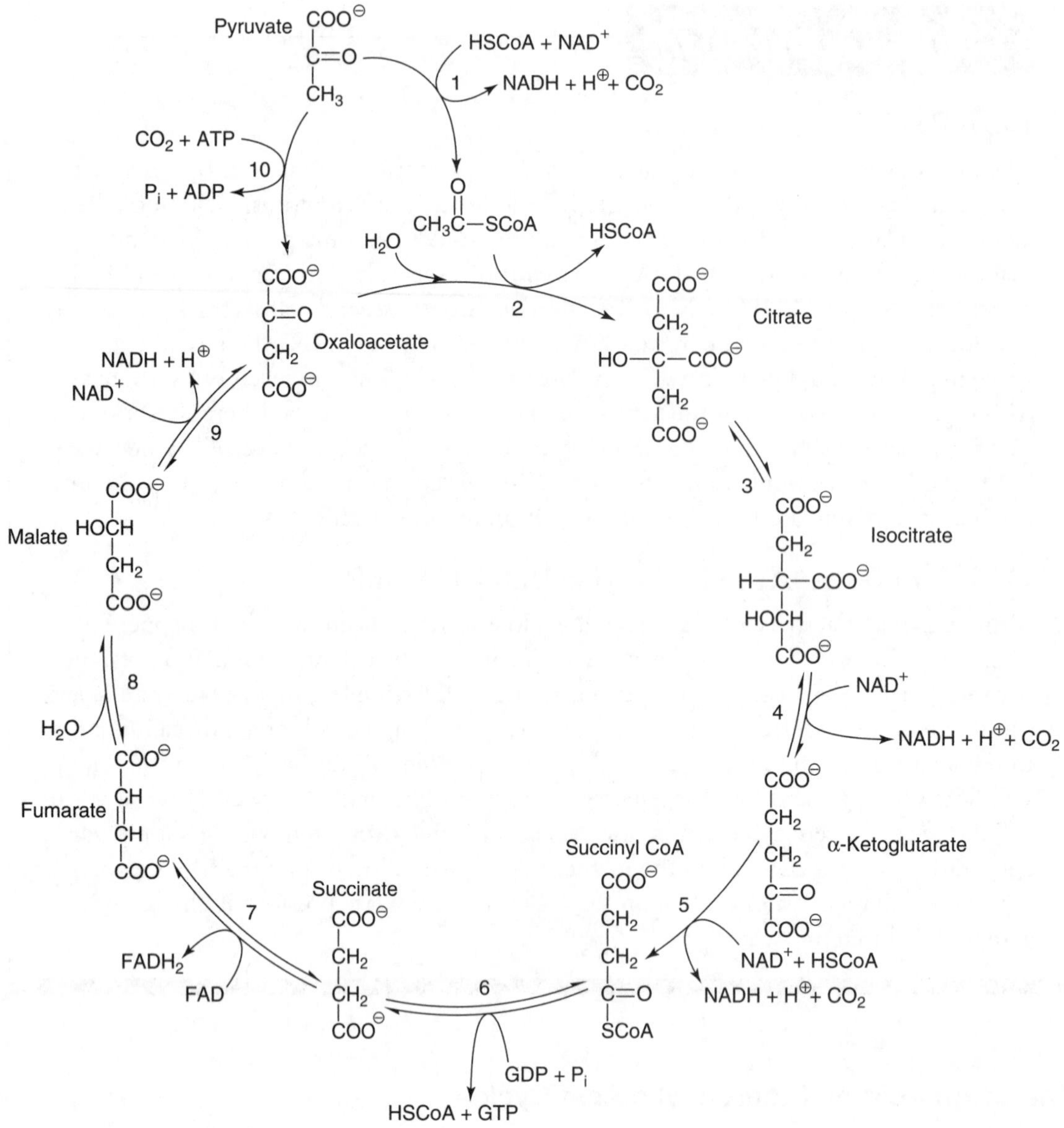

Figure 10-9 The tricarboxylic acid (TCA) cycle—also known as the Krebs or citric acid cycle—with associated reactions.

Reaction Number	Enzyme	Reaction Catalyzed
1*	Pyruvate dehydrogenase	Oxidation of pyruvate to acetyl-CoA; co-generation of NADH from NAD^+
2	Citrate synthase	Condensation of oxaloacetate with acetyl-CoA
3	Aconitase	Isomerization of citrate to isocitrate

Table 10-3 Enzymes in or Associated with the TCA Cycle

*These steps from Figure 10-9 are not, strictly speaking, in the TCA cycle proper, but they are closely associated with it.

Reaction Number	Enzyme	Reaction Catalyzed
4	Isocitrate dehydrogenase	Oxidative decarboxylation of isocitrate to α-ketoglutarate; co-generation of NADH from NAD^+
5	α-Ketoglutarate dehydrogenase	Oxidative decarboxylation of α-ketoglutarate to succinyl-CoA; co-generation of NADH from NAD^+
6	Succinate thiokinase	Hydrolysis of thioester to release succinate from succinyl-CoA; co-generation of GTP from GDP
7	Succinate dehydrogenase	Oxidation of succinate to fumarate; flavoprotein is subsequently regenerated by reduction of coenzyme Q
8	Fumarase	Hydration of fumarate to give malate
9	Malate dehydrogenase	Oxidation of malate to oxaloacetate; co-generation of NADH from NAD^+
10*	Pyruvate carboxylase	Carboxylation of pyruvate to give oxaloacetate, with consumption of ATP

Table 10-3 Enzymes in or Associated with the TCA Cycle (Continued)

*These steps from Figure 10-9 are not, strictly speaking, in the TCA cycle proper, but they are closely associated with it.

be misled by the depiction of an apparently closed circle in Figure 10-9. There is a net flux of matter (atoms and electrons) through the TCA cycle.

Note the use of NAD^+ (reactions 1, 4, 5, and 9) and FAD (reaction 7) in oxidations. Their presence implies that the TCA cycle operates aerobically; there must be adequate oxygen supplied to the cell to regenerate the pool of NAD^+ that is inside the mitochondrion. This aerobic requirement of the TCA cycle will be discussed later. Also, note the point of generation of a "high energy bond" (a phosphoanhydride), using GTP and not ATP. This phosphoanhydride is energetically equivalent to ATP, however, and can be used to rephosphorylate ADP to make ATP.

Most reactions in the cycle are readily reversible. The two exceptions have large negative ΔG values. These are citrate synthesis and succinyl-CoA synthesis—more on these reactions later.

In eukaryotes, the enzymes of the TCA cycle are located in mitochondria, inside the inner mitochondrial membrane. Succinate dehydrogenase is embedded in the inner mitochondrial membrane; this enzyme will reappear in the discussion of oxidative phosphorylation in Chapter 11.

Regulation

There are several major control points within the TCA cycle (**Figure 10-10**), but no single one can be identified as the single most important point. The control points are as follows:

- The synthesis of citrate from acetyl-CoA and oxaloacetate. This reaction has a large negative $\Delta G'^{\circ}$, which makes it (nearly) irreversible. The enzyme involved is *citrate synthase*. This enzyme is activated by ADP and is inhibited by ATP, citrate, NADH, and succinyl-CoA. Under conditions in vivo, the rate of reaction is usually set by the availability of substrate,

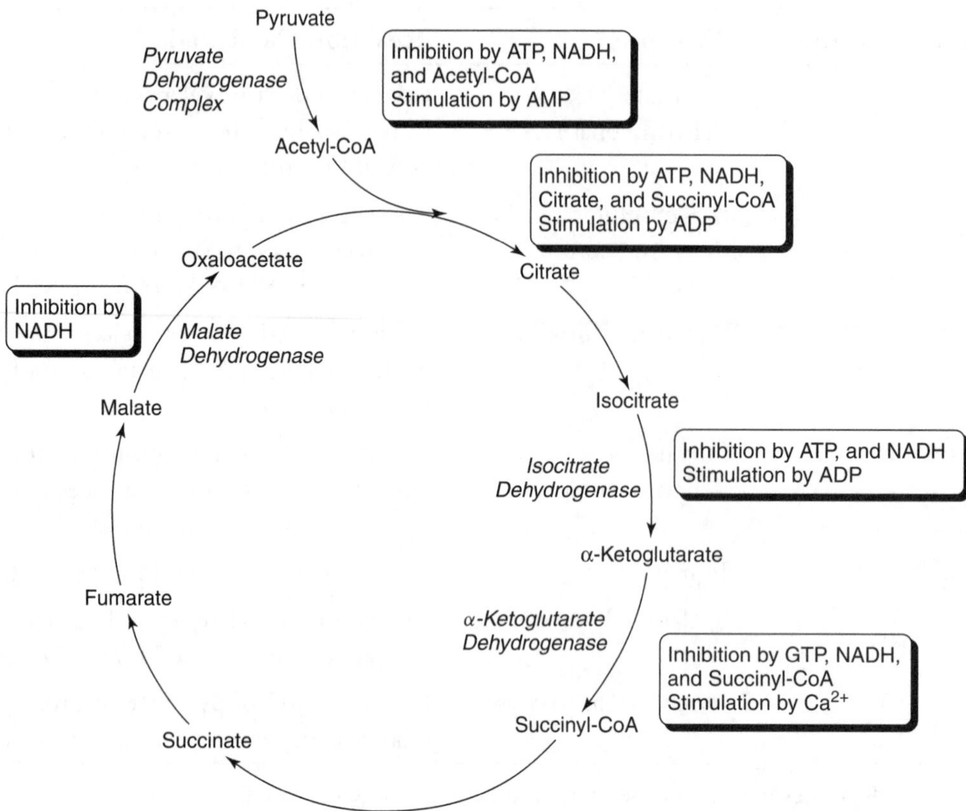

Figure 10-10 Regulation of the TCA cycle.

especially oxaloacetate. Product (that is, citrate) is drawn off by the succeeding TCA cycle reactions almost immediately.

- The conversion of isocitrate to α-ketoglutarate by *isocitrate dehydrogenase*. This enzyme is activated by ADP but inhibited by ATP. The reaction is reversible in vivo, although $\Delta G'^{\circ} = -8$ kJ/mol.
- The conversion of α-ketoglutarate to succinyl-CoA by *α-ketoglutarate dehydrogenase*. This enzyme is inhibited by the product of the reaction, succinyl-CoA, as well as by NADH and GTP. It is activated by calcium ions, Ca^{2+}. This reaction, like the formation of citrate, has a very negative free energy change, so it, too, is nearly irreversible.

Additionally, the TCA cycle is under hormonal control, specifically through thyroid hormones and glucocorticoids. Thyroid hormones generally increase the concentration of Ca^{2+} in mitochondria, which stimulates the activity of α-ketoglutarate dehydrogenase and so increases turnover in the cycle. Thyroid hormones and glucocorticoids also stimulate mitochondrial biogenesis, leading to an overall greater rate of metabolism for cells in the target tissues.

Selected Reactions of the TCA Cycle

Citrate Formation

$$\text{Acetyl-CoA} + \text{Oxaloacetate} + H_2O \rightarrow \text{Citrate} + \text{CoASH}$$

$$\Delta G'^{\circ} = -32.2 \text{ kJ/mol} \qquad (10\text{-}2)$$

Citrate synthase is the catalyst here. The reaction has a Claisen condensation mechanism. The reaction is basically the nucleophilic attack of a carbanion/enolate on the $(\delta+)$ carbon of a carbonyl group. The net result is a C_2 molecule combined with a C_4 molecule, leading to a C_6 molecule.

There is actually an intermediate formed in this reaction, citroyl-CoA, which is not shown; the thioester linkage in this intermediate compound is hydrolyzed by the enzyme immediately after its formation, and the coenzyme and citrate are released to solution. The large negative free energy change is associated with the thioester hydrolysis and release of the CoA moiety; recall that hydrolysis of thioesters is energetically very favorable.

This reaction is sometimes referred to as the "primary pacemaker step," as its rate determines the availability of substrate for succeeding reactions in the cycle. The rate is determined mainly by the availability of acetyl-CoA and oxaloacetate. As noted previously, the enzyme is stimulated by ADP and inhibited by NADH, ATP, citrate, and succinyl-CoA, so it is sensitive to the energy and redox state of the cell, as well as to the abundance of intermediates in the TCA cycle.

The reaction has $\Delta G'^{\circ} = -32.2$ kJ/mol, so it is essentially an irreversible reaction. The release of free energy here draws material from glycolysis (e.g., pyruvate, through the intermediate acetyl-CoA) into the TCA cycle; it also helps to overcome the low natural concentration of oxaloacetate, which would tend to hinder the reaction. This is a rather clever exploitation of what would seem to be "inefficiency" in free energy conservation.

Oxidative Decarboxylation of Isocitrate

$$\text{Isocitrate} + \text{NAD}^+ \rightarrow \alpha\text{-Ketoglutarate} + \text{CO}_2 + \text{NADH} + \text{H}^+$$
$$\Delta G'^{\circ} = -8.4 \text{ kJ/mol} \qquad (10\text{-}3)$$

This reaction is catalyzed by the allosteric enzyme isocitrate dehydrogenase. The binding curve for isocitrate is sigmoidal, indicating positive cooperativity in binding this substrate. The enzyme is inhibited by NADH and ATP, but activated by ADP and Ca^{2+}. Thus it is sensitive to the energy charge of the cell, and this sensitivity helps the cell to maintain its energy supply.

Carboxylation of Pyruvate to Oxaloacetate

$$\text{Pyruvate} + \text{HCO}_3^- + \text{ATP} \rightarrow \text{Oxaloacetate} + \text{ADP} + \text{P}_i \qquad (10\text{-}4)$$

Although this reaction is not itself a part of the TCA cycle, it is intimately connected with it, so we consider it here as effectively a part of the cycle. The carboxylation of pyruvate to form oxaloacetate is catalyzed by *pyruvate carboxylase* (a tetrameric enzyme with four identical subunits) and involves the prosthetic group *biotin* (**Figure 10-11**).

The carboxylation reaction occurs in stages. The first stage is the formation of carboxyphosphate, using bicarbonate and ATP, and generation of carboxybiotin. Here the terminal phosphate group of the ATP is combined with the bicarbonate to form an unstable intermediate, carboxyphosphate (along with ADP), and the carboxyphosphate donates the CO_2 to a nearby biotin moiety to form N^1-carboxybiotin. This activates the carboxyl group for a further transfer reaction.

The second stage is the transfer of the activated carboxyl group onto the substrate pyruvate. It involves a movement of the biotin to place the attached carboxyl group next to a pyruvate molecule bound to a neighboring subunit of the enzyme. In this second active site on the second subunit, the CO_2 is released and the biotin abstracts a proton from the pyruvate molecule to generate pyruvate enolate; the CO_2 then reacts with this enolate and forms the product oxaloacetate.

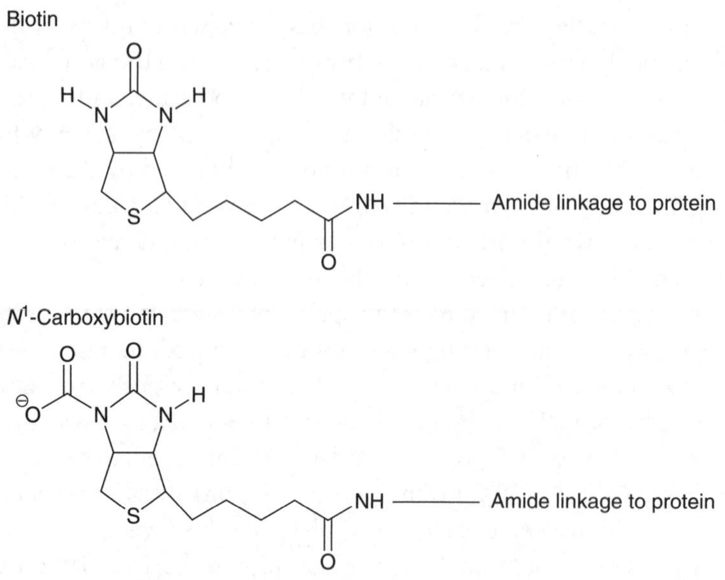

Biotin

NH —— Amide linkage to protein

N^1-Carboxybiotin

NH —— Amide linkage to protein

Figure 10-11 Structures of biotin and carboxylated biotin.

Pyruvate carboxylase is an allosteric enzyme; it is activated by the allosteric effector acetyl-CoA. When supplies of acetyl-CoA are high, this enzyme becomes very active and helps funnel material into the TCA cycle, building up the pool of oxaloacetate. This then helps the cell to make energy (ATP) more rapidly. The reaction is reversible, however, so that there is the possibility of decarboxylating oxaloacetate and forming pyruvate from it.

Biotin is sometimes called vitamin H. The biotin prosthetic group is commonly used to carry activated carboxyl groups. Another important enzyme that uses biotin is acetyl-CoA carboxylase, which catalyzes the formation of malonyl-CoA from acetyl-CoA. This step is a key reaction in the synthesis of fatty acids (see Chapter 13).

Another important route by which oxaloacetate may be formed is through the carboxylation of phospho*enol*pyruvate. This reaction is catalyzed by a different enzyme than the one that operates on pyruvate, however. This alternative route is another way by which the pool of oxaloacetate can be maintained.

Oxidation of α-Ketoglutarate to Succinyl-CoA

$$\alpha\text{-Ketoglutarate} + NAD^+ + CoA \rightarrow \text{Succinyl-CoA} + NADH + CO_2 + H^+$$

$$\Delta G'^\circ = -33.5 \text{ kJ/mol} \qquad (10\text{-}5)$$

This reaction is catalyzed by the α-ketoglutarate dehydrogenase complex (see the earlier discussion of the pyruvate dehydrogenase enzyme complex; there is a strong resemblance between the two enzymes). The overall reaction is analogous to the oxidation of pyruvate to acetyl-CoA and CO_2. The CO_2 leaves the mitochondrion by diffusion. The enzyme here uses the same general mechanism as pyruvate dehydrogenase and the same coenzymes and prosthetic groups.

The enzyme is inhibited by NADH and succinyl-CoA, and is stimulated by Ca^{2+}. The calcium ion signals a general need for more ATP to be made, here serving as an activator of the enzyme. Because NADH and succinyl-CoA are products of the reaction, it is reasonable that when their levels are high, their production should be inhibited.

Note that the product, succinyl-CoA, has high energy thioester bond. This bond will be broken in the next step of the cycle, in the formation of succinate from succinyl-CoA, where the energy is conserved in the form of a phosphoanhydride (as GTP).

Oxidation of Succinate to Fumarate

$$\text{Succinate} + \text{FAD} \rightleftharpoons \text{Fumarate} + \text{FADH}_2$$

$$\Delta G'^{\circ} = 0 \text{ kJ/mol} \qquad (10\text{-}6)$$

This is a reversible reaction, with the oxidation of succinate just balancing the reduction of the flavin group. Although not enough free energy is released in oxidizing succinate to drive the reduction of nicotinamide cofactors, the amount is sufficient for reduction of flavins.

The reaction is catalyzed by *succinate dehydrogenase,* a flavoprotein carrying a covalently bound FAD. This enzyme is bound to the inner mitochondrial membrane and catalyzes a dehydrogenation reaction. Succinate dehydrogenase will appear again in the discussion of oxidative phosphorylation in Chapter 11, where the regeneration of the oxidized flavin will be explained.

Clinical Application

Succinate dehydrogenase (SDH) is a complex formed from four distinct subunits. Subunit A (SDHA) has the active site for conversion of succinate to fumarate; this subunit is a flavoprotein using FAD. Subunit B (SDHB) works with subunits C (SDHC) and D (SDHD) to transfer electrons from the $FADH_2$ formed in the succinate-to-fumarate reaction to an enzyme complex in the electron transport chain (complex II; see Chapter 11). A deficiency in the activity of succinate dehydrogenase is rare but can be quite serious; most of these defects are caused by mutations in SDHA. The symptoms of SDH activity deficiency resemble those of defects in the electron transport chain (not surprising, in view of the close connection of this enzyme to those respiratory complexes), and include neurological and developmental problems. Defects in the other three subunits have been found to be involved in tumor development, specifically in benign, slow-growing tumors of the adrenal gland and related tissues. Interestingly, mutations in the gene for fumarase can also predispose individuals toward development of tumors—specifically uterine and/or cutaneous growths.

Three-Point Attachment Model

The original experiments on the fates of carbon atoms in the TCA cycle gave confusing results. Using ^{14}C-labeled acetate, with the label in the carboxyl group, the expected distribution of the ^{14}C label was half in the α-carboxyl of α-ketoglutarate, and half in the γ-carboxyl, due to the symmetry of the intermediate citrate molecule (isocitrate and α-ketoglutarate are not symmetric molecules). However, all of the label appeared in the γ-carboxyl of α-ketoglutarate. Apparently, in the conversion of citrate to isocitrate, the aconitase enzyme was able to tell one end of a symmetric molecule (citrate) from the other!

How could an enzyme distinguish one end of citrate from the other? The enzyme's surface has three non-equivalent sites: one for binding the OH, one for binding a simple carboxylate, and one for binding an acetate (**Figure 10-12**). Citrate is not optically active, but it can bind to the surface in only one way if it is to make all three contacts simultaneously (the *three-point attachment model*). When bound, the (A) and (B) groups are not sterically equivalent, so (A) and (B) can have different metabolic fates; this discrepancy explains how the aconitase could apparently distinguish one end of a citrate from the other.

The three-point attachment model has been widely used in pharmacology to explain differences in the behavior of stereoisomers of a drug. Having multiple simultaneous contacts of a complex organic molecule with a protein or enzyme may be an important feature in recognition and differential binding of such stereoisomers by receptors. In particular, it may be especially important if one isomer differs in activity from the other.

Anaplerotic Cycle's Role in Biosynthesis

The TCA cycle is connected to other metabolic pathways by anaplerotic reactions. "Anaplerotic" means "filling up," and these reactions allow for excess incoming acetyl-CoA or pyruvate, deficits in pools of amino acids, and other imbalances. Also, other pathways help maintain (refill) the pool of intermediates for the TCA cycle. The net result is to keep the pool of biochemical intermediates at constant concentration. This consistency ensures a constant flow of carbon atoms in and out of the TCA cycle, without interrupting its functioning in helping to generate energy for the cell, and while supplying other pathways at the same time.

Here are some examples of pathways that can draw material from the TCA cycle (**Figure 10-13**):

- Succinyl-CoA can be used in porphyrin biosynthesis (heme groups); it can also be used in the biosynthesis of certain fatty acids.
- α-Ketoglutarate is directly connected by transamination to glutamate, and from there to other amino acids.
- Oxaloacetate is directly connected by transamination to aspartate and to other amino acids.
- Pyruvate is directly connected to the amino acid alanine by a transamination reaction.

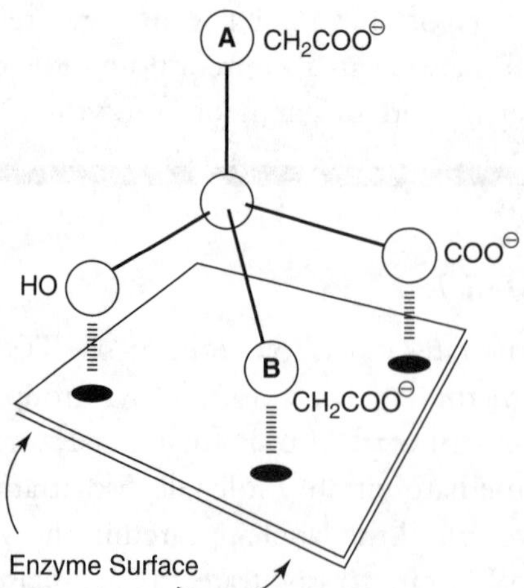

Figure 10-12 Three-point attachment model for citrate.

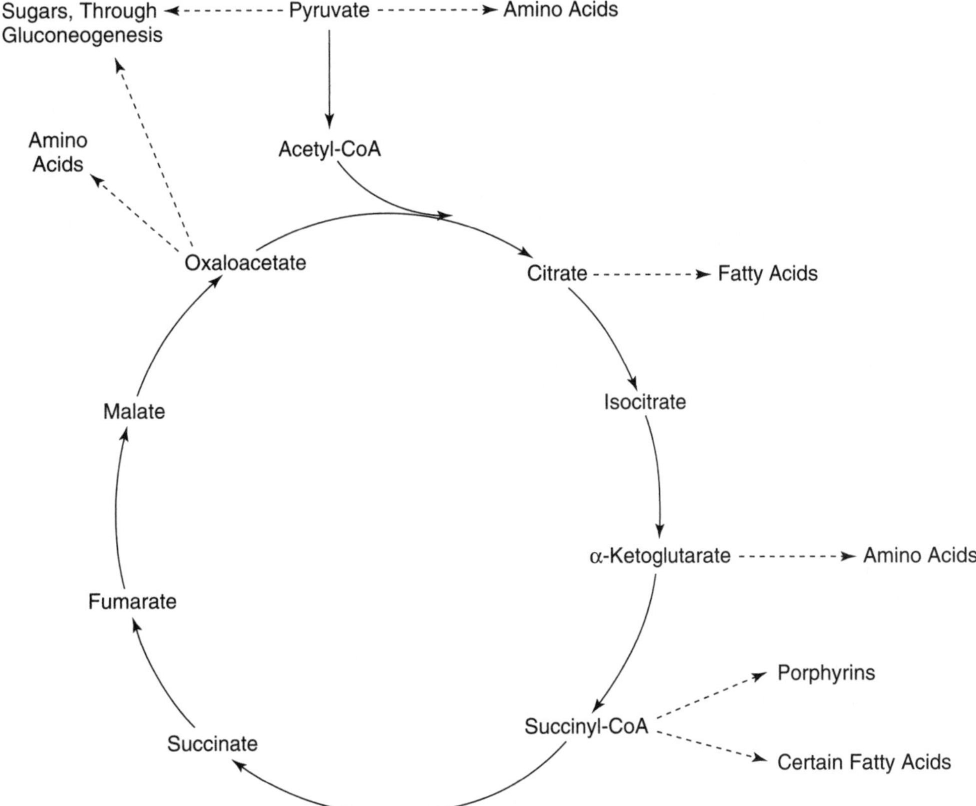

Figure 10-13 Anaplerotic reactions drawing on TCA-cycle intermediates.

- Pyruvate and oxaloacetate can be used in gluconeogenesis.
- Citrate can be exported from the mitochondrion into the cytosol, broken apart into acetyl-CoA and oxaloacete, and the acetyl-CoA used there to help synthesize fatty acids.

Intermediates in the TCA cycle can be replenished by some of the preceding reactions, as well as by the following reactions (**Figure 10-14**):

- Pyruvate can be carboxylated to give oxaloacetate.
- Phospho*enol*pyruvate can be carboxylated to give oxaloacetate (see the earlier material on gluconeogenesis).
- Pyruvate can be reductively carboxylated, at the expense of NADPH, to give malate (catalyzed by the "malic enzyme," a cytosolic enzyme).

Strictly speaking, there is no net synthesis or degradation of intermediates within the TCA cycle. "Outside" reactions are necessary to produce net changes in the level of TCA cycle intermediates. The outside reactions include links to amino acid metabolism, the synthesis of porphyrin, and more. In fact, the TCA cycle serves as a major source of biosynthetic precursors: The intermediates of the TCA cycle are free to move about inside the mitochondrial matrix and to participate in other reactions there, and in some cases even to be transported across the mitochondrial membrane.

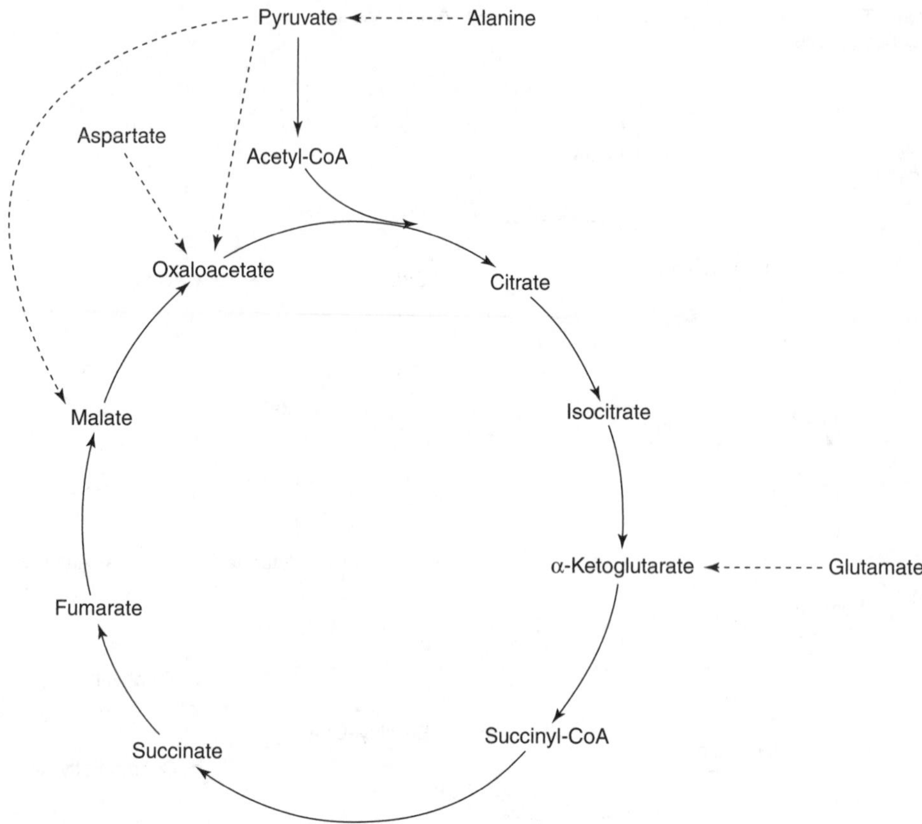

Figure 10-14 Anaplerotic reactions supplying TCA-cycle intermediates.

For example, a large influx of pyruvate can be handled by converting a part of it to oxaloacetate (the reaction is catalyzed by pyruvate carboxylase, as discussed earlier). A secondary cytosolic route uses the malic enzyme (not to be confused with malate dehydrogenase), an enzyme that converts part of the pyruvate to malate, which can then enter the TCA cycle and so generate oxaloacetate.

Requirement for Glucogenic Fuels

Pyruvate is mostly oxidized to acetyl-CoA, but a small amount goes to oxaloacetate (through the action of pyruvate carboxylase). Carbohydrates or glucogenic amino acids give pyruvate; however, fatty acids or ketogenic amino acids do not (they go to acetyl-CoA directly). Recall that oxaloacetate is necessary to "prime" the cycle, because acetyl-CoA cannot enter without it. Thus the entry of ketogenic fuels into the TCA cycle depends on an adequate level of oxaloacetate. As a consequence, ketogenic fuel molecules cannot be oxidized completely without also using up some glucogenic molecules to get oxaloacetate "primers." The body requires an adequate supply of glucogenic molecules to maintain the rate of turnover in the TCA cycle.

In early biochemical studies on diabetic or fasting animals, researchers found that when certain amino acids were fed to the animals, the carbon atoms of the amino acid would appear in glucose or in glycogen (the polymerized form of glucose, discussed in Chapter 9). Such amino acids were termed glucogenic (sometimes "glycogenic," if the study detected the carbon uptake in the form of glycogen). Other amino acids, when fed to the animals, would give rise to ketone bodies (acetone, β-hydroxybutyrate, acetoacetate; see **Figure 10-15**); these ketone bodies would then lead to the formation of acetyl-CoA. These other amino acids were described as ketogenic. See Chapter 13 for more on ketone bodies.

Aerobic Metabolism and TCA Cycle Function

Requirement for Aerobic Conditions

Oxygen is not directly consumed in the TCA cycle. Several redox reactions take place, however, and the TCA cycle does require aerobic conditions to proceed. Why are aerobic conditions required, if no molecular oxygen is directly consumed?

Both NADH and $FADH_2$ are generated by the TCA cycle. These reduced coenzymes/prosthetic groups will later be oxidized in oxidative phosphorylation, using O_2. Turnover in the TCA cycle absolutely requires NAD^+ and FAD; that is, there must be regeneration of the oxidized form of these cofactors.

Furthermore, the pool of NAD^+/NADH inside the mitochondria is compartmentalized, separated by a membrane from the cytosolic pool involved in the glycolytic pathway. There is no exchange between the cytosolic and mitochondrial pools of nicotinamide. Also, there is no lactate dehydrogenase in the matrix to convert pyruvate to lactate, or, therefore, to regenerate NAD^+ from the NADH accumulating in the matrix as the TCA cycle turns over. As a result, it is not possible to run the TCA cycle anaerobically by generating lactate. This situation is very much unlike that found in the glycolytic pathway, where such anaerobic functioning is possible (at least for a brief time).

Because the regeneration of oxidized nicotinamides and flavins is accomplished mainly by the process of coupled electron transport/oxidative phosphorylation, and because this latter process absolutely requires molecular oxygen (O_2) to proceed, aerobic conditions are needed for continued TCA cycle turnover, even though O_2 is not directly used.

Transport of Reducing Equivalents

Cellular oxidation–reduction reactions occurring in the cytosol will generate reduced forms of nicotinamides and flavins, which must be regenerated in the oxidized form to continue normal cellular functioning. The major site of oxidation of these reduced cofactors lies in the mitochondrial matrix, in the four respiratory complexes there. However, the inner mitochondrial membrane is impermeable to NAD^+ or NADH, flavins, and other such molecules. In fact, there are substantial differences in concentration of the nicotinamides across the inner mitochondrial membrane, with the concentration of NADH being higher inside this barrier.

For example, NADH is formed during glycolysis, which occurs in the cytosol, but it is mainly oxidized inside the mitochondrial matrix. Clearly, the cell needs to continually

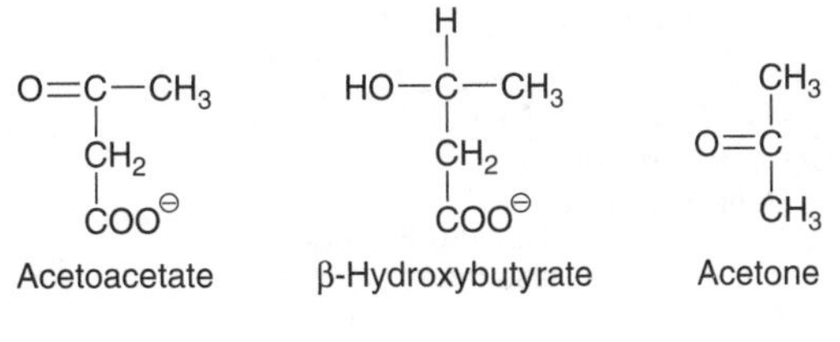

O=C—CH3
CH2
COO⊖
Acetoacetate

H
HO—C—CH3
CH2
COO⊖
β-Hydroxybutyrate

CH3
O=C
CH3
Acetone

Figure 10-15 Ketone bodies.

regenerate NAD^+ in the cytosol to continue glycolysis. How can it do this, if the NADH cannot be directly transferred into the mitochondrial matrix? A temporary solution, discussed earlier, is to use lactate dehydrogenase and perform anaerobic glycolysis. Eventually, however, this process exhausts the cytosolic pool of NAD^+. A longer-term solution, used in higher organisms, is to supplement this activity with the Cori cycle, but this simply transfers the burden from one tissue to another. Somehow the pool of NAD^+ must be regenerated without turning to anaerobic metabolism. The solution here is to transfer only the electrons from NADH across the mitochondrial membrane, not the entire chemical moiety. Transfer of the electrons will regenerate the cytosolic pool of NAD^+. Of course, there must be something in the matrix to accept those electrons.

To perform the electron transfer and regenerate the cytosolic NAD^+, two shuttles for electrons across mitochondrial membranes are used: the *glycerol phosphate shuttle* and the *malate–aspartate shuttle.* Do not confuse these shuttles with the respiratory complexes I through IV, which transfer electrons within the mitochondrion, as will be discussed later.

How the Glycerol Phosphate Shuttle Functions

In the first step of the glycerol phosphate shuttle (**Figure 10-16**), a cytosolic enzyme oxidizes NADH (generated by glycolysis) to NAD^+ and simultaneously reduces DHAP to glycerol 3-phosphate (G3P). In the next step, G3P diffuses through the outer mitochondrial membrane, up to the inner membrane. There it is acted upon by a flavin-containing enzyme and is oxidized back to DHAP. The DHAP is then free to diffuse back out to the cytosol. As this enzyme oxidizes G3P, the reducing equivalents (electrons) are transferred to its bound FAD, forming $FADH_2$. Actually, the flavin is a prosthetic group and does not diffuse about freely, but instead stays more or less permanently attached to the enzyme. Next the reduced flavin on the enzyme gives up its electrons to a membrane-associated mobile electron carrier, coenzyme Q (not shown in Figure 10-16; more details on coenzyme Q will be given in Chapter 11). This donation regenerates

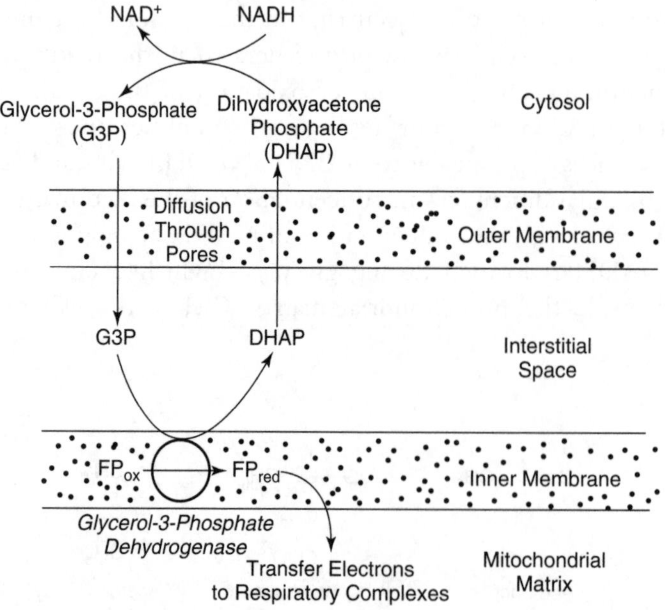

Figure 10-16 Glycerol phosphate shuttle.

the FAD, so the enzyme is ready for the next cycle. The reduced coenzyme Q (QH_2), which is quite nonpolar and thus strongly associated with the lipid bilayer of the membrane, then diffuses away to respiratory complex III, where it is re-oxidized.

How the Malate–Aspartate Shuttle Functions

In the malate–aspartate shuttle (**Figure 10-17**), a cytosolic enzyme oxidizes NADH while simultaneously reducing oxaloacetate to malate (this is not the same enzyme as in the TCA cycle, but the reaction is similar, just run in reverse). The malate diffuses through the outer mitochondrial membrane and encounters a membrane-bound transporter embedded in the inner membrane (the malate–α-ketoglutarate transporter). This transporter specifically carries malate across the membrane, into the mitochondrial matrix. Next, the malate is oxidized to oxaloacetate (by the TCA-cycle enzyme malate dehydrogenase), with simultaneous reduction of NAD^+ to NADH; effectively, the electrons from cytosolic NADH then appear in matrix NADH.

The oxaloacetate gains an amino group from glutamate and becomes aspartate, in a reaction catalyzed by aspartate aminotranferase. The aspartate then is transported out to the interstitial space via the glutamate–aspartate transporter and then diffuses out to the cytosol. The glutamate skeleton, having lost an amino group, becomes α-ketoglutarate, which is likewise transported and diffused out to the cytosol. The reverse of these two reactions then takes place in the cytosol, providing for regeneration of glutamate and oxaloacetate.

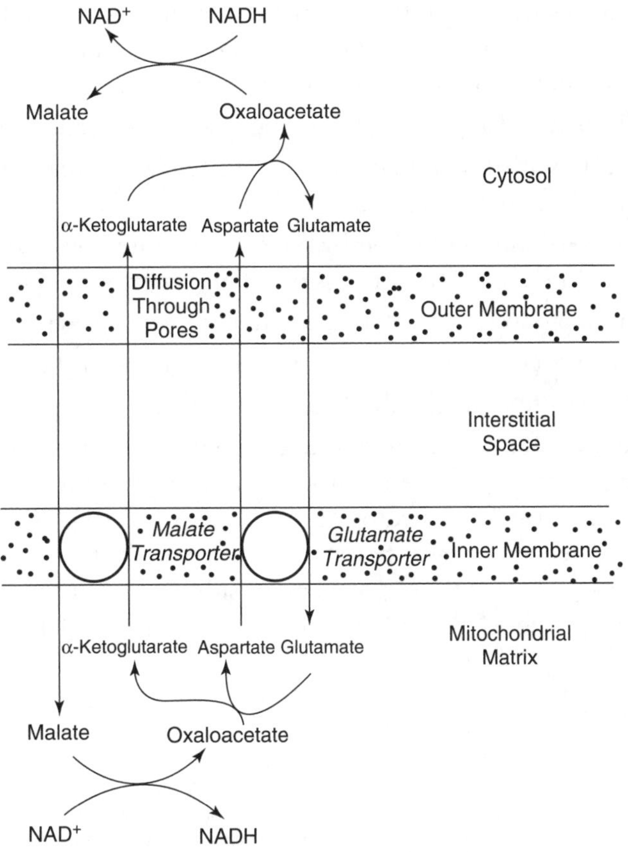

Figure 10-17 Malate–aspartate shuttle.

Are These Shuttles Metabolically Equivalent?

The two shuttle systems show some differences in tissue specificity. The malate–aspartate shuttle is active in liver, kidney, and cardiac muscle tissue. The glycerol phosphate shuttle is active in skeletal muscle and in the brain.

The reactions of the malate–aspartate shuttle are reversible, so what drives the flow of electrons inward toward the matrix is the deficit in the pool of matrix NADH, compared to that in the cytosol. This shuttle will basically shut down when the matrix NADH concentration builds up to too high a level. The reactions of the glycerol phosphate shuttle, however, are not readily reversible: There is no convenient way to go from the reduced coenzyme Q (generated by oxidation of the reduced mitochondrial flavoprotein) back to cytosolic NADH.

The eventual yield of ATP (from oxidation of the reduced coenzyme Q formed) derived from the glycerol phosphate shuttle is lower than that from oxidation of the NADH formed in the matrix by the action of the malate–aspartate shuttle (see Chapter 11 on oxidative phosphorylation). However, because it is not readily reversible, the glycerol phosphate shuttle can transfer reducing equivalents against an unfavorable gradient in $NADH/NAD^+$ concentration ratio across the mitochondrial membrane. Thus this shuttle will keep skeletal muscle functioning aerobically even as NADH builds up in the mitochondrion.

QUESTIONS FOR DISCUSSION

1. Biochemical studies have identified a genetic variant of the E_1 subunit of the pyruvate dehydrogenase complex in which the TPP cofactor is bound more loosely than usual. Patients with this mutant protein are more susceptible to lactic acidemia than normal.
   a. How might such a change in TPP binding lead to the lactic acidemia?
   b. When patients with this mutation were treated with thiamine supplements, their acidemia disappeared. Explain why.
2. Isocitrate dehydrogenase is inhibited by ATP but activated by ADP. Explain this pattern of regulation by ATP and ADP in terms of cellular energy charge maintenance.
3. A new antibiotic is proposed to inhibit the pyruvate dehydrogenase complex (**Figure 10-18**).
   a. Explain why this compound would act as an inhibitor of the PDH complex.
   b. Which other enzymes might also be inhibited by this compound?
4. The oxidative decarboxylation of α-ketoglutarate to succinyl-CoA in the TCA cycle strongly resembles the oxidative decarboxylation of pyruvate to form acetyl-CoA, as catalyzed by the pyruvate dehydrogenase complex. In fact, the TCA-cycle enzyme, α-ketoglutarate dehydrogenase, has the same cofactor requirements and the same general construction from three polypeptide subunits as the pyruvate dehydrogenase complex. Further, one of the subunits in α-ketoglutarate dehydrogenase is identical

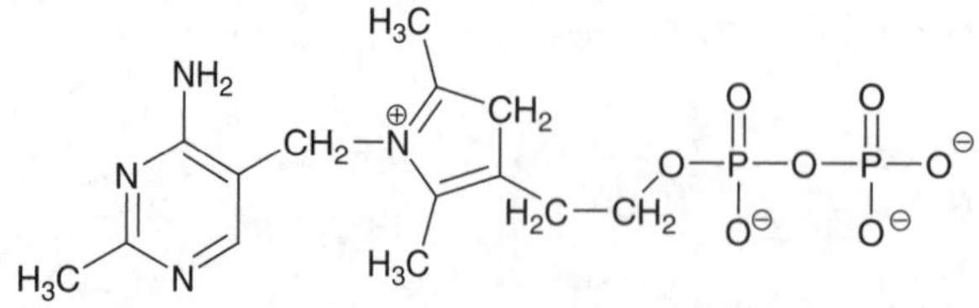

Figure 10-18 Proposed antibiotic for inhibition of the pyruvate dehydrogenase complex.

to the corresponding subunit in the pyruvate dehydrogenase complex. Which subunit would you propose for this identity, and why?

5. In terms of metabolic strategy, explain why the activity of α-ketoglutarate dehydrogenase shifts with NADH concentration, as shown in **Figure 10-19**.
6. The vitamin thiamine must be pyrophosphorylated before it can be used as a cofactor by enzymes. What would be the metabolic consequences of inhibiting the pyrophosphorylation reaction?
7. Phenylephrine is commonly used as a decongestant; it acts at α_1-adrenergic receptors to promote a rise in cytosolic Ca^{2+} levels, among other effects. In turn, the Ca^{2+} ions act as second messengers and cause a general increase in cellular energy production. Suppose a student with a head cold is taking phenylephrine for symptomatic relief.
   a. Which enzymes connected with the TCA cycle would likely respond?
   b. How does their sensitivity to Ca^{2+} lead to greater energy production for the cell?
8. Suppose that the malate–aspartate transporter in the inner mitochondrial membrane were inhibited. What would be the metabolic consequences of such inhibition? Which tissues would be especially at risk?
9. Pyruvate carboxylase forms oxaloacetate from pyruvate, using ATP and bicarbonate. The enzyme is allosterically activated by acetyl-CoA. How is this an example of "feed-forward" metabolic control? How does it help in maintaining activity in both the TCA cycle and gluconeogenesis?
10. Why are mutations frequently fatal if they involve the loss of function of one or another TCA cycle enzyme? Why is the same not true of the glycolytic enzyme, triose phosphate isomerase?
11. Deficiency of pyruvate carboxylase is a rare genetic disease (approximately 1 in 250,000 live births), but it can have quite severe biochemical consequences. If untreated, it can lead to profound mental retardation and an early death.
    a. Deficiency in the activity of the enzyme commonly results in acidosis and elevated blood levels of alanine. Explain why.
    b. One treatment for this condition consists of extra aspartate and citrate in the diet. How would this therapy help to relieve the symptoms?

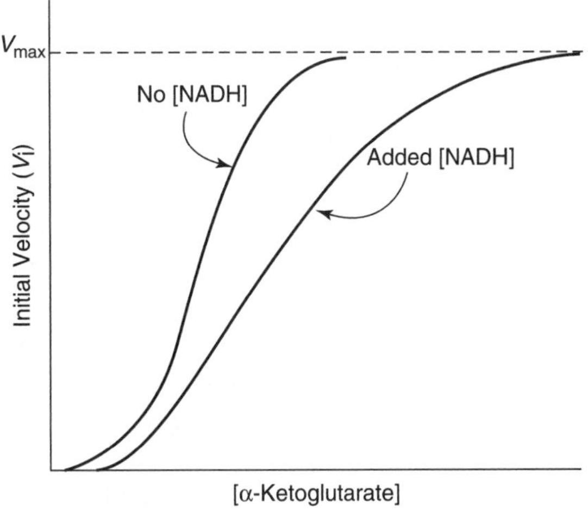

Figure 10-19 Activity of α-ketoglutarate dehydrogenase as a function of substrate and NADH concentrations.

REFERENCES

J.-J. Brière et al. (2006). "Tricarboxylic acid cycle dysfunction as a cause of human diseases and tumor formation," *Am. J. Physiol. Cell Physiol.* 291:C1114–C1120.

O. E. Owen, S. C. Kalhan, and R. W. Hanson. (2002). "The key role of anaplerosis and cataplerosis for citric acid cycle function," *J. Biol. Chem.* 277:30409–30412.

M. S. Patel and L. G. Korotchkina. (2006). "Regulation of the pyruvate dehydrogenase complex," *Biochem. Soc. Trans.* 34:217–222.

P. L. Pedersen. (1993). "An introduction to the mitochondrial anion carrier family," *J. Bioenerg. Biomemb.* 25:431–434.

M. Pithukpakorn. (2005). "Disorders of pyruvate metabolism and the tricarboxylic acid cycle," *Molec. Gen. Metab.* 85:243–246.

J. E. Walker. (1992). "The mitochondrial transporter family," *Curr. Opin. Struct. Biol.* 2:519–526.

Z. H. Zhou et al. (2001). "The remarkable structural and functional organization of the eukaryotic pyruvate dehydrogenase complexes," *Proc. Natl. Acad. Sci. USA* 98:14802–14807.

CHAPTER 11

Respiratory Complexes and ATP Synthesis

Learning Objectives

1. Define and use correctly the following terms: *respiration, electron transport chain, respiratory chain, respiratory complex, proton pump, oxidative phosphorylation, coenzyme Q/ubiquinone, heme, non-heme iron, iron–sulfur complexes, cytochrome, ATP synthase, F_0–F_1 ATPase, stalk domain, headpiece, binding change model, chemiosmotic model, electrochemical potential, proton gradient, vectorial organization, P/O ratio,* and *uncoupling agent.*
2. Describe the organization of a typical mitochondrion, listing and locating membranes, enzymes, respiratory complexes, the F_0–F_1 complex, and important transporter proteins.
3. List the respiratory complexes of mitochondria in appropriate order, along with intermediate electron carriers. Note which complexes are proton pumps.
4. Compare the entry of electrons to the respiratory chain via complex I versus complex II. Explain the consequences for generation of cellular energy.
5. List compounds that block electron transport, noting their sites of action. Explain the consequences for the cell.
6. Explain the chemiosmotic model of oxidative phosphorylation. List examples of energy conversions involving proton gradients.
7. State the biochemical function of the F_0–F_1 complex, relating it to the chemiosmotic model and the flow of protons. Describe the structure of the F_0–F_1 complex, and relate this structure to the binding-change model and catalytic cooperativity.
8. Explain how uncoupling agents can interfere with ATP generation and how they can be used for thermogenesis.

Respiratory Complexes

Overview

Turnover in the TCA cycle generates a great deal of reduced nicotinamides and flavins in the mitochondrial matrix. This process is augmented by the shuttles for reducing equivalents, described in Chapter 10, that bring in electrons from the cytosolic pool of reduced nicotinamides. The main question now is, How does the body oxidize these reduced cofactors and capture their free energy?

Ultimately, the electrons from NADH or $FADH_2$ will be passed to molecular oxygen, O_2, in a process referred to as *respiration*. In fact, a chain or set of redox reactions, under tight control, performs this process. The very complicated, membrane-embedded enzymes that perform the redox reactions in this chain are referred to as *respiratory complexes*. Some auxiliaries—namely, a small membrane-bound protein and a bilayer-embedded small molecule—serve to transport electrons between these respiratory complexes. The entire collection of respiratory complexes plus these auxiliaries is called the *electron transport chain* (ETC) or *respiratory chain*. Some (but not all) of the respiratory complexes are *proton pumps*; they expel H^+ to the cytosol as they perform redox reactions. However, these respiratory complexes themselves do not make ATP.

As the redox reactions in the ETC occur, they release free energy. This energy is stored temporarily in a gradient of protons and electrical voltage across the inner mitochondrial membrane; this gradient arises through the proton-pumping action of the respiratory complexes. An enzyme complex—quite distinct from the respiratory complexes that perform redox—will then use this stored free energy to make ATP through the phosphorylation of ADP, inside the mitochondrial matrix. This is *not* substrate-level phosphorylation, the kind of process that occurs in glycolysis, but is instead an entirely different process with an entirely different enzyme complex. The combination of mitochondrial ATP synthesis and oxidation of nicotinamides and flavins is called *oxidative phosphorylation*. Oxidative phosphorylation is the major source of ATP for aerobic organisms.

The inner membrane of mitochondria is the site of oxidative phosphorylation. The proteins here are carefully ordered for efficiency. They are isolated from the rest of the cell—an excellent example of compartmentalization in metabolism.

Flow of Electrons in Respiration

Electrons are transferred through a series of carriers, including flavins, non-heme iron compounds, hemes, and quinones. The arrows in **Figure 11-1** show the direction of electron flow. This diagram is not meant to indicate that, for example, NADH is somehow transformed into molecular oxygen, O_2. Instead, electrons are transferred from NADH, through a variety of intermediates, onto O_2, while NADH is oxidized to form NAD^+. (The fate of succinate is covered in material on the TCA cycle.) Note that O_2 is not a product; rather, it accepts electrons from complex IV to form water.

Important Coenzymes and Prosthetic Groups

Coenzyme Q

The small molecule *ubiquinone* (also called *coenzyme* Q, or simply Q for short) is one of the intermediate electron carriers in the respiratory chain. It is known as "ubiquinone" because it is ubiquitous in cells. It also participates in some other redox reactions, notably in the oxidation of fatty acids (see Chapter 13) and in the action of glycerol 3-phosphate dehydrogenase on glycerol 3-phosphate (see Chapter 11's discussion of the glycerol phosphate shuttle). In this

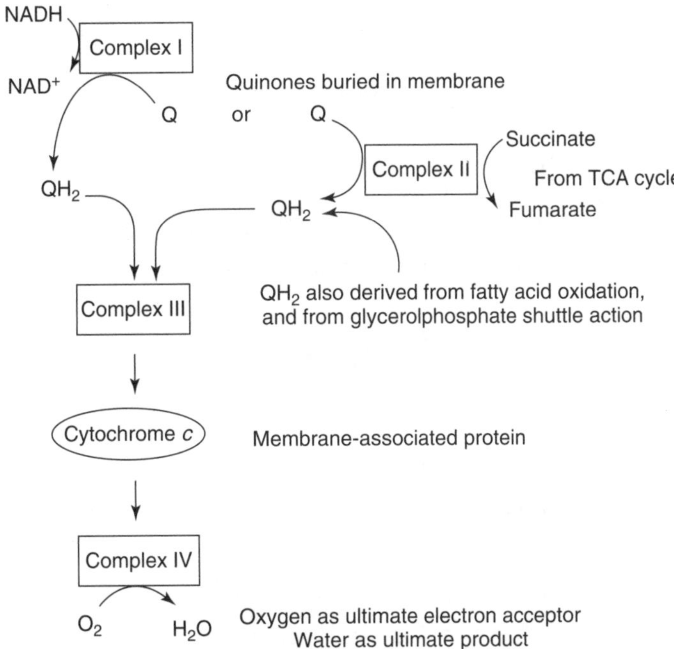

Figure 11-1 The flow of electrons in respiration, from NADH or coenzyme Q down to O_2, the ultimate electron acceptor.

way the electron-shuttling action of ubiquinone links the main respiratory chain to other metabolic pathways.

Coenzyme Q has a quinone structure (**Figure 11-2**). The quinone/semiquinone/quinol forms of this compound allow one-electron transfers between it and single-electron donors or acceptors, but overall the compound can carry two electrons.

Isoprenoid units attached to the ring structure form a hydrophobic tail, suitable as an "anchor" to hold it in a lipid bilayer. This kind of anchoring allows the compound to undergo rapid lateral diffusion in the bilayer, so that electrons are quickly transferred to the next complex. In the electron transport system of the mitochondrion, coenzyme Q is the only electron carrier that is free to move about in this way; the other electron carriers are bound to proteins.

Hemes and Cytochromes

Heme groups are not proteins but rather prosthetic groups, used here for electron transfer (which is quite distinct from their role in myoglobin and hemoglobin, where these groups bind and release molecular oxygen). Their distinctive feature is the tetrapyrrole ring surrounding a central Fe atom (**Figure 11-3**). Heme groups are surrounded by hydrophobic side chains of the protein to which they are attached. Small differences in the surrounding chemical groups can change the local electric field, thereby yielding slight differences in reduction potentials for electron transfer at these heme groups. The details of the mechanism by which electrons pass to and from the heme group remain unclear.

The *cytochromes* are a family of heme-containing proteins involved in electron transfer and redox reactions. They are highly colored, thanks to the strong absorption of visible light by the associated heme groups. Three families of cytochrome proteins exist, denoted as cytochrome *a*, cytochrome *b*, and cytochrome *c*. The families are distinguished by their respective differences in their absorption spectra in the visible range.

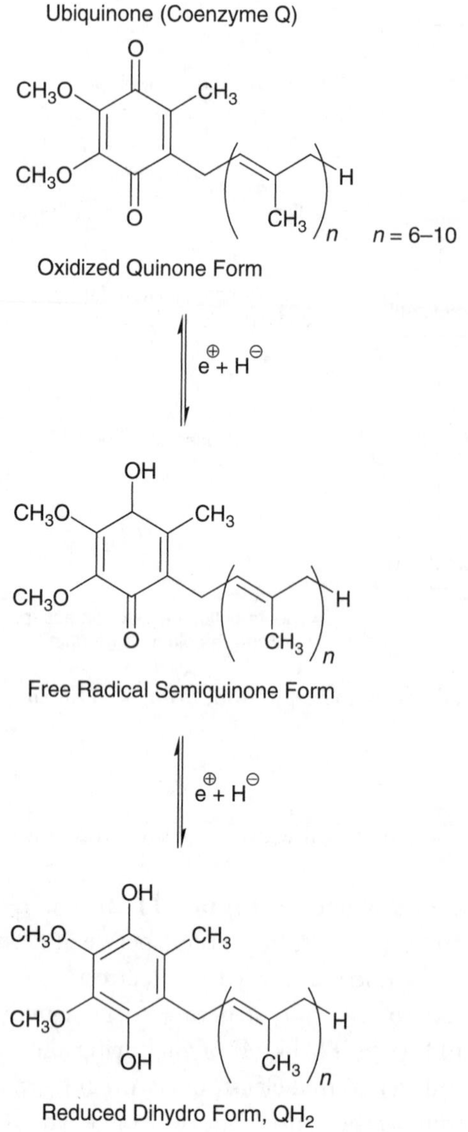

Figure 11-2 Forms of coenzyme Q (ubiquinone), showing the one-electron transfers in going from the oxidized quinone form, through the semiquinone radical, to the reduced dihydroquinone.

The cytochrome *a* family (abbreviated cyt *a*) noncovalently, but tightly, binds its heme group; an example of this type of cytochrome is found in the structure of the enzyme cytochrome *c* oxidase. (Somewhat confusingly, this enzyme contains subunits of the cytochrome *a* family, but its substrate is a cytochrome *c* protein.) Subscripts on the letter denote different members of the protein family (e.g., cyt *a* and cyt a_3).

The *b* family of cytochromes (cyt *b*) have the same heme as in the oxygen transporter protein hemoglobin. These cytochromes perform various functions: They are electron carriers in several systems. Like the cytochrome *a* proteins, the cytochrome *b* proteins also hold their heme groups noncovalently but tightly.

The *c* family of cytochromes (cyt *c*) differ here in that they form a covalent linkage to their heme group. Members of this family are ubiquitous one-electron transfer agents involved in many different systems.

A.

H_3C $HC{=}CH_2$

H_3C CH_3

$N \rightarrow Fe \leftarrow N$

$^{\ominus}O$—$C(=O)$—H_2C—H_2C $HC{=}CH_2$

$^{\ominus}O$—$C(=O)$—H_2C—H_2C CH_3

B.

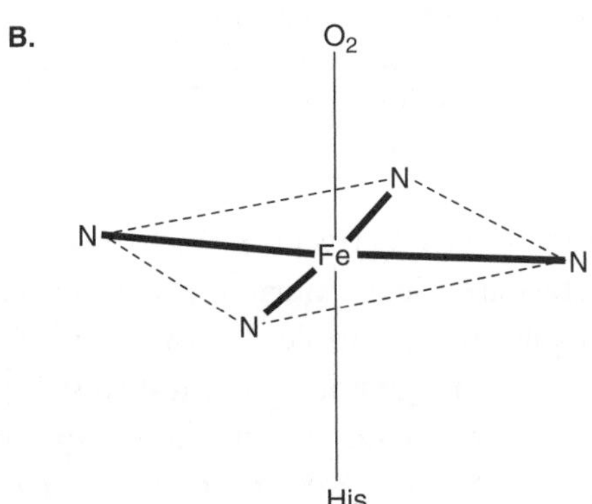

Figure 11-3 Hemes are tightly bound prosthetic groups. **A.** A heme group, composed of a central iron atom surrounded by a tetrapyrrole ring; note the dative bonding of the nitrogens to the central iron atom. The ring substituent groups differ depending on the biological source. **B.** The octahedral complex around iron in hemoglobin. The iron atom has a fifth point of ligation to the nitrogen from a histidine side chain; in oxygenated hemoglobin, the iron's sixth ligation point holds a molecule of oxygen.

As for the general structure of the cytochrome proteins, their charged groups generally are found on the outside of the protein. The distribution of these charged groups is, in fact, a key factor in recognition and binding among them.

Of particular interest in studying the flow of electrons in respiration is the protein known simply as cytochrome *c*. This protein is not a respiratory complex, but does transfer electrons (one at a time, using its single heme group) between respiratory complexes III and IV. Cytochrome *c* is a soluble globular protein located on the external face of the inner mitochondrial membrane. It remains closely associated with the membrane.

Other cytochrome proteins are found in the liver and play very important roles in the metabolism of drugs, biosynthesis of certain hormones, and other processes necessary to the body's proper functioning. An example is the set of enzymes known as cytochrome P-450 (named after their characteristic absorption of visible light around 450 nm).

Iron–Sulfur Complexes

Iron–sulfur (Fe-S) *complexes*, also referred to as *non-heme iron complexes*, contain one, two, or four Fe atoms in complex with sulfides. The sulfides may be of inorganic type, or they may come from the sulfhydryl group of Cys residues (**Figure 11-4**). These clusters have been found in both membrane-bound enzymes (the respiratory complexes to be discussed) and soluble enzymes such as aconitase (in the TCA cycle).

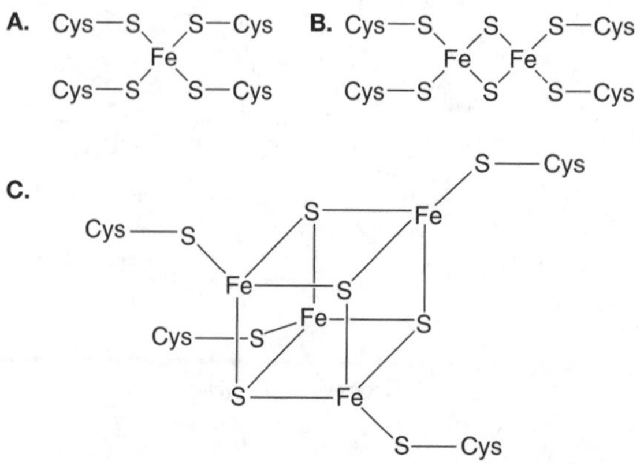

Figure 11-4 Iron–sulfur complexes are prosthetic groups involved in electron transfer reactions. The sulfur atoms may be a part of the side chain of cysteine residues or they may be inorganic sulfur. **A.** Simple single iron atom center. **B.** Center with two sulfur atom bridges and two iron atoms. **C.** Complex center with four iron atoms and four bridging sulfur atoms.

The iron atoms in these clusters cycle between +2 and +3 oxidation states; one electron is transferred at a time. The clusters are usually buried inside proteins, well away from contact with solvent water or dissolved solutes (e.g., molecular oxygen, with which they might react too readily). Bound clusters do not exchange with unbound clusters; they are prosthetic groups.

In addition to their service in redox reactions, such iron–sulfur clusters may help to stabilize the enzyme's conformation and protect it against proteolytic attack. They may also serve as detectors of exogenous iron, dioxygen (O_2), superoxide anion (O_2^-), and possibly nitric oxide.

Respiratory Complex (Electron Transfer) Proteins and Their Function

Overall, four multisubunit enzyme complexes are found in the ETC, respiratory complexes I through IV, plus the intermediate electron carriers coenzyme Q and cytochrome *c*.

NADH–Q Reductase: Complex I

Figure 11-5 gives a schematic view of the function of complex I. This complex transfers electrons from NADH to coenzyme Q, forming NAD^+ and QH_2, and pumps protons out of the mitochondria. The net reaction can be written as follows:

$$\mathrm{NADH} + \mathrm{H^+} + \mathrm{Q} \rightarrow \mathrm{NAD^+} + \mathrm{QH_2} \qquad (11\text{-}1)$$

This is not the whole story, however, because a certain number of protons are actually consumed or taken up from the matrix, while others are released ("pumped") toward the cytosolic side of the inner mitochondrial membrane. Because the inner mitochondrial membrane is typically polarized, with a transmembrane electrical potential of approximately 0.2 volt, the convention is to refer to the N (negative) and P (positive) sides of the membrane. By extension, protons on the negative (or matrix) side of the membrane can be identified with a subscript N, while those outside the matrix, on the positive side, can be labeled with a subscript P. Thus a better representation of the action of this complex would be

$$\mathrm{NADH} + 5\,\mathrm{H_N^+} + \mathrm{Q} \rightarrow \mathrm{NAD^+} + \mathrm{QH_2} + 4\,\mathrm{H_P^+} \qquad (11\text{-}2)$$

This expression shows that four protons are expelled for each molecule of NADH that is oxidized to NAD^+, two protons (with two electrons) are attached to coenzyme Q, and five protons are taken up from the matrix as NADH is oxidized.

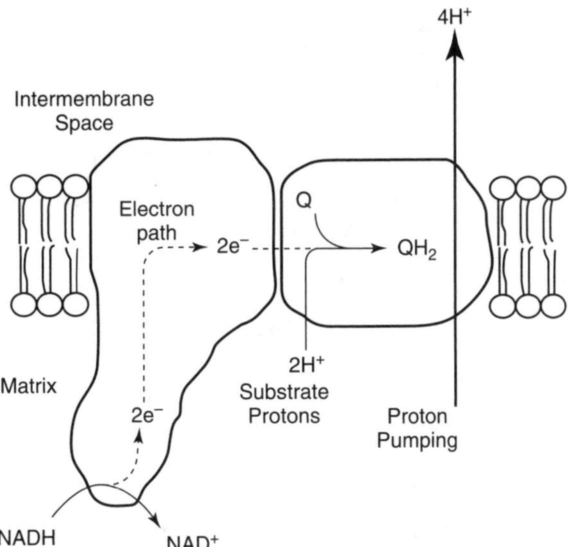

Figure 11-5 Schematic for respiratory complex I. NADH is oxidized to NAD^+, with concomitant reduction of the coenzyme Q quinone to the dihydroquinol QH_2. In the process, four protons are expelled and five protons are taken up from the matrix.

Complex I is a flavoprotein that uses FMN. It also contains non-heme iron centers (Fe-S complexes). The route for electron transfer proceeds from NADH to FMN, then goes through several iron–sulfur centers, and finally reaches coenzyme Q. The flavin moiety can, of course, accept two electrons from NADH (which strictly donates electrons in pairs), then donate them, one at a time, to the Fe-S centers and on to coenzyme Q.

This very large and complex enzyme has multiple subunits (42 polypeptide chains are involved), some of which are buried in a lipid bilayer in the mitochondrion. Thus it is very difficult to purify intact, functional enzyme for crystallization and structure determination. The structure of the membrane-bound "foot" has yet to be determined in detail.

Notice that ATP does not appear in either of the preceding chemical reactions. Complex I helps to make ATP by coupling proton pumping to the phosphorylation reaction performed by a distinct ATP synthase complex, but complex I itself does not make ATP.

Succinate–Q Reductase: Complex II

Complex II transfers electrons, but it does not act as a proton pump (**Figure 11-6**). There is no coupling to ATP synthesis here because this complex is not a proton pump. This is the same enzyme discussed earlier in association with the TCA cycle. The reaction catalyzed by complex II is

$$\text{Succinate} + \text{Q} \rightarrow \text{Fumarate} + \text{QH}_2 \qquad (11\text{-}3)$$

The prosthetic groups here are FAD, heme molecules, and FeS centers, with one subunit being a cytochrome *b* with a heme group. The FAD cycles between oxidized and reduced forms as the complex acts on succinate from the TCA cycle; **Figure 11-7** summarizes the net transfer of electrons from succinate to coenzyme Q.

QH_2–Cytochrome c Reductase: Complex III

Complex III contains *b*- and *c*-type cytochromes as well as an iron–sulfur center. It also has a binding site for the protein cytochrome *c*, located on the outer side of the mitochondrial membrane.

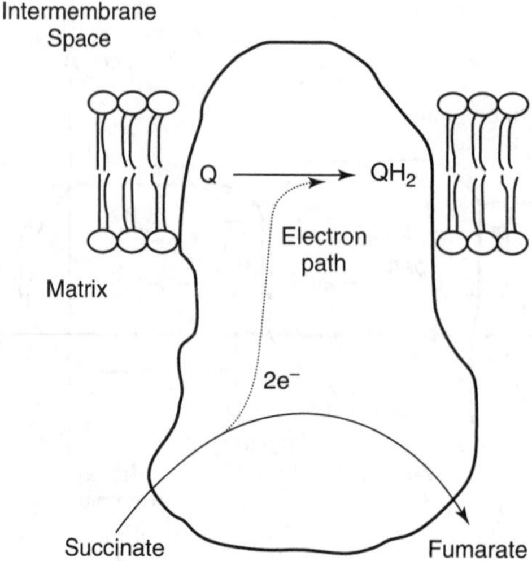

Figure 11-6 Respiratory complex II. Succinate is oxidized to fumarate, with concomitant reduction of a flavin prosthetic group (not shown); subsequently, the reduced flavin is oxidized to reduce a molecule of coenzyme Q. No protons are pumped by this complex.

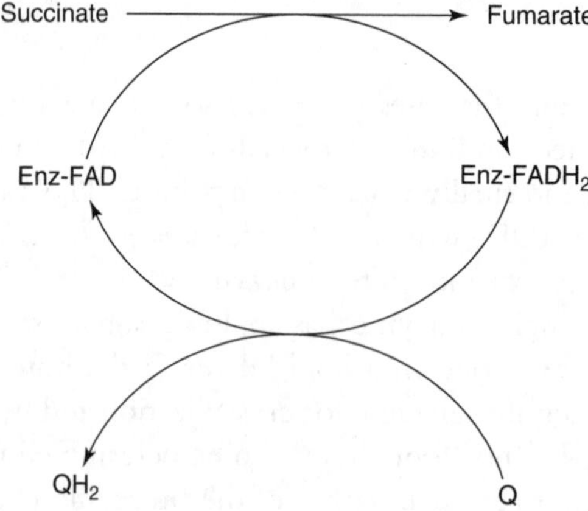

Figure 11-7 The reaction cycle for complex II. Note how the flavin group is regenerated after each cycle of electron transfers. A similar cycle operates in the flavoenzyme that converts glycerol 3-phosphate to dihydroxyacetone phosphate, as part of the glycerol phosphate shuttle system.

This respiratory complex acts as a proton pump (**Figure 11-8**). ATP synthesis is coupled to electron passage through this complex, due to proton pumping by the complex. It is thought to expel four protons per molecule of QH_2 oxidized to the quinone form. As in the case of complex I, some protons are taken up from the matrix, while others are expelled into the interstitial space:

$$QH_2 + 2\text{ cyt } c_{(ox)} + 2H_N^+ \rightarrow Q + 2\text{ cyt } c_{(red)} + 4\ H_P^+ \tag{11-4}$$

The electrons from the oxidation of QH_2 are passed over to the carrier protein, cytochrome *c*. Each oxidation of coenzyme Q releases two electrons, while the heme group of cytochrome *c* can accept only one electron. Hence two molecules of cytochrome *c* must be reduced in order to fully oxidize QH_2.

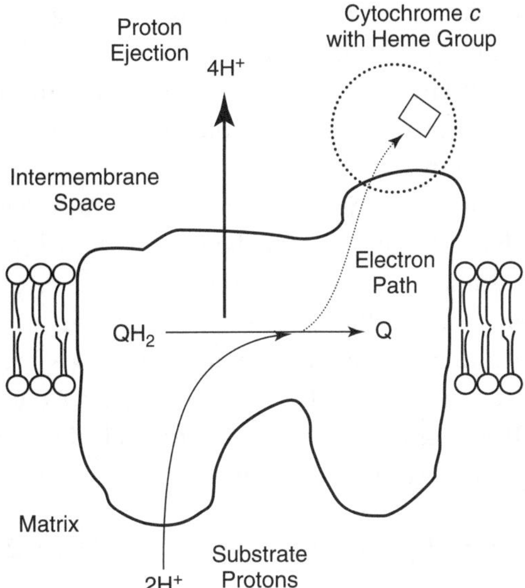

Figure 11-8 Respiratory complex III. QH_2 is oxidized and the electrons are passed one at a time to two successive molecules of cytochrome *c*; four protons are expelled in the process, while two protons are taken up from the matrix.

Cytochrome c Oxidase: Complex IV

This complex transfers electrons and pumps protons (**Figure 11-9**). It is the last ("terminal") complex in the respiratory chain. ATP synthesis is coupled to proton pumping action by this complex. The proton pump mechanism is not clear, but it probably involves conformational changes in key residues that accept and donate protons as electrons are transferred from group to group within the complex. The crystal structure shows movement of a key aspartate residue

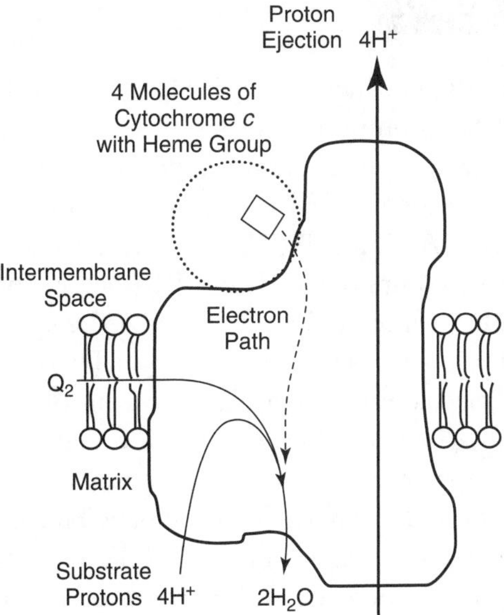

Figure 11-9 Respiratory complex IV. Four successive molecules of cytochrome *c* pass their electrons to the reaction center, where a molecule of O_2 is reduced to two molecules of water. Four protons are expelled per molecule of O_2, while eight protons are taken up from the matrix.

upon a change in the oxidation state of the O_2 reduction site, with a change in pK_a and the state of ionization. Overall, two protons are expelled per pair of electrons consumed in forming a water molecule. Alternatively, one can view this outcome as expulsion of *four* protons per molecule of O_2 consumed (producing *two* molecules of water), which would require the consumption of *two* pairs of electrons.

Notable prosthetic groups in this complex are two different heme groups (denoted *a* and a_3) and two copper ions. It also has a binding site for the protein cytochrome *c*, on its outer face.

As noted earlier, the ultimate electron acceptor in the respiratory chain (that is, the last compound in the chain to be reduced) is O_2. Reduction of molecular oxygen leads to formation of water; H_2O is a reduced form of oxygen, given that it has gained electrons. This reduction is performed by complex IV. The reduction site in complex IV catalyzes a four-electron reduction of O_2. It is highly unusual to see four electrons participating in a reaction; one or two electrons being transferred in a reaction is far more common.

$$4 \text{ cyt } c_{(\text{red})} + 8\, H^+_N + O_2 \rightarrow 4 \text{ cyt } c_{(\text{ox})} + 4\, H^+_P + 2\, H_2O \qquad (11\text{-}5)$$

Notice that four separate molecules of reduced cytochrome *c* are called upon here to bring in those four electrons. Also, while four protons are expelled per molecule of O_2 consumed, another eight protons are taken up from the matrix.

The mechanism by which this reduction–oxidation reaction takes place is not understood completely. Complex IV has both Fe and Cu atoms, and evidence favors the involvement of Cu in the reaction mechanism. It does seem clear that the four-electron reduction is done sequentially, not simultaneously, and it is performed by cycling over several intermediate states of reduction–oxidation of the iron and copper atoms, probably with the oxygen atoms forming peroxide intermediates.

Clinical Application

Reactive oxygen species (ROS), such as $O_2^{\cdot -}$, H_2O_2, and $OH^{\cdot}$, are generated as by-products of the normal functioning of the respiratory complexes. These oxygenated intermediates are highly reactive—they are free radicals—and so would be very injurious to the cell if they were released, potentially causing damage to cellular membranes, proteins, and nucleic acids. Additionally, ROS can attack iron–sulfur centers, which could potentially inactivate complexes I, II, and III (the enzyme aconitase in the TCA cycle also has an iron–sulfur center and would likewise be subject to attack). Given the severe consequences of these actions for the cell, especially for energy production by the mitochondrion, cellular mechanisms are available to control and deal with ROS.

Superoxide anion can arise from side reactions involving complex I and CoQ. Also, peroxide intermediates are presumably formed as a part of the normal functioning of complex IV, and these ROS could be released by accident. Free metal ions, especially those of iron, in the mitochondrion can convert H_2O_2 to $OH^{\cdot}$ radicals by the Fenton reaction. Disruption of the transport of such metal ions can produce severe disease; Friedrich's ataxia is an example. This disease is a result of a mutation in the protein, frataxin, that is responsible for transporting iron out of the mitochondrion. With the loss of function of frataxin, iron accumulates and catalyzes the production of $OH^{\cdot}$ radicals, leading to inactivation of respiratory complexes. The end result is progressive damage to the cell. Nerve and cardiac cells are especially vulnerable, such that the characteristic symptoms of Friedrich's ataxia range from difficulties in walking or in speech to heart disease.

Superoxide anion can be detoxified by a mitochondrial enzyme, superoxide dismutase (which contains the unusual cofactor of a manganese metal atom), which converts it to hydrogen peroxide. In turn, hydrogen peroxide is converted to water by the enzymes catalase and glutathione peroxidase. The body also produces uric acid as an end product of purine catabolism (see Chapter 15), which acts as a general scavenger of free radicals. Further, the body has several specialized systems that function to repair or replace damaged molecules. They include various proteases and peptidases to cleave oxidized proteins, phospholipases, and acyltransferases to remove oxidized parts of membrane lipids and replace damaged fatty acids, and DNA repair systems that cut out damaged DNA segments and replace them.

Dietary components that act to reduce the levels of free radicals are called antioxidants. These molecules include coenzyme Q, vitamin E, β-carotene, and vitamin C. They may offer limited benefit to patients who are suffering from diseases related to production of excess levels of reactive oxygen species.

Action of ATP Synthase in Oxidative Phosphorylation

The *ATP synthase* of the mitochondrion is the enzyme that is mainly responsible for ATP synthesis from ADP and P_i in metabolism. Under normal conditions—that is, a transmembrane pH gradient with a higher proton concentration on the cytosolic side—this enzyme makes ATP from ADP. This synthesis is tightly coupled to the flow of electrons through respiratory complexes down to O_2, the process that generates the proton gradient in the first place. Its mechanism of action involves concerted conformational changes in multiple subunits, and it depends strongly on transmembrane gradients in both pH and electrical potential to phosphorylate ADP to ATP.

Structure of ATP Synthase ($F_0 - F_1$ Complex, Complex V)

The ATP synthase is a massive complex that has a structure that has been highly conserved in evolution; the bacterial form is very similar to that in the mitochondria and chloroplasts of eukaryotes. In the mitochondria of eukaryotes, this complex is embedded in the inner mitochondrial membrane; in bacteria, it is embedded in the cell membrane. It is composed of a multitude of polypeptide chains—there are at least 21 polypeptide chains in the bacterial form from *E. coli*. The two main domains in the complex (**Figure 11-10**) are denoted as F_0 and F_1, and the ATP synthase is sometimes referred to simply as the *F_0-F_1 ATPase* or F_0-F_1 enzyme complex.

The F_1 Domain

The F_1 domain is located on the matrix side of the inner membrane, projecting inward into the matrix, and it can be reversibly dissociated from the intact F_0-F_1 complex. The F_1 domain contains multiple subunits, with the stoichiometry of $\alpha_3\beta_3\gamma\delta\varepsilon$ for the bacterial enzyme; the

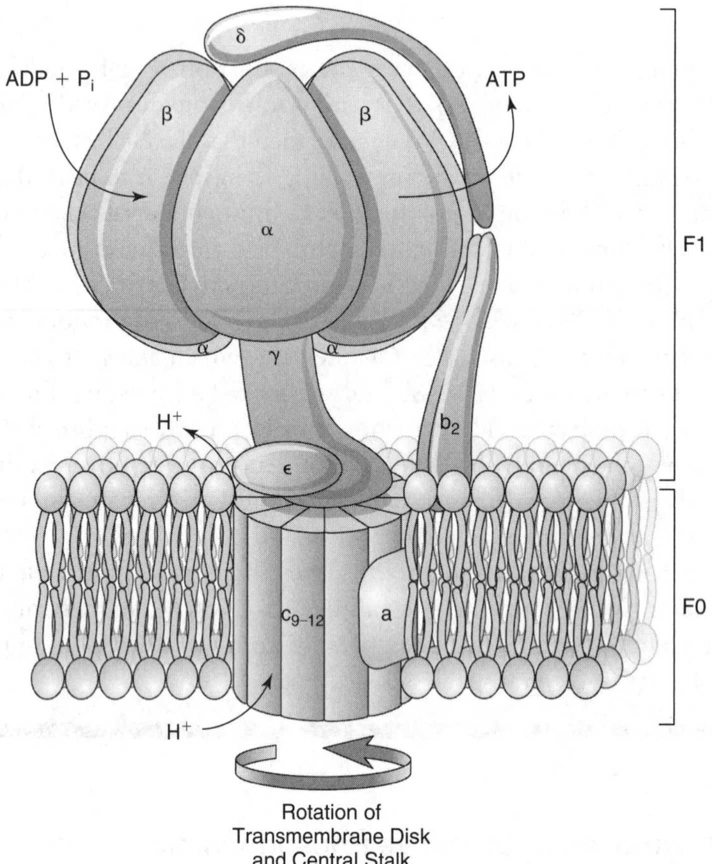

Figure 11-10 The F_0–F_1 ATP synthase. This figure depicts the overall structure of a bacterial enzyme; the eukaryotic mitochondrial form is similar. The F_0 domain, composed of α, β, and c subunits, is embedded in the membrane. The F_1 domain, composed of the α, β, γ, δ, and ε subunits, is peripheral; the catalytic sites are located in each of the three β subunits.

Source: Adapted with permission from S. T. Cole and P. M. Alzari. (2005). "TB—A new target, a new drug." *Science* 307:214–215. Copyright AAAS 2005.

mitochondrial form is more complex and the stoichiometry less certain. When isolated as a soluble protein, the F_1 domain can serve as a very active ATPase. In the intact complex, F_1 acts as an ATPase if there is no $[H^+]$ gradient across the membrane or if the gradient is in the wrong direction. Its *headpiece* contains a catalytic hexamer of subunits, with a stoichiometry of $\alpha_3\beta_3$.

The F_0 Domain

The F_0 domain is an integral membrane protein, also with multiple subunits; for *E. coli,* the stoichiometry is ab_2c_{9-12}. F_0 spans the membrane, and acts as a transmembrane channel for protons. The action as a proton channel is under strict control: F_0 will not let protons pass unless conditions are right.

As seen in electron micrographs, there is a "stalk-like" structure that connects the F_1 headpiece to the membrane-embedded F_0. This *stalk domain* is composed of the δ, γ, and ε subunits of the F_1 domain, along with the b polypeptide chain of the F_0 domain. This stalk protrudes inward, into the mitochondrial matrix. The function of the stalk is that of mechanical coupling of cation passage to substrate turnover (catalysis of phosphorylation). Some subunits of the stalk are sensitive to antibiotics.

ATP synthesis occurs at sites located on the β subunits of the F_1 region of the enzyme. The minimum stable complex of subunits, isolated as a separate enzyme, has the composition $\alpha_3\beta_3\gamma$. X-ray crystallography has shown that the α and β subunits form a hexameric ring, with the α and β subunits alternating in position around the ring. The γ subunit has one end inserted into the central cavity of the hexameric ring; its other end makes contact with the F_0 domain, specifically the c subunits there. The central γ subunit rotates inside the ring formed by the hexameric $\alpha_3\beta_3$ structure. The rotation is driven by the passage of protons through the c subunits of the F_0 domain; these c subunits are thought to change conformation as protons are passed from one subunit to the next. **Figure 11-11** has a close-up view of the proposed proton-driven rotation mechanism.

ATP Synthesis

The overall reaction for ATP synthesis is

$$ADP^{3-} + P_i^{2-} + H^+ \rightarrow ATP^{4-} + H_2O \qquad (11\text{-}6)$$

Note the expulsion of water as the phosphoanhydride bond is formed. This phosphoryl transfer reaction uses an "in-line" mechanism, involving a pentacovalent intermediate in the form of a trigonal bipyramid (**Figure 11-12**).

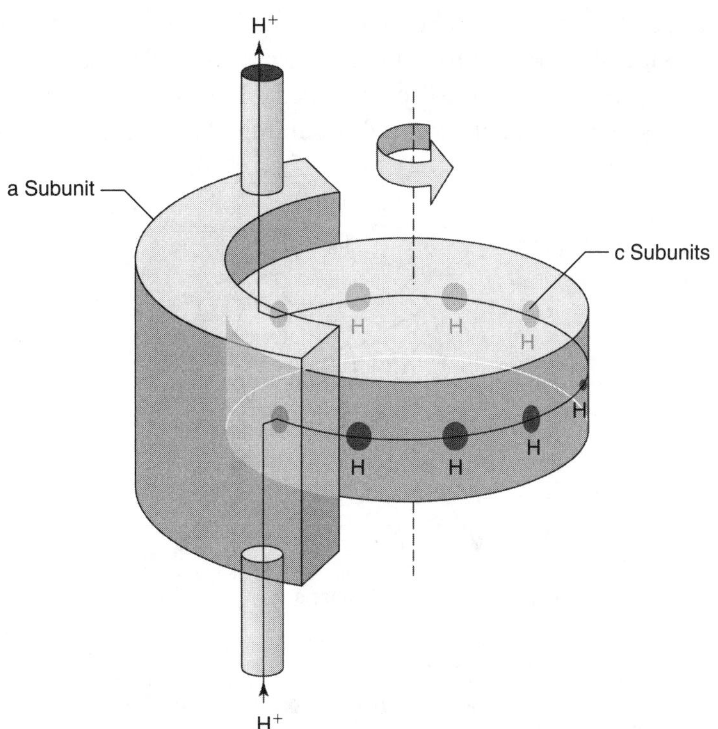

Figure 11-11 Detail of the membrane-embedded domain of the ATP synthase, showing a proposed mechanism for proton passage and rotation of the enzyme. Ten to twelve c subunits form a ring, with the α subunit to the side. Protons enter the α subunit from the outside, then pass to α c subunit to force a conformational change and rotation of the entire assembly, and finally exit from another site on the a subunit to the matrix side of the membrane.

Source: Adapted with permission from D. Stock, A. G. W. Leslie, and J. E. Walker. (1999). "Molecular architecture of the rotary motor in ATP synthase," *Science* 286:1700–1705. Copyright AAAS 1999.

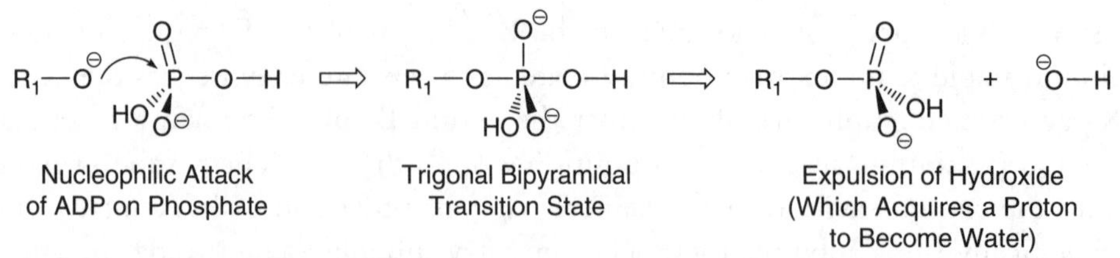

Nucleophilic Attack of ADP on Phosphate ⟹ Trigonal Bipyramidal Transition State ⟹ Expulsion of Hydroxide (Which Acquires a Proton to Become Water)

Figure 11-12 Phosphorylation of ADP to form ATP involves nucleophilic attack of the ADP terminal phosphate on inorganic phosphate, and a trigonal bipyramidal transition state.

Magnesium is required for activity because the enzyme uses Mg^{2+} complexes of ADP and ATP, not the "naked" nucleotides. This reaction goes steeply "uphill" in terms of free energy, at +30.5 kJ/mol under standard conditions. This free energy must be supplied by running "downhill" some other process that is coupled to the synthesis of the phosphoanhydride. That downhill process is the favorable entry of protons from outside the mitochondrial matrix, into the matrix. The later section on the chemiosmotic model discusses this topic in more detail.

Binding Change Mechanism

As proposed by Paul Boyer, the *binding change model* of the ATP synthase's action explains a variety of kinetic, equilibrium, and structural observations on the enzyme. It involves highly cooperative, sequential changes in subunit conformation in the F_1 domain that are tightly coupled to the passage of protons through the F_0 region of the complex.

Figure 11-13 presents a highly schematized "bottom-up" view of the F_1 domain, emphasizing the β subunits and the central γ subunit. The actual catalytic site is on the β

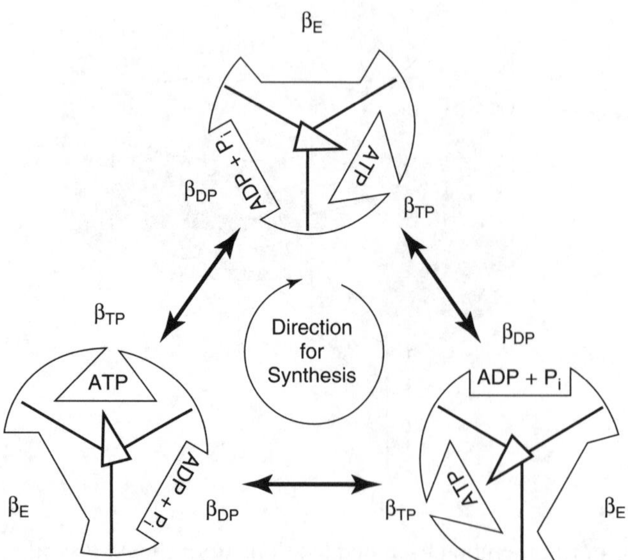

Figure 11-13 The binding change mechanism for ATP synthesis by the F_0–F_1 ATP synthase, emphasizing the catalytic role of the β subunit. Individual subunits change conformation successively from β_E to β_{DP} to β_{TP} and back to β_E. The conformational change is highly cooperative among the three subunits in the F_1 domain. Also shown is the 120° rotation of the γ subunit (central triangle) that enforces the directionality of the conformational change.

subunit, for a total of three catalytic sites per F_1 domain. Not shown are the rest of the rotor and F_0 pieces of the enzyme.

The three catalytic sites have different conformations, which have been verified through determination of the crystal structure of the enzyme. By convention, the three conformations are distinguished by their affinities for ATP or ADP (and P_i), and the state of occupancy of the active site. The β_{TP} conformation binds ATP with high affinity and is likely the state or conformation that can reversibly synthesize or hydrolyze ATP. The β_{DP} conformation binds ADP loosely. The β_E conformation has an empty site; it does not have either ATP or ADP bound, but it is the change in this subunit's conformation that presumably utilizes the free energy from proton passage through the F_0 domain, with this subunit going to a state that can bind ADP and P_i with high affinity.

There is an orderly progression through the conformations for a given subunit as ATP is synthesized: β_E to β_{DP}, then β_{DP} to β_{TP}, then β_{TP} back to β_E. The units appear to change conformation in a concerted cooperative way, together. Rotation of the central γ subunit is clockwise in Figure 11-13 and is the direction for ATP synthesis; counterclockwise rotation would result in ATP hydrolysis. Direct observation of an isolated and specially labeled ATP synthase headpiece assembly has shown that, in fact, the entire F_1 domain can rotate in steps of 120°, one third of a circle. There is some evidence that this rotation is broken down into substeps of 30–60°.

The synthetic process starts with the binding of ADP and inorganic phosphate to the subunit in the β_E conformation. There is already a molecule of ATP bound tightly at an adjacent subunit, which is in the β_{TP} conformation, and the third subunit is in the β_{DP} conformation, holding molecules of ADP and inorganic phosphate.

As ADP binds to the empty site, this site changes conformation somewhat and increases its affinity for inorganic phosphate. It appears that the γ subunit rotates by 30–60° during this change. As phosphate enters the site, conformational changes are triggered in the other two subunits; the ATP is released from one of them (this subunit now takes up the β_E conformation), and the other subunit proceeds to the β_{TP} conformation, driving the reaction of ADP with P_i to form ATP. During this process the γ subunit rotates further, so that there is an overall 120° rotation. Completion of two more such catalytic cycles, with synthesis of two more molecules of ATP, will return the β subunits to their original conformational states and the γ subunit to its original direction and position.

The ATP synthase can reverse its action and act as an ATPase, hydrolyzing ATP back to ADP and P_i. The mechanism for ATP hydrolysis is just the reverse of that for synthesis. Whether the enzyme acts to synthesize or hydrolyze ATP depends on the direction of spontaneous movement of protons. Spontaneous inward movement into the mitochondrial matrix (such as when the pH is more acidic outside the matrix, and the matrix is relatively alkaline) favors ATP synthesis. It is possible to reverse this movement, however, under unusual physiological or laboratory conditions.

Proton Electrochemical Free Energy and ATP Synthesis

The phosphorylation of ADP to ATP costs energy—approximately 30.5 kJ/mol in the standard state. Where does this free energy come from? Recall that electron transport through respiratory complexes is a downhill process in terms of energy: Reducing oxygen to water is overall a favorable process when coupled to the oxidation of fuel molecules. The free energy released as the electrons pass along the respiratory chain is used, at least partially, to pump protons out of the mitochondrial matrix. This pumping itself is an uphill process, so that the protons on the outside of the inner membrane are at a higher concentration and a higher voltage than those inside the membrane. In other words, the "outside" protons have a higher free energy than those inside. When those outside protons move back inside, they give up that free energy. In the case of the ATP synthase, that release of free energy drives the unfavorable phosphorylation of ADP to ATP.

The *electrochemical potential* of H^+ refers to the free energy for that species. This free energy has two components: (1) a concentration difference (i.e., the ratio of concentrations across the membrane) and (2) the transmembrane potential (i.e., the voltage across the membrane). The free energy change for movement of protons across the membrane is sometimes referred to as the *proton gradient*, abbreviated sometimes as Δp. The term "proton gradient" is somewhat misleading, however, because it overlooks the important role of a voltage difference across the membrane in determining the overall free energy change needed for movement of protons across the mitochondrial membrane.

The electrochemical potential of protons is used in a variety of biochemical processes where free energy is needed to drive the process, including (1) heat production; (2) flagellar rotation; (3) active transport of a variety of substances across membranes (e.g., sugars, amino acids, ions); (4) NADPH synthesis; and, of course, (5) ATP synthesis. Other processes can be coupled to transmembrane concentration gradients or voltages, as discussed in Chapter 5.

Recall a basic relation for electrical voltage, concentrations across a membrane, and free energy differences, for moving a charged species (an ion) from an initial concentration and voltage, to a final concentration and voltage:

$$\Delta G = RT \ln\left(\frac{C_{\text{final}}}{C_{\text{initial}}}\right) + zF\Delta V \quad \Delta V = V_{\text{final}} - V_{\text{initial}} \qquad (11\text{-}7)$$

Here z is the ion's valence, F is the Faraday constant (96,480 joules/volt-equivalent), R is the gas constant (8.314 Joules/mole-Kelvin), and ΔV is the voltage difference.

A pH gradient exists and can be detected across mitochondrial membranes. The matrix side is less acidic (more alkaline) than the area outside the membrane (the cytosolic side). There is also typically a voltage difference ΔV across the membrane of 0.18 to 0.22 V, with the matrix being at a lower voltage (more negative voltage) than the cytosolic side. This difference arises due to excess cations outside (on the cytosolic side) and excess anions inside (on the matrix side). Together, the concentration difference and the voltage difference generally make it favorable to bring protons "inside" from outside the mitochondrial membrane; that is, ΔG is negative for proton movement from "outside" to "inside." This negative free energy difference is exploited to drive the unfavorable formation of a phosphoanhydride bond, in making ATP from ADP and P_i.

Thermodynamics and ATP Yield

The Complete Oxidation of Glucose Can Produce (Approximately) 30 ATP

The vast majority of this ATP (26 molecules out of 30, using some conventional or "textbook" estimates) is generated in oxidative phosphorylation. **Table 11-1** details the process of accounting for the ATP generated by primary metabolism.

The overall process of digesting glucose is approximately 32% efficient in conserving free energy. The complete combustion of glucose is highly exothermic:

$$\text{Glucose} + 6\ O_2 \rightarrow 6\ CO_2 + 6\ H_2O \quad \Delta G'^{\circ} = -2870\ \text{kJ/mol} \qquad (11\text{-}8)$$

Reaction	ATP Yield per Glucose
Glycolysis (glucose to pyruvate; cytosolic process)	
Phosphorylation of glucose	−1
Phosphorylation of fructose 6-phosphate	−1
Dephosphorylation of 2 molecules of 1,3-bisphosphoglycerate	+2
Dephosphorylation of 2 molecules of phosphoenol pyruvate	+2
Formation of 2 NADH in the cytosol (see shuttle cost, below)	
Pyruvate to acetyl-CoA (inside mitochondria)	
Formation of 2 NADH	
TCA cycle (inside mitochondria)	
Formation of 2 GTP from 2 succinyl-CoA	+2
Formation of 6 NADH from oxidation of 2 molecules each of isocitrate, α-ketoglutarate, and malate	
Formation of 2 $FADH_2$ by oxidation of 2 molecules of succinate	
Oxidative phosphorylation (inside mitochondria)	
Oxidation of 2 NADH from glycolysis; each yields 1.5 ATP due to shuttle cost	+3
Oxidative decarboxylation of 2 molecules of pyruvate; each yields 2.5 ATP (no shuttle cost)	+5
Oxidation of 2 $FADH_2$ from the TCA cycle; each yields 1.5 ATP	+3
Oxidation of 6 NADH from TCA cycle; each yields 2.5 ATP	+15
Net Yield per Glucose	+30

Table 11-1 ATP Yield from the Complete Oxidation of Glucose

Given that 30 moles of ATP will store 916 kJ and that 916/2,870 = 0.32, we have an efficiency of 32% in trapping the energy as ATP. This may seem inefficient, but actually this is rather good, especially in comparison to mechanical combustion systems, such as automobile engines.

P/O Ratios

The *P/O ratio* is defined as the moles of inorganic phosphate (P_i) incorporated into ATP (or GTP, or some other nucleotide triphosphate) per mole of atomic oxygen consumed (not O_2, but O, as in H_2O) in respiration. Various models for coupling electron transport to phosphorylation give different P/O ratios, leading to different estimates of how many ATP molecules are synthesized as the result of one or another step in the oxidative pathways. Actual measurements of the P/O ratio for mitochondria can test these models, allowing us to discard those that make wrong predictions. Recent evidence is that the P/O ratios are non-integral (see Table 11-1 and the discussion of the chemiosmotic model in the next section). Older chemical models that predicted integral values for P/O ratios are inadequate to explain the non-integral experimental values, and these models have since been discarded.

If the phosphorylation reactions were directly coupled to electron transport, we would expect integers for the values of the ratio, given that chemical reactions are normally stoichiometric, with integers. Conversely, indirect coupling could give non-integer P/O ratios; the experimental evidence of non-integer ratios further supports the idea of indirect coupling.

Chemiosmotic Coupling

Summary of the Chemiosmotic Model

Electron transport through respiratory complexes releases free energy, and the complexes must somehow expel or pump H^+ out of the matrix. Ejection of H^+ sets up a difference (gradient) in pH. This factor, with transport of other ions (e.g., K^+, Na^+, Cl^-), also sets up a transmembrane electrical potential ΔV. This difference in pH and in voltage allows for storage of energy. ΔpH combined with ΔV drives ATP synthesis (performed by the F_0–F_1 complex) as protons flow back through a channel in the ATP synthase complex.

The *chemiosmotic model* assumes *vectorial organization* of electron carriers (respiratory complexes and their adjuncts, such as ubiquinone and cytochrome *c*), such that electron transfer follows a definite order of intermediate carriers (that is, electron transport starts with complex I and electron transport ends at complex IV). The model also assumes unidirectional H^+ release by certain of these carriers; release is to the outside of the mitochondrion only. Here, the term "vectorial" means the transfer of electrons between carriers has a sense of direction; it does not occur between just any randomly chosen pair of electron carriers. It also implies a sense of direction to the net transfer of protons outward from the mitochondrial matrix. Moreover, the electron carriers are considered to be distinct from sites where phosphorylation (ATP synthesis) occurs. This is the basis for saying that there is indirect coupling, via the membrane potential and $[H^+]$ concentration differences, of electron transfer and ATP synthesis.

Details of the Chemiosmotic Model

Figure 11-14 summarizes the current version of the chemiosmotic model for the coupling of respiration to ATP synthesis. Respiratory complexes I, III, and IV are transmembrane proteins that can eject protons from the matrix across the inner mitochondrial membrane. Complex II is on the inner side of the membrane, and the cytochrome *c* protein is on the outer side. Glycerol 3-phosphate dehydrogenase (which, like complex II, passes electrons to coenzyme Q, and is also a flavoprotein) is on the outer side of the membrane (not shown in Figure 11-14).

Some key points related to this model are the following:

- Coenzyme Q (symbol Q) is buried in the lipid bilayer of the membrane.
- Cytochrome *c* (circle in Figure 11-14) is held on the outer side of the membrane.
- The ATP synthase is a distinct protein complex, different from all of the respiratory complexes.
- Complex I ejects four protons as it oxidizes one molecule of NADH.
- Complex II is not a proton pump.
- Complex III ejects four protons as it oxidizes one molecule of QH_2.
- Two protons are ejected per atom of oxygen (not per molecule of O_2!) that is used to make one molecule of water, in complex IV. Note carefully that consumption of a molecule of oxygen would result in ejection of four—not two—protons here.

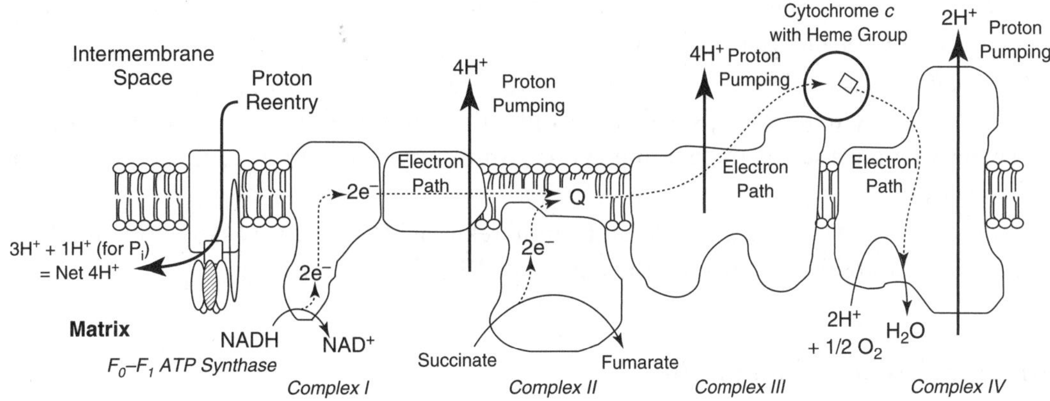

Figure 11-14 The chemiosmotic model. Proton pumping by respiratory complexes as they pass electrons down to molecular oxygen will generate a transmembrane electrical potential and gradient in proton concentration, which the F_0–F_1 ATP synthase uses to drive ATP synthesis. Note the stoichiometry of proton pumping and oxygen reduction by complex IV, and the accounting of proton entry through the F_0–F_1 ATP synthase.

Overall, the oxidation of a molecule of NADH, releasing two electrons, results in one water molecule being formed and half of an O_2 molecule being consumed; the corresponding number of protons pumped for this process would be 10 (= 4 + 4 + 2, from complexes I, III, and IV). For the oxidation of succinate (or of glycerol 3-phosphate by the flavoenzyme of the glycerol phosphate shuttle), the number of protons pumped would be 6 (= 4 + 2, from complexes III and IV).

ATP synthesis by the F_0– F_1 ATP synthase is accompanied by proton reentry into the matrix. Currently it is thought that the ATP synthase requires three protons to accomplish one synthetic cycle. Another proton is brought into the matrix when inorganic phosphate is imported from the cytosol, along with the exchange of ADP for ATP across the inner membrane. Thus a total of four protons enter the matrix per molecule of ATP synthesized.

This model is the basis for the consensus P/O ratios of 2.5 for NADH and 1.5 for succinate used in Table 11-1. If 10 protons are expelled per NADH oxidized, and 4 protons brought in, then the P/O ratio for NADH oxidation is 10/4 or 2.5. For succinate oxidation, the ratio would be 6/4 or 1.5.

Clinical Applications

Poisons of Respiration

Several kinds of inhibitors of oxidative phosphorylation exist:

- *Agents that block electron flow.* These may act at different points in the electron transport chain. Rotenone and amytal inhibit electron transfer to CoQ in complex I. Antimycin acts on complex III and inhibits it. CN^-, N_3^-, and CO act on complex IV; they bind to heme and inactivate it.
- *Agents that inhibit phosphorylation.* Oligomycin blocks the F_0−F_1 ATP synthase by binding to a particular peptide subunit in the stator unit. Using a different mechanism entirely, arsenate substitutes for phosphate in the phosphorylation reaction, but is spontaneously and rapidly hydrolyzed after being joined to ADP. In this way, ATP synthesis is again foiled.
- *Proton transporters.* These compounds upset the H^+ gradient across the inner mitochondrial membrane, and "uncouple" proton pumping/transport from ATP synthesis; hence they

may be referred to as *uncoupling agents*. See the discussions later in this chapter for examples of dinitrophenol and gramicidin A.

- *Other ion transporters.* These agents upset the voltage difference across the inner membrane—for example, by transferring small cations like K^+ across the membrane. Such compounds may also be regarded as uncoupling agents. An example is valinomycin (discussed later in this section).
- *Translocase inhibitors.* Atractyloside and bongkrekic acid (**Figure 11-15**) both inhibit the ATP–ADP translocase, blocking the export of ATP from the matrix.

Antibiotic Action of Gramicidin A

Gramicidin A is a polypeptide that buries itself in the membrane and creates a pore through which ions (e.g., protons) can pass (**Figure 11-16**). Thus pore formation destroys the proton gradient (and also the voltage difference across the membrane). The cell cannot make ATP or perform other processes dependent on the proton gradient, so the cell dies.

The pore is formed by a head-to-head dimerization of two chains of Gramicidin A. Each of these chains coils up in a helix, with the nonpolar side chains oriented into the lipid bilayer and the polar amide linkages to the interior of the helix. The nonpolar outside of the helix helps hold it in the bilayer, while the polar interior can hold cations and pass them across the bilayer.

Gramicidin A contains two "unnatural" types of amino acids, notably the D isomers (not the "natural" L isomers) of leucine and valine.

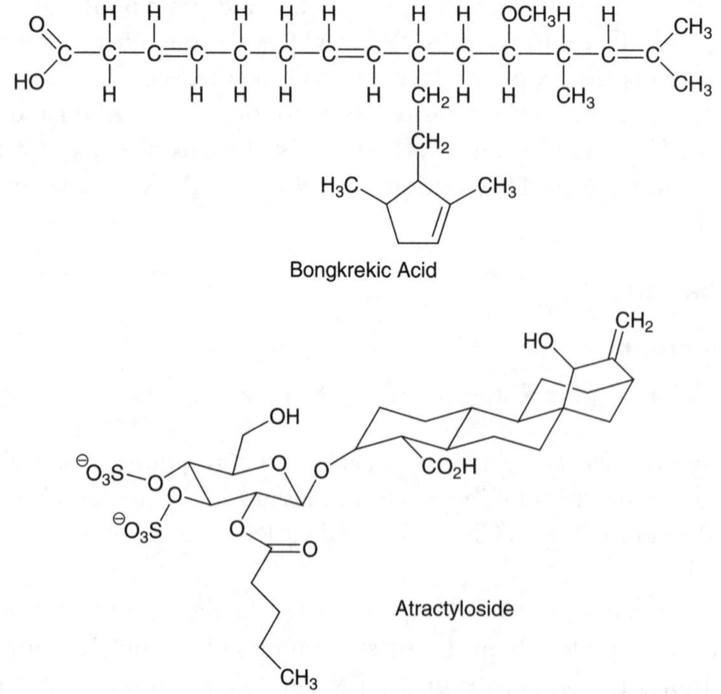

Bongkrekic Acid

Atractyloside

Figure 11-15 Inhibitors of the ATP–ADP translocase, bongkrekic acid and atractyloside, reduce ATP synthesis by blocking the entry of the substrate ADP into the matrix and the release of ATP to the cytosol.

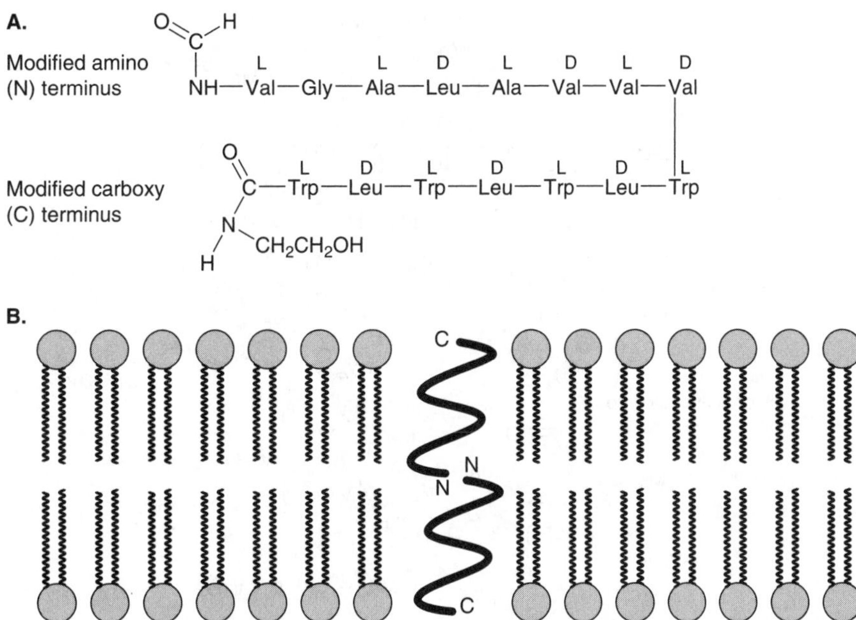

Figure 11-16 Gramicidin A is an antibiotic peptide that dimerizes to form transmembrane pores. Cations may pass through these pores, destroying the transmembrane pH and voltage gradients and leading to inhibition of ATP synthesis. **A.** Amino acid sequence; note the unusual D isomers. **B.** Head-to-head dimerization within a bilayer leads to pore formation; N denotes amino terminus, C denotes carboxy terminus.

Antibiotic Action of Valinomycin

Valinomycin is an ion carrier: It binds and transports potassium ions across the lipid bilayer, thereby destroying the voltage gradient (**Figure 11-17**). In Figure 11-17, note how unnatural amino acids are used (hydroxyisovalerate and D-valine), along with some residues of lactate, to form a cyclic structure that can wrap around a single potassium cation. In the presence of valinomycin, electron transport (respiration) can continue, but ATP synthesis will be impaired, because the agent reduces or destroys the transmembrane voltage difference that is important for driving ATP synthesis.

Weight-Reduction Aids

The ingestion of dinitrophenol (DNP) has been used in schemes for weight reduction. DNP transports protons back inside the mitochondrion, without driving action by the F_0–F_1 ATP synthase. The key is that the neutral phenol can diffuse across the membrane, but it ionizes in the alkaline interior of the mitochondrial matrix and releases a proton (**Figure 11-18**). Electron transport occurs as usual ("respiration," including the consumption of O_2). However, the proton concentration gradient is partially or completely destroyed, depending on the dose of DNP. Little or no phosphorylation occurs; that is, ATP synthesis is blocked in the mitochondrion. Thus respiration or electron transport is uncoupled from phosphorylation; DNP is a prime example of an uncoupling agent.

The free energy of ionization of the DNP, together with the free energy of moving the (released) proton across the membrane into the matrix, is favorable. However, this free energy has not been trapped by the formation of ATP because the protons did not pass through the F_0–F_1 ATP synthase and did not drive its action on ADP + P_i to make ATP. Instead, the free

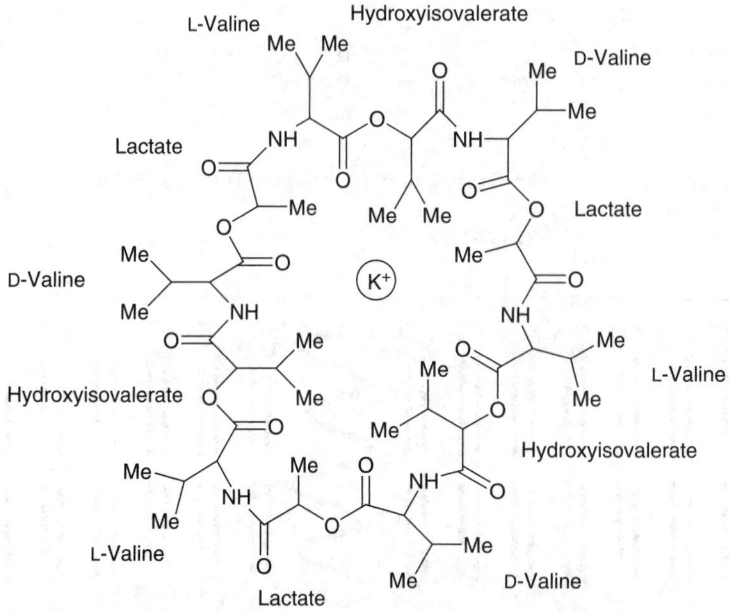

Figure 11-17 Valinomycin is a cyclic oligomer, formed from lactate and from regular and unusual amino acids, that can bind and carry potassium ions across membranes. This process reduces the transmembrane voltage gradient (but not the pH gradient) and inhibits ATP synthesis.

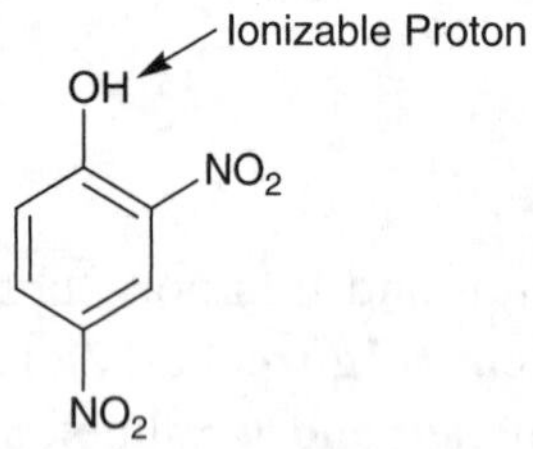

Figure 11-18 2,4-Dinitrophenol is an uncoupling agent that inhibits ATP synthesis by upsetting the transmembrane gradients in terms of both voltage and pH.

energy appears as heat in the surroundings, raising the local temperature, so a fever results. Little or no ATP is then made in the mitochondrion (even though electron transport continues as usual), so the cell depends on glycolysis and the TCA cycle for ATP. This process leads to rapid depletion of carbohydrate and lipid stores, with ensuing loss of weight.

Ischemia and ATP Hydrolysis

In ischemia, a tissue is deprived of sufficient oxygen (as in a stroke or heart attack), and the cells turn to anaerobic sources for ATP. This process generates acids like lactate and pyruvate. If their concentrations build up to any appreciable degree, the proton-motive force across the mitochondrial membrane will collapse. It then becomes important to shut down the ATP synthase, so that it will not reverse itself and become an ATPase. A special inhibitory protein, IF_1, binds to and inhibits two ATP synthase complexes, simultaneously. It acts this way as a dimer, and it only dimerizes when the pH drops below approximately 6.5 in the matrix. This acid pH would arise only during some pathological condition, as with ischemia.

Brown Fat

Brown fat is a type of adipose tissue, found mainly in newborns, that serves to generate heat without shivering. Its brown color comes from the large numbers of mitochondria in the cells; the mitochondrial respiratory complexes, of course, have cytochrome prosthetic groups, which absorb light and produce the brown color.

The heat is generated by the uncoupling of respiration in these cells, which contain a special uncoupling protein called thermogenin. The uncoupling protein is a transmembrane protein extending across the inner mitochondrial membrane. It serves as a channel for protons to enter the mitochondrial matrix without forcing them to first pass through the ATP synthase complex. This bypassing of the ATP synthase does not lead to ATP synthesis, but it does release free energy, in the form of heat. In turn, this heat raises the temperature of the cell, and helps the newborn to maintain homeostasis with respect to temperature.

QUESTIONS FOR DISCUSSION

1. Cyanide is very toxic; it binds to heme groups quite avidly and blocks oxygen binding.
   a. Which proteins in the electron transport chain of mitochondria are potential targets for cyanide poisoning?
   b. Why would a mildly toxic dose of cyanide produce a lactic acidosis?
   c. Brain and heart tissues are those most sensitive to cyanide toxicity. Why?
   d. A common emergency treatment for cyanide intoxication is intravenous sodium nitrite combined with sodium thiosulfate. Nitrite is an oxidizing agent, capable of converting heme iron from Fe(II) to Fe(III); it oxidizes hemoglobin to methemoglobin. How would this reaction help to restore function to the electron transport chain? What would be the function of the thiosulfate?
2. Antimycin blocks the transfer of electrons from respiratory complex III to cytochrome *c* in the electron transport chain. What effect would this inhibition have on ATP synthesis in the cytosol?
3. The compound 3-nitropropionic acid specifically inhibits respiratory complex II. Compare its structure to that of succinate, and propose a mechanism for this inhibition.
4. The anthracycline quinone known as doxorubicin (Adriamycin) is widely used in cancer chemotherapy; it intercalates into the DNA double helix and interferes with DNA polymerase and RNA polymerase, leading to an arrest of the cell cycle. This compound is also well known for its cardiotoxicity. The cardiotoxicity is thought to be due to metabolism of the parent quinone to the corresponding semiquinone free radical, which generates highly reactive free-radical species (such as the superoxide anion) while the semiquinone is recycled back to the quinone form (**Figure 11-19**).
   a. Vitamin E is thought to help reduce the toxic effects of this cardiotoxicity. Propose a mechanism for this effect.
   b. Complex I of the electron transport chain has been proposed as the major site of anthracycline reduction in mitochondria. Figure 11-19 shows a single-electron reduction of doxorubicin to the semiquinone radical. Review the passage of electrons through complex I and the redox chemistry of nicotinamides, and then propose how

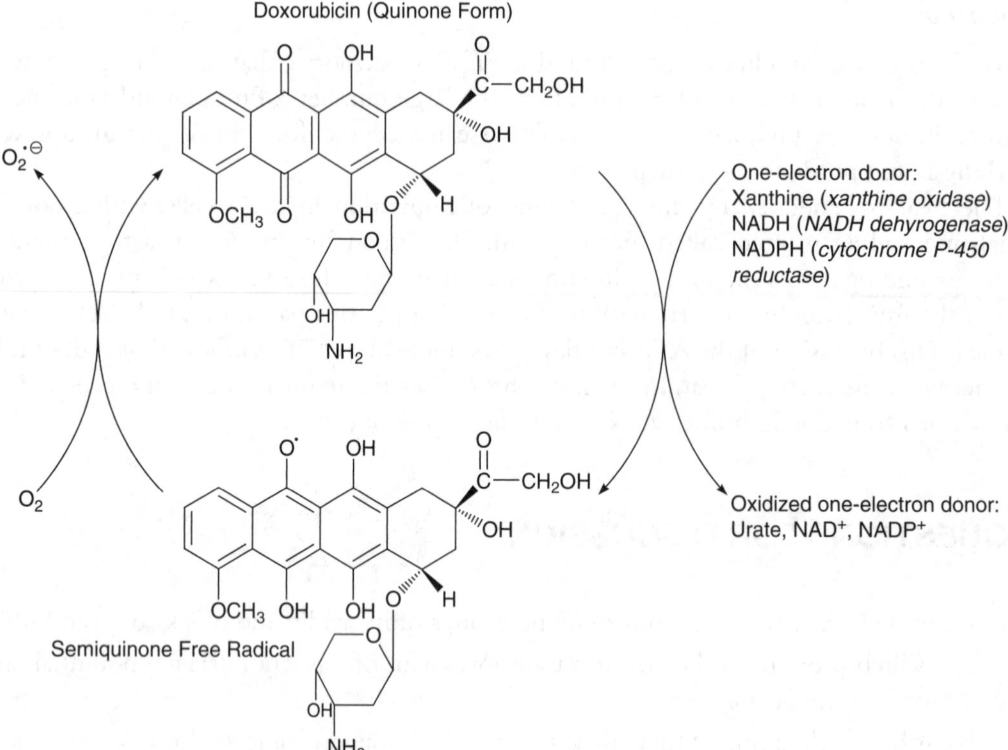

Figure 11-19 Reduction–oxidation cycle for doxorubicin, showing formation of a highly reactive superoxide radical anion.

the electrons could pass from NADH to doxorubicin, in view of the fact that NADH does not donate electrons one at a time.

c. The standard reduction potential for the one-electron reduction of doxorubicin to the semiquinone is −0.32 volt at pH 7, relative to the normal hydrogen electrode. Under which conditions (if any) can oxidation of NADH by complex I drive the one-electron reduction of doxorubicin?

5. Inhibition of ATP synthase activity would understandably lead to depletion of ATP. It may also lead to imbalance in pH homeostasis. Explain why.
6. Experiments on ATP hydrolysis by the F_0–F_1 ATP synthase have led to insights into the mechanism for ATP synthesis. Measurements of the rate of ATP hydrolysis were first done with sub-stoichiometric amounts of Mg·ATP. These rate experiments showed very tight binding of the first ATP and very slow release of the products of ADP and P_i, as if the reaction were taking place at only one occupied site per enzyme molecule. When the experiments were repeated using much higher concentrations of Mg·ATP, the rates of product ADP and P_i release were greatly enhanced, by a factor of about 10^5. How is this outcome consistent with cooperative interactions among the three active sites on the enzyme?
7. Pentachlorophenol has been widely used as a wood preservative and insecticide. It is no longer available to the general public, however, because of concerns over its toxic effects. Symptoms in exposed humans include very high fever, sweating, and liver damage. How does pentachlorophenol produce these symptoms?

8. In a recent review, the authors assert that a proton motive force of only 150 millivolts across the mitochondrial membrane is sufficient to drive ATP synthesis.
   a. How much free energy is released by the translocation of four protons through the ATP synthase?
   b. In fact, the amount of free energy released from this process seems to be in great excess over that needed to form ATP from ADP and P_i if the concentrations inside the mitochondrion matched those of the standard biochemical state. Why, then, does the excess occur?
9. Ascorbic acid (ascorbate; vitamin C) is a strong reducing agent; the oxidation occurs in stepwise fashion, with the compound losing one electron at a time, eventually leading to the formation of dehydroascorbic acid. Thus ascorbic acid can donate electrons to cytochrome *c*, one electron at a time, forming dehydroascorbic acid as the ultimate oxidized product. If respiratory complexes I and II were blocked by suitable inhibitors, how many molecules of ATP could be made per ascorbate molecule oxidized?
10. Besides the routes through respiratory complexes I and II, there are two other major routes by which electrons can be passed to ubiquinone.
    a. One of these involves glycerol 3-phosphate dehydrogenase, which oxidizes glycerol 3-phosphate to DHAP and passes the electrons via a FAD moiety to ubiquinone. This flavoprotein is bound to the outer leaflet of the inner mitochondrial membrane, and is an important player in the glycerol phosphate shuttle (its counterpart is the cytosolic enzyme of the same name that oxidizes NADH to reduce DHAP to glycerol 3-phosphate). Why does this route lead to the synthesis of only 1.5 ATP molecules per 1 molecule of glycerol 3-phosphate oxidized?
    b. The second major alternative route starts inside the mitochondrial matrix, with the oxidation of fatty acids. Through a series of flavoproteins, the electrons from fatty acid oxidation are passed to ubiquinone. The breakdown of a 16-carbon fatty acid such as palmitic acid will generate 7 molecules of $FADH_2$, whose pairs of electrons can be passed to ubiquinone by this route. How many ATP molecules, in total, could be generated from these seven $FADH_2$ molecules?

REFERENCES

R. K. Nakamoto, D. J. Ketchum, and M. K. Al-Shawi. (1999). "Rotational coupling in the F_0F_1 ATP synthase," *Annu. Rev. Biophys. Biomol. Struct.* 28:205–234.

M. Saraste. (1999). "Oxidative phosphorylation at the *fin de siècle*," *Science* 283:1488–1494.

L. Sazanov. (2007). "Respiratory complex I: Mechanistic and structural insights provided by the crystal structure of the hydrophilic domain," *Biochemistry* 47:2275–2288.

D. Stock, A. G. W. Leslie, and J. E. Walker. (1999). "Molecular architecture of the rotary motor in ATP synthase," *Science* 286:1700–1705.

T. Tsukihara et al. (1996). "The whole structure of the 13-subunit oxidized cytochrome *c* oxidase at 2.8 Å," *Science* 272:1136–1144.

D. Xia et al. (1997). "Crystal structure of the cytochrome bc_1 complex from bovine heart mitochondria," *Science* 277:60–66.

V. Yankovskaya et al. (2003). "Architecture of succinate dehydrogenase and reactive oxygen species generation," *Science* 299:700–704.

CHAPTER 12

Other Pathways of Carbohydrate Metabolism

Learning Objectives

1. Define and use correctly the following terms: *glucose 6-phosphate dehydrogenase, transketolase, stages 1 and 2 of pentose phosphate path, glutathione, sulfhydryl buffer, glutathione reductase, hemolytic anemia, glucuronic acid, glucuronides, glycoprotein, Wernicke-Korsakoff syndrome,* and *bilirubin.*
2. Describe the role of the pentose phosphate pathway, noting important products, intermediates, and precursors in this pathway (e.g., fructose 6-phosphate, ribose 5-phosphate, NADPH). Identify the two stages in this pathway. Note the different modes of operation of the pathway, its connection to cellular demands for energy and reducing power, and the availability of substrate.
3. Recognize the compound glutathione, and describe its multiple biochemical roles in the cell. Explain how levels of reduced and oxidized glutathione are related to NADPH levels in the cell. Describe how this phenomenon offers protection against malaria and how it affects the action of antimalarial compounds such as pamaquine.
4. Describe the role of UDP-activated intermediates in the synthesis of complex carbohydrates. Explain why nucleotide sugars often appear as intermediates in the interconversion of sugars and in the biosynthesis of complex carbohydrates. Describe the role of pyrophosphorylases in the syntheses of complex carbohydrates.
5. Describe how glucuronic acid is made. Explain how and where glucuronic acid plays a role in the cell. Recognize the structures of glucuronic acid and *N*-acetylglucosamine.
6. List several common complex carbohydrates. List several common glycoproteins and identify their functions.
7. Describe the symptoms and common biochemical cause of Wernicke-Korsakoff syndrome. Describe the treatment for this disease.
8. Explain how sugars are linked to proteins via asparagine and serine or threonine.
9. Describe differences in the glycolipids contributing to the different blood group antigens. Explain the biochemical basis for these differences.

Pentose Phosphate Pathway

The pentose phosphate path is also known as the phosphogluconate pathway, hexose monophosphate shunt, and pentose phosphate shunt (**Figure 12-1**). This pathway is principally responsible for producing NADPH for biosynthetic reactions (anabolism) and pentoses for nucleic acids (e.g., ribose 5-phosphate).

Like glycolysis, the pentose phosphate path oxidizes glucose. Instead of producing NADH, however, it produces NADPH and a mix of sugar–phosphates and intermediates related to

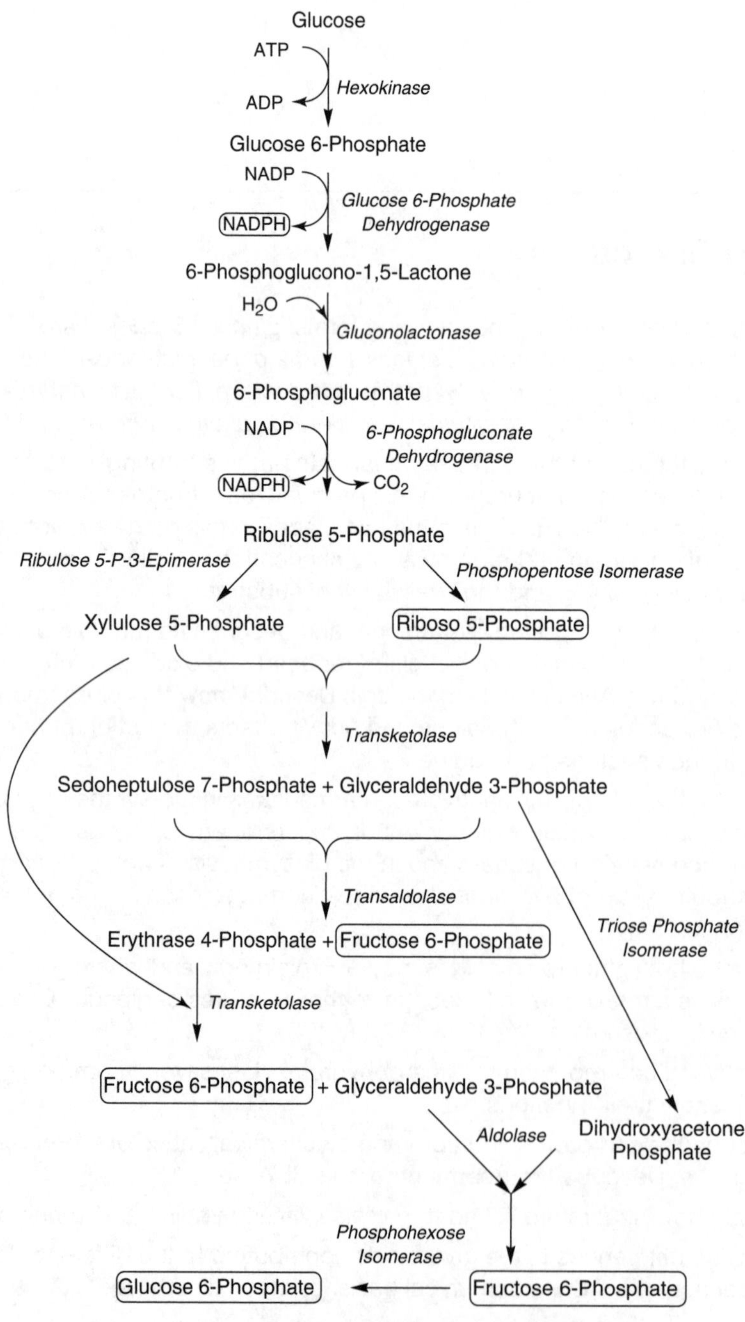

Figure 12-1 The pentose phosphate pathway. Glucose enters and is oxidized to provide NADPH and ribose 5-phosphate. The path shares enzymes and intermediates with glycolysis.

glycolysis. The enzymes of this pathway are cytosolic, located in the liver, in adipose tissue, and in other tissues. The "shunt" terminology arises from the fact that this is not the major path for the oxidation of glucose; instead, it is a relatively minor pathway for the oxidation of glucose (approximately 10% in adipocytes, but near 0% in muscle).

Summary of the Pathway

A Major Source of Reducing Power for Biosynthesis

In both glycolysis and the pentose phosphate pathway, glucose is oxidized to CO_2 in the cytoplasm, with trapping of electrons and hydrogen in form of reduced nicotinamides. In the pentose phosphate pathway, those reduced nicotinamides are NADPH. This pathway is the principal source of reducing power for biosynthesis in chemotrophs. There are, however, other sources of NADPH in the cytoplasm—namely, cytosolic NADP-linked malate and isocitrate dehydrogenases (the mitochondrial forms of these enzymes appeared briefly earlier in this book, in the discussion of the TCA cycle). Overall, the pentose phosphate pathway is very active in adipose tissue and in liver and kidney cells; it is also quite important for red blood cells. This high level of activity is linked primarily to consumption of NADPH in fatty acid synthesis in those metabolically active tissues, but there is also a linkage to protection against oxidative damage (see the material later in this chapter on glutathione). The pathway does not contribute much in muscle, where little or no synthesis of fatty acids takes place.

Reactions

The pentose phosphate path has several reactions and compounds in common with glycolysis (compare stages I and II of glycolysis and the reactions here involving glyceraldehyde 3-phosphate and dihydroxyacetone phosphate). Also, there is linkage through the enzymes transketolase and transaldolase, which help convert (excess) ribose 5-phosphate into glycolytic intermediates.

The path has two stages. *Stage I* involves the oxidation of glucose to CO_2, forming ribulose 5-phosphate; it is also where NADPH is generated. *Stage II* recombines the carbon skeletons and feeds them back to stage I for further reaction; it is also where ribose 5-phosphate is formed. Stage II is where most of the branching in the pathway arises. The rate of the process through the various branches is controlled by cellular demands for NADPH, ATP, and/or ribose 5-phosphate.

Glucose 6-phosphate dehydrogenase is a key enzyme in this cascade of events. It catalyzes the committed step; its catalytic action is regulated by levels of $NADP^+$. Overall regulation of the pathway is accomplished in large part by controlling the amount of this enzyme. Its cellular concentration can rise 10-fold as the organism goes from the "starved" state to the "fed" state.

Note the use of thiamine pyrophosphate (TPP) as a cofactor in the enzyme *transketolase*. This enzyme appears more than once in stage II of the pentose phosphate pathway. It catalyzes the removal of a two-carbon unit from a ketose and its transfer to an aldose. The mechanism here is similar to that used in the oxidative decarboxylation of pyruvate in the enzymatic action by the E_1 subunit of the pyruvate dehydrogenase complex, and it involves the ability of the thiazole ring of TPP to form a carbanion, which can then attack carbonyl groups. Refer back to Chapter 10 for further details on the role of TPP in the pyruvate dehydrogenase complex and its mechanism.

Modes of Operation

Very crudely, there are four modes of operation of the pentose phosphate path (**Table 12-1**). For example, rapidly dividing cells are synthesizing large amounts of nucleic acid—both DNA and RNA—so they need a great deal of ribose 5-phosphate to make the precursor nucleotides

Condition	Response
Rapidly dividing cells; need for much more ribose 5-P than NADPH	Convert most of the glucose 6-P through fructose 6-P, and glyceraldehyde 3-P, to yield ribose 5-P
Balanced need for NADPH and ribose 5-P	Mostly form two NADPH and one ribose 5-P, using the oxidative branch
High demand for NADPH, little demand for ribose 5-P or ATP	Oxidize glucose completely to CO_2, by recycling ribose 5-P back to glucose 6-P, repeatedly
Growth, with high biosynthesis demands for NADPH and ATP	Use ribose 5-P to make pyruvate, then oxidize the pyruvate Also, feed glyceraldehyde 3-P and fructose 6-P into the glycolytic pathway, for ATP

Table 12-1 Four Modes of Operation for the Pentose Phosphate Pathway

(a good deal of NADPH is also produced this way). By adjusting the flow through the pathway to favor this particular output, the cell adjusts its metabolism for cell division. In a different setting, mature cells may have need for more protection against oxidative attack by free radicals or molecular oxygen, which calls for less ribose 5-phosphate but a great deal of NADPH. Under these circumstances, the cell does not draw off the ribose 5-phosphate, but instead further metabolizes it, thereby generating small fragments that are recombined in stage II to form new glucose molecules. (Of course, the atoms are not the same as those of the first glucose to enter the pathway, due to the oxidative decarboxylation in stage I.) The new glucose molecules can then be fed back to and degraded by stage I enzymes to yield more NADPH. This sort of "recycling" can continue until the original glucose is fully converted to CO_2.

The possibilities for rechanneling metabolic flow through stage II permit the cell to have a very flexible response, with different levels of output, depending on cellular conditions and demands. In actuality, cellular operation is probably a mixture of two or more of these modes, with the proportions varying according to cellular demands and the availability of substrate.

Glutathione and NADPH

Structure and Function of Glutathione

Glutathione is an important tripeptide with a free —SH group (**Figure 12-2**); thus a commonly used abbreviation for this compound is GSH. The free thiol undergoes redox readily. When it is oxidized in detoxification reactions, the product is a dimeric form of the peptide, held together by a disulfide bridge. This dimer is denoted as GSSG.

Two Important Roles for Glutathione

Action as a Sulfhydryl Buffer

Glutathione, which is present in a wide variety of cells at high concentrations (0.1 to 10 mM), acts as a reservoir of reducing power to maintain the proper oxidation state of key biochemicals. Its action here is analogous to the action of acid–base buffers, which help to stabilize the pH of a solution; hence glutathione can be described as a *sulfhydryl buffer*. Glutathione maintains the

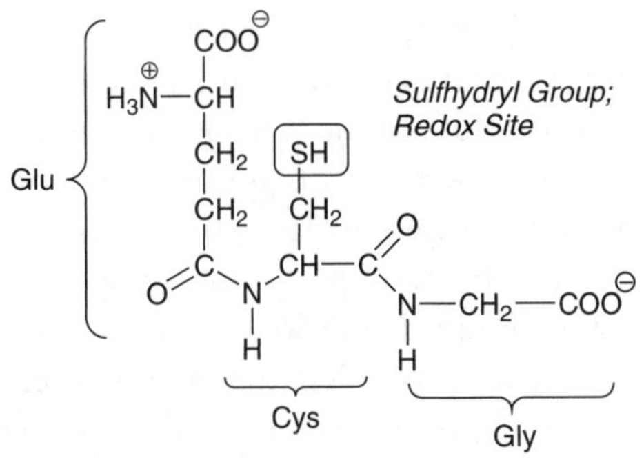

Figure 12-2 Glutathione structure. This tripeptide has a redox-active thiol group.

side chains of Cys residues of hemoglobin and other proteins in the reduced state (in the form with the side chains having a free thiol —SH, not as —S—S— or other oxidized forms).

Detoxification of Dangerous Oxidants

Oxidants such as peroxides would cause extensive cellular damage to structural proteins and enzymes, nucleic acids, and biomembrane components. To avoid this outcome, they must be quickly scavenged from the cell before they cause major harm. Glutathione can readily react with them in a redox reaction, to inactivate them:

$$2\ \text{GSH} + \text{R—O—O—H} \rightarrow \text{GSSG} + \text{H}_2\text{O} + \text{ROH} \qquad (12\text{-}1)$$

When glutathione is oxidized, it forms —S—S— bridges (disulfide form, GSSG). In this form it cannot detoxify oxidants or reduce Cys thiols in proteins. The thiol (reduced) form of glutathione must be regenerated from the disulfide form by the action of *glutathione reductase,* which uses NADPH as a source of electrons. In fact, in red blood cells, this function is a major role for NADPH. The reaction is

$$\text{GSSG} + \text{NADPH} + \text{H}^+ \rightarrow 2\ \text{GSH} + \text{NADP}^+ \qquad (12\text{-}2)$$

Protection Against Hemolysis

NADPH is formed through the pentose phosphate pathway. Disruptions of the pathway will, of course, reduce the level of available NADPH. Lower levels of NADPH lead to lower levels of (reduced) glutathione. Such a decrease can become an especially acute problem for red blood cells, which cannot generate reduced glutathione by other paths. This problem translates into less protection for the cell against oxidants in general. For red blood cells, sulfhydryl groups on the hemoglobin molecules may be oxidized, which will destabilize the hemoglobin and cause it to denature and aggregate. This aggregation of hemoglobin can lead to hemolysis (rupture of the cell membrane) and, therefore, to *hemolytic anemia.*

Enzyme Deficiency and Malarial Protection

A deficiency in glucose 6-phosphate dehydrogenase activity lowers NADPH levels, which in turn means that less glutathione is present in the reduced form. This deficiency leaves cells more susceptible to oxidant attack; red blood cells are especially be susceptible to hemolysis. This particular enzyme deficiency is widespread (hundreds of millions of people have reduced activity in this enzyme), and several types of it are possible.

The lower activity of glucose 6-phosphate dehydrogenase may act as protective device against plasmodial parasites that attack red blood cells, such as those causing malaria. These parasites require a reduced form of glutathione. Thus, if the red blood cell has less reduced glutathione, then the parasite has less chance to replicate and continue infection. In this way, the mutation offers some protection against malaria. Of course, the red blood cells are now in danger of hemolysis because the hemoglobin is not as well protected against oxidation. The protective effect of this apparently deleterious biochemical mutation (loss of activity in glucose 6-phosphate dehydrogenase) parallels the hemoglobin-S mutation that leads to sickle cell trait, where again the danger of hemolysis is balanced against the protection against malarial infection.

Clinical Application

Certain drugs increase levels of toxic peroxides—for example, pamaquine, an antimalarial agent (**Figure 12-3**). In the absence of sufficient reduced glutathione, treatment with pamaquine may cause hemolysis and anemia. Compounds in certain foods (e.g., in fava beans) may also produce the same effects. If unchecked, the symptoms may become severe and lead to death.

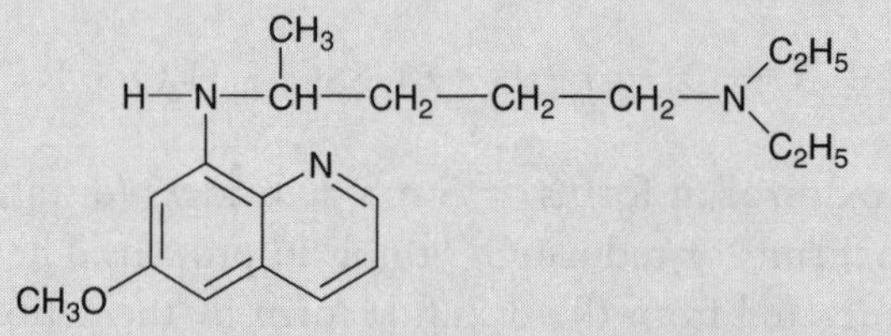

Figure 12-3 Pamaquine is representative of a set of compounds that are used to combat malaria. These agents interfere with the parasite's ability to detoxify hemoglobin digestion by-products.

Metabolism of Complex Carbohydrates

As noted in connection with glycolysis, the body can use a variety of hexoses besides glucose as fuel. These hexoses are derived from enzymatic hydrolysis of polysaccharides taken in through the diet (see Chapter 8). Generally these other hexoses require conversion to glucose or fructose (or phosphorylated derivatives of these sugars) before entering an oxidative pathway. Also, these interconversions often use a UDP moiety as an activating group. Furthermore, the cell can use activated sugars to make new, more complicated chains of sugars, so-called complex carbohydrates. The synthesis of glycogen was discussed earlier, in Chapter 9. Here we return to some of the carbohydrates covered in Chapter 2, to discuss details of their biosynthesis.

Biosynthesis of Complex Carbohydrates

In the term *complex carbohydrate*, "complex" means some form of polysaccharide. These molecules include lactose, starch, sucrose, pectin, chondroitin, hyaluronic acid, blood group antigens, and many more. Such complex carbohydrates are often synthesized using nucleotide sugars as intermediates, much as was seen with the synthesis of glycogen. Most often it is the UDP–sugar that is used, but other nucleotide sugars (with, for example, ADP and GDP) play roles as well.

Nucleotide sugars are used as intermediates in this biosynthesis process for three reasons: (1) the nucleotide is an excellent leaving group, (2) the nucleotide moiety provides a good recognition point for channeling such metabolites into the correct pathways, and (3) the free energy of hydrolysis of the sugar–nucleotide is comparable to that for hydrolysis of ATP. When a good leaving group is available, there is a lower energy barrier and the kinetics are faster; with a very favorable free energy of hydrolysis, the system gains a favorable equilibrium constant for a coupled reaction, so there is more formation of product.

Nucleotide sugars are synthesized from the phosphorylated sugar and the nucleotide triphosphate, much as was seen previously with the synthesis of UDP–glucose. In general, the reaction is

$$\text{Hexose 1-P} + \text{NTP} \rightarrow \text{NDP-hexose} + \text{PP}_i \qquad (12\text{-}3)$$

This is the route to ADP–glucose, dTDP–glucose, and GDP–mannose, for example. The enzymes catalyzing these reactions are pyrophosphorylases. Subsequent biochemical reactions use these activated sugars to make sucrose, lactose, and other complex carbohydrates.

General Synthetic Paths to Complex Carbohydrates

The reactions in the biosynthesis pathways for complex carbohydrates (**Figure 12-4**) are the opposite of "digestion," or stage I of catabolism. We omit most of the details; we have already seen the pathway leading to glycogen in Chapter 9.

Some of these products are short oligomers (e.g., sucrose is a simple heterodimer of glucose and fructose), some are of intermediate length (e.g., the blood group antigens), and others are quite long polymers (e.g., starch). Some involve groups other than carbohydrates (e.g., the blood group antigens are linked to a lipid, forming a *glycolipid*; see Chapter 2).

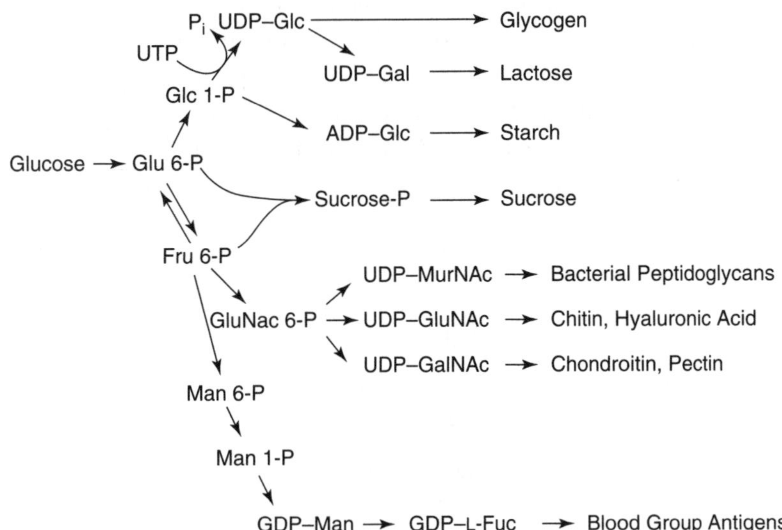

Figure 12-4 The routes to different complex carbohydrates, from simple disaccharides to complex polymers. Note the use of common intermediates.

Note the use of ADP as an activating group in the synthesis of starch. Starch is a storage form of glucose used by plants. There are two general forms of starch. The first is amylose, in which the glucose residues are joined in a linear chain (no branches) by $\alpha(1 \rightarrow 4)$ linkages. The second is amylopectin, which also has $\alpha(1 \rightarrow 4)$ linkages between glucose units, but is branched similarly to glycogen, with occasional $\alpha(1 \rightarrow 6)$ linkages.

Glucuronic Acid and N-Acetylglucosamine

N-Acetylglucosamine

As discussed in Chapter 2, amino sugars are important building blocks of several different types of biopolymers found in connective tissue, and they play key roles in cell surface recognition moieties used by the immune system, among other functions. *N*-Acetylglucosamine (NAG; **Figure 12-5**) is the most common amino sugar in these biopolymers.

Through a series of sequential steps, for NAG the nitrogen in the amino group is derived from glutamine, and the acetyl group is derived from acetyl-CoA, (**Figure 12-6**). The amino sugar–phosphate is then acetylated and converted to the UDP derivative. Note the appearance here of acetyl-CoA again, a reminder of how intimately metabolic pathways are intertwined.

Glucuronic Acid

Glucuronic acid is an oxidized form of glucose, formed by the enzymatic oxidation of UDP–glucose (**Figure 12-7**). With *N*-acetylglucosamine, it forms hyaluronic acid, or hyaluronate, an ionic polymer (**Figure 12-8**). Hyaluronate is composed of repeating disaccharide units of glucuronic acid and *N*-acetylglucosamine (see Chapter 2). Solutions of hyaluronic acid are clear and viscous; they are a major constituent of both the vitreous humor of the eye and the synovial fluid in joints (serving there as a lubricant). Hyaluronate is also a component of cartilage and tendons.

Glucuronic acid is important in the metabolism of drugs and other exogenous substances. In particular, it is used to form *glucuronides*. In a glucuronide, glucuronic acid is covalently joined (conjugated) with another compound (e.g., drugs, bilirubin) to help in their excretion or detoxification by improving the overall aqueous solubility of the compound.

Glycoproteins

Table 12-2 lists some of the main classes of *glycoproteins* and their biological roles (also see Chapter 2). In glycoproteins, oligosaccharides (short chains of sugars directly linked to one another) are attached to the protein. Some carbohydrate groups are used as recognition features to direct the protein after synthesis to the appropriate cellular location; in other cases, the carbohydrate chain plays a direct structural role (e.g., in keratan sulfate and chondroitin sulfate for connective tissues such as cartilage and ligaments). The sugar residues may be modified in

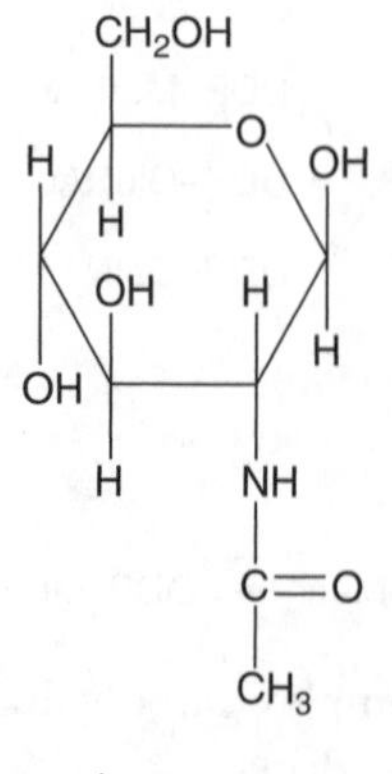

Figure 12-5 Structure of *N*-acetylglucosamine.

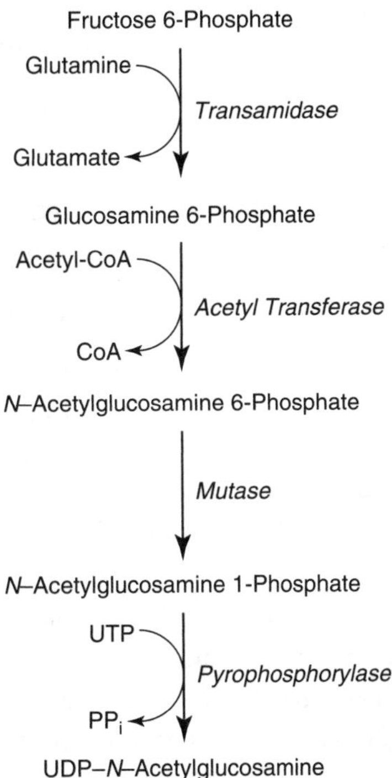

Figure 12-6 The route from fructose to *N*-acetylglucosamine starts with fructose 6-phosphate and ends with the easily hydrolyzed UDP derivative of *N*-acetylglucosamine.

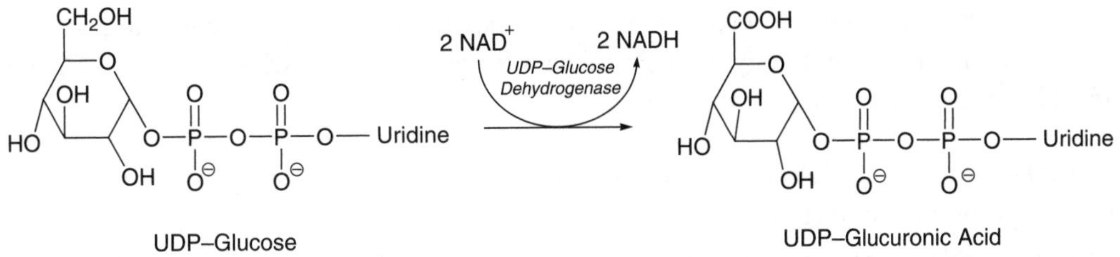

UDP–Glucose $\xrightarrow{\text{UDP–Glucose Dehydrogenase; } 2\ NAD^+ \rightarrow 2\ NADH}$ UDP–Glucuronic Acid

Figure 12-7 Glucuronic acid is formed via UDP derivatization of glucose, followed by oxidation (linked to two sequential reductions of NAD^+), and then release of the oxidized sugar.

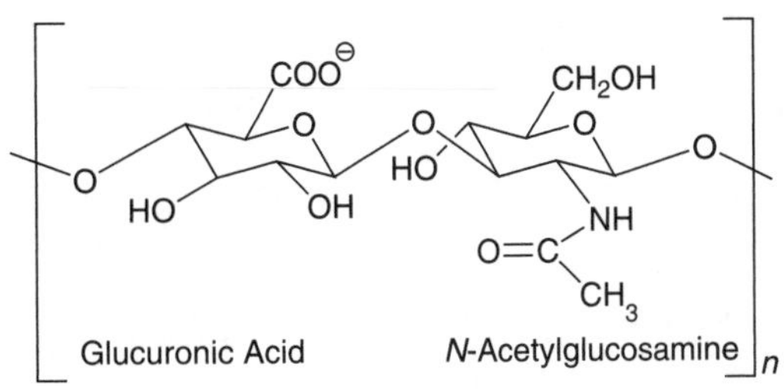

Glucuronic Acid — *N*-Acetylglucosamine

Figure 12-8 Hyaluronic acid is a copolymer of alternating residues of glucuronic acid and *N*-acetylglucosamine.

Name	Function
Collagen	Structural, connective tissue
Mucopolysaccharides	Structural, connective tissue
Enzymes (e.g., ribonuclease B, prothrombin)	Catalytic activity regulation
Hormones (e.g., thyroglobulin, erythropoietin)	Intercellular communication and control
Glycophorin	Erythrocyte membrane structure
HLA antigens	Immune system regulation
γ-Globulins	Immune system recognition/regulation
Fibrinogen	Blood clotting

Table 12-2 Selected Glycoproteins and Their Presumed Functions

a number of ways: They may have amino or acetyl or sulfate groups attached, and they may be oxidized to produce carboxylic acid moieties, and so on.

Glycosaminoglycans are polysaccharides used by bacterial and animal cells to form a protective but porous coating. They are composed of repeating disaccharide units, with each unit containing an amino sugar that is either *N*-acetylglucosamine or *N*-acetylgalactosamine. Either or both of the two sugars may be further modified, by oxidation, sulfation, or other means.

Certain extracellular proteins, called *proteoglycans* or *mucopolysaccharides*, carry sulfated glycosaminoglycans. They constitute a large class of glycoproteins. Some of these polymers act as a sort of glue or cement, holding tissues and cells together. Others are involved in blood clotting (e.g., the anticoagulant heparin), and still others in cell-to-cell signaling and signal transduction, recognition of pathogens, and more. A number of rather severe (but relatively rare) genetic diseases are associated with deficiencies in formation or breakdown of mucopolysaccharides or glycosaminoglycans.

The structure and terminology of sugar linkages for glycoproteins were covered in Chapter 2. **Figure 12-9** recapitulates the essentials:

- *N*-Linked sugars are generally attached through a side-chain nitrogen on an asparagine (Asn) residue of the protein.
- *O*-Linked sugars are generally attached through the oxygen atom on the side chain of a serine (Ser) or threonine (Thr) residue.

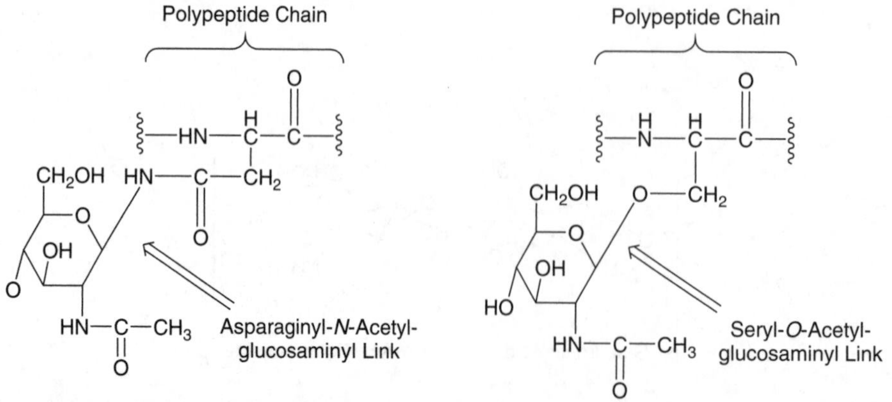

Figure 12-9 *N*-Linked sugars are attached to proteins through asparaginyl residues; O-linked sugars are attached through residues such as serine or threonine.

Clinical Application

UDP–glucuronate can be reacted with an exogenous or endogenous compound, in a reaction catalyzed by UDP–glucuronyltransferase (abbreviated as UGT). Attachment of the glucuronic acid moiety improves the aqueous solubility of the compound, due to the ionized carboxylate on the glucuronyl moiety. This increase in solubility is important for drug detoxification, steroid excretion, and bilirubin excretion.

Bilirubin Excretion

Bilirubin derives from the breakdown of hemoglobin, specifically the heme group. The catabolism of hemoglobin goes through opening of the tetrapyrrole ring, leading to a dark-green-pigmented protein, verdoglobin. The protein is digested back to amino acids and the tetrapyrrole is liberated as biliverdin. The liver converts the biliverdin to bilirubin monoglucuronide and diglucuronide, first by reducing the biliverdin (a greenish pigment) to bilirubin (a yellowish pigment) and then by conjugating the bilirubin with one or two molecules of glucuronic acid (**Figure 12-10**). This transformation improves the solubility of bilirubin and aids in its excretion.

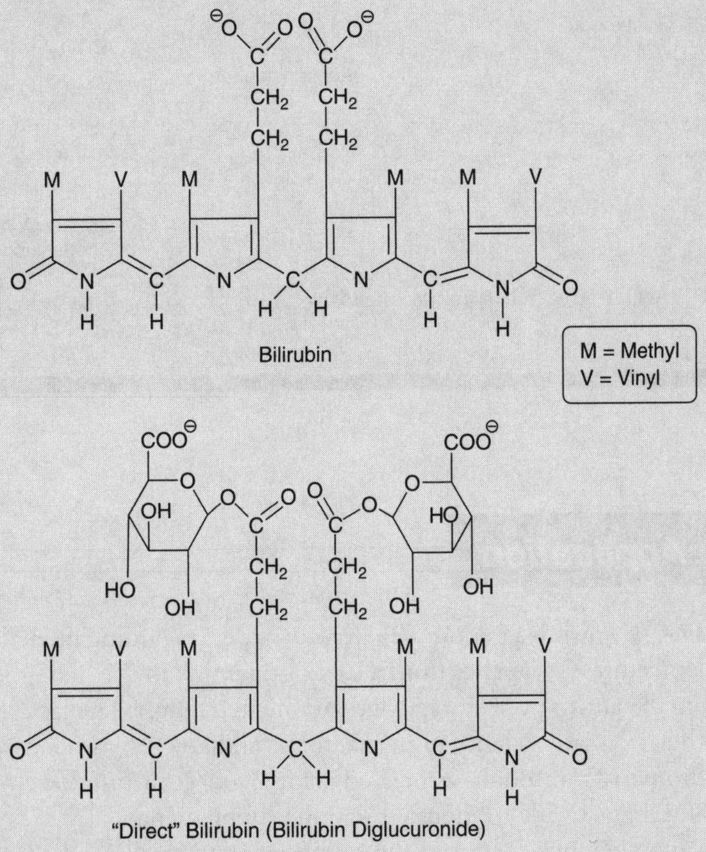

Bilirubin

M = Methyl
V = Vinyl

"Direct" Bilirubin (Bilirubin Diglucuronide)

Figure 12-10 The solubility, and hence the excretion, of bilirubin is improved by attaching residues of glucuronic acid.

(Continued)

In newborns, the activity of the UGT enzyme is low and can take a few days to develop. In the meantime, bilirubin builds up in the newborn's bloodstream, leading to physiological jaundice. The characteristic yellow skin and eye color associated with jaundice stems from the accumulation of bilirubin in the blood.

Acetaminophen Excretion

As an example of drug conjugation, the common pain-relief drug acetaminophen is conjugated with glucuronic acid (**Figure 12-11**) to improve its solubility and aid in its excretion via the urine. Note the attachment of the glucuronide moiety via the phenolic group on the acetaminophen. This kind of ester formation is a common feature of drug metabolism and excretion.

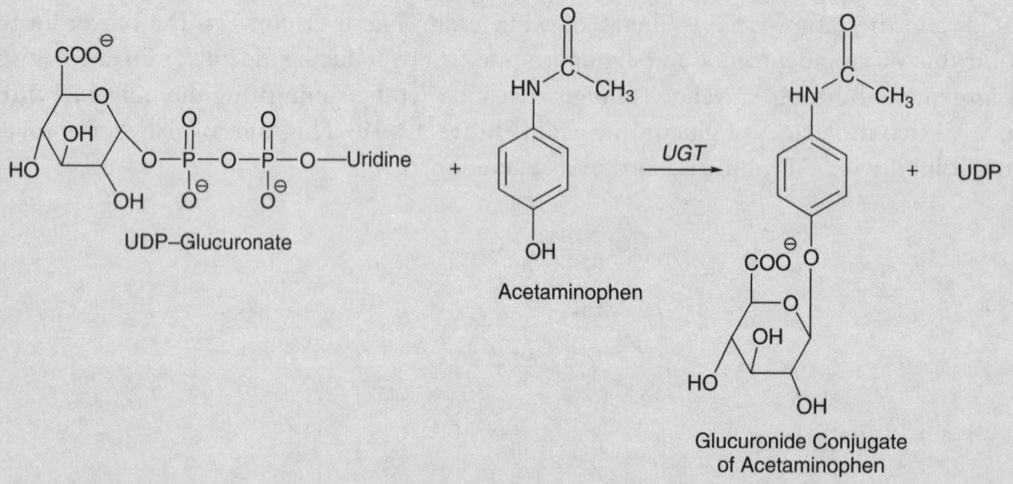

UDP–Glucuronate + Acetaminophen —UGT→ Glucuronide Conjugate of Acetaminophen + UDP

Figure 12-11 Acetaminophen is metabolized by the body to form the glucuronide, which is readily excreted.

Clinical Application

Wernicke-Korsakoff syndrome is a neuropsychiatric disorder (including mental disturbances, ataxia, and other features) that arises from a lack of thiamine in the diet, poor absorption of thiamine from the gut, or poor storage of thiamine in the liver. The lack of thiamine (as TPP) impairs the enzymatic activity of transketolase and key dehydrogenases. Wernicke-Korsakoff syndrome is commonly associated with alcoholism or a malnourished state. Sufferers respond dramatically to dietary thiamine supplements.

There is some evidence for a genetic component to this disease. Transketolase in susceptible persons has been shown to bind TPP much less tightly, and the circulating level of TPP is simply not high enough to drive the cofactor onto the enzyme. Without the necessary bound cofactor, the enzyme is catalytically inactive.

QUESTIONS FOR DISCUSSION

1. The only known way for cells to generate $NADP^+$ is from NAD^+ through a phosphorylation catalyzed by NAD kinase. What would be the consequences of a mutation in this kinase that reduced its catalytic ability?
2. Suppose that a defect reduced the activity of the enzyme transaldolase. For each of the four modes of operation of the pentose phosphate path, list possible consequences of such a defect.
3. Primaquine is an antimalarial drug that can generate reactive oxygen species. Would it be a safe drug to administer to a patient who has a deficiency in the activity of the enzyme glucose 6-phosphate dehydrogenase? Explain your choice.
4. Crigler-Najjar syndrome is a rare autosomal disorder in the excretion of bilirubin, resulting in high circulating blood levels of free bilirubin. A deficiency in which of the following enzymes would cause this disorder? Explain your choice.
   a. Glutathione reductase
   b. Galactose 1-P uridyl transferase
   c. UDP–glucuronosyltransferase
   d. Glucose 6-phosphate dehydrogenase
5. Identify sites on the following drugs where the enzyme UDP–glucuronosyltransferase might act.
   a. Aspirin
   b. Chloramphenicol
6. Neonates can show an inability to excrete the antibiotic chloramphenicol, resulting in "gray baby syndrome." How might this disorder be related to a deficiency in the activity of the enzyme UDP–glucuronosyltransferase?
7. Suppose that a patient has a mutated form of transketolase that is defective in binding TPP; the defective enzyme binds the cofactor about one-tenth as well as does the wild-type enzyme. Which symptoms might the patient exhibit? How might they be treated?
8. Why isn't the pentose phosphate path very active in muscle tissue, compared to adipose tissue?

REFERENCES

T. Feizi. (1990). "The major blood group ABO(H) determining genes are isolated," *Trends Biochem. Sci.* 15:330–331.

C. G. Gahmberg and M. Tolvanen. (1996). "Why mammalian cell surface proteins are glycoproteins," *Trends Biochem. Sci.* 21:308–311.

A. Meister. (1988). "Glutathione metabolism and its selective modification," *J. Biol. Chem.* 263:17205–17208.

T. W. Sedlak et al. (2009). "Bilirubin and glutathione have complementary antioxidant and cytoprotective roles," *Proc. Natl. Acad. Sci. USA* 106:5171–5176.

N. M. Senozan and C. A. Thielman. (1991). "Glucose 6-phosphate dehydrogenase deficiency," *J. Chem. Educ.* 68:7–10.

K. R. Taylor and R. L. Gallo. (2006). "Glycosaminoglycans and their proteoglycans: host-associated molecular patterns for initiation and modulation of inflammation," *FASEB J.* 20:9–22.

CHAPTER 13

Lipid Metabolism

Learning Objectives

1. Define and use correctly the following terms: *lipoproteins, lipase, lipolysis, chylomicrons, acyl carrier protein, phosphopantetheine, malonyl-CoA, acetyl-CoA carboxylase, citrate shuttle, fatty acid synthase, pernicious anemia, carnitine, β-oxidation, α-oxidation, ω-oxidation, carnitine palmitoyl transferase, cobalamin (Vitamin B_{12}), Refsum disease, ketone bodies,* and *ketogenesis.*
2. Describe the process by which lipids are taken up by the body, including the hydrolytic steps and the role of lipases.
3. Recognize the structures of carnitine, ketone bodies, and cobalamin.
4. Explain how fatty acids are stored as a fuel reserve by the body. Relate the structure of triacylglycerols (triglycerides) to their ability to store metabolic energy.
5. Describe the process of lipolysis, noting important reactions, enzymes, cellular locations, and mechanisms of regulation.
6. Describe the β-oxidation pathway for fatty acids, noting important cofactors. Relate the production of acetyl-CoA here to the need for oxaloacetate for complete oxidation of fatty acids via the TCA cycle, and to the production of ketone bodies.
7. Describe the role of carnitine in the transport of fatty acyl moieties into the mitochondrial matrix by the acylcarnitine:carnitine antitransporter. Note the roles of CPT1 and CPT2; describe how CPT1 is sensitive to malonyl-CoA and how this characteristic relates to cellular demand for energy.
8. Describe how the cell breaks down fatty acids with an odd number of carbon atoms. Connect this process to the metabolism of succinyl-CoA in the TCA cycle. Explain how catabolism of fatty acids with an odd number of carbons might be useful when carbohydrates are missing or depleted in the diet. Predict and explain the consequences of a defect in the catabolism of such fatty acids, including the relationship to methylmalonic aciduria.
9. Explain the molecular basis for pernicious anemia. List symptoms of this disease, and relate them to the underlying biochemical defect.
10. Explain how ketone bodies arise, and relate them to the pathology of diabetes mellitus.

11. Describe the biochemistry of the synthesis of fatty acids. Note starting materials and necessary cofactors, and identify the cellular location of the synthetic apparatus.
12. Describe the committing step for fatty acid biosynthesis, naming the enzyme and discussing the regulation of its activity. Compare the short-term and long-term regulation of fatty acid biosynthesis.
13. Explain why the synthesis of fatty acids costs energy. Connect fatty acid biosynthesis to the pentose phosphate pathway and the role of NADPH.
14. Explain how palmitate serves as a precursor for other fatty acids. Describe briefly how fatty acid chains may be elongated beyond palmitate, how they may have carbon–carbon double bonds or chain branches incorporated, and how they may be converted to fatty alcohols. Note how the absence of certain enzymes in humans makes particular fatty acids "essential."
15. Sketch the biosynthesis of triglycerides from fatty acids.
16. Sketch the biosynthesis of membrane phospholipids from fatty acids. Explain the role of cytidine nucleotides in the biosynthesis of membrane phospholipids. Describe the role of the endoplasmic reticulum as a location for membrane lipid biosynthesis.
17. Sketch the biosynthesis of cholesterol starting from acetyl-CoA, noting the key intermediate hydroxymethylglutaryl-CoA. List several biochemical roles for cholesterol, noting key metabolites. Recognize the structure of cholesterol.
18. Describe the citrate shuttle, and explain its role in the biosynthesis of lipids from carbohydrates, noting especially the role of membrane compartmentalization.
19. Describe how phytanic acid may be degraded through α-oxidation, followed by β-oxidation. Relate Refsum disease to a defect in α-oxidation.

Uptake and Storage of Lipids

Dietary fat (triglycerides) provides a major share of energy for the body. As a consequence, the transport, storage, and release of these lipids is of central importance in understanding energy metabolism in the body. Cholesterol is needed for modulating biomembrane fluidity and flexibility; in addition, it is important as a precursor to the steroid hormones and to the bile acids that help to solubilize dietary lipids. The uptake and distribution of dietary cholesterol is also of major importance; there is a strong connection between circulating cholesterol levels and diseases of the circulatory system. The body has a rather intricate set of processes for absorbing, distributing, and storing these two classes of lipids.

Lipid Uptake from the Digestive Tract: Lipoproteins

Dietary intake of fatty acids is mostly in the form of triglycerides (typically 20–40% of dietary calories). The process of digestion starts with secretion of bile (a mixture of bile salts, phosphatidylcholine, and cholesterol) into the digestive tract. Bile combines with dietary lipids to form micelles in a process called emulsification; the micelles hold the otherwise insoluble lipids in suspension. The micelles are then attacked by hydrolytic enzymes (*lipases*) in the digestive tract: pancreatic lipase, cholesteryl esterase, and a phospholipase. Pancreatic lipase partially hydrolyzes triglycerides to the 2-monoglyceride and free fatty acids; cholesteryl esterase cleaves the ester linkage joining cholesterol to a fatty acid and releases the free fatty acid and free cholesterol; and phospholipase acts to hydrolyze the ester linkage between a fatty acid chain and the glycerol–phosphate backbone of a phospholipid. The fatty acids and 2-monoglycerides are then absorbed by mucosal cells, through passive diffusion. Inside the mucosa, there is resynthesis of the fatty acids into triglycerides. This breakdown and resynthesis is necessary because triglycerides themselves diffuse very poorly into mucosal cells. The triglycerides and the absorbed cholesterol are then secreted via the lymph into the blood, in association with phospholipids and certain proteins (apolipoproteins) that strongly associate with lipids, with the macromolecular aggregates forming what are called *lipoproteins*.

Lipoprotein aggregates are roughly spherical or discoidal in shape, with a core of very nonpolar lipids surrounded by a monolayer of phospholipids, together with the apolipoprotein polypeptide chains. The protein chains help to solubilize the lipids and provide recognition features for directing the lipoprotein particle to one or another cellular target.

Five major classes of lipoprotein particles have been identified. **Table 13-1** summarizes the major physical features and functions of the lipoprotein particles, and **Table 13-2** describes their composition. *Chylomicrons* are large particles—composed mainly of triglycerides, but also cholesterol and phospholipids along with apolipoprotein B48—that are synthesized in intestinal mucosal cells. Their major function is to transport dietary triglycerides to adipose tissue and to muscle; they also transport dietary cholesterol from the gut to the liver. Very-low-density lipoproteins (VLDL) are predominantly triglycerides but also contain appreciable amounts of cholesterol, cholesterol esters, and phospholipids. They function mainly to transport endogenous triglycerides (e.g., those derived from storage sites in the body, not from the diet) and cholesteryl esters from the liver to outlying tissues. Low-density lipoproteins (LDL) are mainly cholesterol esters and phospholipids; they transport cholesterol to a wide variety of tissues. Intermediate-density lipoproteins (IDL) have a high proportion of endogenous cholesterol esters. These particles help to transport endogenous cholesterol either for uptake by the liver or for conversion to LDL. High-density lipoproteins (HDL) are composed of phospholipids and cholesterol esters, but contain a higher proportion of protein than the other lipoproteins; they

Lipoprotein class	Size (nm)	Density Range (g/mL)	Major Function
Chylomicron	100–1000	<0.94	Dietary triglyceride transport
Very low density (VLDL)	30–80	0.94 to 1.006	Endogenous triglyceride transport
Intermediate density (IDL)	25–30	1.006 to 1.019	Endogenous cholesterol transport, triglyceride transport
Low density (LDL)	20–25	1.019 to 1.063	Endogenous cholesterol transport
High density (HDL)	5–12	1.063 to 1.21	Removal of cholesterol from tissues outside the liver

Table 13-1 Plasma Lipoprotein Characteristics and Function

Lipoprotein Class	Major Apoliproteins	Major Lipid Components
Chylomicrons	Apo A-I, apo A-II, apo A-IV, apo B-48, apo C-I, apo C-II, apo C-III, apo E	Triglycerides and phospholipids
VLDL	Apo B-100, apo C-I, apo C-II, apo C-III, apo E	Triglycerides, phospholipids, cholesterol, and cholesterol esters
IDL	Apo B-100, apo C-I, apo C-II, apo C-III, apo E	Composition intermediate between VLDL and LDL; triglycerides notably depleted
LDL	Apo B-100	Cholesterol esters, phospholipids, triglycerides, cholesterol
HDL	Apo A-I, apo A-II, apo A-IV, apo C-I, apo C-II, apo C-III, apo D, apo E	Phospholipids and cholesterol esters

Table 13-2 Composition of Major Lipoprotein Classes

help to remove cholesterol from tissues outside the liver and transfer cholesterol esters to other lipoprotein particle classes. Additionally, chylomicron fragments, which are composed mainly of cholesterol esters from the diet, transport cholesterol to the liver for uptake.

LDL accounts for approximately two-thirds of total serum cholesterol. High levels of LDL are associated with atherosclerosis, or "hardening of the arteries." Atherosclerosis derives from the accumulation of arterial plaques (fatty deposits in the lining of the artery) that can eventually lead to blockage of the artery and to coronary heart disease if the artery so affected passes through cardiac tissue. LDL is certainly a necessary part of the lipid transport system, but its association with coronary heart disease has led to its popular characterization as the "bad" lipoprotein (it is, of course, a misnomer to refer to LDL as "bad cholesterol"). Conversely, HDL is thought to aid in the removal of cholesterol from arterial wall plaques and so to reduce the risk of atherosclerosis—hence its reputation as the "good" lipoprotein.

Lipid Transport and Distribution

Lipids enter the circulation via the thoracic duct, which is part of the lymph system. Enterocytes form and secrete chylomicrons into the duct. When they are first secreted, these particles carry just apolipoprotein B48; once in the bloodstream, however, the chylomicrons gain additional lipoproteins (apo E and apo C-II). While circulating, the chylomicrons are also acted upon by lipoprotein lipase, an enzyme that splits off fatty acids from triglycerides. The liberated fatty acids are picked up by serum albumin, which is responsible for the major part of transport of free fatty acids. Free fatty acids are taken up by muscle cells and by adipocytes for use as fuel (muscle) or for synthesis into triglycerides for storage (adipose tissue).

As a chylomicron is depleted of triglycerides, its density increases but its size decreases; the remnant chylomicron fragments are taken up by liver cells through receptor-mediated endocytosis (apo E is the ligand for the receptor). Liver cells break apart the remnant fragments and recycle the lipids, adding endogenous lipids as well, to form VLDL particles that are released into the circulation. VLDL particles carry apo E and apo C-II, but they have apo B-100 instead of apo B-48. As with chylomicrons, lipoprotein lipase degrades the triglycerides in the VLDL particles, converting them to the smaller and denser IDL species. Further action on triglycerides—this time by hepatic lipase—reduces the size even more, and the particle transfers its complement of apo C-II to HDL particles. The result is LDL: lipoprotein particles that are composed mainly of cholesterol esters and that carry only the apo B-100 lipoprotein. These particles can be taken up by receptor-mediated endocytosis by cells expressing a receptor for the apo B-100 lipoprotein. In this way, cholesterol is delivered to a wide variety of tissues for use in synthesizing and maintaining cell membranes. **Figure 13-1** sketches the overall process.

As noted earlier, fatty acids serve as a primary metabolic fuel for the cell; thus the triglycerides and free fatty acids delivered to peripheral tissues are either degraded to produce energy or (as triglycerides) stored in fat droplets in adipose tissue, as a deposit against future demands for energy. Cholesterol, however, is not degraded as a fuel. Its accumulation beyond a certain level can be cytotoxic, because a sufficiently high level of free cholesterol can disrupt cell membranes. To avoid this problem, cholesterol must be carried away from peripheral tissues for disposal. This "reverse transport" is accomplished by HDL.

HDL particles are made by both liver and intestinal cells. As secreted from these cells, the HDL particles are small, disc-shaped objects. They carry some phospholipid and apo A-I. These particles are very good at picking up unesterified cholesterol from peripheral cells. The cholesterol is then esterified by lecithin–cholesterol acyltransferase (LCAT). As the esterified cholesterol accumulates, the particle swells and becomes spherical. The particle also acquires a complement of apo C-II and apo E from VLDL and IDL. The cholesterol esters of HDL can be transferred to VLDL, IDL, and LDL, in a process mediated by cholesterol ester transfer protein. These latter classes of particles all carry apo B, so they can be taken up by the LDL receptors on liver cells. HDL itself can be taken up by liver cells as well, but investigation has shown

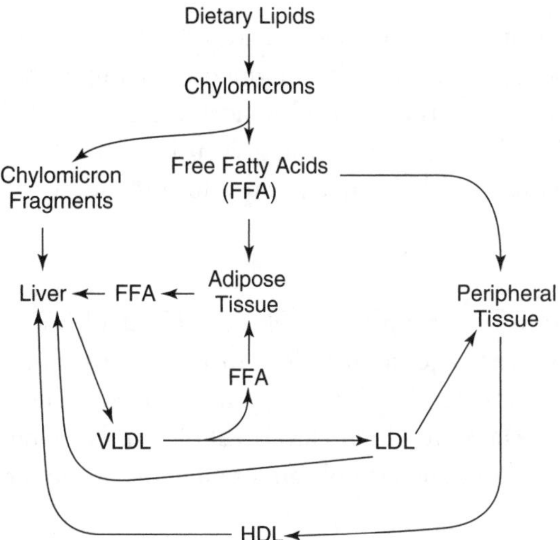

Figure 13-1 Summary of transport of lipids by lipoprotein particles. Dietary lipids enter the circulation as chylomicrons. Some of these fatty acids go to adipose and peripheral tissues, while fragments of the chylomicron are recycled in the liver and released as VLDL. VLDL loses fatty acids to adipose and peripheral tissues, becoming denser and smaller, and ending as LDL or as fragments (IDL; not shown); both VLDL and LDL deliver cholesterol to peripheral tissues. VLDL fragments and LDL are recycled to the liver and taken up by receptor-mediated endocytosis. HDL is responsible for reverse transport of cholesterol from peripheral tissues and is taken up by the liver by receptor-mediated endocytosis.

that the bulk of cholesterol from HDL enters the liver cells indirectly, through the shuttling of cholesterol esters from HDL to VLDL, IDL, and LDL.

Fatty Acid Storage in Adipocytes

Adipocytes (fat cells) are the obvious storage site for fatty acids. Under the light microscope one can see visible droplets of fat (triglycerides) inside adipocytes. Their structure consists of a very nonpolar core of triglycerides and sterol esters, with a surface layer of phospholipids and some associated proteins that block access of cellular enzymes to the fat droplet and that provide some regulatory control over the release of the lipids. Other cell types can also possess fat droplets—notably muscle cells, where the fat droplets are often found in close proximity to mitochondria, the organelles that will use the fatty acids for energy production.

Why store energy as triglycerides? And why use fatty acids as energy-storage molecules? Storing metabolic energy in this way provides a number of advantages:

- Fatty acids are highly reduced (many $—CH_2—$ groups), which means that they can be oxidized to release much more energy than partially oxidized fuels like sugars.
- Fatty acids tend to pack closely together, thereby excluding molecules of water (unlike sugars, which tend to stay highly hydrated). Thus fatty acids are relatively "dense" in terms of energy stored, compared to sugars.
- The triglyceride form puts three alkyl chains in close proximity to one another and promotes self-aggregation instead of individual solvation. That is, it promotes fat droplet formation, which is a good choice for compact storage.
- The glycerol "backbone" can also be used as fuel; nothing is wasted.
- Aggregation into droplets effectively reduces osmotic stress on the cell (similar to the use of glycogen for storage of glucose).

There are two main sources of fatty acids in adipocytes: They can enter as fatty acids from the circulation or they can be synthesized from glucose. In adipocytes, glucose is broken down to DHAP and pyruvate. Pyruvate is converted to acetyl-CoA, which then enters the fatty acid biosynthetic pathway. DHAP is also used for glycerol 3-phosphate synthesis. **Figure 13-2** summarizes the overall passage of these metabolites through adipocytes.

Cholesterol Storage

The storage and distribution of appropriate levels of cholesterol is a physiological problem. The aqueous solubility of cholesterol is extremely low, that of cholesterol esters even lower. Thus, in an aqueous environment, cholesterol will strongly tend to associate with other lipids, forming hydrophobic, nonpolar aggregates. Too high a level of cholesterol in a membrane will unfortunately tend to disrupt the membrane, so cholesterol cannot safely be sequestered for storage by building it up in biomembranes.

Cholesterol can be exchanged fairly readily by contact between lipoprotein particles and cell membranes, especially those lining the walls of blood vessels. Even so, its concentration in the bloodstream must be kept low, to avoid accumulation of the cholesterol in those cells lining blood vessels. Here the properties of cholesteryl esters come to the fore. These esters are even more hydrophobic than is cholesterol itself. Moreover, the esterified cholesterol is a larger molecule, which does not readily penetrate and cross biomembranes. Thus the cholesteryl esters in a lipoprotein particle are not so readily exchanged into the membranes of cells lining blood

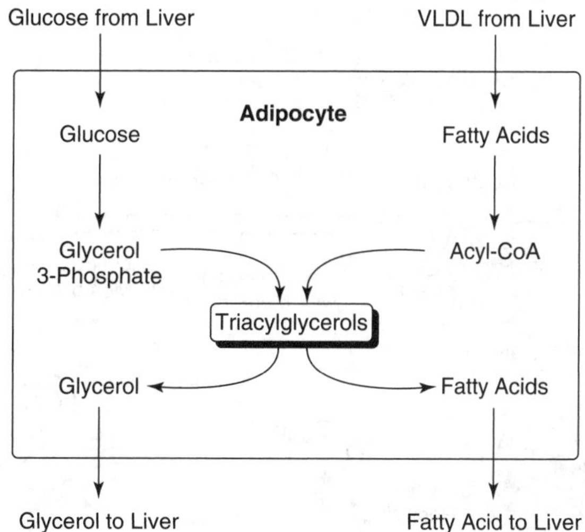

Figure 13-2 Metabolic flow through adipocytes. Lipids may enter the cell and be directly incorporated into stores of triglycerides, or lipids may be synthesized in situ from glycolytic intermediates. Stored triglycerides can be locally hydrolyzed to release free fatty acids and glycerol.

vessels; instead, these cholesteryl esters are taken up by cells when the lipoprotein particle is endocytosed.

The general process is illustrated in **Figure 13-3**. The lipoprotein makes contact with a specific receptor protein on the surface of the cell. The cell membrane folds around the receptor–lipoprotein complex and pinches it off to form a vesicle. The vesicle then fuses with degradative organelles called lysosomes. The lysosomes contain hydrolytic enzymes that break down the cholesterol esters to release the cholesterol and fatty acids; these molecules may be further metabolized inside the cell. The lipoprotein receptors are recycled to the plasma membrane for reuse by the cell, while the lipoproteins may be digested to amino acids and used locally.

While many types of cells can endocytose lipoprotein particles and thus take up cholesterol and triglycerides, the liver plays a major role in regulating the circulating level of cholesterol. First, the liver is the major site of cholesterol biosynthesis. Thus, even in the absence of dietary cholesterol, the body can still maintain enough cholesterol for proper functioning. Second, the liver actively regulates the level of lipoprotein particles transporting cholesterol, through uptake of LDL particles by endocytosis and release of VLDL particles. VLDL particles transport triglycerides and esterified cholesterol, whereas LDL particles are mostly responsible for cholesterol transport.

After endocytosis of an LDL particle by a liver cell, the lipoprotein receptors are recycled to the outer surface of the cell, as described previously. The incoming free cholesterol is esterified by acyl-CoA:cholesterol acyltransferase (ACAT), and the cholesteryl esters are stored as droplets (in association with triglycerides) inside the cell. Also, the incoming cholesteryl esters undergo a process of ester hydrolysis and re-esterification with a different fatty acid. The fatty acids attached to cholesteryl esters in LDL particles are typically polyunsaturated (e.g., linoleate). Upon uptake of the LDL particle, they are removed and replaced with mono-unsaturated fatty acids (for example, with oleate). These processed cholesteryl esters, with the attached mono-unsaturated fatty acids, serve as the storage form for cholesterol in liver cells. The stored cholesteryl ester depot can then be drawn upon as needed to supply constituents for VLDL particles for release to the circulation.

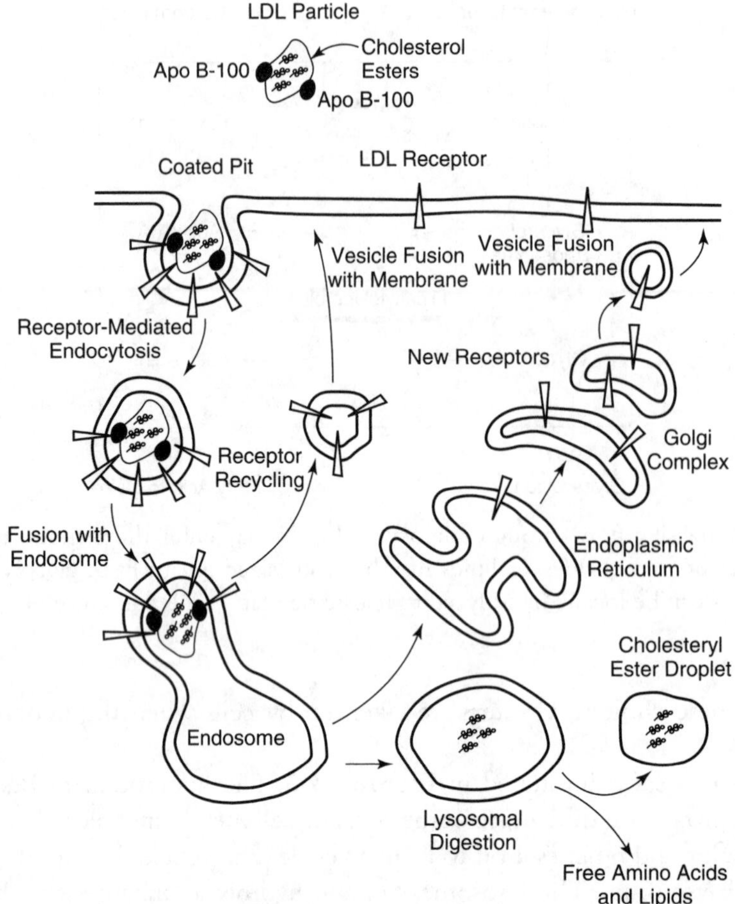

Figure 13-3 Uptake of LDL particles by receptor-mediated endocytosis. Binding is followed by endocytosis and fusion with lysosomes. Receptor proteins are recycled to the plasma membrane, while other proteins are digested to amino acids; fatty acids and cholesterol are liberated. Cholesterol and cholesterol esters are targeted to the endoplasmic reticulum or stored as droplets. Synthesis and processing of new receptors occur in the endoplasmic reticulum and the Golgi complex.

Fatty Acid Catabolism

The release of fatty acids and their subsequent controlled oxidation is a primary source of metabolic energy for the cell. The process of fatty acid release from triglyceride deposits (called lipolysis) is under hormonal control, which coordinates metabolism in different tissues according to demands for energy. Further control is exerted during the oxidation process, a process called β-oxidation.

The enzymes for β-oxidation are located in the mitochondrial matrix. Fatty acids or their CoA esters cannot cross the inner mitochondrial membrane without using a special transport mechanism involving the carrier molecule carnitine and the enzymes carnitine palmitoyl transferases 1 and 2. After transport, oxidation of the fatty acid occurs by removal of two-carbon units sequentially, as acetyl-CoA. Much of the catalytic action involves the β-carbon of the fatty acid chain—hence the description of the process as β-oxidation.

Fatty acid metabolism is intimately tied to carbohydrate metabolism. The acetyl-CoA generated from the breakdown of carbohydrates can be used for lipid biosynthesis, although the route is circuitous and involves export of the carbons from the matrix into the cytosol, via citrate.

Lipolysis and Its Regulation

In adipose tissues, the droplets of triglycerides (which may also contain esters of cholesterol and related compounds) are normally covered by a monolayer of phospholipids and proteins. These help to stabilize the fat droplet and protect it from the loss of its constituent lipids. When energy is needed by the body, hormones are released that stimulate the mobilization of these fat droplet stores of triglycerides. The protective protein coating is removed, and the triglycerides are hydrolyzed to release free fatty acids that can be transported through the bloodstream to tissues that need metabolic energy.

Lipolysis is the initial event in the breakdown of triglycerides inside adipocytes. This ester hydrolysis of the fatty acids linked to glycerol (**Figure 13-4**) is catalyzed by a hormone-sensitive lipase. In turn, the activity of the hormone-sensitive lipase is regulated by several hormones. Epinephrine, norepinephrine, glucagon, and adrenocorticotropic hormone (ACTH) all stimulate the activity, while insulin inhibits it. The general order of events leading to lipolysis is as follows (**Figure 13-5**):

1. Stimulatory hormones bind to a G-protein–coupled receptor on the outside of the cell, and stimulate adenylyl cyclase.
2. The stimulated adenylyl cyclase produces high intracellular levels of cAMP. As the level of cAMP rises, it stimulates activity of various protein kinases (cAMP acts here as a "second messenger").
3. A kinase phosphorylates the lipase and so activates it.
4. The phosphorylated, activated lipase proceeds to catalyze hydrolysis of triglycerides, and lipolysis results.

This pattern is very similar to that seen in glycogen breakdown, with the use of protein phosphorylation and second messengers.

Insulin produces its inhibitory actions by binding to a different kind of receptor on the outside of the cell—namely, a receptor-tyrosine kinase. The extracellular domain of this receptor binds insulin, while the intracellular domain has an enzymatic active site that phosphorylates tyrosines on proteins. The activated receptor initiates a cascade of steps that eventually leads to inhibition of the lipase. The pattern resembles that for inhibition of glycogen breakdown.

As an aside, the body produces several kinds of lipase, not all of which are sensitive to hormones. Some are secreted into the gastrointestinal tract, to aid in the breakdown of dietary fat (e.g., pancreatic lipase); some are extracellular and act on lipoprotein particles to release the fatty acids from triglycerides (e.g., lipoprotein lipase, which is activated by apolipoprotein C-II, a component of chylomicrons); and some are intracellular and act on internal stores of

$$R_2{-}\overset{\overset{O}{\|}}{C}{-}O{-}CH(CH_2{-}O{-}\overset{\overset{O}{\|}}{C}{-}R_1)(CH_2{-}O{-}\overset{\overset{O}{\|}}{C}{-}R_3) + 3\,H_2O \xrightarrow{\textit{Lipase}} \left\{\begin{array}{l} R_1{-}\overset{\overset{O}{\|}}{C}{-}OH \\ R_2{-}\overset{\overset{O}{\|}}{C}{-}OH \\ R_3{-}\overset{\overset{O}{\|}}{C}{-}OH \end{array}\right. + \begin{array}{c} CH_2OH \\ | \\ CHOH \\ | \\ CH_2OH \end{array}$$

Figure 13-4 Breakdown of triglycerides (lipolysis) releases one molecule of glycerol and three fatty acids per triglyceride molecule.

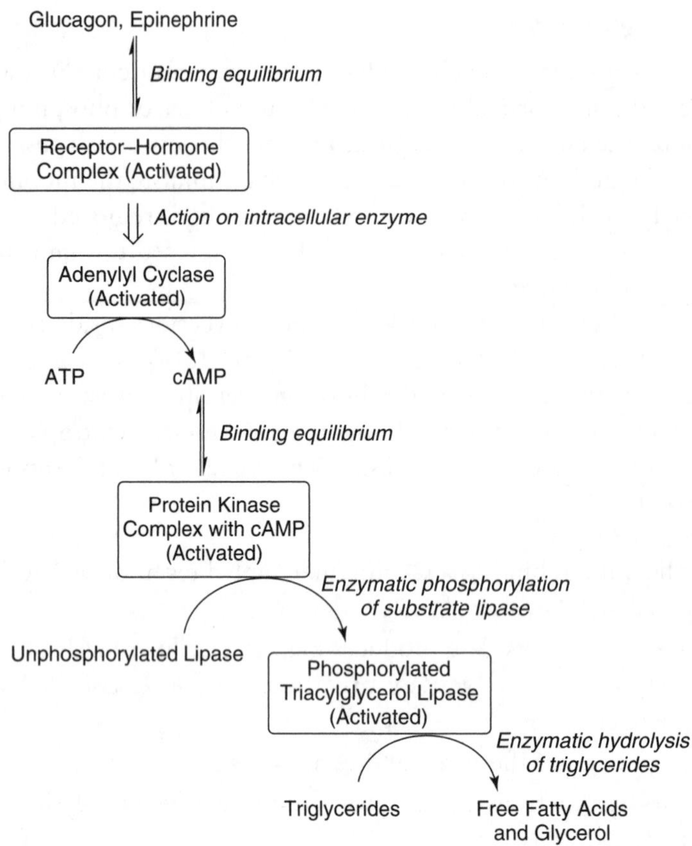

Figure 13-5 Hormonal stimulation of lipolysis starts with hormone binding to an extracellular domain of a receptor. This process initiates the release of the second messenger cAMP and starts a cascade of protein phosphorylations. Eventually it activates a lipase that will hydrolyze triglycerides.

triglycerides (e.g., the hormone-sensitive lipase of adipocytes, which is responsible for releasing free fatty acids from lipid droplets).

Fate of the Products: Fatty Acids and Glycerol

Glycerol goes to the glycolytic pathway; it enters as DHAP after undergoing phosphorylation and participating in a redox reaction (it may also become a precursor for gluconeogenesis). Fatty acids enter a special oxidative pathway, generating reduced nicotinamides that subsequently can be used to generate ATP. This special pathway (β-*oxidation*) first cleaves the fatty acid into two-carbon fragments and then oxidizes them.

Fatty acids are transported from fatty tissue through the circulation as free fatty acids, not as triglycerides. The solubility of free fatty acids is not very high. Serum albumin plays an important role here because it can form a complex with fatty acids and because a single albumin molecule can carry more than one fatty acid molecule. Glycerol also leaves adipose tissue; these cells lack the enzyme glycerol kinase, which is needed to prepare the glycerol for entry to glycolytic pathway. Because glycerol is quite soluble, there is no problem in transporting it through the circulation.

Role of Carnitine

Free fatty acids or acylated CoA molecules can diffuse across the outer mitochondrial membrane through pores, but the inner membrane poses a barrier to their passage. This barrier keeps all of the enzymes of β-oxidation localized to the mitochondrial matrix and plays an important role in regulating overall cell metabolism. To get acyl groups across the barrier, the cell uses a helper molecule, *carnitine,* and an associated specialized system of enzymes and transporters.

Carnitine forms an ester linkage with the acyl group of a fatty acid. This reaction is catalyzed by *carnitine palmitoyl transferase 1* (CPT1). This enzyme does not use free fatty acids as substrate, but instead acts on acylated CoA to generate *O*-acylcarnitine (**Figure 13-6**). Palmitic acid is commonly the fatty acid supplying the acyl group here—hence the "palmitoyl" in the enzyme's name—but the enzyme will also work on other long-chain acyl groups attached to CoA.

CPT1 is embedded in the outer mitochondrial membrane (**Figure 13-7**) and is an enzyme sensitive to the levels of *malonyl-CoA*. It has two subunits: a catalytic subunit with the active

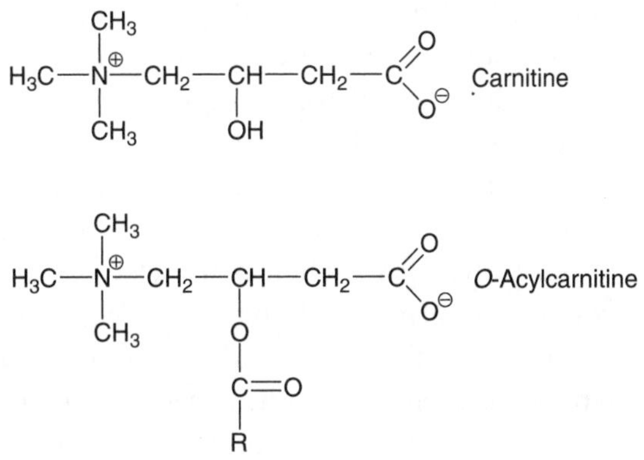

$$H_3C-\overset{CH_3}{\underset{CH_3}{N^{\oplus}}}-CH_2-\underset{OH}{CH}-CH_2-C(=O)O^{\ominus}$$ Carnitine

$$H_3C-\overset{CH_3}{\underset{CH_3}{N^{\oplus}}}-CH_2-\underset{O-C(=O)-R}{CH}-CH_2-C(=O)O^{\ominus}$$ *O*-Acylcarnitine

Figure 13-6 Structures of carnitine and *O*-acylated carnitine.

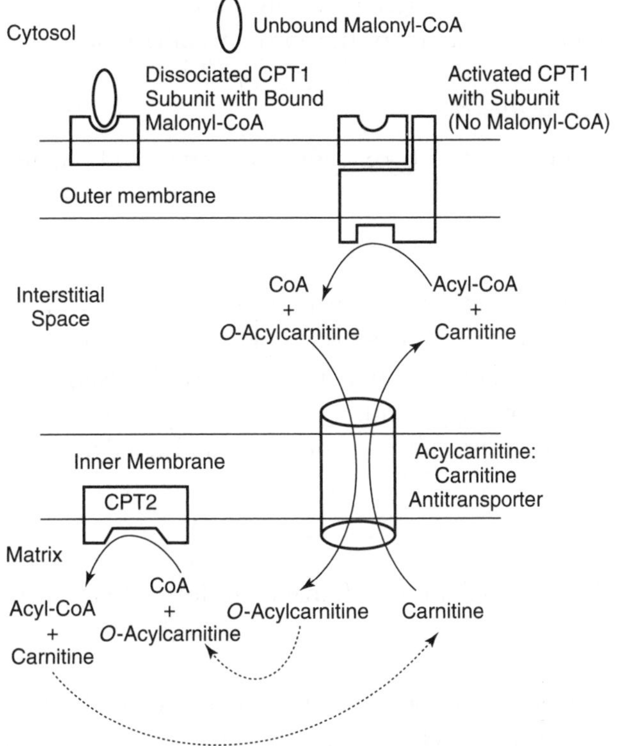

Figure 13-7 Actions of carnitine-palmitoyl transferases CPT1 and CPT2, showing the effects of malonyl-CoA on the activity of CPT1 (the antitransporter for carnitine and *O*-acyl carnitine that spans the inner mitochondrial membrane) and the re-formation of acylated CoA in the matrix by CPT2.

site, and a regulatory subunit with a binding site for malonyl-CoA. Malonyl-CoA will reappear shortly in the discussion of fatty acid biosynthesis; it is a key intermediate in that process, and its cytosolic level provides an indirect measure of the readiness of the cell to perform fatty acid biosynthesis. If levels of malonyl-CoA are high, then the cell most likely is ready to carry out fatty acid biosynthesis; that is, the cell has sufficient energy for biosynthesis. Under these conditions, there should be no need for breaking down fatty acids, so β-oxidation should be reduced. One obvious way to do so is to stop the importation of fatty acids into the mitochondrion for β-oxidation.

Prevention of the entry of fatty acids is accomplished by inhibiting the action of CPT1 through binding of malonyl-CoA to the regulatory subunit. The catalytic subunit of CPT1 has its active site on the inside toward the interstitial space, away from the cytosol, while the regulatory subunit has its binding site oriented toward the cytosol. For the catalytic subunit to be active, it must be associated with the regulatory subunit.

When the regulatory subunit has bound a molecule of malonyl-CoA, it dissociates from the catalytic subunit; the catalytic subunit now becomes inactive. Thus, when malonyl-CoA is abundant (signifying the readiness to perform fatty acid synthesis), the system will shut down. However, the enzyme becomes active again when malonyl-CoA levels drop and the bound malonyl-CoA dissociates from the regulatory subunit and so permits reassociation of catalytic and regulatory subunits. As a result of this process, the system becomes sensitive to cellular demands for oxidation of fatty acids compared to its capacity to make fatty acids.

The *O*-acylcarnitine can now be transported across the inner mitochondrial membrane by a special transporter. This particular transporter actually is an antitransporter: As it brings in a molecule of *O*-acylcarnitine, it expels a molecule of carnitine. Once past the inner membrane, the *O*-acylcarnitine is acted upon by a second enzyme, CPT2. It removes the carnitine (for recycling to the interstitial space via the antitransporter) and attaches the acyl group to a molecule of CoA. Now the acyl-CoA becomes a substrate for the apparatus of β-oxidation.

β-*Oxidation Reaction Sequence*

Figure 13-8 diagrams one round of β-oxidation of a fatty acid. There are four reactions in the sequence.

Oxidation

The oxidation step resembles the succinate-to-fumarate reaction in the TCA cycle. It involves action by a flavoenzyme, followed by electron transfer to CoQ through a special electron-transferring flavoprotein (not shown in the figure). Note the *trans* geometry of the double bond, as opposed to the *cis* geometry found in most naturally occurring unsaturated fatty acids. This *trans* fatty acid is only an intermediate, however, and does not normally accumulate to appreciable amounts.

Hydration

The second step resembles the hydration of fumarate to form malate in the TCA cycle.

Oxidation

The third step is a standard redox reaction, the oxidation of an alcohol to a ketone. It resembles the TCA cycle conversion of malate to oxaloacetate (a β-keto ester). Note the use of a nicotinamide cofactor here, in contrast to the first oxidation of the sequence.

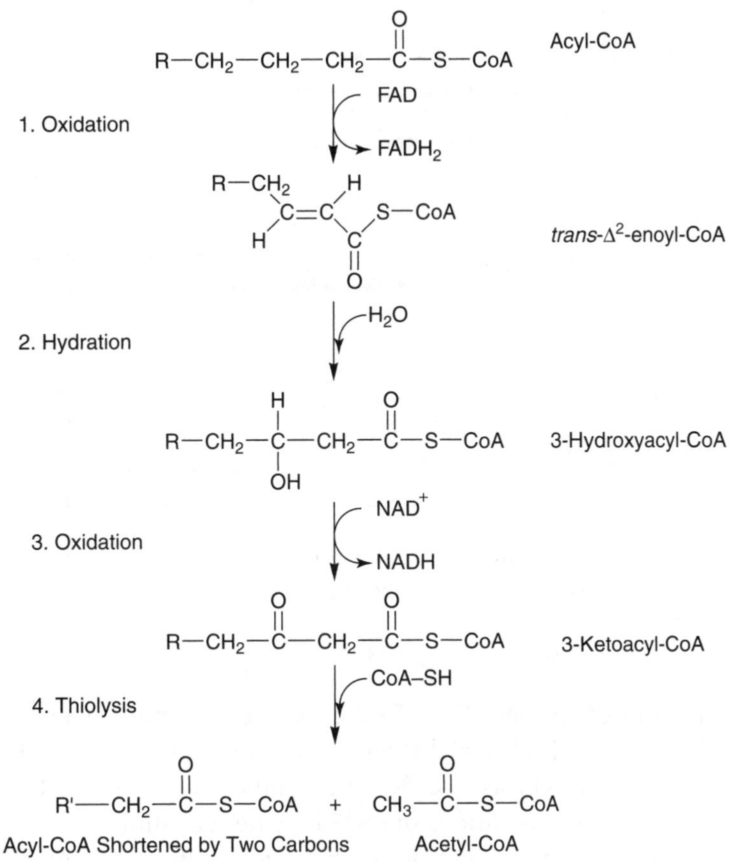

$$R{-}CH_2{-}CH_2{-}CH_2{-}\overset{O}{\overset{\|}{C}}{-}S{-}CoA$$ Acyl-CoA

1. Oxidation (FAD → $FADH_2$)

trans-Δ^2-enoyl-CoA

2. Hydration (H_2O)

$$R{-}CH_2{-}\underset{OH}{\overset{H}{C}}{-}CH_2{-}\overset{O}{\overset{\|}{C}}{-}S{-}CoA$$ 3-Hydroxyacyl-CoA

3. Oxidation (NAD^+ → NADH)

$$R{-}CH_2{-}\overset{O}{\overset{\|}{C}}{-}CH_2{-}\overset{O}{\overset{\|}{C}}{-}S{-}CoA$$ 3-Ketoacyl-CoA

4. Thiolysis (CoA–SH)

$$R'{-}CH_2{-}\overset{O}{\overset{\|}{C}}{-}S{-}CoA \quad + \quad CH_3{-}\overset{O}{\overset{\|}{C}}{-}S{-}CoA$$

Acyl-CoA Shortened by Two Carbons — Acetyl-CoA

Figure 13-8 The process of β-oxidation. A fatty acid, as the activated acyl-CoA thioester, is sequentially broken down into molecules of acetyl-CoA.

Thiolysis

Thiolysis involves a nucleophilic attack on an activated carbonyl by an incoming thiol, with displacement of the two-carbon fragment as acetyl-CoA. The fatty acid chain has been shortened now by two carbons. The chain can be cycled through repeated rounds of β-oxidation until the R group is simplified to H or CH_3.

Each round of β-oxidation generates one molecule each of $FADH_2$, NADH, and acetyl-CoA. Because all of the reactions are contained in the mitochondrial matrix, they use only mitochondrial CoA; the cytosolic pool of CoA is not involved here.

Oxidation of Fatty Acids with an Odd Number of Carbons

Fatty acids with an odd number of carbons can undergo β-oxidation just as well as those with an even number of carbon atoms, except that at the last round of the process. We are left with a molecule of acetyl-CoA and a molecule of propionyl-CoA, instead of two molecules of acetyl-CoA. Further metabolism of the propionyl-CoA requires some special enzymes and a special cofactor, derived from *vitamin* B_{12}.

Figure 13-9 shows how propionyl-CoA is converted to succinyl-CoA (this molecule is also formed in the breakdown of several amino acids), so that it can be metabolized to

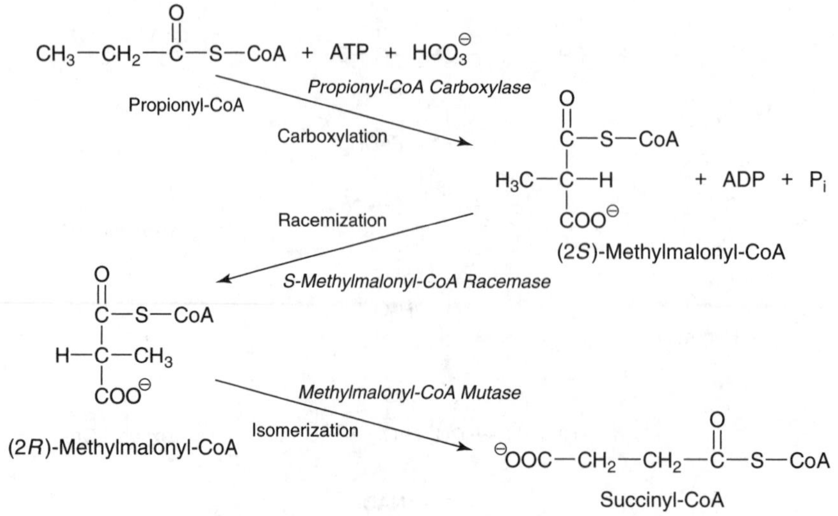

$CH_3-CH_2-C(=O)-S-CoA + ATP + HCO_3^{\ominus}$

Propionyl-CoA

Propionyl-CoA Carboxylase

Carboxylation

$H_3C-CH(COO^{\ominus})-C(=O)-S-CoA$ + ADP + P_i

(2*S*)-Methylmalonyl-CoA

Racemization

S-Methylmalonyl-CoA Racemase

$H-C(CH_3)(COO^{\ominus})-C(=O)-S-CoA$

(2*R*)-Methylmalonyl-CoA

Methylmalonyl-CoA Mutase

Isomerization

$^{\ominus}OOC-CH_2-CH_2-C(=O)-S-CoA$

Succinyl-CoA

Figure 13-9 Conversion of propionyl-CoA to succinyl-CoA, a process involving the B_{12}-dependent isomerization of (2*R*)-methylmalonyl-CoA to succinyl-CoA.

yield energy. Metabolism of succinyl-CoA in the TCA cycle will generate one NADH, one GTP, and one $FADH_2$. Note, however, the earlier consumption of one ATP molecule in the carboxylation reaction. Also, this process leads to net synthesis of oxaloacetate in the TCA cycle, which can be important under conditions of carbohydrate starvation.

In the pathway leading to succinyl-CoA, note the shift of a hydrogen atom and a (—CO—S CoA) unit, a very unusual isomerization (**Figure 13-10**). This isomerization requires a coenzyme, which is derived from *cobalamin* (Cbl). In cobalamin, a cobalt metal ion is held at the center of four pyrrole units, forming a corrin ring; the structure resembles that of porphyrin. The coenzyme form of interest to us is AdoCbl (5′-deoxyadenosylcobalamin). It has two substituents, R and B, in the fifth and sixth coordination positions, respectively, on the cobalt, where the B substituent is dimethylbenzimidazole ribonucleotide and the R substituent is a deoxyadenosyl group (**Figure 13-11**). The precursor, called vitamin B_{12} or cobalamin proper, has a cyanide ligand in place of the deoxyadenosyl group. The cobalt–carbon bond is unusually long and rather labile as a result, enabling the action of the coenzyme in catalyzing isomerizations and methyl transfers.

Vitamin B_{12} is synthesized only by micro-organisms, not by plants or animals, and is an essential vitamin, although only rather small amounts are needed for good health. Vitamin B_{12} also plays a role in amino acid and folate metabolism, in the conversion of homocysteine to cysteine, where it helps to catalyze a methyl transfer reaction (see Chapter 14).

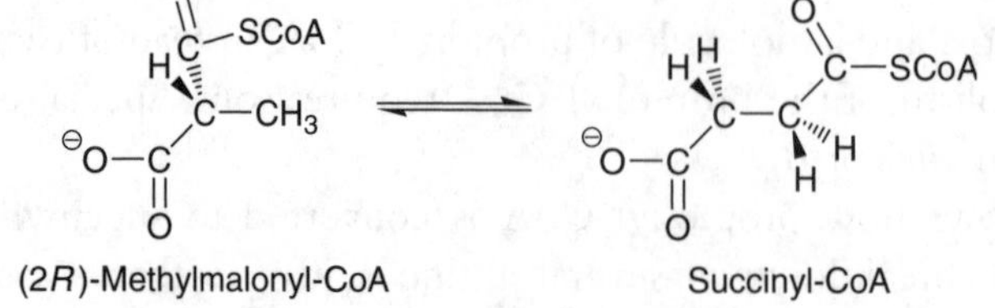

(2*R*)-Methylmalonyl-CoA ⇌ Succinyl-CoA

Figure 13-10 Detail of the stereochemistry of the B_{12}-dependent isomerization.

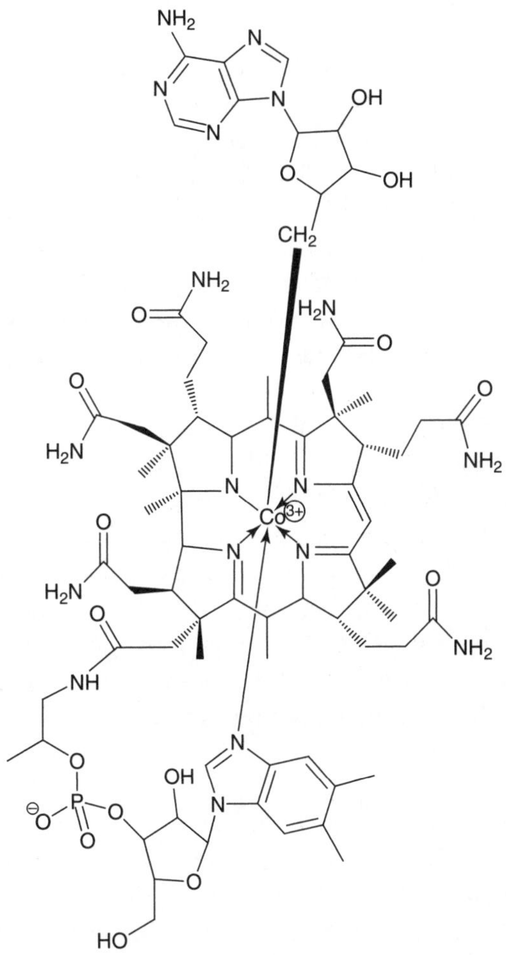

Figure 13-11 Structure of coenzyme B_{12} as AdoCbl. A central atom of cobalt is surrounded by a tetrapyrrole ring, with dative bonds connecting the cobalt and several nitrogens of the ring. A dimethylbenzimidazole ribonucleotide substituent appears at the cobalt's fifth coordination position ("B"), and a deoxyadenosyl moiety at the sixth position ("R").

Clinical Application

Dietary sources of vitamin B_{12} are mainly meat, eggs, and dairy foods; vegetables are not a sufficient source. For this reason, strict vegans need to supplement their diet with this vitamin to maintain proper levels for good health.

The stomach secretes a glycoprotein ("intrinsic factor") that binds cobalamin. The cobalamin–intrinsic factor complex then binds to a specific receptor in the lining of the ileum, and Cbl is actively transported across the membrane after its detachment from intrinsic factor by a releasing factor. Transport through the blood to tissues occurs via a complex with a transporter protein, transcobalamin II (transcobalamin I binds Cbl but is not responsible for delivery to tissues). This complex is taken up via receptor-mediated endocytosis by peripheral tissues; the complex is then degraded within a lysosome,

(Continued)

and the Cbl released to the cytoplasm. Subsequent enzymatic action converts it to the active cofactor by methylation to form methylcobalamin, or by adenosylation to form AdoCbl. Methylcobalamin is used as a cofactor in the conversion of homocysteine to methionine (see Chapter 14), while AdoCbl is the form involved in the conversion of L-methylmalonyl-CoA to succinyl-CoA.

The disease of *pernicious anemia* arises when uptake of this vitamin from the gut is impaired owing to a lack of intrinsic factor. The adjective "pernicious" is used because, in the days before the discovery of treatments, the disease was fatal. The adjective is still retained to distinguish this particular cause of anemia from other disorders in Cbl uptake and metabolism.

Symptoms of pernicious anemia include megaloblastic anemia, damage to myelinated nerve cells, and peripheral neuropathy (with this disease, the neurological deficits may appear in the absence of any anemia). A deficiency in Cbl affects all rapidly dividing tissues because DNA synthesis is impaired (Cbl is needed for recycling folate, another cofactor used in making thymidine for DNA; see Chapter 15). The production of red blood cells is especially affected: Large, immature cells (megaloblasts) are released that are dysfunctional. Cbl deficiency also affects the production of the myelin membrane of certain nerve cells and leads to the development of neuropathy. Because of the linkage of Cbl metabolism with folate metabolism, dietary supplementation with folate can "mask" the symptoms of Cbl deficiency, relieving the anemia (but not, unfortunately, the neuropathy).

Pernicious anemia can be treated by injections of vitamin B_{12}. Once the body's stores of the vitamin have been replenished parenterally, treatment can continue with oral dosing with the vitamin. Daily requirements for the vitamin are quite low, and even very inefficient uptake of the vitamin from the gut will usually suffice to maintain health.

Other Oxidative Systems for Fatty Acids

Trans-Cis Isomerization

For further metabolism, unsaturated fatty acids must have their *cis* double bonds isomerized to the *trans* form (recall that a *trans* isomer appears as an intermediate during β-oxidation); a special enoyl-CoA isomerase accomplishes this task. Additionally, the position of the double bond may have to be shifted, to permit β-oxidation to proceed.

α-Oxidation

α-*Oxidation* attacks the α-carbon (carbon 2 in the chain), releasing the carboxylate carbon 1 as CO_2. This minor pathway, which is found in peroxisomes, shortens the fatty acid chain one carbon at a time, and not by two carbons as in β-oxidation. This sort of attack on the chain is important if the β-carbon of the chain cannot be attacked as in regular β-oxidation. Certain plant-derived fatty acids contain methyl groups in this position, and they constitute an appreciable fraction of daily dietary intake of lipids. To dispose of them, the body uses α-oxidation instead of β-oxidation.

A defect in the α-oxidation pathway leads to *Refsum disease*, which is characterized by the buildup of phytanic acid (derived from phytol, a terpene found in leafy green vegetables; see

Figure 13-12). Refsum disease results in a number of neurological upsets, and its main treatment consists of restriction of dietary intake of phytol. Figure 13-12 also shows in general how fatty acids with branches (usually simple methyl groups) from whatever source can be further metabolized, after a round of α-oxidation. Notice here the production of propionyl-CoA, which is converted to succinyl-CoA by the pathway sketched in Figure 13-9.

ω-Oxidation

ω-*Oxidation* is another minor pathway that attacks the ω-carbon (at the nonpolar end of the fatty acid) and converts it to a carboxyl. This process gives a dicarboxylic acid that can then be activated with CoA at one end or the other, for entry into the β-oxidation pathway.

Atmospheric Oxidation

Polyunsaturated fatty acids are susceptible to attack by molecular oxygen, through nonenzymatic reactions that give lipid peroxides. This process produces rancid butter, for example. In vivo, the degradation of these oxidized fatty acids can yield malondialdehyde, which can cross-link proteins and cause other cellular damage. Lipid peroxide formation has been implicated in a number of diseases (e.g., cancer, atherosclerosis).

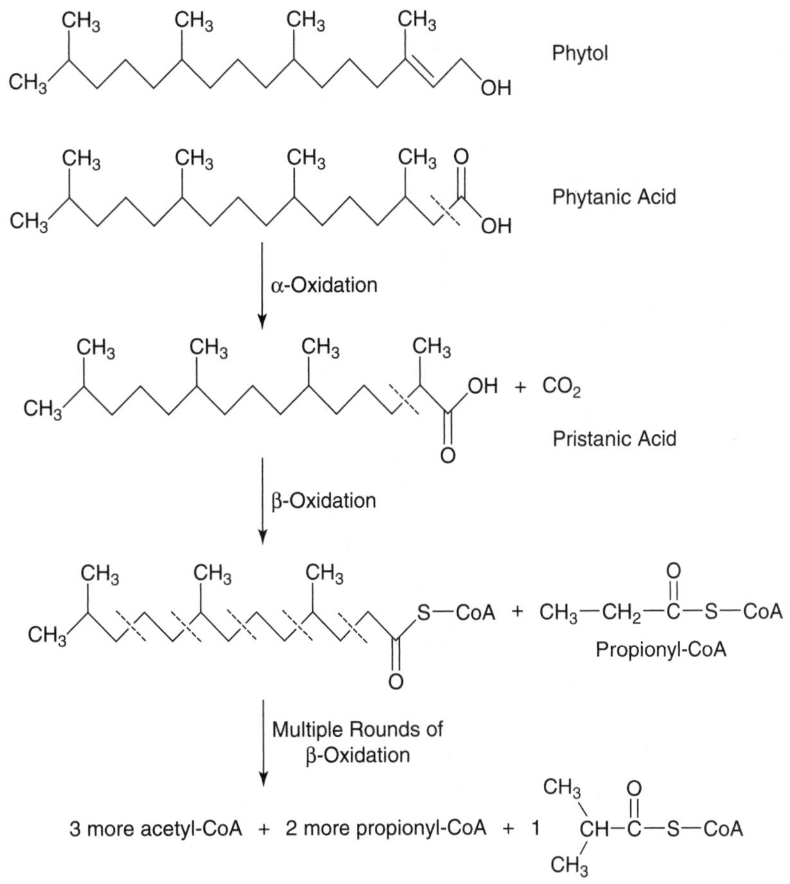

Figure 13-12 Structures of the "branched" lipids, phytol and phytanic acid, and the process of oxidation of such lipids. The presence of the methyl group on the β-carbon blocks normal β-oxidation. A preliminary round of α-oxidation (chain cleavage indicated by the dashed lines) resolves this problem and enables β-oxidation to proceed.

Ketone Bodies and Their Oxidation

Ketogenesis is the biochemical process leading to the synthesis of *ketone bodies*. Ketone bodies (acetoacetate, β-D-hydroxybutyrate, and acetone) can arise under conditions where carbohydrate intake is restricted or absent. Ketone bodies result from the breakdown of lipids. They can be oxidized and serve as a (partial) replacement for glucose in cells that are metabolically active, such as nerve cells. The physiological condition of ketosis results when ketone bodies build up in the bloodstream; ketosis is associated with the disease known as diabetes. Unusually high levels of circulating ketone bodies can produce acidosis, a dangerous physiological state.

Ketogenesis

The liver is the primary organ generating ketone bodies. Both acetoacetate and β-D-hydroxybutyrate are formed in the mitochondria of the liver, from acetyl-CoA (**Figure 13-13**). Acetone is produced by spontaneous (nonenzymatic) decarboxylation of acetoacetate as well as by enzymatic reaction involving acetoacetate decarboxylase.

Note an important intermediate in ketogenesis here: 3-hydroxy-3-methylglutaryl CoA (HMG CoA). Its synthesis is the rate-limiting step in ketogenesis from acetyl-CoA, and the

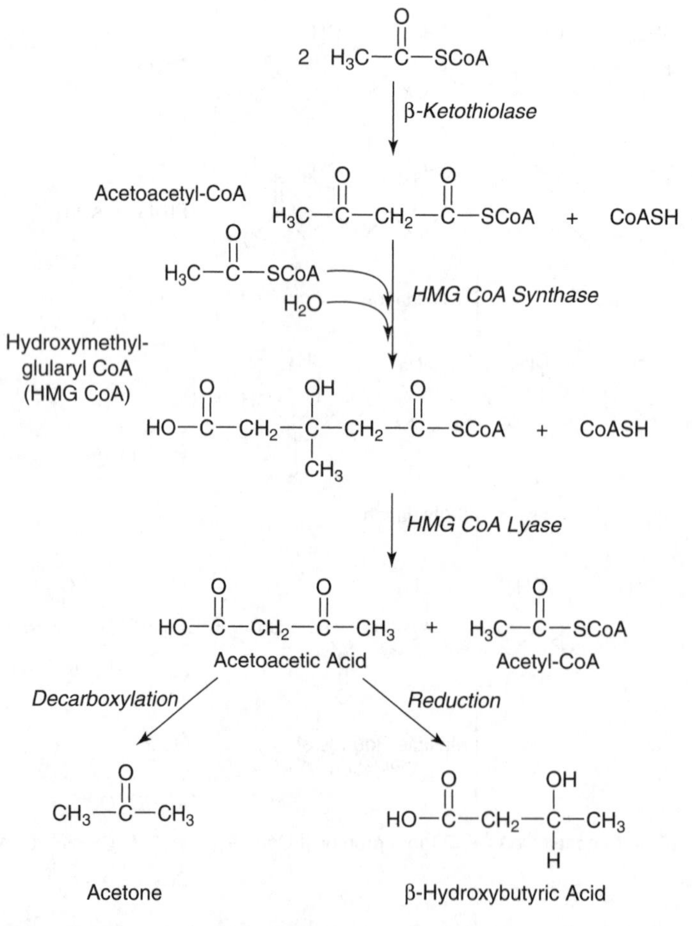

2 $H_3C-C(=O)-SCoA$

β-Ketothiolase

Acetoacetyl-CoA: $H_3C-C(=O)-CH_2-C(=O)-SCoA$ + CoASH

$H_3C-C(=O)-SCoA$, H_2O → HMG CoA Synthase

Hydroxymethyl-glularyl CoA (HMG CoA): $HO-C(=O)-CH_2-C(OH)(CH_3)-CH_2-C(=O)-SCoA$ + CoASH

HMG CoA Lyase

$HO-C(=O)-CH_2-C(=O)-CH_3$ Acetoacetic Acid + $H_3C-C(=O)-SCoA$ Acetyl-CoA

Decarboxylation → $CH_3-C(=O)-CH_3$ Acetone

Reduction → $HO-C(=O)-CH_2-C(OH)(H)-CH_3$ β-Hydroxybutyric Acid

Figure 13-13 Origin of the ketone bodies. Condensation of two molecules of acetyl-CoA yields acetoacetyl-CoA; hydrolysis of the thioester here gives acetoacetate. Addition of a third acetyl-CoA gives hydroxymethylglutaryl CoA (HMG CoA—a key intermediate in the biosynthetic route to cholesterol); lyase action produces acetoacetate, which leads either to β-hydroxybutyrate or (via decarboxylation) to acetone.

liver is the only organ that contains large quantities of the enzyme responsible for catalyzing this step; thus ketone body generation is the responsibility of the liver. Synthesis of the enzyme catalyzing this step is induced by fatty acids. HMG CoA is also a precursor to cholesterol, and the steps leading to ketone body generation are the same as those leading to cholesterol biosynthesis. However, these processes take place in different cellular locations, with ketone bodies arising from liver mitochondrial action, and cholesterol biosynthesis involving enzymes in the cytosol and the endoplasmic reticulum.

Why Ketone Bodies Arise

Acetyl-CoA enters the TCA cycle if sufficient oxaloacetate is available. If not, acetyl-CoA is diverted to form ketone bodies, which enter the blood and then are degraded in peripheral tissues. Cardiac muscle, skeletal muscle, and the renal cortex can use ketone bodies directly, and the brain can adapt to use them as fuel.

The conditions under which appreciable amounts of ketone bodies are formed are low carbohydrate intake (lipid only, or complete starvation) and diabetes. Under low carbohydrate intake conditions, gluconeogenesis in the liver will be stimulated as part of the body's attempt to maintain blood levels of glucose for those tissues (e.g., nerve cells) that are most dependent on glucose for energy. In the absence of incoming carbohydrate, gluconeogenesis can proceed by using as precursors the carbon chains from certain amino acids ("glucogenic" amino acids) as well as the glycerol derived from triglyceride breakdown. To spare the limited amount of glucose that can be supplied through gluconeogenesis for the sensitive tissues, the body will turn to fatty acid catabolism for energy. This process does, of course, generate ample amounts of acetyl-CoA inside the mitochondria. The further metabolism of this pool of acetyl-CoA may meet a roadblock, however. If pyruvate is unavailable from, for example, carbohydrate breakdown, the liver cells cannot make oxaloacetate for gluconeogenesis without seriously depleting the TCA-cycle intermediates, especially oxaloacetate. Recall that entry of acetyl-CoA to the TCA cycle requires oxaloacetate; thus removal of oxaloacetate for gluconeogenesis would compromise TCA cycle functioning. To support gluconeogenesis, then, the acetyl groups should not be oxidized in the liver in the usual way. Instead, the acetyl moieties are diverted into ketone bodies, which can be transported in the blood and oxidized in extrahepatic tissues (e.g., muscle, brain).

Also, under these conditions, the level of malonyl-CoA drops. As will be discussed later in this chapter malonyl-CoA is derived from acetyl-CoA by carboxylation through the action of the enzyme acetyl-CoA carboxylase (ACC). The activity of ACC is sensitive not only to the overall energy level of the cell but also to the level of the pool of TCA-cycle intermediates through citrate's effect on ACC activity. If either the energy level or the level of the TCA-cycle pool drops, then ACC activity will drop, and consequently less malonyl-CoA will be made. The drop in malonyl-CoA levels will relieve inhibition of CPT1 (carnitine palmitoyl transferase 1, which is inhibited by malonyl-CoA), so that fatty acids will now enter mitochondria and undergo β-oxidation, which will build up the pool of acetyl-CoA. In this way the body adapts to a lipid-rich, carbohydrate-poor diet; a similar adaptation occurs during starvation conditions.

Ketone Body Catabolism

Ketone bodies can replace glucose as a fuel for cells. The ketone bodies are quite water soluble and easily transported through the blood from the liver (the principal site of their synthesis) to muscle, nerve cells, and other sites where they can be used as fuel. (Acetone also has a high vapor pressure and is easily exhaled, leading to the characteristic "chemical" or "fruity" breath odor

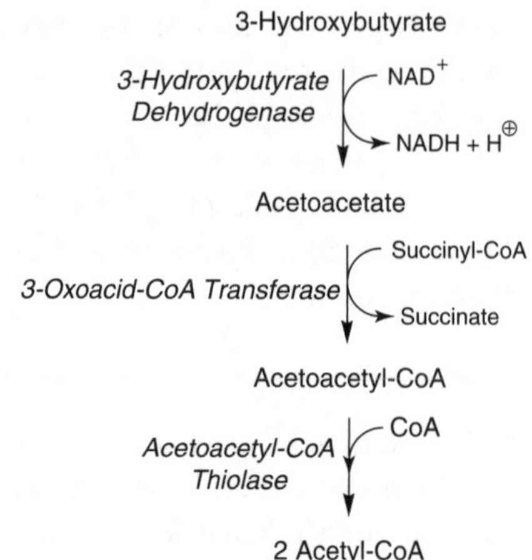

Figure 13-14 Reconversion of ketone bodies to acetyl-CoA for use as fuel in peripheral tissues. The liver lacks the enzyme 3-oxoacid-CoA transferase, so it cannot use ketone bodies as fuel.

of someone in ketosis.) Upon entering the nonhepatic tissues, the ketone bodies are converted in a series of reactions to acetyl-CoA, which can then enter the TCA cycle and help generate energy for the cell. These reactions are shown in **Figure 13-14**. The first and third reactions are the same as those in the production of ketone bodies; the middle reaction, however, is not. In fact, this second reaction catalyzes the rate-limiting step in the conversion process. Moreover, the enzyme that catalyzes this step is not expressed in liver tissue, although it is otherwise widely present, which explains why the liver itself does not consume ketone bodies.

Clinical Application

Ketosis

Ketosis is caused by an unusually high concentration of ketone bodies in the bloodstream, defined by a blood level between 0.3 and 7.0 mmol/L. It develops when the body is starved for carbohydrates (specifically glucose) during prolonged fasting or starvation. It can also be induced by a diet that excludes most or all carbohydrates and replaces them with fat. Ketosis is commonly associated with the disease of diabetes mellitus.

In the absence of dietary carbohydrates, the body tends to metabolize fatty acids (from triglycerides) and amino acids (from protein) instead of glucose. The breakdown of triglycerides to release glycerol, combined with the catabolism of certain amino acids, will generate precursors for gluconeogenesis. This activity occurs primarily in the liver, and is the way that the body attempts to maintain blood glucose levels for the demands of nerve cells, muscle, and other tissues. However, the glucose that can be supplied this way is limited (especially the amount that can be derived from the glycerol from triglycerides). Under conditions of starvation, its restriction will result in muscle wasting as body protein is used to supply gluconeogenic precursors.

As detailed earlier, the breakdown of fatty acids leads to acetyl-CoA. Because of the lack of carbohydrates, however, it cannot enter the TCA cycle as it would normally. Instead, the acetyl-CoA is converted to ketone bodies by the liver, which exports them to peripheral tissues as an energy source in place of the missing glucose. Excess ketone bodies in the bloodstream will be filtered out by the kidneys and excreted in the urine, a condition called ketonuria. The dissolved ketone bodies will exert an osmotic effect on the kidneys, causing the excretion of more urine than usual. This imbalance can lead to severe disease states if body stores (and hence serum levels) of ions such as sodium, potassium, and phosphate become depleted; obviously, dehydration can be an issue as well.

Ketone bodies are organic acids, and as such will naturally tend to acidify their environment. If the concentration of these organic acids in the bloodstream exceeds the buffering capacity of intracellular and extracellular fluids, the blood pH will drop below pH 7.3. This is an acidosis; in particular, because of its origin it is termed ketoacidosis. Among other effects, the acidosis will reduce the oxygen-carrying capacity of erythrocytes, so it can be a very serious medical condition.

Diabetes Mellitus

In diabetes mellitus, the urine contains high levels of glucose and is sweet ("mellitus" means "honey" in Latin). Diabetes insipidus is a very different disorder—a pituitary disorder that directly affects kidney function. There is no unusual level of glucose in the urine in diabetes insipidus; instead, the urine is insipid, and has no taste.

Diabetes mellitus has two forms or types. In type 1 diabetes, the β-cells of the pancreas are gone; no insulin is produced. This results in too much sugar in the blood (hyperglycemia), because insulin normally promotes transport of glucose into cells from blood. Type 1 diabetes is controlled by daily injections of insulin. A current hypothesis suggests that this disease is a derangement of the immune system in which the immune system attacks pancreatic β-cells, acting as if the cells were "foreign." Given that this defect occurs typically early in life, this form of diabetes is sometimes referred to as the juvenile-onset form.

In type 2 diabetes, a normal amount of insulin is synthesized and, more importantly, is secreted. However, either it is not released fast enough when blood sugar rises or the target tissues have a reduced responsiveness to insulin (insulin resistance), or both. This condition typically arises later in life ("adult-onset" form), and it is often controllable through diet and exercise without insulin injection.

In either case, the body acts as if it were starved for energy because glucose is not being taken up by tissues. Metabolic pathways will shift their output in ways very similar to those seen under conditions of extended fasting or starvation, resulting in ketosis. A common side effect of diabetes mellitus is dehydration, due to ketone and sugar excretion through the urine. Also, the high circulating levels of sugar lead to non-enzymatic glycosylation of hemoglobin and other proteins. In fact, the stable glycosylated product hemoglobin A_{1c} is used diagnostically to obtain information about the severity of the hyperglycemia.

Unfortunately, one of the complications of diabetes mellitus can be ketoacidosis, when the ketosis becomes too extreme. This outcome is more common with type 1 (juvenile-onset) diabetes mellitus than with type 2 (adult-onset) disease. Severe cases of ketoacidosis necessitate admission to the hospital for treatment. A first measure to

(Continued)

treat this condition is administration of intravenous isotonic saline solution to correct the dehydration, to restore the balance among the various dissolved ions, and to reverse the acidosis and the ketosis. In cases of diabetic ketoacidosis, patients may also need intravenous insulin.

Recall that acetone results from the decarboxylation of acetoacetate. The resulting "chemical" smell on the breath can unfortunately be confused with alcohol intoxication. In extreme cases, this problem may be further compounded by mental disorientation of the diabetic who may be suffering from extreme ketoacidosis.

Fatty Acid Biosynthesis

Fatty acid biosynthesis occurs mainly in the cytosol (recall that fatty acid oxidation occurs mainly inside mitochondria). The biosynthetic reactions are nearly the reverse of the degradation reactions in β-oxidation. However, there are different cofactor requirements:

- The enzymes in biosynthesis use $NADP^+$/NADPH instead of NAD^+/NADH (a characteristic of biosynthesis in general).
- A special thiol, acting to carry acyl groups, here replaces the CoA that is used in β-oxidation. This special thiol is found on the *acyl carrier protein* (*ACP*). ACP has a *4′-phosphopantotheine* (**Figure 13-15**) prosthetic group; recall that pantothenic acid is part of coenzyme A. The sulfhydryl moiety of this prosthetic group serves as a site for acyl group attachment.

The fatty acid chain is built up by successive addition of two-carbon units. Thus fatty acids usually have an even number of carbon atoms. The two-carbon units are derived from acetyl-CoA, which in turn is produced in the cytosol through the action of the citrate shuttle, bringing out carbons from the mitochondrial matrix.

Reaction Sequence

Initially two acetate units (from the acetyl-CoA pool) are used to start the process. One is transferred to a thiol site on the synthetic complex (*fatty acid synthase*, abbreviated as *FAS*), while the other is first activated by carboxylation to form malonyl-CoA and then attached to a second thiol site, close by on the FAS complex. These acyl moieties are combined (in several steps, involving a decarboxylation of the malonyl group; details are not covered here) to make a butyrate thioester attached at that second thiol site (butyryl ACP). At this point, the first thiol site is vacant. Another malonyl unit is passed to this first thiol site, and the adjacent acyl groups are joined, with the product remaining attached at the second thiol site. This process is repeated multiple times to elongate the carbon chain, using several more molecules of malonyl-CoA.

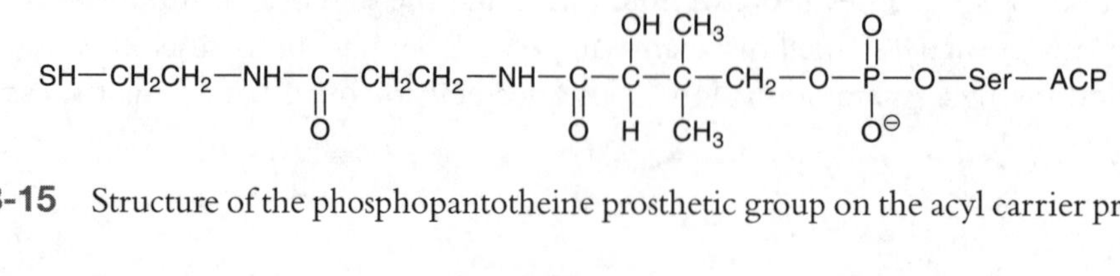

$$\mathrm{SH{-}CH_2CH_2{-}NH{-}C({=}O){-}CH_2CH_2{-}NH{-}C({=}O){-}C(OH)(H){-}C(CH_3)_2{-}CH_2{-}O{-}P({=}O)(O^{\ominus}){-}O{-}Ser{-}ACP}$$

Figure 13-15 Structure of the phosphopantotheine prosthetic group on the acyl carrier protein (ACP).

Typically the process terminates when the chain reaches a length of 16 carbons (corresponding to a molecule of palmitic acid).

Figure 13-16 summarizes the reactions involved in the overall synthesis of palmitate. Notice the consumption of four reducing equivalents in each step, as two carbons are added to the chain (four moles of electrons per one mole of ethyl moiety added). These come from the oxidation of NADPH; each NADPH molecule can donate two electrons, and two NADPH molecules are used in each step.

Figure 13-17 presents further details of the reaction sequence, including the formation of malonyl-CoA from acetyl-CoA, along with the subsequent decarboxylation step, the joining of the acyl moieties to form a longer (but not fully saturated) chain, and the chemical process to convert that longer chain to the saturated form. For simplicity, Figure 13-17 shows the scheme for prokaryotes; in mammalian cells, the ACP is actually a part of the same polypeptide chain as the other enzymatic activities.

Carboxylation of Acetyl-CoA

The first step is catalyzed by *acetyl-CoA carboxylase* (*ACC*), an enzyme that is entirely separate from the FAS complex. In a reaction driven by ATP hydrolysis, acetyl-CoA is carboxylated to give malonyl-CoA. The carboxylase has a required cofactor, biotin, and the activity of this enzyme is highly regulated (its regulation is covered later in this chapter).

Loading the Fatty Acid Synthase

Next comes the transfer of the respective acyl moieties from coenzyme A to the acyl carrier protein. The acetyl transferase activity loads the acetyl moiety onto ACP, and the malonyl

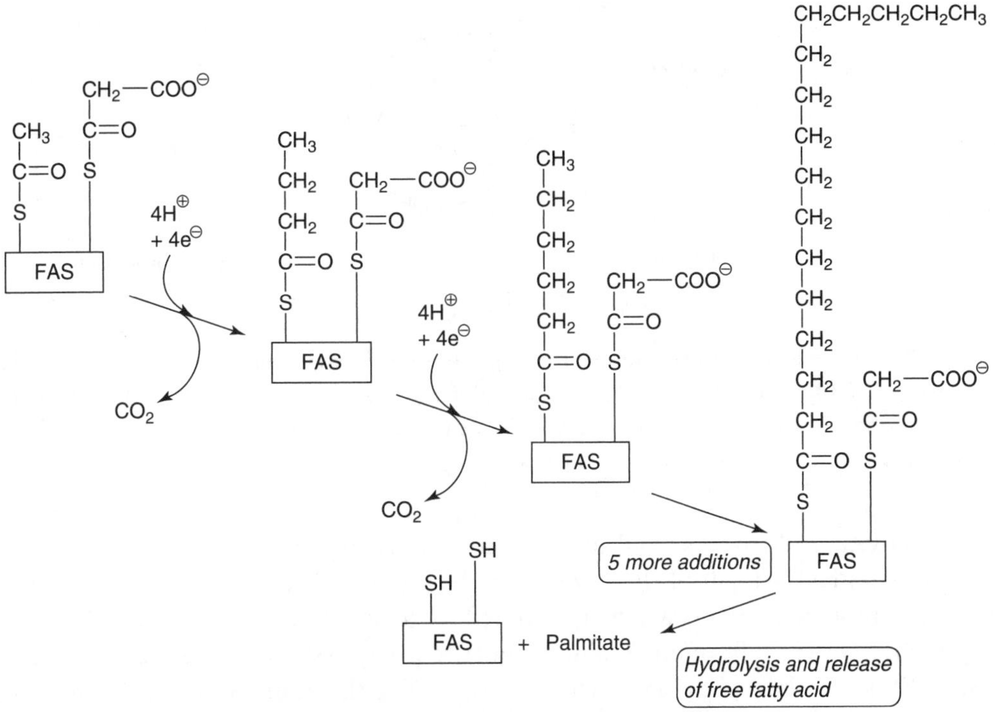

Figure 13-16 Summary of the reactions leading to the synthesis of palmitic acid, showing the seven rounds of synthesis needed for this C-16 fatty acid.

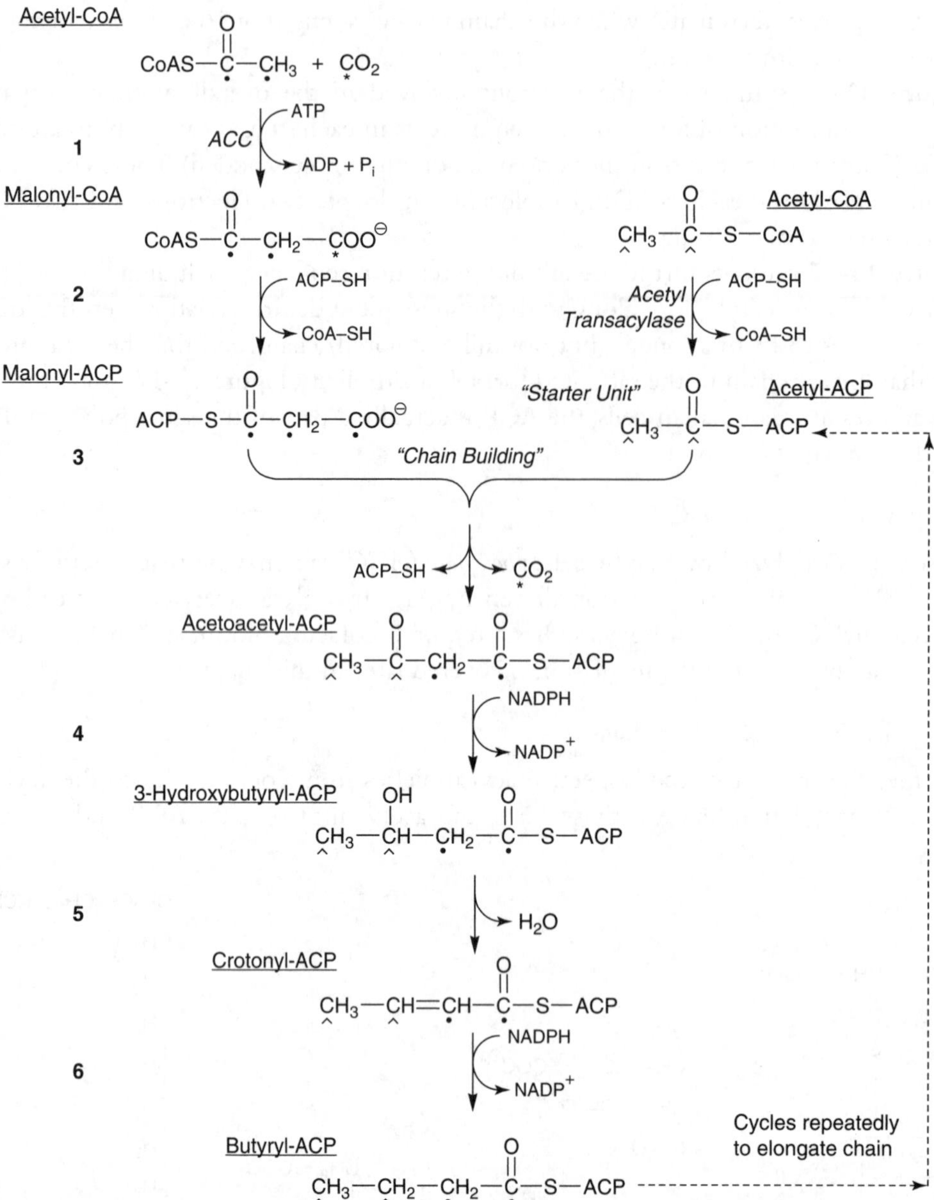

Figure 13-17 Details of a single round of chain extension in the synthesis of a fatty acid, starting from acetyl-CoA, CO_2, and malonyl-CoA. Formation of malonyl-CoA is not catalyzed by the fatty acid synthase, but rather by a separate enzyme, acetyl-CoA carboxylase. The symbols ^, ★, and • indicate the sources and fates of carbons from these precursors.

transferase activity loads the malonyl moiety (after the acetyl moiety has moved to a second site). In the mammalian form of the enzyme, both of these activities are located in the same (bifunctional) protein domain, which is denoted as malonyl-acetyl transferase (MAT). The acetyl group is transferred from the ACP to a thiol site (a key cysteine residue) at the β-ketoacyl synthase (KS) active site, on the fatty acid synthase. After this transfer, the malonyl moiety is loaded onto the ACP. Note that both a malonyl moiety and an acetyl moiety are now attached, ready for the next step (the synthase is "loaded," ready to start chain elongation). The site of attachment of the acetyl group is sometimes referred to as the "starter" site.

Condensation

The third step is the condensation of the malonyl group with the acetyl starter unit. The KS activity will catalyze the condensation of these two acyl groups to form a β-ketoacyl intermediate that is bound to the ACP. (In subsequent rounds of chain building, the starter unit is replaced by the elongated chain from the immediately previous round.) This condensation reaction proceeds via decarboxylation of the malonyl moiety, generating a carbanion that readily attacks the carbonyl group on the starter acetyl unit. The carbon dioxide generated in this way then leaves. Also, the thiol group that carried in the malonyl moiety leaves. (In the bacterial system, the entire ACP protein dissociates from the complex; for the mammalian FAS, the ACP is a domain of the same polypeptide chain as the rest of the FAS, so in this case this domain rotates away from the active site.) The elongated acyl moiety—now four carbons in length—remains attached to the FAS complex. Release of the CO_2 helps to drive the reaction.

First Reduction

The fourth step is catalyzed by a β-ketoacyl reductase (KR) activity that uses NADPH to reduce the 3-keto group to the corresponding alcohol.

Dehydration

The fifth step is catalyzed by a dehydratase (DH) to give a carbon–carbon double bond, with *trans* geometry.

Second Reduction

A second reductase (an enoyl reductase, or ER) acts here, again using NADPH, but now giving the saturated alkyl chain, which is still attached via a thioester link to the ACP. This butyryl chain occupies the starter site, and in a repetition of steps 3 through 6 the chain will be elongated, using a fresh malonyl group (made and brought in as described in steps 1 and 2).

The entire cycle is repeated until a sufficiently long alkyl chain is made. For humans, this will generally be a chain with 16 carbons (a palmitoyl chain). At this point, the thioester link is hydrolyzed by the thioesterase (TE) site, releasing the free fatty acid and regenerating the intact ACP.

Fatty Acid Synthase Structure and Activities

The eukaryotic form of the FAS enzyme is a dimer of identical polypeptide chains (**Figure 13-18**), with the chains crossing each other to form a rough "X". Each chain has multiple activities. The compact arrangement of the active sites makes for efficient transfer of intermediates from one catalytic site to the next. The bacterial form of FAS is dissimilar in that it is an aggregate of several different polypeptide chains, each with only a single enzymatic activity.

Overall Reaction for Palmitic Acid Synthesis

$$\text{Acetyl-CoA} + 7\ \text{Malonyl-CoA} + 14\ \text{NADPH} + 14\ \text{H}^+$$
$$\rightarrow \text{Palmitic acid} + 8\ \text{CoA} + 14\ \text{NADP}^+ + 6\ \text{H}_2\text{O} + 7\ \text{CO}_2 \qquad (13\text{-}1)$$

One acetyl unit enters this pathway directly, while the rest (e.g., 7 more units for palmitic acid synthesis) come in as malonyl-CoA. An energy cost is incurred in the carboxylation required as well as in the redox reactions; note the use of ATP in step 1 and of NADPH in steps 4 and 6 in Figure 13-17. For the synthesis of a C-16 fatty acid, the process would use 7 ATP molecules

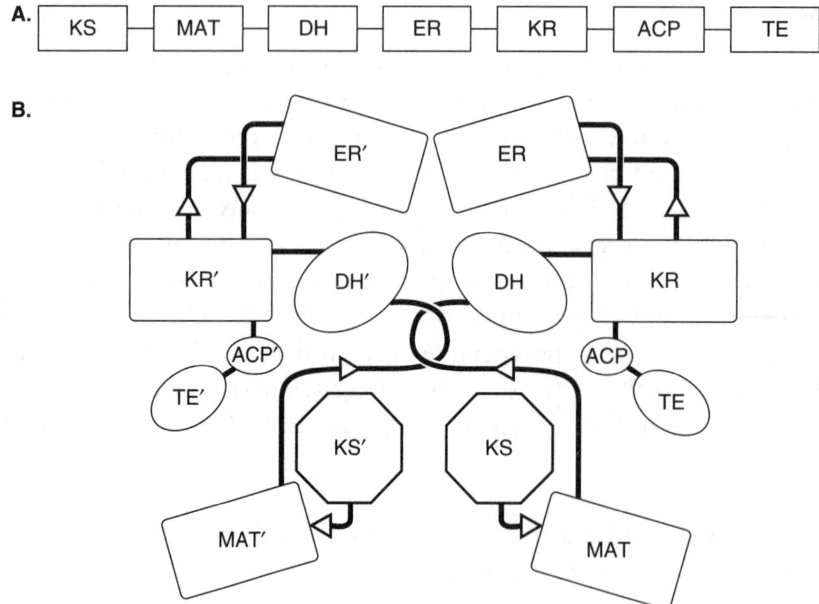

Figure 13-18 **A.** The arrangement of domains in a single subunit of the eukaryotic fatty acid synthase complex. **B.** The enzyme is an intertwined dimer of identical subunits that form a rough "X" shape; arrowheads indicate the direction of the respective polypeptide chains. Domain/active site abbreviations used: TE, thioesterase; ACP, acyl carrier protein; KR, ketoacyl reductase; ER, enoyl reductase; DH, dehydratase; MAT, malonyl acetyl transferase; KS, β-ketoacyl synthase. Superscript primes indicate domains from the second subunit chain.

Source: Modified from the representation of the mammalian fatty acid synthase in T. Maier, M. Leibundgut, and N. Ban. (2008). "The crystal structure of a mammalian fatty acid synthase," *Science* 321:1315–1322.

(not 8) and 14 NADPH molecules. The decarboxylation reaction and loss of CO_2 help drive the condensation, as partial compensation for the ATP consumption.

Regulation of Fatty Acid Biosynthesis

Short-term regulation of fatty acid biosynthesis involves hormonal signals and enzyme cascades. Control is exerted on both the FAS complex and on the enzyme acetyl-CoA carboxylase. Short-term regulation (on a time scale of minutes) is sensitive to immediate energy demands. For this purpose, the enzymes use citrate as an indicator of cellular energy supplies. Their state of phosphorylation, which depends on ATP levels, also provides sensitivity to energy levels. Long-term control of fatty acid metabolism (adaptive control, over days or weeks) is exerted by relative rates of enzyme synthesis and degradation, principally of the fatty acid synthase itself as well as of acetyl-CoA carboxylase.

Acetyl-CoA Carboxylase

The enzyme acetyl-CoA carboxylase (not the FAS enzyme) catalyzes the formation of malonyl-CoA from acetyl-CoA. This can be considered the committed step in fatty acid biosynthesis.

Catalysis

Acetyl-CoA carboxylase (ACC) catalyzes the carboxylation of acetyl-CoA in a biotin-dependent, two-step reaction:

$$\text{ATP} + \text{HCO}_3^- + \text{ACC-biotin} \rightarrow \text{ACC-biotin-CO}_2^- + \text{ADP} + \text{P}_i \qquad (13\text{-}2)$$

$$\text{ACC-biotin-CO}_2^- + \text{Acetyl-CoA} \rightarrow \text{ACC-biotin} + \text{malonyl-CoA} \qquad (13\text{-}3)$$

The ACC enzyme uses biotin as a cofactor to acquire and donate carboxyl groups (**Figure 13-19**). Carboxylation on biotin takes place preferentially at the N-1 nitrogen, probably due to steric effects. The carboxyl group comes from carbonyl phosphate, synthesized by another enzyme system.

Carbonyl phosphate is an unstable intermediate, derived from a reaction involving bicarbonate and the γ-phosphate on ATP. In **Figure 13-20,** the N-1 nitrogen is depicted in the midst of a nucleophilic attack on the highly activated carbonyl of carbonyl phosphate, generating N^1-carboxybiotin. The carboxyl group is now activated. **Figure 13-21** shows how it becomes attached to acetyl-CoA to form malonyl-CoA.

Forms of the Enzyme

The bacterial form of ACC, which has multiple subunits made up from multiple gene products, is under study for development of antibiotics, as the bacterial forms are quite distinct from the eukaryotic forms. The enoyl-ACP reductase (the FabI protein in bacteria) is one major target. Isoniazid, which inhibits this enzyme, is used in treating tuberculosis. Triclosan,

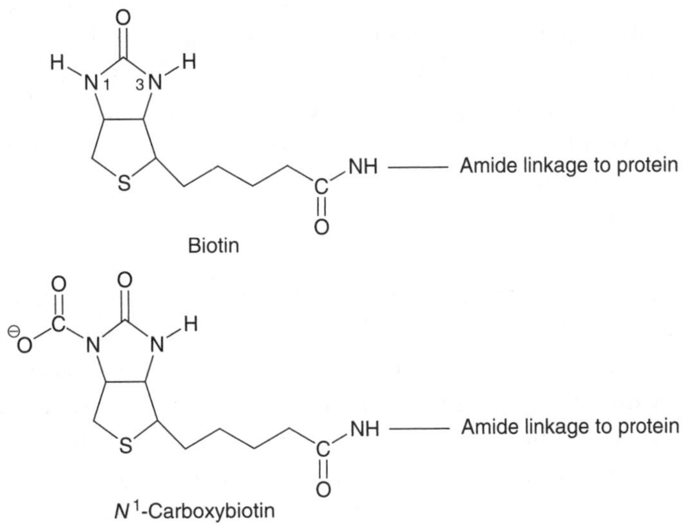

Amide linkage to protein

Biotin

Amide linkage to protein

N^1-Carboxybiotin

Figure 13-19 Structure of biotin and its carboxylated form.

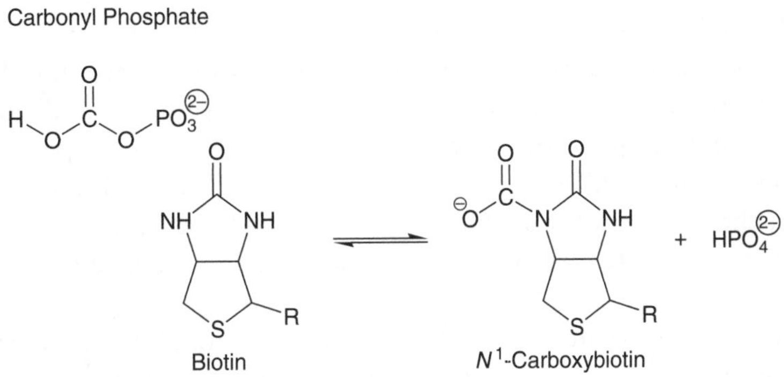

Carbonyl Phosphate

Biotin

N^1-Carboxybiotin

Figure 13-20 Activation of a carboxyl group in the form of carboxybiotin.

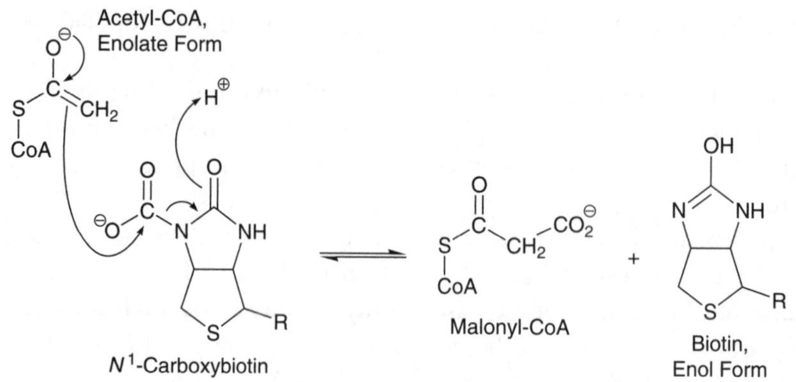

Figure 13-21 Formation of malonyl-CoA by carboxylation of acetyl-CoA, with biotin as the donor of the activated carboxyl group.

which also inhibits it, is used widely as an antibacterial agent. Plant ACC is similar to the bacterial form, and several inhibitors of plant ACC have been developed for use as herbicides.

Two distinct forms of mammalian ACC exist, with distinct genes, amino acid sequences, and tissue-specific expression. Most of the older studies of ACC focused on what is now designated as ACC-β (sometimes denoted as ACC-2) from the liver. It is also the major form expressed in skeletal and cardiac muscle. The other isoform, designated as ACC-α (or ACC-1), predominates in white adipose tissue but is also found in substantial amounts in the liver. Studies of the molecular weight of the active form of ACC imply that the smallest form in vivo is a dimer, either a homodimer or a heterodimer of the two isoforms.

Regulation

Malonyl-CoA is required for fatty acid (FA) biosynthesis, and its formation by ACC is the committed step toward FA biosynthesis. FA biosynthesis, which uses NADPH, is an energy-demanding process (principally through its dependence on the oxidation of glucose in the pentose phosphate pathway, where the required amounts of NADPH are generated). The enzyme ACC can, therefore, be expected to be under strict regulation to provide a flexible response to cellular demands for FA biosynthesis versus energy generation by oxidizing fatty acids. Acetyl-CoA is also a precursor for cholesterol biosynthesis, whose pathway is primarily regulated by the enzyme HMG CoA reductase, and which is also under tight regulation. Similarly, malonyl-CoA is required in some specialized lipid biosynthetic pathways, such as elongation of fatty acids to form eicosanoids (arachidonic acid, especially) and sphingolipids.

The regulation of ACC is complicated and not yet fully understood. Citrate allosterically activates the phosphorylated forms of both ACC-α and ACC-β, so it acts as a "feed-forward" activator. Glutamate also can activate both forms of the enzyme. These allosteric effectors seem to promote polymerization of the activated, phosphorylated enzyme; however, ACC-β does not seem to respond this way as much as does ACC-α. Depolymerization (and loss of activity) can be induced by malonyl-CoA, Mg^{2+} ion, and ATP. Fatty acids (such as palmitic acid) attached to CoA act as inhibitors in vitro. However, older textbooks tend to overemphasize the roles of fatty acyl-CoA and citrate as the immediate fast-acting regulators of ACC activity.

Both ACC-α and ACC-β are regulated by phosphorylation. Insulin and glucose increase ACC activity with concomitant loss of enzyme phosphorylation. Glucagon causes a modest increase in ACC phosphorylation, as does epinephrine, so both of these hormones increase enzyme inhibition. As yet, the pathways from these various hormone receptors to the kinases and phosphatases acting in vivo on ACC have not been completely worked out.

It does appear certain, however, that the major kinase acting on ACC is the AMP-dependent protein kinase (AMPK). This kinase is *not* a cAMP-dependent enzyme but instead is regulated by binding of 5′-AMP, which activates it. The enzyme is also subject to phosphorylation by a "kinase kinase," which itself has not yet been characterized in detail. Both phosphorylation and AMP binding appear to be necessary for activation of the AMPK enzyme. Regulation of AMPK by levels of 5′-AMP means that the enzyme is sensitive to the relative levels of ATP versus AMP in the cell; that is, the cellular energy charge regulates the activity of AMPK, rather than hormone signaling.

ACC is dephosphorylated by protein phosphatase 2A, which activates it. A different phosphatase acts on AMPK: protein phosphatase 2C. **Figure 13-22** summarizes this cycle, along with the citrate action that stimulates ACC activity. Notice the use of an AMP-activated protein kinase to regulate the activity. This kinase plays a role in other metabolic pathways, making them sensitive to the energy charge in the cell.

Citrate Shuttle

The *citrate shuttle* is the route (**Figure 13-23**) by which two-carbon fragments, derived from metabolism of carbohydrates, amino acids, or fatty acids, can be moved from the mitochondrial matrix out into the cytosol, where fatty acid synthesis takes place. Once again, we see the use of compartmentalization—this time for regulation of the opposing processes of fatty acid breakdown and synthesis. Notice how the citrate is first made inside the mitochondrion, then broken apart once it crosses the membrane into the cytosol.

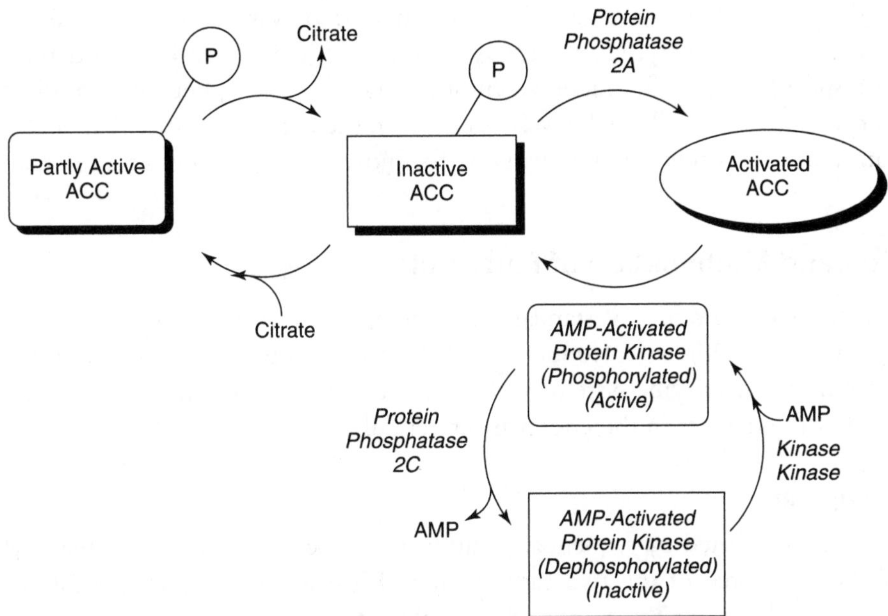

Figure 13-22 Regulation of the activity of acetyl-CoA carboxylase (ACC) by citrate and by phosphorylation. Citrate activates the enzyme; phosphorylation inhibits it. Phosphorylation is linked to an AMP-dependent kinase.

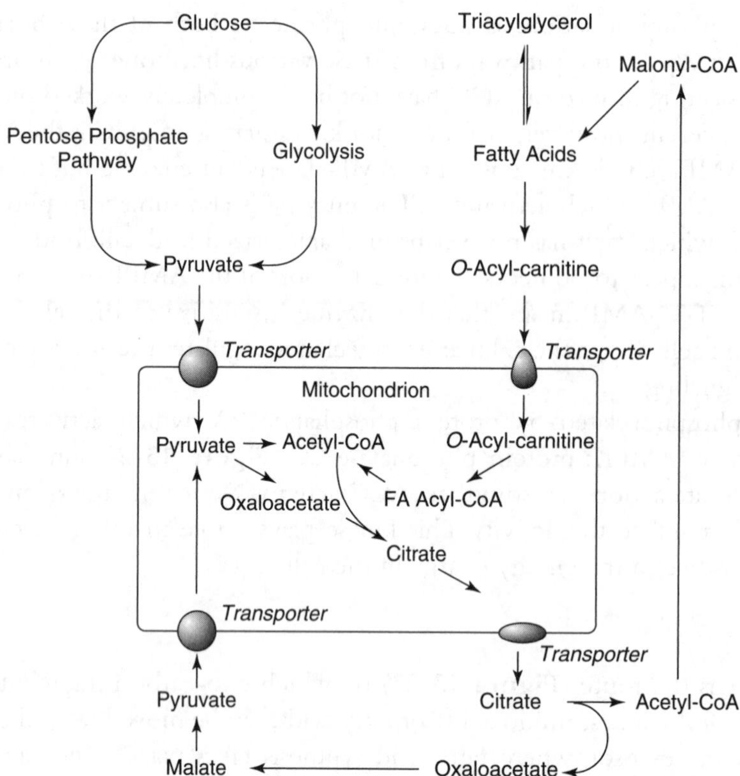

Figure 13-23 The citrate shuttle. Citrate can shuttle carbons, derived from carbohydrate, out to the cytosol from the mitochondrial matrix. The carbons appear there as acetyl-CoA, which can be used for fatty acid biosynthesis in the cytosol.

Recall that citrate may act as an allosteric effector of various enzymes in the cytosol, notably as an activator of acetyl-CoA carboxylase for fatty acid biosynthesis, and as an activator of fructose bisphosphatase-1 in gluconeogenesis. Citrate is serving here as an indicator of the general energy state of the cell: High levels of citrate in the cytosol indicate that energy supplies are abundant and that conditions are favorable for biosynthetic processes that demand energy input.

Elongation and Modification of Fatty Acids

Palmitate is the major product of standard fatty acid synthesis by the FAS complex. Longer chains (e.g., C-18, C-20) or introduction of functional groups (double bonds, hydroxyl moieties) require other enzyme systems and special reactions. To a large extent, these reactions are associated with enzymes in the endoplasmic reticulum.

Chain Elongation

Palmitate may be elongated by sequential addition of two-carbon units, with malonyl-CoA or acetyl-CoA as the source of the two-carbon units (**Figure 13-24**). The elongation reactions resemble those catalyzed by the FAS complex, using the same four-step pattern of thioester activation, reduction of the carbonyl group, dehydration, and reduction of the carbon–carbon double bond. NADH or NADPH provides the reducing equivalents, depending on the tissue and cellular site of the reactions. Reactions occur in the mitochondria or in the endoplasmic reticulum.

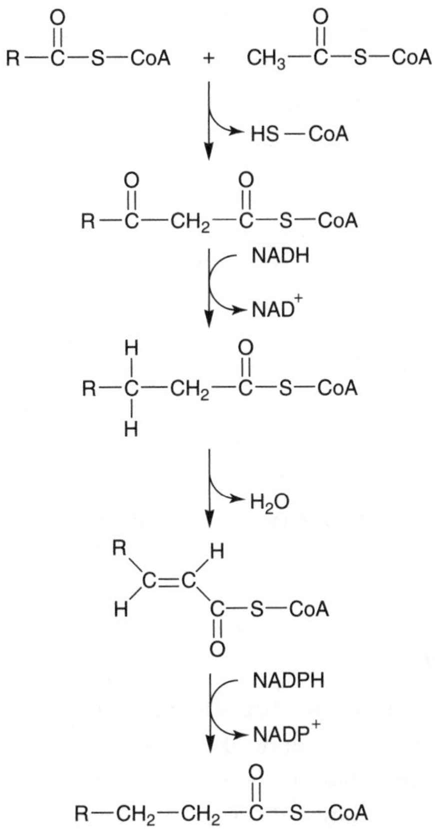

$$R{-}\overset{O}{\overset{\|}{C}}{-}S{-}CoA \;+\; CH_3{-}\overset{O}{\overset{\|}{C}}{-}S{-}CoA$$

$$\downarrow \; \rightarrow HS{-}CoA$$

$$R{-}\overset{O}{\overset{\|}{C}}{-}CH_2{-}\overset{O}{\overset{\|}{C}}{-}S{-}CoA$$

$$\downarrow \; NADH \rightarrow NAD^+$$

$$R{-}\underset{H}{\overset{H}{C}}{-}CH_2{-}\overset{O}{\overset{\|}{C}}{-}S{-}CoA$$

$$\downarrow \; \rightarrow H_2O$$

$$(R)(H)C{=}C(H){-}\underset{O}{\underset{\|}{C}}{-}S{-}CoA$$

$$\downarrow \; NADPH \rightarrow NADP^+$$

$$R{-}CH_2{-}CH_2{-}\overset{O}{\overset{\|}{C}}{-}S{-}CoA$$

Figure 13-24 Elongation of a fatty acid chain by a specialized synthase, not the FAS complex. The pattern of reactions is similar to that found in regular fatty acid synthesis.

Desaturation

Formation of monoenoic acids occurs in the endoplasmic reticulum, where mixed-function oxidases simultaneously oxidize the fatty acid (introducing the double bond) and oxidize NADPH. The result is the formation of a *cis* double bond, in a position at least six carbons removed from the end of the chain (giving an ω-6 fatty acid, for example). Polyunsaturated fatty acids (with *cis* double bonds) are formed by a combination of chain elongation reactions and desaturation reactions. These products include arachidonic acid, which is important as a precursor for prostaglandins and thromboxanes. **Figure 13-25** summarizes the overall pattern of chain elongation and chain desaturation leading to production arachidonic acid and other substances. In humans, certain of these reactions do not occur—notably, the desaturation of oleate to linoleate, and linoleate to α-linolenate; this is the basis for declaring linoleate and α-linolenate to be "essential" in the diet.

Branched-Chain Fatty Acids

Branched-chain fatty acids are rare in higher animals, but are relatively common in plants. The "branch" is a methyl group, which is introduced when methylmalonyl-CoA is used instead of malonyl-CoA in a chain-elongation reaction (for examples, see the structures of phytol and phytanic acid in Figure 13-12). This type of reaction may occur pathologically in humans when there is a deficiency of vitamin B_{12} in the diet (recall that vitamin B_{12} is involved in the conversion of methylmalonyl-CoA to succinyl-CoA, which can then enter the TCA cycle).

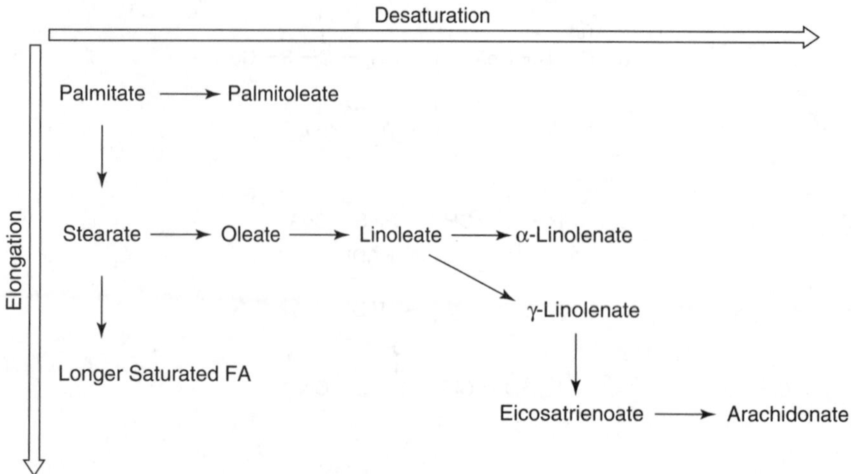

Figure 13-25 The pattern of chain elongations and desaturations leading to key long-chain fatty acids with double bonds.

Reduction to Fatty Alcohols

The fatty acid may be reduced in a NADPH-dependent process to form the corresponding fatty alcohol. This reaction occurs in the endoplasmic reticulum. The fatty alcohols may then be incorporated into certain phospholipids. Fatty alcohols are found in skin oil, ear wax, and other substances, where they function as lubricants and as barriers to water and to bacteria.

Triglyceride and Membrane Lipid Biosynthesis

The biosynthesis of fatty acids leads directly to the products triglycerides and membrane lipids. These are energy-requiring processes, using activated intermediates. Triglyceride biosynthesis uses fatty acids activated with CoA as well as phosphorylated glycerol. Phospholipid biosynthesis employs nucleotide-activated intermediates, with two different pathways leading to the final product. Sphingolipid biosynthesis uses the intermediate sphingosine en route to ceramide; glycosphingolipid formation involves the attachment of short chains of sugars.

Triglyceride Biosynthesis

Activated fatty acids are used to make phosphatidic acid, from which triglycerides and various phospholipids may be derived. In particular, triglycerides are synthesized from activated fatty acids and a phosphorylated three-carbon molecule, either DHAP or glycerol 3-phosphate. The activated fatty acid is in the form of an acyl-CoA; the reaction is catalyzed by acyl-CoA synthetase:

$$RCO_2^- + ATP + CoASH \rightarrow RCO\text{-}SCoA + AMP + PP_i + H_2O \qquad (13\text{-}4)$$

Note the appearance of AMP and pyrophosphate as products. Free energy is, of course, stored in the thioester linkage. Nevertheless, because the pyrophosphate group is readily hydrolyzed, the product side of the reaction is favored.

In eukaryotes, the synthesis of phosphatidic acid is mainly associated with the endoplasmic reticulum, but also occurs in mitochondria. It involves two sequential acylations of glycerol 3-phosphate, using the activated fatty acids and forming the intermediate lysophosphatidic acid. Glycerol 3-phosphate can be derived either from glycerol itself or by reduction of dihydroxyacetone phosphate (DHAP; see **Figure 13-26**). An alternative route to phosphatidic acid is via the phosphorylation of a diacyl glycerol.

In triglyceride formation, phosphatidic acid is dephosphorylated to the diacyl glycerol; the available hydroxyl group is then acylated using an activated acyl group, giving finally the triglyceride (Figure 13-26). The three fatty acids used here may all be distinct and different from one another. For example, the first may be palmitic, the second myristic, and the third linoleic acid (**Figure 13-27**).

Membrane Lipids from Fatty Acids

Membrane Phospholipids

Membrane phospholipids are synthesized by two routes. Some of the enzymes here are found in the cytosol, whereas others are associated with the endoplasmic reticulum. **Figure 13-28** compares the biosynthesis of phosphatidylserine to that of phosphatidylcholine.

In the first case, the path starts with phosphatidic acid, which is activated by attachment of a cytidine moiety (from the nucleotide cytidine triphosphate, or CTP) to give cytidine diphosphodiacylglycerol (CDP-diacylglycerol). A pyrophosphate group is displaced in this reaction, and its subsequent hydrolysis favors product formation at this point. This is similar to the use of UTP to activate sugars in biosynthesis, forming the UDP–sugar conjugate and releasing pyrophosphate. Next, cytidine monophosphate is displaced as a phosphoester link is made to the hydroxyl group on serine; the product (phosphatidylserine) has a phosphodiester link joining the serine to the glycerol backbone.

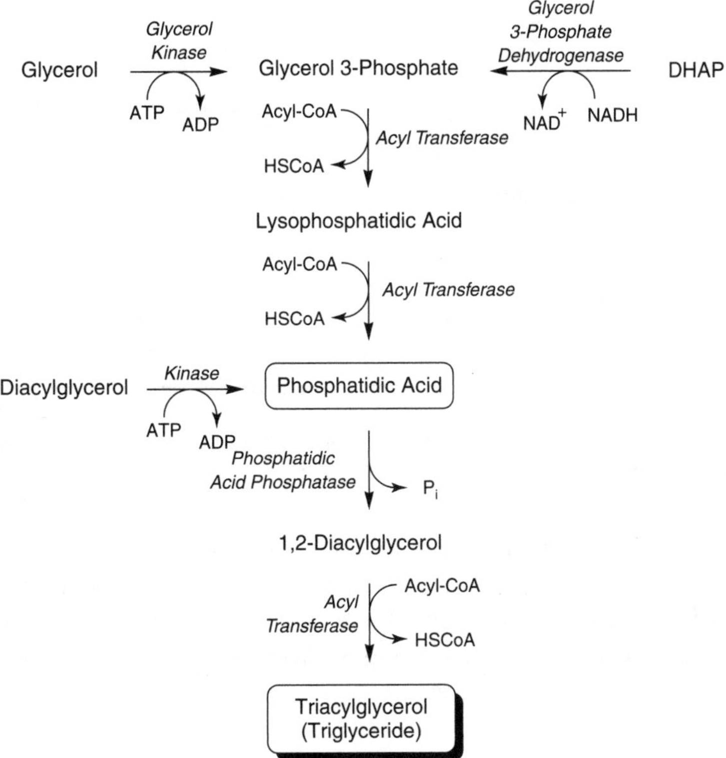

Figure 13-26 Reaction pathway leading from glycerol 3-phosphate to phosphatidic acid and on to triglycerides.

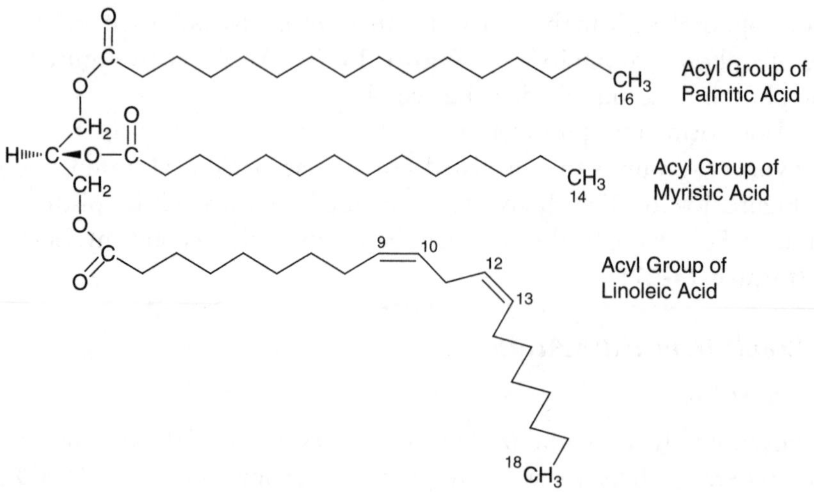

Acyl Group of Palmitic Acid

Acyl Group of Myristic Acid

Acyl Group of Linoleic Acid

Figure 13-27 A triglyceride showing glycerol esterified with three different fatty acids.

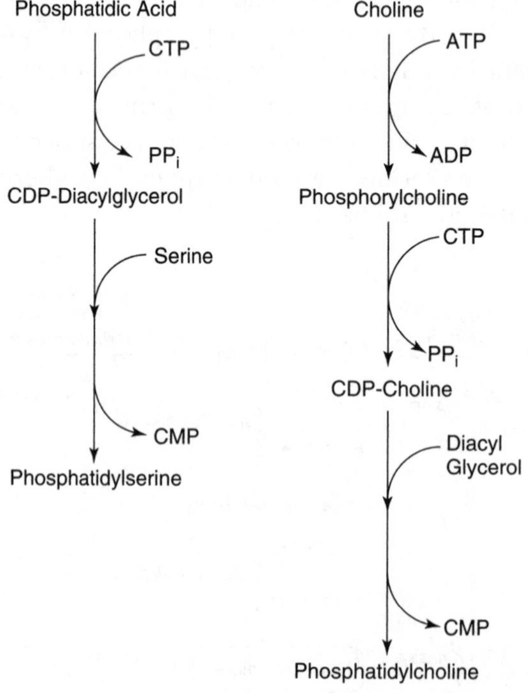

Figure 13-28 Biosynthesis of phospholipids, showing two different patterns of usage of the activating nucleotide, cytidine triphosphate.

The second route to membrane phospholipids starts with activation of the future head group—in this case, choline—by phosphorylation at the expense of ATP. Next, a cytidine moiety (from CTP) is attached, and again there is displacement of pyrophosphate to form CDP-choline. Finally, the activated head group is attached to a diacylglycerol via a phosphate link, and the activating CMP group leaves.

Sphingolipids

The biosynthesis of sphingolipids follows a different path. The process starts with the synthesis of sphingosine. **Figure 13-29** shows the route from palmitoyl-CoA to sphingosine. Serine is attached, via decarboxylation, to the activated fatty acid; this reaction is dependent on pyridoxal

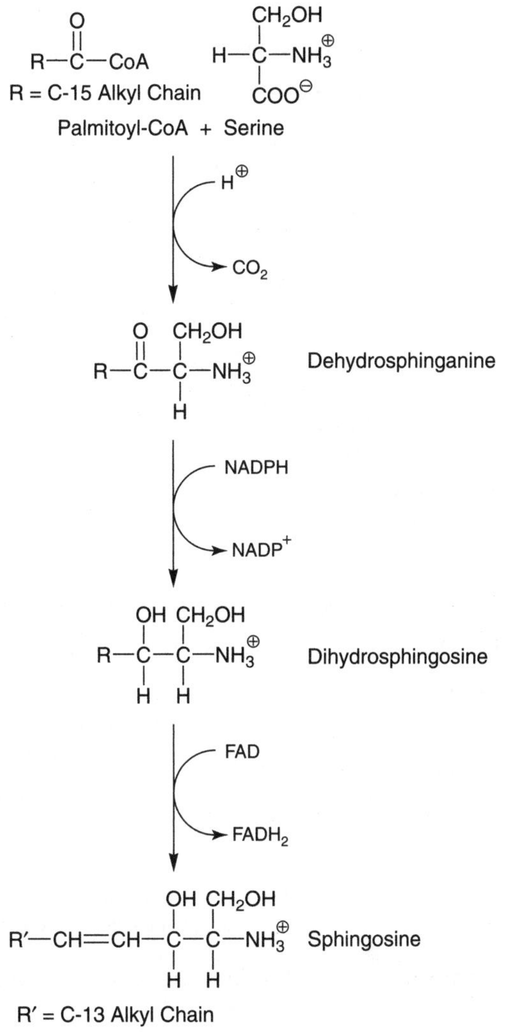

$R{-}C({=}O){-}CoA$ $\quad$ $H{-}C(CH_2OH)(COO^{\ominus}){-}NH_3^{\oplus}$

R = C-15 Alkyl Chain

Palmitoyl-CoA + Serine

$H^{\oplus}$ → CO_2

$R{-}C({=}O){-}C(H)(CH_2OH){-}NH_3^{\oplus}$ Dehydrosphinganine

NADPH → $NADP^+$

$R{-}C(OH)(H){-}C(H)(CH_2OH){-}NH_3^{\oplus}$ Dihydrosphingosine

FAD → $FADH_2$

$R'{-}CH{=}CH{-}C(OH)(H){-}C(H)(CH_2OH){-}NH_3^{\oplus}$ Sphingosine

R′ = C-13 Alkyl Chain

Figure 13-29 Biosynthesis of sphingosine.

phosphate, a cofactor that will be discussed in Chapter 14. Two successive redox reactions then follow—first a reduction using NADPH, and then an oxidation using FAD.

The sphingosine so synthesized is only an intermediate and does not accumulate appreciably. It is used to make ceramide (**Figure 13-30**), by attachment of a fatty acid chain to the amino group of the sphingosine core. Sphingomyelin results when a phosphorylcholine is transferred from phosphatidylcholine to the hydroxyl group on ceramide. Sphingomyelin is a major membrane component in some cells and organelles, and contributes to membrane rigidity.

If one or more sugars are linked in this position instead, the result is a glycosphingolipid (Figure 13-30). If only a single sugar is attached, the compound is called a cerebroside. However, more sugars may be attached to the terminal monosaccharide, including modified sugars such as acetylgalactosamine and *N*-acetylneuraminic acid (also known as sialic acid). These complex glycosphingolipids in cell membranes are oriented so that the saccharide moieties project outside the cell; they are important extracellular features for cell–cell recognition (e.g., in the immune system for blood group antigens).

The initial phases of sphingolipid synthesis (e.g., with dihydrosphingosine and ceramide) are associated with the endoplasmic reticulum. More complex sphingolipids (e.g., sphingomyelin or glucosylceramide) are elaborated from these precursors in the Golgi apparatus.

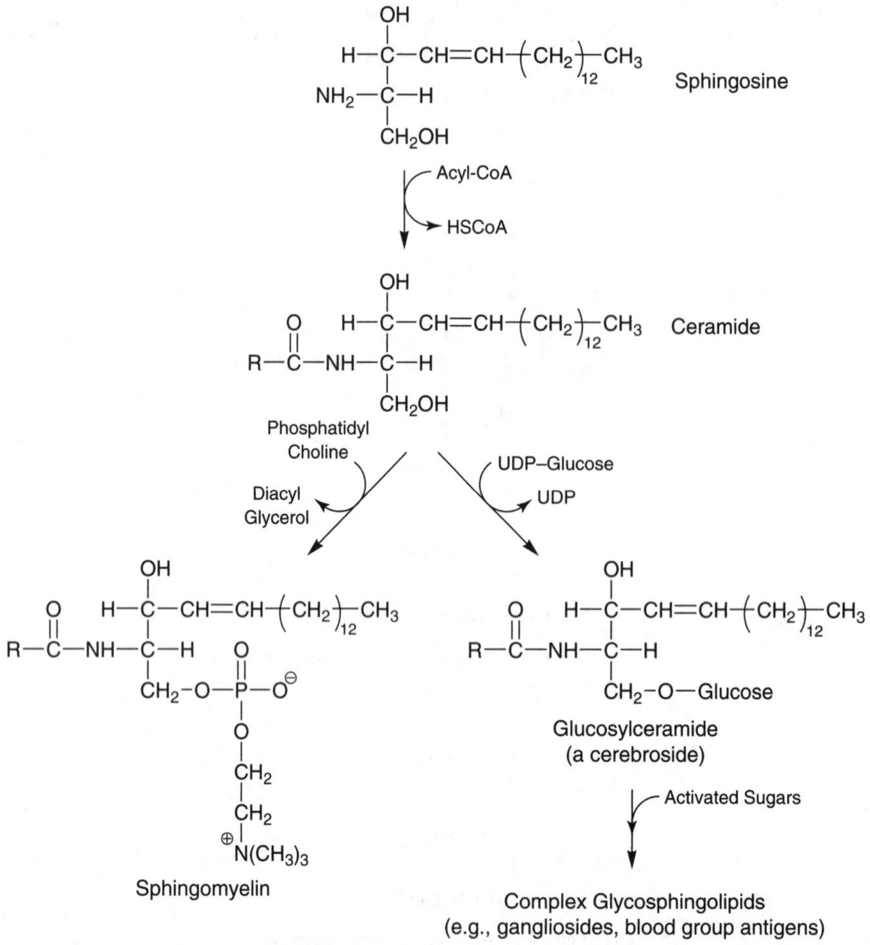

Figure 13-30 The route from sphingosine through ceramide, to sphingomyelin, glucosylceramide, and complex gangliosides.

Cholesterol Metabolism

Cholesterol and its acyl esters are highly hydrophobic and tend to shy away from contact with water and form lipid bilayers and micelles. As a membrane constituent, cholesterol embeds itself between phospholipids in the lipid bilayer of the membrane, orienting its hydroxyl group toward the aqueous phase. Cholesterol stabilizes the alkyl chains of the neighboring phospholipids in an extended conformation, thereby helping to stiffen and make more viscous (less fluid) the bilayer structure. These characteristics can be important factors in the organization of the bilayer into regions that are fluidized and those that are rigid (e.g., lipid rafts). Fluidized regions allow membrane bending and the relatively rapid and free motions of embedded proteins, cofactors, and other materials, while rigidified regions restrict those motions and resist bending or folding.

Cholesterol metabolites are important in their own right. The uptake and digestion of lipids from the diet would not be possible without their solubilization by the bile salts, which are the principal catabolic metabolites of cholesterol. Although the steroid hormones count for much less of the catabolism of cholesterol, their functions as communication agents are essential to proper growth, development, and health.

Biosynthesis of Cholesterol

Although a significant amount of cholesterol is derived from diet (mainly from cholesterol-rich foods such as meat, eggs, and dairy products), the body also synthesizes cholesterol readily. The liver is the main organ for cholesterol biosynthesis, although other tissues synthesize it as well (e.g., glands that produce steroid hormones).

Biosynthesis of cholesterol takes place in the endoplasmic reticulum and starts from the common precursor, acetyl-CoA. Condensation of two acetyl-CoA moieties leads (through the key intermediate hydroxymethylglutaryl-CoA) to mevalonate (**Figure 13-31**). From mevalonate, two pyrophosphorylated intermediates are made: isopentenyl pyrophosphate and dimethylallyl pyrophosphate. Condensation of a total of six of these activated units gives the polyunsaturated compound squalene, which then in a series of ring closures give the steroid nucleus. Next, some hydride transfers and methyl group rearrangements yield lanosterol. Lanosterol undergoes three demethylations, a shift in the position of the double bond in the ring system, and saturation of the double bond in the alkyl tail, to give cholesterol (**Figure 13-32**).

Cholesterol biosynthesis is feedback regulated at the step catalyzed by the enzyme HMG CoA reductase, which catalyzes the rate-limiting step in the pathway. Increases in intracellular cholesterol also tend to reduce transcription of the gene for HMG CoA reductase. Dietary cholesterol serves to inhibit HMG CoA reductase and to reduce synthesis of the enzyme. Turnover (degradation) of this enzyme is relatively rapid. Thus, with the combined effects of direct enzyme inhibition and indirect loss of enzyme level, within a matter of hours the overall biosynthetic activity in the liver can drop quite appreciably.

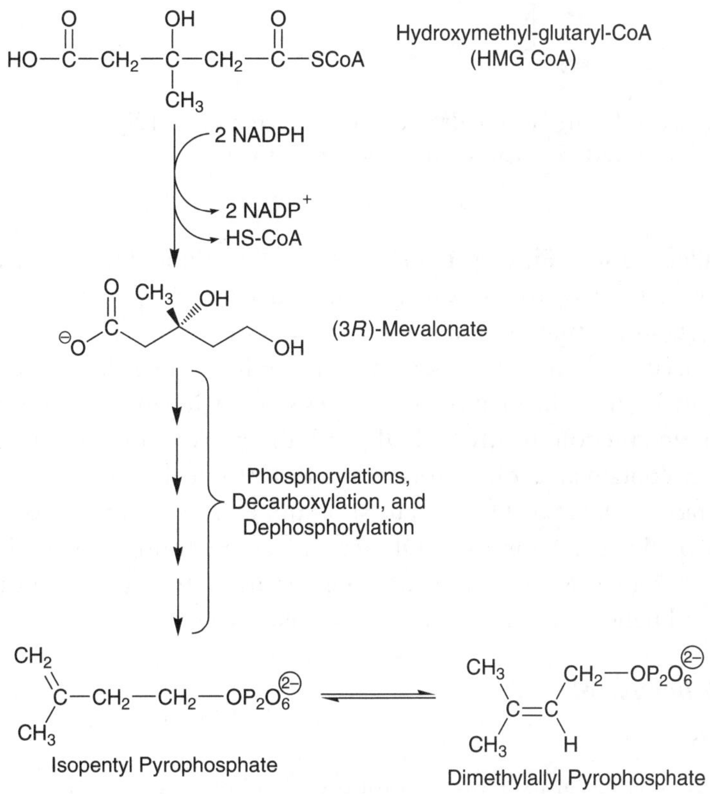

Hydroxymethyl-glutaryl-CoA (HMG CoA)

2 NADPH → 2 $NADP^+$, HS-CoA

(3*R*)-Mevalonate

Phosphorylations, Decarboxylation, and Dephosphorylation

Isopentyl Pyrophosphate ⇌ Dimethylallyl Pyrophosphate

Figure 13-31 The route from HMG CoA to isopentenyl pyrophosphate and dimethylallyl pyrophosphate.

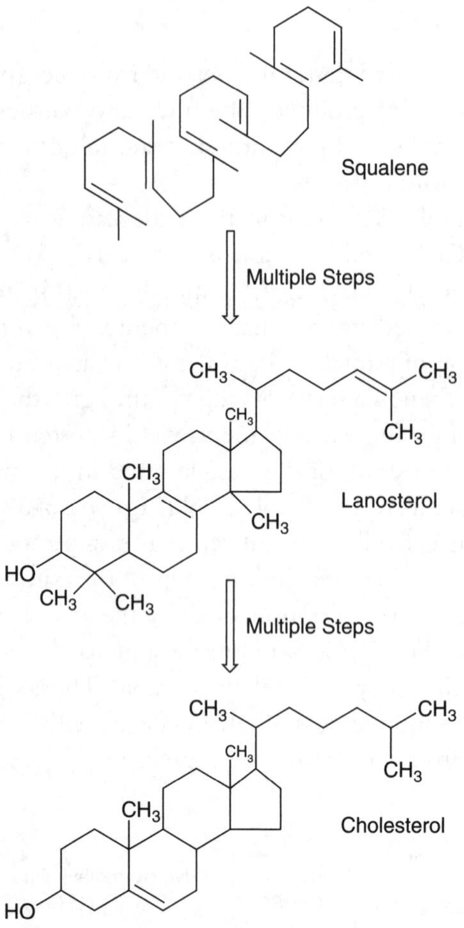

Squalene

Multiple Steps

Lanosterol

Multiple Steps

Cholesterol

Figure 13-32 Squalene, formed by condensation of units of dimethylallyl pyrophosphate and isopentenyl pyrophosphate, is converted to lanosterol, which leads to cholesterol.

The drugs called statins (**Figure 13-33**) specifically inhibit HMG CoA reductase and, therefore, block cholesterol synthesis. When combined with an appropriate diet that restricts cholesterol intake, statin therapy can reduce serum cholesterol appreciably.

Newly synthesized cholesterol is exported from the liver through the circulation to other tissues where it can be used in membrane synthesis or in hormone biosynthesis. Transport occurs via lipoproteins, predominantly by LDL, with the cholesterol in the form of a fatty acid ester. These particles contain an apolipoprotein, apo B-100, which is specifically recognized and bound by cell-surface receptors (LDL receptors) on the plasma membrane of nonliver cells.

Transcription of the gene for the LDL receptor is responsive to levels of cholesterol. Decreases in cholesterol levels result in greater gene transcription, more synthesis of the LDL receptor protein, and hence greater uptake of cholesterol from serum.

Metabolites of Cholesterol

Fatty Acid Esters

Cholesterol can be esterified at its hydroxyl group with a fatty acid (often oleate or linoleate, in humans). Esterification may be catalyzed intracellularly by an acyl-CoA:cholesterol transferase (ACAT), with the acyl-CoA as a co-substrate. Alternatively, in serum the fatty acid moiety

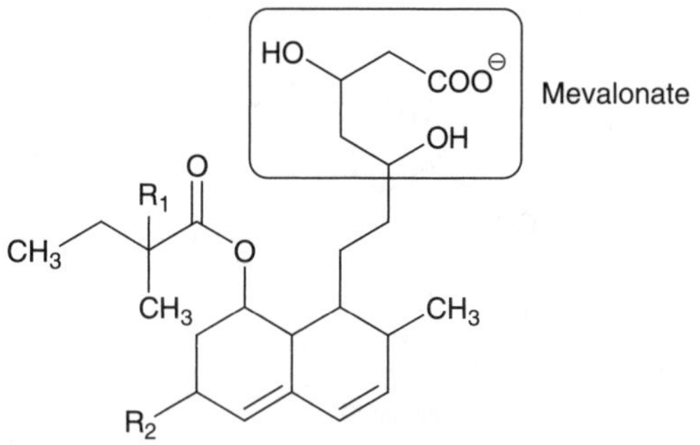

R_1	R_2	
CH_3	CH_3	Simvastatin (Zocor)
H	OH	Pravastatin (Pravachol)
H	CH_3	Lovastatin (Mevacor)

Figure 13-33 Statins inhibit production of HMG CoA reductase and reduce cholesterol synthesis. Part of their structure resembles the enzyme's substrate, mevalonate.

may be transferred from phosphatidylcholine, in a reaction catalyzed by lecithin-cholesterol acyltransferase (LCAT). The serum reaction takes place mainly within HDL particles and helps to trap newly synthesized cholesterol inside the particle.

Much of the cholesterol in lipoprotein particles is present as the acly ester. Cholesterol esters are prominent components of LDL particles; lesser amounts are present in VLDL and HDL (**Table 13-2**).

Bile Acids

Bile acids are a major component of bile, the digestive fluid secreted by the gallbladder into the digestive tract. Three major bile acids are cholate (cholic acid), glycocholate, and taurocholate (**Figure 13-34**); they are synthesized from cholesterol in the liver and then transported to the gallbladder for secretion. Cholate is made, as cholyl-CoA, in several steps from cholesterol. Reaction with glycine gives glycocholate, which is the major digestive bile acid. Alternatively, reaction of cholyl-CoA with taurine (a catabolite of the amino acid cysteine) gives taurocholate. Bile acids are effective biological detergents, as they contain both nonpolar groups (the sterol ring system) and a polar region (the ionic acid groups). In aqueous solution, bile salts form micelles into which nonpolar lipids will dissolve. The micelles transport the lipids and expose them to the action of lipases for digestion.

Humans do not have the capacity to degrade the steroid rings, so cholesterol and other sterols are excreted with the ring system intact. Because of their poor aqueous solubility, sterols are excreted via the feces.

Hormones

Steroid hormones can be categorized into three general classes: sex hormones, glucocorticoids, and mineralocorticoids. Sex hormones are involved in sexual maturation and reproduction; glucorticoids help to regulate gluconeogenesis and the immune response; and mineralocorticoids help to control reabsorption of small ions in the kidney (e.g., Na^+, Cl^-, and bicarbonate).

All steroid hormones are derived from pregnenolone. Pregnenolone is obtained from cholesterol by removing most of the hydrocarbon chain attached to its D ring (**Figure 13-35**).

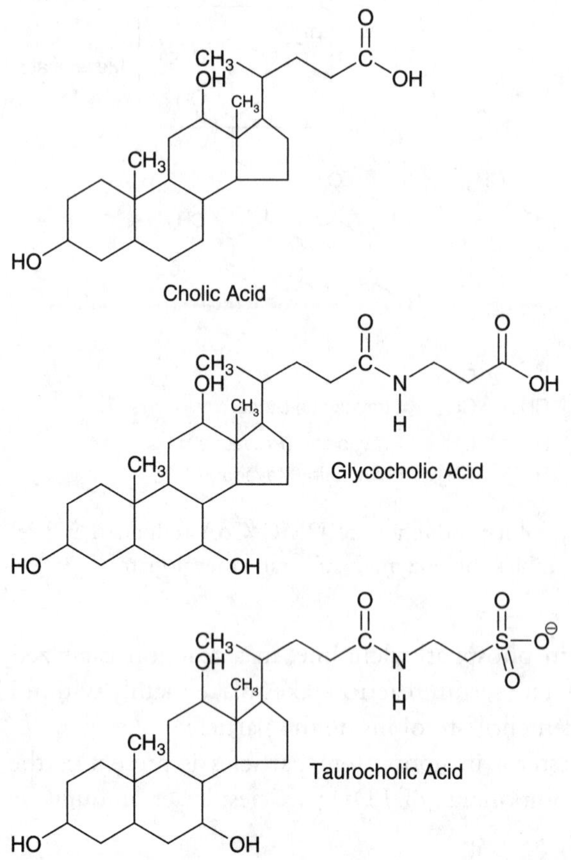

Cholic Acid

Glycocholic Acid

Taurocholic Acid

Figure 13-34 Common bile acids, which act as solubilizing agents for lipid emulsification.

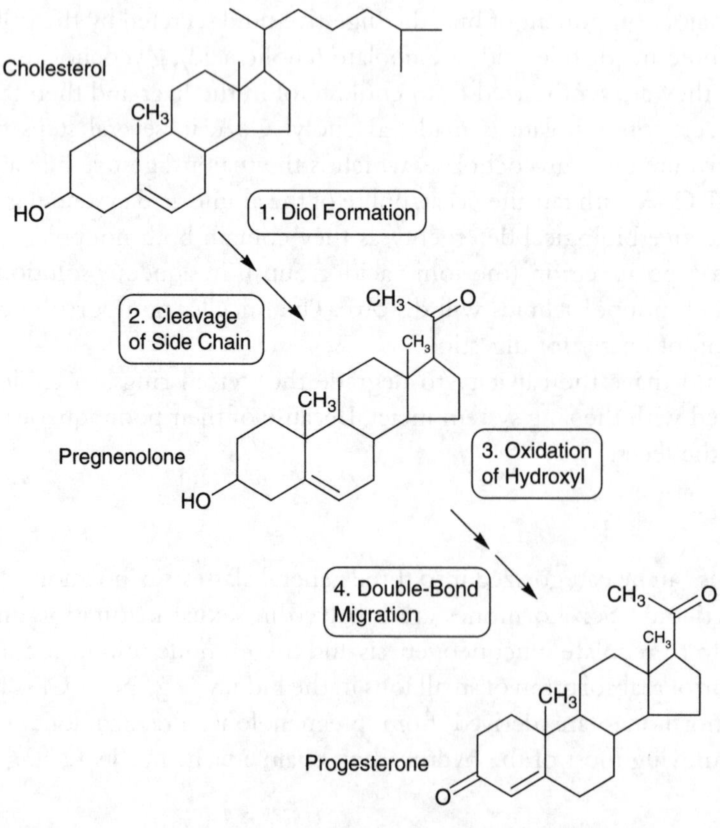

Cholesterol

1. Diol Formation

2. Cleavage of Side Chain

Pregnenolone

3. Oxidation of Hydroxyl

4. Double-Bond Migration

Progesterone

Figure 13-35 The route from cholesterol to progesterone.

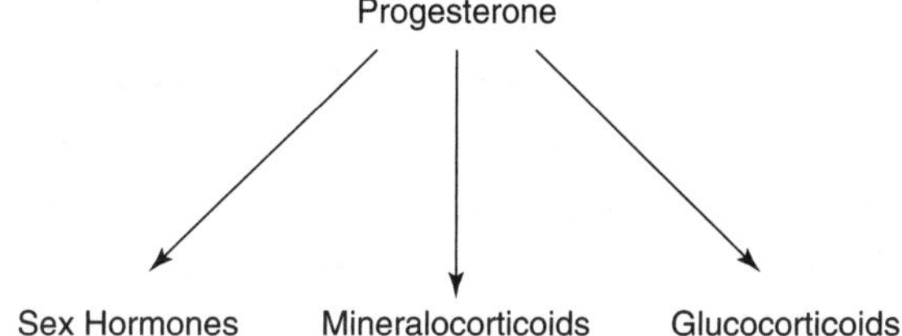

Figure 13-36 Progesterone is the precursor to the sex hormones, glucocorticoids, and mineralocorticoids.

Progesterone is then derived from pregnenolone by oxidizing the 3-hydroxyl group to a ketone and shifting the double bond's position. **Figure 13-36** shows the general derivation from progesterone of the sex hormones (e.g., testosterone, estradiol), glucocorticoids (e.g., cortisol, the principal glucocorticoid), and mineralocorticoids (e.g., aldosterone, the principal mineralocorticoid).

QUESTIONS FOR DISCUSSION

1. Why might spinach be banned from the diet of a patient who has Refsum disease?
2. Suppose that you lived in the far north and had to spend the winter living on a diet of whale blubber. Explain why the concentration of ketone bodies in your blood would increase. Then explain why supplementing your diet with soda crackers might be a good idea.
3. Patients with methylmalonic aciduria have a high level of methymalonic acid in their blood and urine. Explain why a vegan diet, with little or no intake of vitamin B_{12}, might lead to this condition.
4. Studies on cultured fibroblasts from certain patients' skin, emphasizing the cells' ability to metabolize phytanic acid, demonstrated the incompetence of the cells to metabolize this lipid. When the same cell cultures were given pristanic acid, however, the pristanic acid was metabolized at a normal rate (see Figure 13-12 for the chemical structures of phytanic and pristanic acids). What is the enzymatic defect responsible for the inability of these cells to metabolize phytanic acid?
5. In Figure 13-12, explain the presence of propionyl-CoA and 2-methylpropionyl-CoA, in addition to acetyl-CoA, as end products of the oxidation of phytanic acid.
6. Humans are unable to synthesize biotin, so they depend on dietary sources to secure enough of the cofactor for maintaining activity of biotin-dependent enzymes. Most dietary biotin is bound to protein and must be released through the action of the pancreatic enzyme biotinidase, which hydrolyzes the amide linkage of biotin to the protein. The free biotin is then absorbed from the gut via a sodium-dependent transport system. However, certain proteins are known to sequester biotin—for example, the egg-white protein avidin, which binds biotin with a binding constant on the order of 10^{12} M^{-1}. What would be the biochemical consequences of a defect in either the activity of the biotinidase enzyme or the activity of the intestinal transporter protein for biotin?
7. Valproic acid (2-*n*-propylpentanoic acid) is used for control of epilepsy and seizures. It is a substrate for the β-oxidation pathway in mitochondria, which may account for 40% or more of the overall metabolism of the drug (30–50% of the drug is excreted in the urine

as the glucuronide conjugate, and 10–20% is oxidatively metabolized by the cytochrome P-450 system). It is important to control levels of valproic acid to avoid toxic side effects.

a. Predict the breakdown products of valproic acid metabolized via the β-oxidation pathway.
b. How might valproic acid block the metabolism of regular fatty acids? Consider inhibition of CPT1 or CPT2 as well as of enzymes directly in the β-oxidation pathway.
c. Gastrointestinal disturbances and weight gain are common side effects of a chronic regimen of valproic acid therapy. Propose connections to the blockages suggested in part b.

8. Why do hepatocytes and adipocytes have a relatively high level of activity of carbonic anhydrase?
9. How might chronic treatment of glaucoma with acetazolamide affect fatty acid biosynthesis?
10. An adult patient complained of exercise-induced muscular pain and stiffness. Laboratory tests showed the patient had a deficiency in carnitine palmitoyltransferase 2. How would this deficiency be related to the symptoms presented by the patient?
11. **Figure 13-37** shows the structures of several statins, all of which are inhibitors of HMG CoA reductase. **Table 13-3** lists thermodynamic properties of these drugs as they bind to the enzyme.
    a. Which drug has the highest affinity for HMG CoA reductase?
    b. Which drug shows the most favorable enthalpy change upon binding?

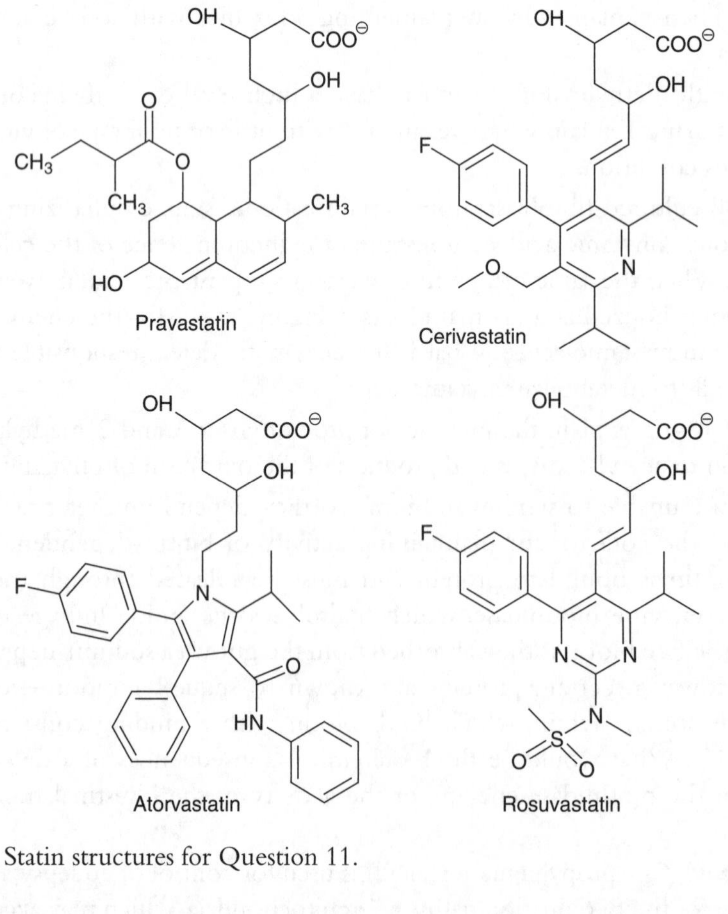

Pravastatin

Cerivastatin

Atorvastatin

Rosuvastatin

Figure 13-37 Statin structures for Question 11.

Compound	ΔG (kJ/mol)	ΔH (kJ/mol)	$-T\Delta S$ (kJ/mol) at 298 K
Pravastatin	−40.6	−10.5	−30.1
Cerivastatin	−47.7	−13.8	−33.9
Atorvastatin	−45.6	−18.0	−27.6
Rosuvastatin	−51.5	−38.9	−12.6

Table 13-3 Thermodynamics of Statin Binding to HMG CoA Reductase

Source: T. Carbonell and E. Freire. (2005). "Binding Thermodynamics of Statins to HMG-CoA Reductase," *Biochemistry* 44:11741–11748.

c. Which drug shows the most favorable entropy change upon binding?
d. For which drugs does the entropy change dominate the binding? What about the enthalpy change?

12. In humans, dietary consumption of *trans* fatty acids (unsaturated fatty acids whose double bonds have the *trans* geometry) increases the activity in plasma of cholesteryl ester transfer protein; this protein is responsible for transferring plasma cholesterol esters from HDL to LDL and VLDL. How could a diet rich in such fatty acids alter the ratio of HDL to (LDL plus VLDL)? What consequences would this effect have for cardiovascular health?
13. Per molecule of ATP produced, which requires more O_2: the catabolism of fatty acids or the catabolism of glycogen?
14. A patient with plasma cholesterol levels greater than 8.5 millimolar was diagnosed with hypercholesterolemia and placed on a cholesterol-free diet for several months. This intervention reduced his plasma cholesterol to just below 8 millimolar. How is it possible that the patient could continue to have such high cholesterol levels despite following this diet?
15. To lose weight, a college student starts an extreme diet, high in processed carbohydrates but in which dietary fat is almost completely eliminated. By the end of the term, the student is complaining of a loss of night vision, skin itchiness and dryness, frequent nose bleeds, and many small skin bruises. How is the diet related to these problems?

REFERENCES

R. W. Bishop and R. M. Bell. (1988). "Assembly of phospholipids into cellular membranes: biosynthesis, transmembrane movement and intracellular translocation," *Annu. Rev. Cell Biol.* 4:579–610.

K. L. Brown. (2005). "Chemistry and enzymology of vitamin B_{12}," *Chem. Rev.* 105:2075–2149.

M. S. Brown and J. L. Goldstein. (1986). "A receptor-mediated pathway for cholesterol homeostasis," *Science* 232:34–47.

R. W. Brownsey et al. (2006). "Regulation of acetyl-CoA carboxylase," *Biochem. Soc. Trans.* 34:223–227.

S. Eaton, K. Bartlett, and M. Pourfarzam. (1996). "Mammalian mitochondrial β-oxidation," *Biochem. J.* 32:345–357.

W.-H. Kunau, V. Dommes, and H. Schulz. (1995). "β-Oxidation of fatty acids in mitochondria, peroxisomes, and bacteria: A century of continued progress," *Prog. Lipid Res.* 34:267–342.

T. N. Lupenko and A. E. Sumner. (2002). "The physiology of lipoproteins," *J. Nucl. Cardiol.* 9:38–49.

T. Maier, M. Leibundgut, and N. Ban. (2008). "The crystal structure of a mammalian fatty acid synthase," *Science* 321:1315–1322.

D. Mozaffarian et al. (2006). "*Trans* fatty acids and cardiovascular disease," *New England J. Med.* 354:1601–1613.

K. J. Payne et al. (2001). "Bacterial fatty-acid biosynthesis: A genomics-driven target for antibacterial drug discovery," *Drug Discovery Today* 6:537–544.

R. R. Ramsay, R. D. Gandour, and R. R. van der Leij. (2001). "Molecular enzymology of carnitine transfer and transport," *Biochim. Biophys. Acta* 1547:21–43.

D. W. Russell and K. D. R. Setchell. (1992). "Bile acid biosynthesis," *Biochemistry* 31:4737–4749.

D. Steinberg et al. (1067). "Refsum's disease: Nature of the enzyme defect," *Science* 156:1740–1742.

F. G. Tafesse, P. Ternes, and J. C. M. Holthuis. (2006). "The multigenic sphingomyelin synthase family," *J. Biol. Chem.* 281:29421–29425.

S. J. Wakil. (1989). "Fatty acid synthase, a proficient multifunctional enzyme," *Biochemistry* 28:4523–4530.

CHAPTER 14

Amino Acid Metabolism

Learning Objectives

1. Define and use correctly the following terms: *essential amino acid, ketogenic amino acid, glucogenic amino acid, nitrogen fixation, transamination, oxidative deamination, Schiff base linkage, aldimine, ketimine, pyridoxal phosphate, hyperammonemia, folate, tetrahydrofolate, folate antagonist, S-adenosylmethionine, urea cycle, carbamoyl phosphate*, N-*acetyl glutamate, carbamoyl phosphate synthetase, phenylketonuria, catecholamine, alcaptonuria*, and *maple syrup urine disease*.
2. Summarize the fate of dietary protein. Explain what happens in general terms to amino acids that are not immediately used in protein biosynthesis. State where in the body the bulk of amino acid metabolism occurs.
3. Explain how and why various amino acids are classified as ketogenic, glycogenic, or both. List the 20 amino acids according to these classifications.
4. Relate the catabolism of glycogenic amino acids to TCA cycle intermediates. Draw a diagram to illustrate the connections.
5. Explain why catabolism of amino acids is increased during periods of fasting. Explain why ketosis may arise during periods of fasting.
6. List the essential amino acids, distinguishing those that may be required for infants or children but not for adults. Explain briefly why the other amino acids are non-essential, in terms of intermediates in the TCA cycle and elsewhere.
7. Describe how glutamate and glutamine are important sources of nitrogens for amino acids and other biochemicals. Briefly relate glutamate synthesis to nitrogen fixation.
8. For the amino acid serine, list several important biochemicals for which it is a precursor (apart from protein synthesis). Do the same for the amino acid glycine.
9. Trace the biosynthetic pathway leading to serine. Explain how the pathway is regulated, and how it is connected to glycolysis.
10. Explain the source of sulfur atoms in Met and Cys.
11. Recognize the structures of *S*-adenosylmethionine and tetrahydrofolate (THF), and indicate the constituent pteridine, glutamate, and *p*-aminobenzoate moieties in THF.

12. Describe how a Schiff base link is formed. Distinguish between an aldimine and a ketimine.
13. Recognize the structures of pyridoxine (vitamin B_6), pyridoxal, pyridoxal phosphate (PLP), and pyridoxamine phosphate (PMP).
14. Describe the process of transamination, noting the role played by Schiff bases involving pyridoxal phosphate. Identify which enzymes are involved, and distinguish their role from that of glutamate dehydrogenase.
15. Explain how serine and threonine lose their amino groups.
16. Describe the reaction catalyzed by glutamate dehydrogenase, and explain its importance. Explain how this enzyme is regulated.
17. Explain the metabolic toxicity of ammonia and describe the possible causes of hyperammonemia, especially in relation to deficiencies in urea-cycle enzymes. Describe possible therapies for hyperammonemia.
18. Describe the urea cycle. Diagram the urea cycle, naming enzymes and intermediates, and noting intracellular locations. Explain the energy requirement for urea cycle functioning. Recognize and draw the structure of urea.
19. Explain regulation of the urea cycle. Describe the role of *N*-acetyl glutamate in short-term regulation, and relate it to the enzyme carbamoyl phosphate synthetase.
20. Describe connections between the TCA cycle and the urea cycle.
21. Explain what a folate antagonist is and how it works, and give examples of such drugs. Relate their mechanism of action to their application as antibiotic and anticancer agents.
22. Describe the most common biochemical defect leading to phenylketonuria. Explain the consequences of this defect, and discuss possible therapies.
23. List several important catecholamines, and explain how they are related biosynthetically to Tyr.
24. Describe the characteristic symptoms and biochemical basis for alcaptonuria and maple syrup urine disease.

Overview of Amino Acid Metabolism

Amino acids are closely connected metabolically, through their carbon skeletons, to the sugar metabolites we have seen in earlier chapters. Amino acid anabolism features many of the same simple metabolic intermediates that we have seen before, such as TCA-cycle intermediates. In amino acid catabolism, the reaction sequences converge on a few terminal pathways—notably, glycolysis and the TCA cycle for the carbon skeletons, and the urea cycle for disposal of the amino nitrogens. **Figure 14-1** is a flowchart summarizing these relationships. Six major biosynthetic families of amino acids exist, and there are 20 different multienzyme catabolic sequences for the naturally occurring 20 amino acids in vertebrates. Many reactions are shared with other biosynthetic paths; the intermediates in amino acid catabolism are often precursors for other biosynthesis products. The role of amino acids in nucleotide biosynthesis, for example, is covered in Chapter 15.

When used as fuel, amino acids must lose their amino groups. The carbon skeleton goes to a variety of small-molecule intermediates: acetyl-CoA, acetoacetyl-CoA, pyruvate, and TCA-cycle intermediates. These intermediates may also be used for biosynthesis. Thus it is possible,

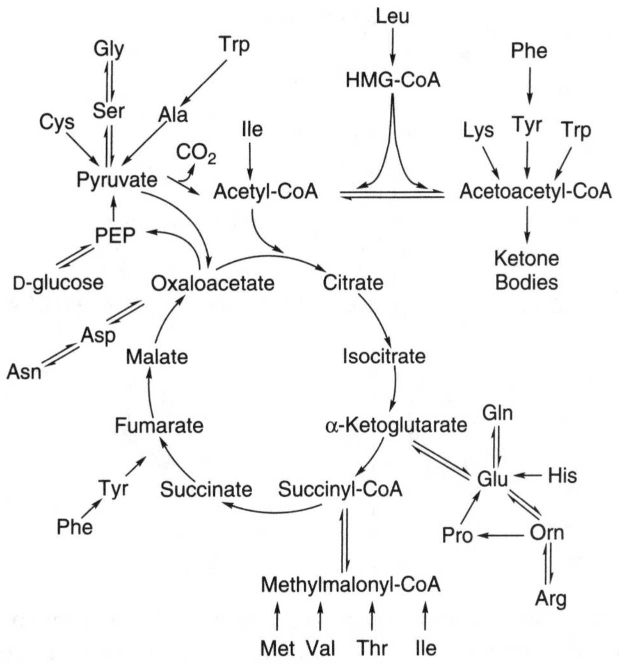

Figure 14-1 Connections of amino acid metabolism to carbohydrate and fatty acid metabolites.

in principle, to make sugars and fatty acids from amino acids. The main metabolic problem is how to deal with the nitrogen (as ammonia) that is generated when the carbon skeleton of the amino acid molecules is used this way. Ammonia is highly toxic to mammals, and a special pathway—the urea cycle—deals with this toxic waste product of metabolism. (Other organisms have other ways of disposing of the ammonia; for example, many marine organisms simply let the ammonia diffuse away into the surrounding water.)

Although defects in the metabolism of amino acids, considered individually, are relatively rare, defects in the excretion of nitrogen are much more common. Because the bulk of nitrogen generation occurs in the liver, pathologies of the liver can lead to upsets in nitrogen excretion, with toxic consequences.

Connections with Human Nutrition

A balanced diet should contain carbohydrates, lipids, and protein. The amino acids derived from protein can be used by the body as fuel (as well as for biosynthesis of proteins, nucleic acids, neurotransmitters, and more), by oxidizing the carbon skeleton. These processes funnel the carbons down to a set of metabolic intermediates we have seen before in the catabolism of carbohydrates and lipids. In this way, the digestion and utilization of some amino acids resembles that of carbohydrates, while for other amino acids there is a fundamental connection to lipid metabolism.

Humans are limited in their capacity to biosynthesize all of the necessary amino acids for proteins. Thus some species of amino acids need to come from diet and can be regarded as essential to maintaining good health.

Digestion of Protein and Amino Acids

Amino acids enter the stomach as proteins. Pepsin breaks them down to peptides. At this stage relatively few free amino acids are present. In the small intestine, pancreatic juice containing digestive enzymes (trypsin, chymotrypsin, carboxypeptidases A and B, and elastase) converts

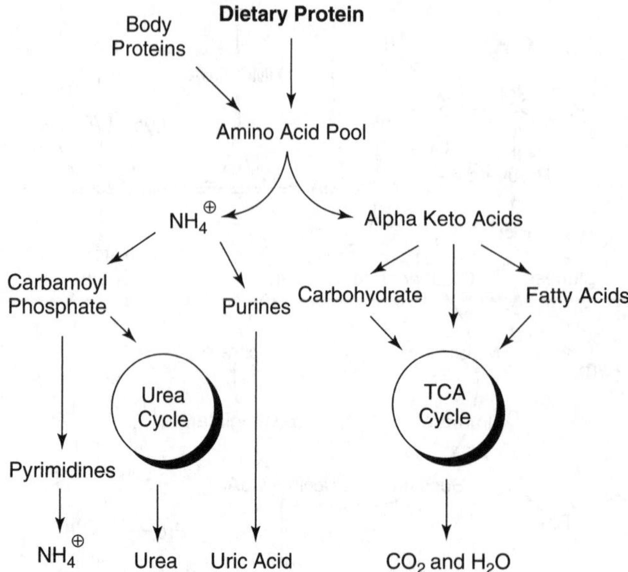

Figure 14-2 Overview of the catabolism of amino acids, from dietary protein to metabolic end products that are excreted. Carbon skeletons from the amino acids are oxidized to generate energy, but may also be used to make carbohydrates and fatty acids. Nitrogen atoms from the amino groups are extracted as ammonia; most nitrogen atoms are excreted as urea, but some may be used in the biosynthesis of nucleotides.

peptides to free amino acids and shorter peptides. Further degradation is also undertaken by enzymes in the intestinal mucosa. Free amino acids are absorbed in the small intestine, then transported to the liver, where $-NH_2$ groups are removed by transamination (discussed later in this chapter). The resulting α-keto acid is then used as fuel or as a biosynthetic intermediate.

Figure 14-2 sketches the pathway by which the absorbed amino acids are broken down to the excreted end products. The nitrogens from the amino acids appear either as ammonia or as uric acid. Note the contribution of the released ammonia to biosynthesis of nucleotides. Note also that the α-keto acid skeleton is broken down to contribute directly to the TCA cycle and energy production; alternatively, it may be processed for carbohydrate or fatty acid biosynthesis.

"Ketogenic" Versus "Glucogenic"

The details of the breakdown of the individual carbon skeletons of all 20 amino acids are beyond the scope of this text. However, amino acids can be classified by the final degradation product of the carbon skeleton and point of entry into the TCA cycle (**Table 14-1**). *Glucogenic amino acids* will form oxaloacetate, pyruvate, α-ketoglutarate, succinyl-CoA, and fumarate. *Ketogenic amino acids* will form, most notably, acetoacetyl-CoA. Depending on the particular amino acid, they may or may not form other carbon compounds that enter the TCA cycle; hence some amino acids are both ketogenic and glucogenic.

When catabolized, the ketogenic amino acids produce ketone bodies. The ketone bodies can be used to produce energy, much as fatty acids can be broken down by β-oxidation. Leu is solely ketogenic (Lys may also belong to this category, according to some authorities), whereas Ile, Phe, Tyr, and Trp are ketogenic but also glucogenic.

The catabolism of glucogenic amino acids produces either TCA-cycle intermediates or pyruvate. These carbon skeletons can then be used to produce energy. They can also be regarded

Solely Ketogenic	Ketogenic and Glucogenic	Solely Glucogenic
Leu	Ile	Ala
	Lys*	Arg
	Phe	Asp
	Trp	Asn
	Tyr	Cys
		Glu
		Gln
		Gly
		His
		Met
		Pro
		Ser
		Thr
		Val

Table 14-1 Catabolic Fates of the Common Amino Acids

*Some authorities classify lysine as solely ketogenic, in addition to leucine.

as precursors of glucose; that is, gluconeogenesis can use the pyruvate, and the TCA-cycle intermediates can all be (eventually) converted to pyruvate via oxaloacetate.

The side chains of amino acids may be cleaved off and metabolized by reactions different from those involving the α-carbon. Thus some carbon atoms may end up as TCA-cycle intermediates, while others go to acetoacetyl-CoA (and thence to ketone bodies).

Starvation and Fasting

Under conditions of fasting or starvation, no carbohydrate intake occurs, so the body is forced to use lipids and protein as fuels. A problem will arise with the body's oxaloacetate levels if no carbohydrate is coming in. An adequate pool of oxaloacetate is important for continued TCA cycle function, but the oxaloacetate pool may be depleted by other metabolic processes under starvation (recall the anaplerotic role of the TCA cycle). Amino acid catabolism can provide oxaloacetate and other TCA-cycle intermediates, using glucogenic amino acids. Thus ATP production can continue in the face of a mild ketosis. The source of the amino acids is skeletal muscle—hence the "wasting away" look of people who have fasted for extended periods.

Essential Amino Acids

Heterotrophs can grow by using a single carbon source to make all amino acids. Blocks in biosynthesis lead to a dietary requirement for one or more amino acids. Humans, unfortunately, are not heterotrophs for all of the amino acids. In humans, 10 of the 20 amino acids can be synthesized in adequate amounts, but the other 10 must be supplied (at least partially) in the diet; these are the *essential* amino acids. **Table 14-2** lists both types of amino acids.

Nonessential	Essential
Alanine	Arginine[*]
Asparagine	Histidine[*]
Aspartic acid	Isoleucine
Cysteine[†]	Leucine
Glutamic acid	Lysine
Glutamine	Methionine[‡]
Glycine	Phenylalanine
Proline	Threonine
Serine	Tryptophan
Tyrosine[†]	Valine

Table 14-2 Essential and Nonessential Amino Acids

[*]Required by growing children only; not essential for healthy adults.

[†]May be required for infants; Tyr is essential if Phe is absent from the diet.

[‡]Additional amounts required if the diet is deficient in Cys.

Tyrosine can be thought of essential when phenylalanine is absent from diet, given that Phe is the direct precursor of Tyr. Arginine is made by mammalian cells, but not in adequate amounts to satisfy demands during growth; histidine may also be required in growing children. In addition, infants may require dietary supplementation for tyrosine and cysteine. Extra methionine may be required as well if the diet is deficient in cysteine.

Here is a useful mnemonic for remembering the essential amino acids:

Any help in learning these little molecules proves truly valuable.

Amino Acid Biosynthesis

While some of the amino acids must be garnered from the diet (the essential amino acids), the body can biosynthesize the others, thanks to connections of the biosynthetic precursors to compounds derived from carbohydrate and lipid metabolism. The nitrogens needed to convert these precursors come themselves from essential amino acids, and their presence ultimately depends on biological nitrogen fixation by bacteria.

Looking beyond humans, it is possible to categorize the biosynthetic pathways for amino acids into six general families. One of these—the pathway for serine—is important in humans not only for its capacity to produce several amino acids besides serine, but also for its connection to the biosynthesis of other important biomolecules, such as phospholipids, purines, hemes, and more.

Source of Nitrogen Atoms

Nitrogen fixation is one of the key processes that make life as we know it possible. Nitrogen fixation, which entails the reduction of N_2 to NH_3, is carried out in the biosphere by bacteria. Bacteria use a special enzyme complex, under anaerobic conditions, to make ammonia. This process requires energy input in the form of ATP, as well as reducing power from either chemical or photochemical reactions.

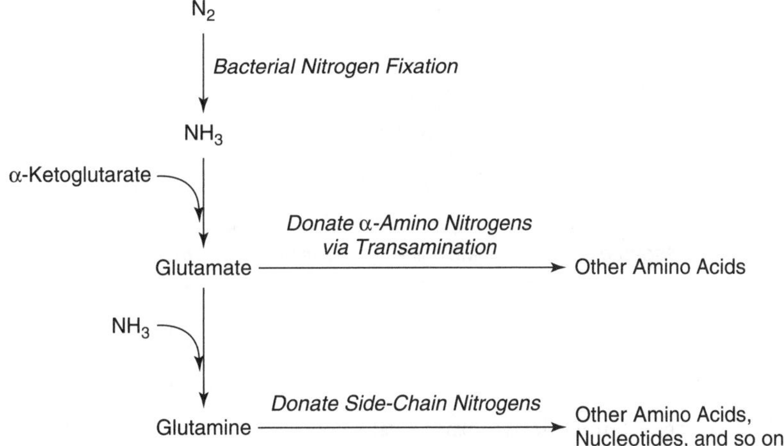

Figure 14-3 Nitrogen fixation as ammonia provides the nitrogen atoms for incorporation into amino acids, and from them, into all manner of biochemicals.

Two key amino acids for incorporation of the ammonia into biochemicals in general are Glu and Gln (**Figure 14-3**). Briefly, Glu is made from ammonia and α-ketoglutarate in a reduction reaction catalyzed by glutamate dehydrogenase, with the reducing power coming from NADPH. Gln is then made from Glu by amidation of the side-chain carboxylic acid using NH_3. Amino groups of most other amino acids derive from glutamate by transamination. Gln donates its side-chain nitrogen in many biosynthetic reactions—for example, in the synthesis of Trp and His, and in the biosynthesis of nucleotides.

Six Families for Biosynthesis

Amino acid biosynthesis can be divided into six families of pathways. Not all of these pathways are fully functional in humans; recall that 10 amino acids are regarded as "essential," meaning that they must be present in the diet in adequate amounts to maintain health. The following figures sketch these pathways, but omit many details.

Glutamate Family

α-Ketoglutarate leads to glutamate, and glutamate is a precursor to glutamine, proline, and arginine (**Figure 14-4**). Only arginine is not made by humans in adequate amounts for growth; in contrast, humans can independently synthesize adequate amounts of Glu, Gln, and Pro. The transamination of α-ketoglutarate to Glu will be covered in detail in a later section of this chapter. The biosyntheses of Pro and of Arg both follow directly from Glu, in multistep pathways.

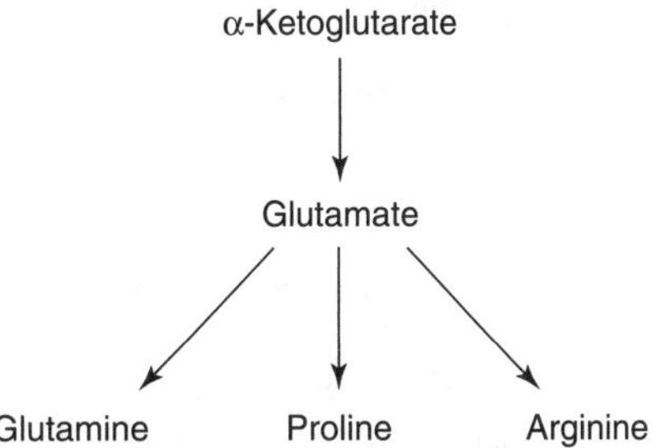

Figure 14-4 The glutamate family, consisting of Glu, Gln, Pro, and Arg, originates from α-ketoglutarate.

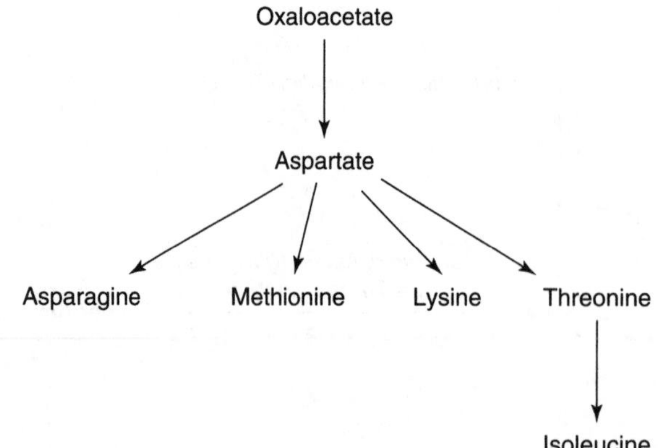

Figure 14-5 The aspartate family derives from oxaloacetate. Asp leads to Asn, Met, Lys, and Thr; Thr leads to Ile.

Aspartate Family

Oxaloacetate (from, for example, the TCA cycle) leads to aspartate, which is a precursor for asparagine, methionine, threonine, and lysine; isoleucine is then derived from threonine (**Figure 14-5**). Humans are not able to synthesize Met, Ile, Thr, or Lys, but they are able to amidate the side-chain carboxyl of Asp to give Asn.

Serine Family

3-Phosphoglycerate leads to serine, which is a precursor for cysteine and glycine (**Figure 14-6**). Humans are able to synthesize adequate amounts of all three amino acids independently. Ser is itself derived from 3-phosphoglycerate, an intermediate in glycolysis.

Alanine Family

Transamination of pyruvate (another link to glycolysis) leads to alanine; other reactions lead to valine and leucine (**Figure 14-7**). In humans, these latter paths are not functional, making consumption of Val and Leu essential as part of a proper diet.

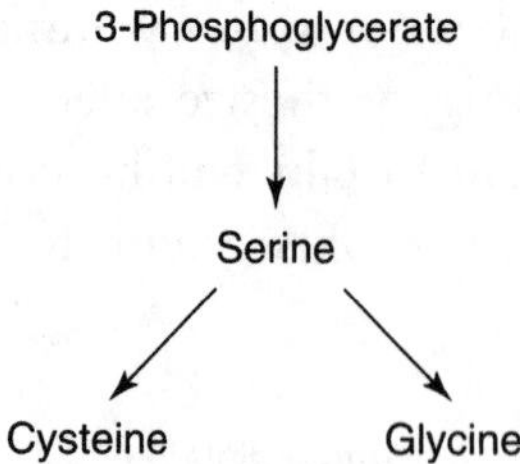

Figure 14-6 3-Phosphoglycerate is the precursor to serine, which in turn is the precursor to Gly and Cys.

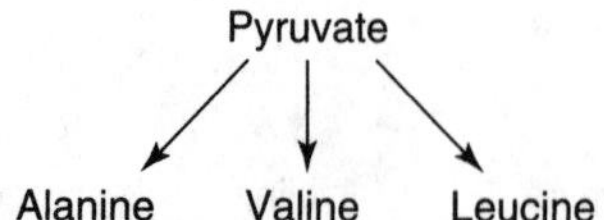

Figure 14-7 Pyruvate is the precursor to several amino acids with aliphatic side chains.

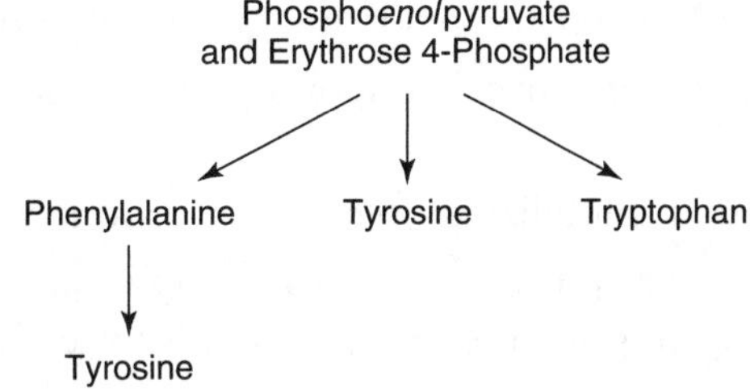

Figure 14-8 The aromatic amino acid family stems from phospho*enol*pyruvate and erythrose 4-phosphate. Note that there are two possible routes to Tyr: (1) directly from these two precursors or (2) indirectly through Phe. Humans have only the latter capability.

Aromatic Amino Acids

Phosphoenolpyruvate (PEP) and erythrose-4-phosphate are precursors to the aromatic amino acids phenylalanine, tyrosine, and tryptophan (**Figure 14-8**). Humans cannot synthesize Phe or Trp by themselves, but if adequate amounts of Phe are present in the diet, humans can convert this amino acid to Tyr. An important genetic disease, phenylketonuria (discussed later in this chapter), involves this latter conversion.

Histidine

Histidine is made from ATP and ribose-5-phosphate (**Figure 14-9**). While humans are quite capable of synthesizing ribose 5-phosphate (recall the pentose phosphate path), the further conversion to His is blocked in humans, making His one of the essential amino acids.

Details of Biosyntheses in the Serine Family

Instead of trying to cover in detail all the different pathways for amino acid synthesis, we will look at only one family of amino acids, related by their common pathways of anabolism: the serine family. The serine family includes Ser, Gly, and Cys, and the metabolism of Ser and Cys is closely connected to that of Met. Also, many biosynthetic paths use either Ser or Gly as a precursor. The biochemical importance of serine can be seen from its use in the following processes:

- The synthesis of phospholipids (attachment via its hydroxyl group, as an "alcohol," to the phosphate group)
- The synthesis of the amino acid cysteine; Ser is a precursor to Cys
- The donation of a methyl group for forming methionine (in organisms that can synthesize Met)

Additionally, the glycine member of the serine family is used in the biosynthesis of the following compounds:

- Purines (adenine, guanine), used in nucleic acids and in enzymatic cofactors (e.g., adenine in NADH)

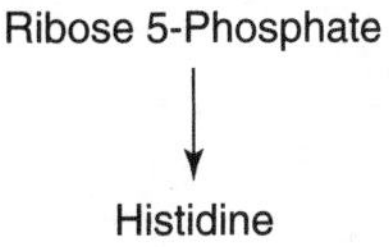

Figure 14-9 The histidine family has only one member, His.

- Porphyrin or porphyrin-like rings, such as heme groups, chlorophyll, or coenzyme B_{12}
- Creatine, whose phosphate derivative is important as an energy storage intermediate in muscle
- Bile acids, which are used in solubilizing lipids for digestion
- Glutathione, a compound that protects against metabolic stress by reducing peroxides or free radicals and by conjugating with toxic compounds for easier excretion

Lastly, cysteine, with its reactive thiol, is an important component of glutathione that offers protection against reactive peroxides and other oxidative species. It is also used in the biosynthesis of coenzyme A, and appears as a precursor to taurine (used to make a bile acid derivative, taurocholic acid).

Figure 14-10 presents the synthetic path to serine from 3-phosphoglycerate. Key points to note here include these relationships:

- The 2-hydroxyl on 3-phosphoglycerate is oxidized to a keto group, with hydride transfer to NAD^+.
- Glutamate donates an amino group to the 2-keto group by transamination.

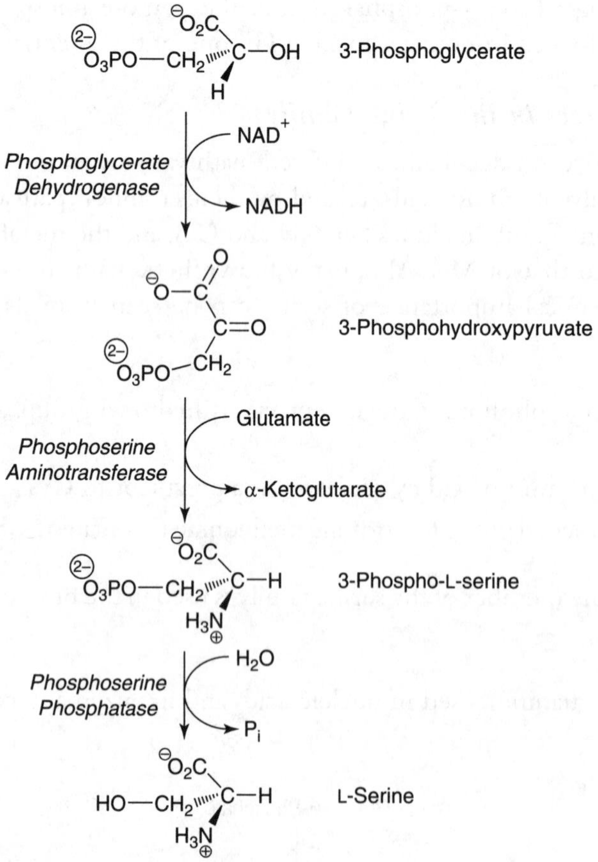

3-Phosphoglycerate

Phosphoglycerate Dehydrogenase (NAD^+ → NADH)

3-Phosphohydroxypyruvate

Phosphoserine Aminotransferase (Glutamate → α-Ketoglutarate)

3-Phospho-L-serine

Phosphoserine Phosphatase (H_2O → P_i)

L-Serine

Figure 14-10 Biosynthesis of serine.

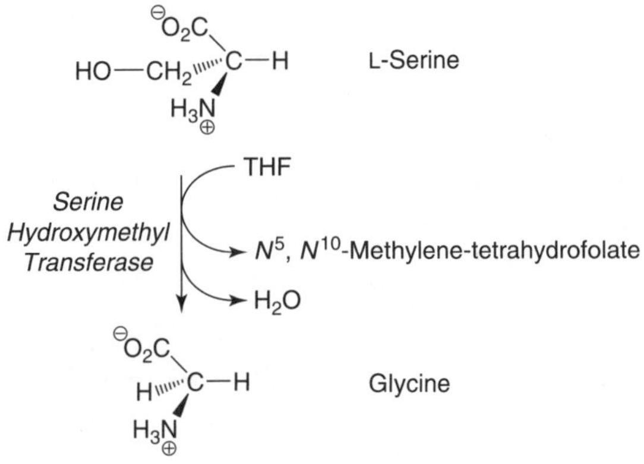

Figure 14-11 Glycine is derived from serine in a complicated reaction requiring the cofactor tetrahydrofolate (THF).

- There is a standard dephosphorylation to produce serine.
- The committed step involves the dehydrogenase. In bacteria, there is allosteric regulation by the end product serine, an example of feedback inhibition.

Serine contributes to a number of other important biomolecules.

Glycine Synthesis

Glycine synthesis is a complex single-step reaction, catalyzed by serine hydroxymethylase, with pyridoxal phosphate and tetrahydrofolate as cofactors (see **Figure 14-11**; more on these cofactors later in the chapter). Additionally, vertebrates can synthesize glycine directly from ammonia and carbon dioxide, with the help of these same cofactors, along with NADH as a source of reducing power.

Cysteine Synthesis

In bacteria and plants, the source of the sulfur in Cys is originally inorganic sulfate. A special pathway in bacteria and plants converts sulfate (SO_4^{2-}) to sulfide (S^{2-}), which will form the sulfur found in cysteine. The sulfide reacts with *O*-acetylserine (made by acetylation of serine with the acetyl group coming from acetyl-CoA), the acetyl group is displaced and leaves as acetate (a good leaving group), and the result is attachment of the sulfur on the amino acid's side chain, giving cysteine.

Animals do not have this capability. Instead, they obtain the sulfur for Cys indirectly from Met (recall that Met is an essential amino acid for humans, but Cys is not). Animals use Met to make *S*-adenosylmethionine, an important cofactor in methyl donation reactions (more on these reactions in the section on folate and *S*-adenosylmethionine). The methyl donation reactions convert the *S*-adenosylmethionine to *S*-adenosylhomocysteine, which is hydrolyzed to release homocysteine. Animals can then use Ser to scavenge the homocysteine, making Cys and α-ketobutyrate. In this way, the sulfur atom in Cys is derived from the homocysteine, which obtained it from the essential amino acid methionine. At the same time, the carbon skeleton in Cys is derived from Ser (**Figure 14-12**).

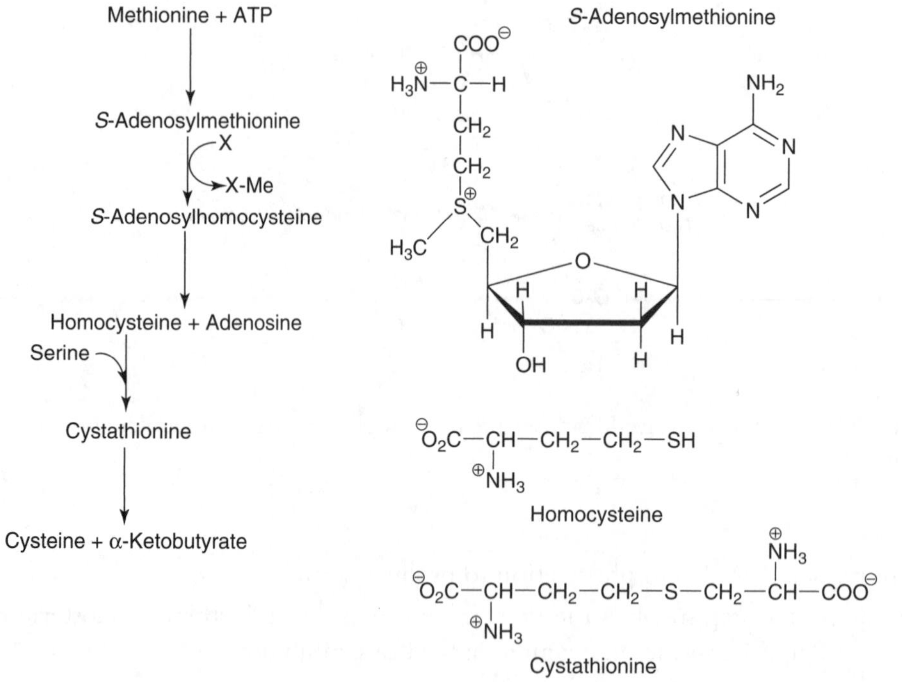

Methionine + ATP → S-Adenosylmethionine → (X → X-Me) S-Adenosylhomocysteine → Homocysteine + Adenosine → (Serine) Cystathionine → Cysteine + α-Ketobutyrate

S-Adenosylmethionine

$^{\ominus}O_2C-CH(NH_3^{\oplus})-CH_2-CH_2-SH$

Homocysteine

$^{\ominus}O_2C-CH(NH_3^{\oplus})-CH_2-CH_2-S-CH_2-CH(NH_3^{\oplus})-COO^{\ominus}$

Cystathionine

Figure 14-12 The route from Met to Cys leads through the formation of *S*-adenosylmethionine, to homocysteine and cystathionine. Here X represents a general methyl-acceptor compound.

Catabolism of Amino Acids: Transamination and Formation of α-Keto Acids

The catabolism of most amino acids starts with a common reaction, transamination, which removes the nitrogen from the amino acid and prepares the remaining carbon skeleton for oxidative processing. The mechanism of transamination uses a cofactor derived from vitamin B_6, and employs a reversible covalent linkage of substrate to cofactor called a Schiff base linkage.

α-Ketoglutarate Accepts Nitrogens and Glutamate Releases Ammonia

The initial step in the catabolism of amino acids is the removal of the amino group from the substrate amino acid. The amino group is transferred onto an acceptor compound, α-ketoglutarate, in a reaction called *transamination*. The substrate carbon chain becomes an α-keto acid, while the α-ketoglutarate that acquires the amino group becomes glutamate.

The glutamate is then recycled to α-ketoglutarate in a different reaction entirely, one that oxidatively deaminates the glutamate. In humans, this reaction takes place primarily in the liver. It recycles the glutamate back to α-ketoglutarate and permits continued turnover in the cycle. The general "funneling" of the amino nitrogens to glutamate allows a single enzyme system (e.g., glutamate dehydrogenase) to perform *oxidative deamination* in the liver, rather than the liver cells having to synthesize many different enzymes, each one geared toward oxidative deamination of a different amino acid. Also, this single oxidative deamination enzyme (glutamate dehydrogenase) can then be tightly regulated, for greater control and efficiency. **Figure 14-13** shows how this recycling of α-ketoglutarate and glutamate proceeds.

The enzymes called transaminases catalyze the transfer of $-NH_2$ groups from the substrate amino acids onto α-ketoglutarate, thereby forming glutamate and the corresponding α-keto acid. Many different transaminases are known (more than 50); they are generally of broad

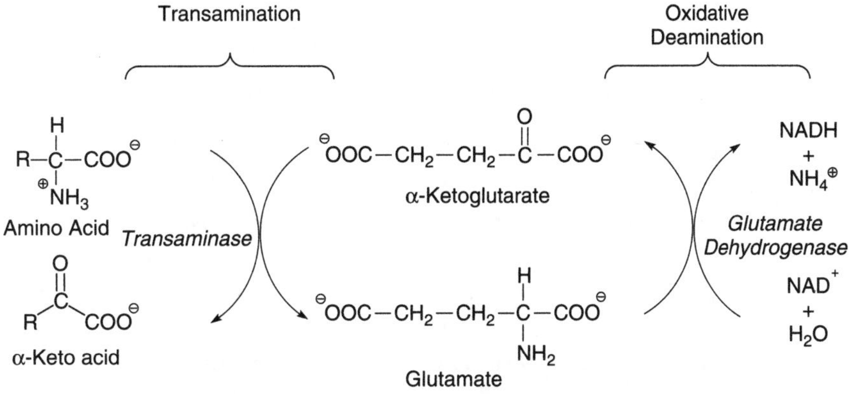

Figure 14-13 Overview of the reaction cycle by which nitrogen is extracted from amino acids and released as ammonia. For most amino acids, transamination converts them to the corresponding α-keto acid and passes the amino group to the acceptor α-ketoglutarate to make glutamate. Glutamate is then oxidatively deaminated by a different enzyme system, which leads to the release of ammonia and the regeneration of α-ketoglutarate.

specificity for amino acids, but specifically require α-ketoglutarate as the $—NH_2$ acceptor. In the transamination reaction, they release glutamate (the result of α-ketoglutarate accepting the $—NH_2$ groups) and the α-keto acid corresponding to the carbon skeleton of the original amino acid. The equilibrium constant for transamination is approximately 1, so this is generally a freely reversible reaction. All transaminases have the same cofactor requirement—namely, *pyridoxal phosphate (PLP)*.

Two amino acids can be directly deaminated, serine and threonine. They do not undergo this process of transamination, but instead undergo a dehydration to the corresponding α-keto acid. The enzymes here also use PLP but the mechanism is different; it is discussed later in this chapter.

Role of Vitamin B_6

Pyridoxine is the vitamin form of the cofactor vitamin B_6. The vitamin must be activated by enzymes in the body to generate the actual cofactor pyridoxal phosphate; pyridoxine oxidase generates the aldehyde pyridoxal, and a kinase attaches the 5′-phosphate group. **Figure 14-14** shows these various forms of this cofactor.

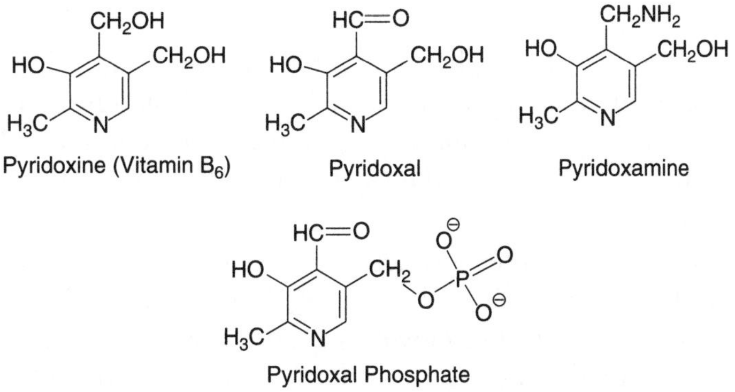

Figure 14-14 Vitamin B6 and related compounds. Pyridoxal phosphate is the cofactor used by transaminases.

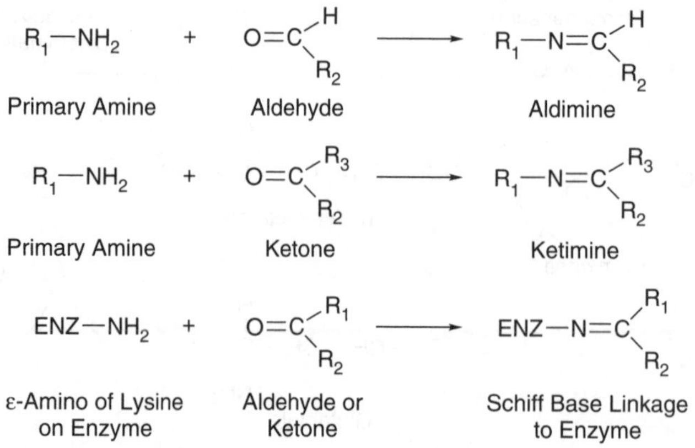

$$R_1{-}NH_2 + O{=}C(H)R_2 \longrightarrow R_1{-}N{=}C(H)R_2$$

Primary Amine, Aldehyde, Aldimine

$$R_1{-}NH_2 + O{=}C(R_3)R_2 \longrightarrow R_1{-}N{=}C(R_3)R_2$$

Primary Amine, Ketone, Ketimine

$$ENZ{-}NH_2 + O{=}C(R_1)R_2 \longrightarrow ENZ{-}N{=}C(R_1)R_2$$

ε-Amino of Lysine on Enzyme, Aldehyde or Ketone, Schiff Base Linkage to Enzyme

Figure 14-15 Formation of Schiff bases (aldehydes form aldimines, ketones form ketimines), and linking of the ϵ-amino group of an enzyme's lysine to the carbonyl of a ketone or aldehyde.

PLP is a cofactor for many enzymes, including the transaminases, for aldolase (in glycolysis), for several amino acid decarboxylases, and for various amino acid racemases (for interconversion of the D and L isomers). PLP is also a cofactor in the enzyme glycogen phosphorylase; here, however, it is probably the phosphate group (and not the aldehyde) that is catalytically important, in acid–base catalysis.

Schiff base linkages are a key part of the mechanism by which PLP operates in the transamination of amino acids, as well as in amino acid decarboxylases and racemases. A Schiff base linkage is a covalent linkage, involving imine formation between a free primary amino group and a carbonyl group. When the carbonyl group comes from an aldehyde or ketone, the compounds so formed are called *aldimines* or *ketimines*, respectively (**Figure 14-15**). In proteins, the ε-amino group on the side chain of a lysine residue is often used to form a Schiff base link to a suitable aldehyde or ketone.

Mechanism of Transamination

Schiff base linkages can be reversed much more easily than might be expected for a typical covalent bond. This flexibility is an important factor in the mechanism of action of the transaminases. The key points in the mechanism are summarized here:

- Transaminase binds pyridoxal phosphate in a Schiff base link to a Lys residue of the enzyme (the attachment is to the ε-amino group of the Lys). This binding forms an aldimine (an "internal aldimine," in which the linkage is internal to the enzyme). The PLP is held in place by several other interactions with groups surrounding the active site of the transaminase (**Figure 14-16**).
- As a new substrate molecule enters the active site, its amino group displaces the $\varepsilon{-}NH_2$ of the active site Lys. Then a new Schiff base link is formed to the α-amino group of the substrate, as the active site Lys moves aside; the result is an "external" aldimine, in which the linkage is to the substrate, not the enzyme (**Figure 14-17**). This reaction involves closure of the cleft of the active site and a major conformational change in

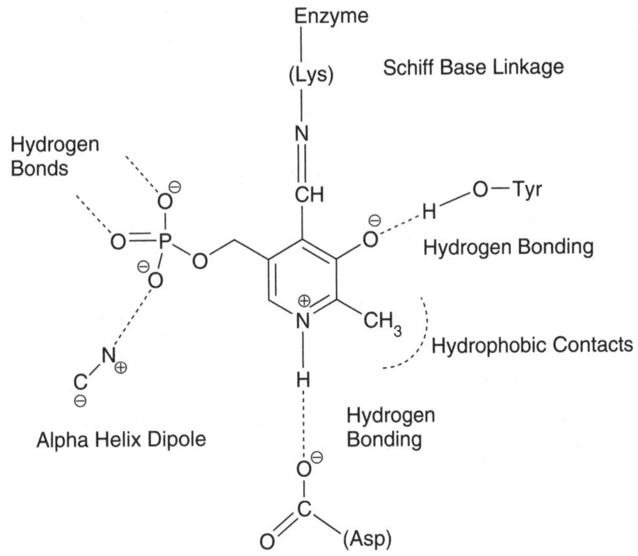

Enzyme
(Lys)
Schiff Base Linkage
Hydrogen Bonds
O–Tyr
Hydrogen Bonding
Hydrophobic Contacts
Alpha Helix Dipole
Hydrogen Bonding
(Asp)

Figure 14-16 Pyridoxal phosphate is held in the active site of a transaminase by multiple interactions, including a Schiff base link to a lysine residue, various hydrogen bonds and electrostatic interactions, and hydrophobic contacts.

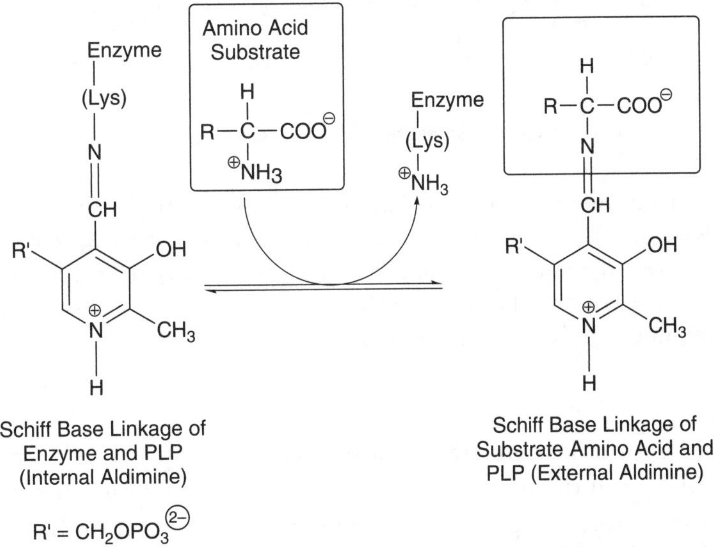

Figure 14-17 The initial step in the transamination reaction. An incoming amino acid displaces a lysine residue in the enzyme's active site (for emphasis, a box encloses the amino acid residues).

the enzyme. **Figure 14-18** shows how the cofactor eases the barrier to reaction of the bound amino acid.

- An electronic rearrangement in the external aldimine results in shifting the double bond to form a ketimine (**Figure 14-19**).
- This reaction is followed by hydrolysis to generate pyridoxamine monophosphate (PMP) and an α-keto acid (continuing in Figure 14-19). This α-keto acid is released into solution. The nitrogen from the amino acid has gone to the pyridoxal moiety to form PMP. The PMP is held by the enzyme and is not released.

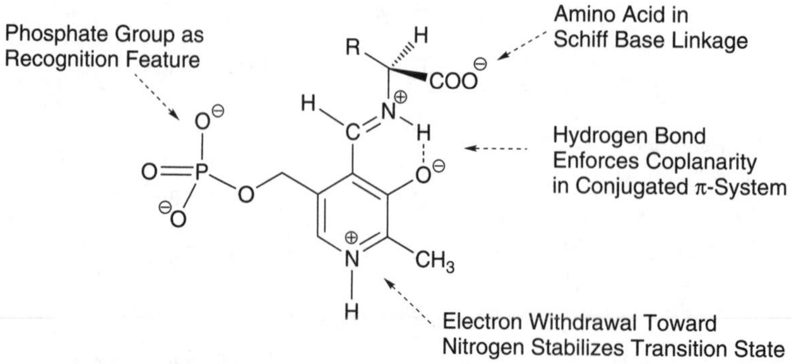

Figure 14-18 Pyridoxal phosphate helps to catalyze the transamination reaction. Note the role of the positive charge on the ring nitrogen in withdrawing electron density, as well as the planarity of the bonding arrangement, which helps to stabilize the transition state.

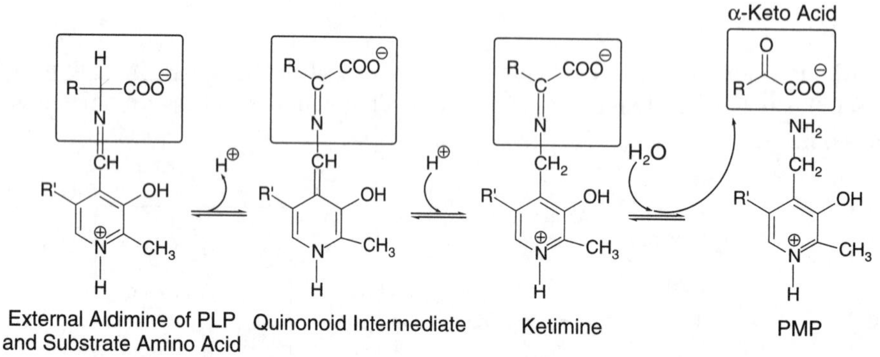

Figure 14-19 Later steps in transamination. The amino group is transferred onto the cofactor (forming PMP) with release of a keto acid. To regenerate the original cofactor–enzyme state, the reaction steps would now be reversed, with an incoming keto acid (specifically, α-ketoglutarate) forming first a ketimine, then an external aldimine. The enzyme then releases an amino acid (specifically, glutamate) to carry away the amino nitrogen from the first amino acid.

- PMP combines with α-ketoglutarate in a reversal of the steps just described. The amino group from PMP (from the first amino acid) now moves over onto the carbon skeleton of the α-ketoglutarate, forming glutamate. The net result is transfer of this amino group from an amino acid onto a pyridoxal cofactor, and then onto α-ketoglutarate. The glutamate so formed is released, while regenerating the PLP–enzyme complex.

All of these reactions are reversible. After releasing the α-keto acid, with the nitrogen captured on PMP, the enzyme regenerates itself by binding α-ketoglutarate and reversing the steps. The nitrogen ends up transferred onto the carbon skeleton of the α-ketoglutarate, creating a molecule of glutamate that is then released. This is an example of a ping-pong enzymatic mechanism: The enzyme cycles back and forth, transferring nitrogens from amino acids onto α-ketoglutarate and forming glutamate. **Figure 14-20** schematically shows this ping-pong mechanism, and emphasizes the recycling of the PLP group of the enzyme.

Notice how the cell makes use of a common amino acid, glutamate, and a common TCA-cycle intermediate, α-ketoglutarate; this is a good example of biochemical economy. Glutamate appears over and over again in biochemistry. Apart from its role as a building block in proteins

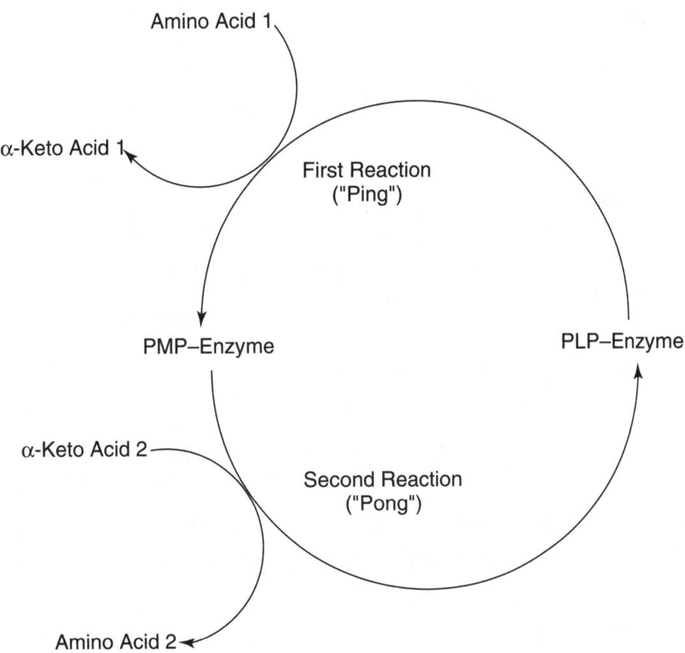

Figure 14-20 The transaminase mechanism is a good example of a double-displacement, or "ping-pong," mechanism. First one substrate forms a complex and reacts with the enzyme, and a first product is released while the enzyme is chemically altered in some fashion; then a second substrate enters the active site and reacts, generating a second product and regenerating the original state of the enzyme.

and peptide hormones, it acts as an important nitrogen carrier, as described here. It is also a neurotransmitter, of course, and one of the three amino acids in the important cellular redox component, glutathione. Another role it plays is as a "tail" on the pteridine group in folate. Moreover, glutamate serves as an osmoprotectant and protein stabilizer in bacteria subjected to stress from high salt concentrations. It is also used in the food industry as a flavor-enhancing agent.

Direct Deamination of Serine and Threonine

Both serine and threonine carry a hydroxyl group on their side chain, on the β-carbon. They can undergo a pyridoxal phosphate–catalyzed β-elimination, losing the amino group. The net reactions are as follows:

$$\text{Serine} \rightarrow \text{Pyruvate} + \text{Ammonia} \qquad (14\text{-}1)$$

$$\text{Threonine} \rightarrow \alpha\text{-Ketoglutarate} + \text{Ammonia} \qquad (14\text{-}2)$$

Threonine has two other pathways for breakdown. First, it may be converted to glycine and acetaldehyde, and the acetaldehyde may then be converted to acetyl-CoA. Second, it can be oxidized at the β-carbon, then decarboxylated, to yield aminoacetone. Aminoacetone can be oxidatively deaminated, giving methylglyoxal, and eventually lactate.

Figure 14-21 illustrates two of the routes for preparing these amino acids for entry into the TCA cycle.

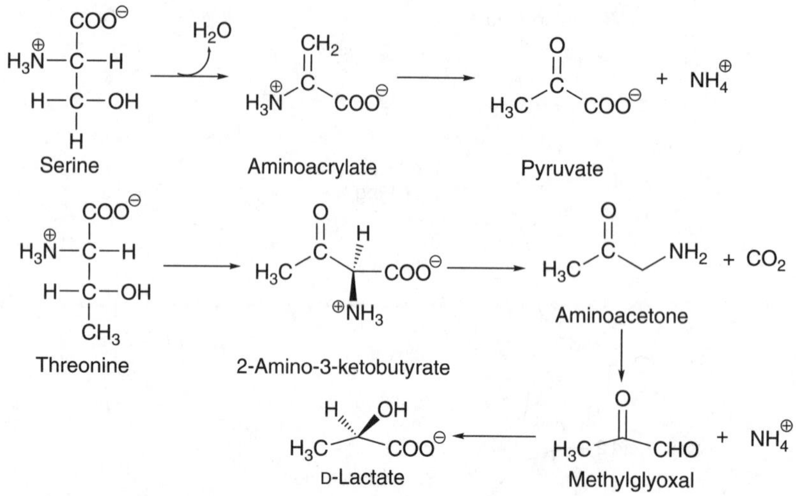

Serine → Aminoacrylate → Pyruvate + NH_4^+

Threonine → 2-Amino-3-ketobutyrate → Aminoacetone + CO_2

Aminoacetone → Methylglyoxal + NH_4^+ → D-Lactate

Figure 14-21 Both serine and threonine can be deaminated, releasing ammonia, without undergoing transamination. The eventual carbon skeleton products (pyruvate, lactate) can then be used for energy generation.

Oxidative Deamination and Ammonia Toxicity

The nitrogens collected through transamination reactions pass through a common metabolic intermediate, the amino acid glutamate and its corresponding keto acid, α-ketoglutarate. The glutamate is recycled to α-ketoglutarate, accompanied by loss of the nitrogens in the form of ammonia. Ammonia is toxic, and its disposal presents a major metabolic problem to the body.

Glutamate Dehydrogenase and Oxidative Deamination

In the liver, amino groups from various amino acids are collected in glutamate. Then the glutamate is deaminated (not transaminated), specifically by glutamate dehydrogenase. The overall reaction is

$$\text{Glu} + \text{NAD(P)}^+ + H_2O \rightarrow \alpha\text{-Ketoglutarate} + NH_4^+ + \text{NAD(P)H} \qquad (14\text{-}3)$$

Note the release of the amino group as NH_4^+. The enzyme glutamate dehydrogenase prefers NAD^+ but will accept $NADP^+$ as a cofactor. This acceptance is unusual, given that most enzymes are quite specific for one or the other of the nicotinamide coenzymes. Notice again that this is not a transamination reaction, so there is no PLP here—instead, we have NAD^+ or $NADP^+$.

In animals, the reaction summarized in Equation 14-3 takes place primarily in the liver, in the mitochondrial matrix. The glutamate dehydrogenase is a hexamer of identical subunits. It acts in the direction of deamination of glutamate. (In bacteria, the corresponding enzyme is specific for NADPH and catalyzes the formation of glutamate—just the reverse of the animal enzyme.)

Regulation

The glutamate dehydrogenase enzyme is under tight regulation. It has several allosteric effectors that make it sensitive to the energy charge of the cell as well as the demand for reducing power: The compounds NADH, ATP, and GTP inhibit the enzyme, whereas ADP and GDP

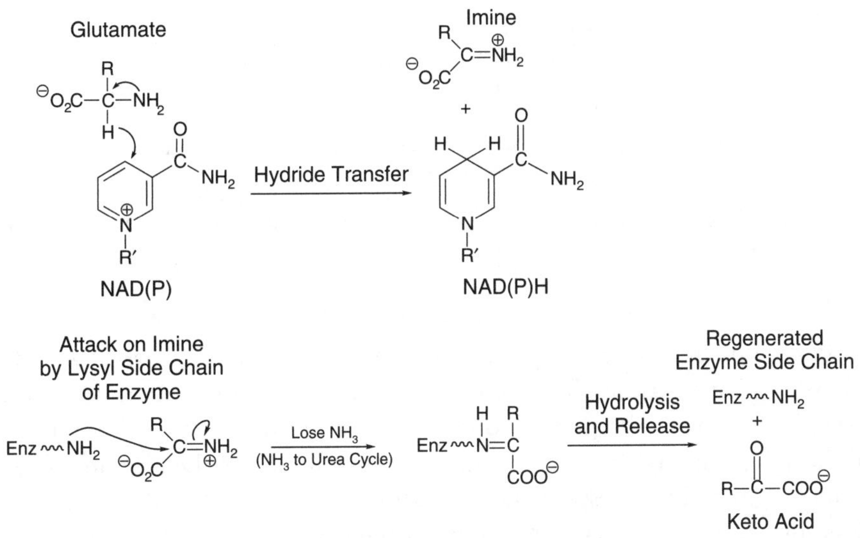

Figure 14-22 Oxidative deamination of glutamate by glutamate dehydrogenase involves hydride transfer to a nicotinamide cofactor, then release of ammonia, and finally generation of the keto acid α-ketoglutarate.

stimulate its activity. When the energy charge is high, the enzyme is inhibited, the glutamate concentration increases, and amino acids generally will not be deaminated for use as fuel. Instead, the amino acids can be diverted into biosynthetic pathways—for example, for protein synthesis. When the energy charge is low and there is a demand for energy in the cell, the enzyme is stimulated. This activity tends to reduce the glutamate concentration and raise the concentration of α-ketoglutarate. The α-ketoglutarate (and some of the α-keto acids generated by the action of transaminases) can then enter the TCA cycle, providing for energy production. Overall, this pattern of regulation of the enzyme enables the cell to use amino acids as fuel when energy is needed, but to avoid generation of toxic ammonia (which is metabolically expensive to excrete) when there is no need to break down amino acids for energy.

Mechanism

In the first step of the reaction, glutamate loses a hydride to NAD^+, generating the imine shown in **Figure 14-22**, along with the reduced nicotinamide. In the second step, the terminal amino group of a lysine side chain on the enzyme attacks the electron-deficient carbon of the imine, thereby displacing the imino group as ammonia (which goes to the urea cycle; see the next section). The lysine forms a Schiff base link here to the carbon chain of the former glutamate. Finally, hydrolysis of the Schiff base occurs; the carbon chain is released as the α-keto acid, α-ketoglutarate; and the free lysyl residue of the enzyme is regenerated, so that the enzyme is ready for another catalytic cycle.

Ammonia Toxicity

As mentioned earlier, ammonia is extremely toxic to cells. This toxicity is related to the reductive amination of α-ketoglutarate, which is the reverse of oxidative deamination of glutamate (**Figure 14-23**). A high serum level of NH_4^+ (*hyperammonemia*) drives the reaction toward glutamate and depletes α-ketoglutarate. The lack of α-ketoglutarate then interferes with turnover of the TCA cycle. Eventually the production of NADH and ATP declines. Brain cells are particularly vulnerable to ammonia's toxic effects; high NH_4^+ levels can cause cerebral

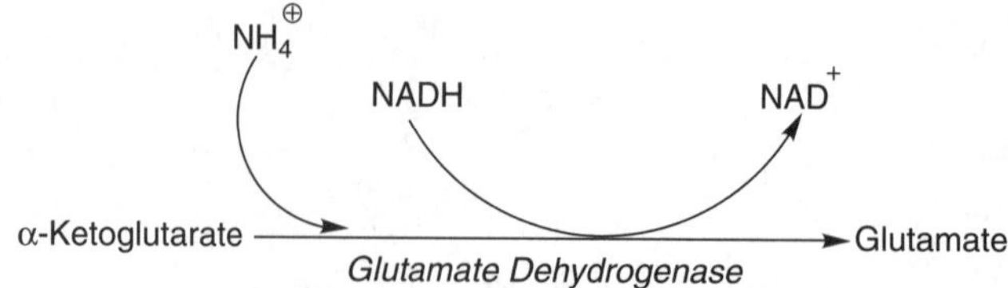

Figure 14-23 High levels of ammonia can reverse the normal conversion of glutamate to α-ketoglutarate, with toxic consequences.

edema with concomitant blurred vision, tremors, weakness, seizures, coma, and death. Other effects of high levels of ammonia include elevated glutamine concentrations in the blood (as the body tries to eliminate nitrogens through this compound), and swelling and edema due to the osmotic effect of high solute (ammonia) concentrations. Depletion of glutamate by its conversion to glutamine is especially important in nerve cells, where glutamate and its derivative γ-aminobutyric acid (GABA) are neurotransmitters.

Hyperammonemia can be caused by liver damage (e.g., due to viral or drug-induced hepatitis) or by genetic defects in the enzymes responsible for nitrogen excretion. Treatment for severe hyperammonemia may involve hemodialysis, which seeks to eliminate the ammonia directly from the bloodstream. The patient may also be given sodium benzoate or phenylacetate—both are compounds that accept nitrogens and then are excreted. This treatment takes advantage of so-called latent pathways of nitrogen excretion, where amino acids (bearing nitrogens, of course) are conjugated to the exogenous benzoate or phenylacetate; this arrangement improves the solubility of the aromatic compound and eases its excretion via the kidney. Over the long term, the patient should reduce protein intake in the diet and spread protein consumption out over time. In some cases the diet may also need to be supplemented with extra arginine and citrulline; see the material on the urea cycle later in this chapter to understand the basis for this approach.

Biochemistry and Physiology of Ammonia Transport in the Body

In peripheral tissues, ammonia can be generated by the breakdown of nucleotides or polyamines, or from amino acids that are being used as fuel locally. Of course, the body faces the problem of how to transport the toxic ammonia molecules from these peripheral tissues to central organs where the nitrogen can be safely converted to urea for excretion. In the peripheral tissues, the free ammonia is used with glutamate to make glutamine in an ATP-consuming reaction catalyzed by glutamine synthetase. The nontoxic glutamine is then released into the bloodstream and carried to the liver, kidneys, or intestines, where the enzyme glutaminase removes the amide nitrogen and releases it as ammonia. The ammonia so generated in the kidneys or intestines is quickly transported through the bloodstream to the liver, where it will enter the urea cycle.

Another solution to the ammonia elimination problem is to join together the metabolism of glucose with that of alanine. Glucose is metabolized in muscle to pyruvate. This α-keto acid corresponds to alanine; thus, if amino acid carbon chains are to be burned as fuel by muscle, they can donate their amino groups (via glutamate) to the pyruvate, generating alanine. Alanine, which is not toxic, can be transported through the blood to the liver, where it undergoes transamination and gives up the nitrogen atoms collected from the peripheral tissues. The transamination yields pyruvate, which can be used by the liver in gluconeogenesis to make more glucose. The liver disposes of the nitrogen through the urea cycle.

The enzyme catalyzing the transamination reaction (in muscle and in liver) is alanine transaminase or alanine aminotransferase, abbreviated as ALT in clinical chemistry. Automated clinical methods have been developed to test for ALT. Because this enzyme normally is contained inside cells and does not appear in the bloodstream, its presence in serum indicates that damage has occurred to muscle, liver, or other tissues.

An especially important example here is the use of branched-chain amino acids (valine, isoleucine, leucine) for fuel by skeletal muscle, brain, kidney, and adipose tissue. Interestingly, these three amino acids are not metabolized primarily by the liver but instead are metabolized extensively in these peripheral tissues. (As an aside, these three amino acids are popular with serious athletes as dietary supplements and are thought to enhance both endurance and strength.) The amino acids are first transaminated to yield the corresponding α-keto acid, and the carbon chains are then oxidatively decarboxylated to give the corresponding acyl-CoA derivative. This latter reaction is catalyzed by the enzyme branched-chain α-keto acid dehydrogenase, an enzyme very similar to pyruvate dehydrogenase and α-ketoglutarate dehydrogenase.

Urea Cycle

Mammals "solve" the problem of ammonia toxicity by converting it to urea, a soluble nitrogenous compound that is much less toxic than ammonia. However, the conversion has an energetic cost. The urea cycle uses energy (ATP, in forming *carbamoyl phosphate*) to remove the toxic ammonia in the form of urea.

Figure 14-24 presents the *urea cycle*. Unlike the TCA cycle, this set of reactions spans the inner mitochondrial membrane, with key reactions taking place both in the mitochondrial

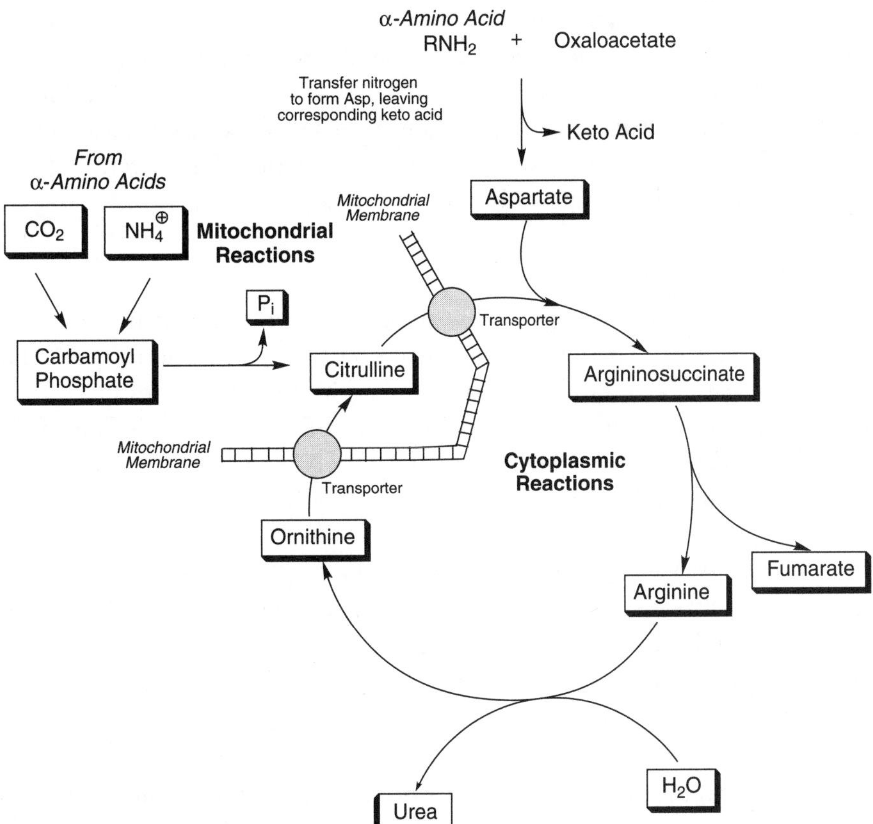

Figure 14-24 Schematic view of the urea cycle.

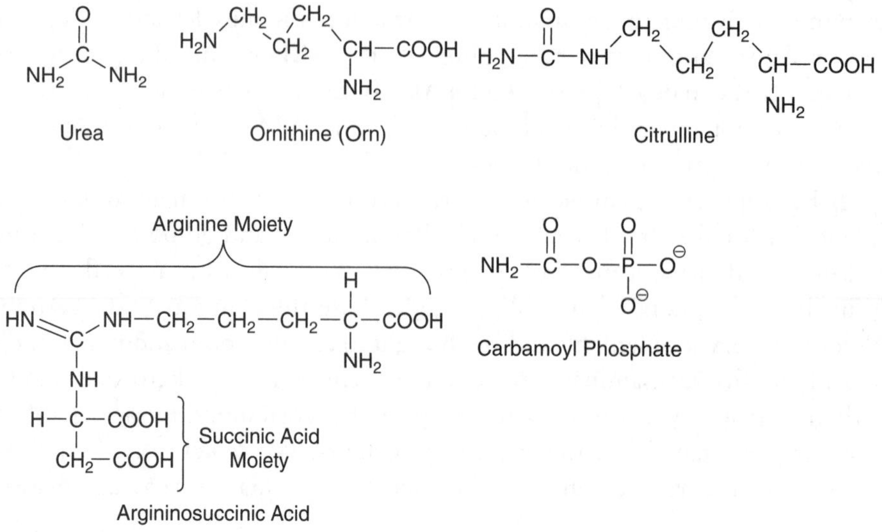

Urea
Ornithine (Orn)
Citrulline
Arginine Moiety
Carbamoyl Phosphate
Succinic Acid Moiety
Argininosuccinic Acid

Figure 14-25 Compounds involved in the urea cycle.

matrix and in the cytosol. Inside the matrix, the toxic ammonia (generated from the action of glutamate dehydrogenase on glutamate) is combined with CO_2 to form carbamoyl phosphate. This compound reacts with ornithine, an unusual amino acid not commonly found in proteins, to form citrulline, another unusual amino acid (see Chapter 3). Citrulline is transported across the inner membrane by a specific transmembrane carrier; in the cytosol, it reacts with available aspartate to form argininosuccinate. This compound is then split to release fumarate (note that this reaction occurs on the cytosolic side of the membrane) and arginine. The side chain of arginine is then hydrolyzed to release urea and to regenerate a molecule of ornithine, which can then be transported into the matrix to complete the cycle. The urea that is released in the cytosol is quite soluble, and is carried via the bloodstream to the kidneys for excretion. **Figure 14-25** shows the structures of the key compounds in this pathway.

Linkage of Urea Cycle to TCA Cycle

The TCA cycle and (a part of) the urea cycle share the same subcellular compartment—the matrix of the mitochondrion. These pathways are also linked by common intermediates or by-products. Finally, one pathway produces energy while the other consumes it.

Breakdown of argininosuccinate forms arginine and fumarate. If the fumarate enters the matrix, then in the TCA cycle the cell can convert it (via malate) into oxaloacetate. Now oxaloacetate has four possible fates:

- React with acetyl-CoA to give citrate (the next step in the TCA cycle)
- Undergo decarboxylation to give pyruvate (which can enter the TCA cycle after being processed to an acetyl group by pyruvate dehydrogenase)
- Enter gluconeogenesis to give glucose (which is an anaplerotic use of the TCA cycle)
- Be transaminated to give aspartate, which can be fed back to the urea cycle

The α-ketoglutarate (produced by oxidative deamination of glutamate) also connects the excretion of nitrogen to the TCA cycle. Thus the urea cycle is closely linked at multiple points to the TCA cycle.

Carbamoyl Phosphate

Formation of carbamoyl phosphate and citrulline occurs inside the inner mitochondrial membrane, while the other reactions of the urea cycle occur in the cytosol. This is another example of compartmentalization.

Carbamoyl phosphate is synthesized from ammonia and bicarbonate by the enzyme *carbamoyl phosphate synthetase* (CPS):

$$NH_4^+ + HCO_3^- + 2\ ATP \rightarrow \text{Carbamoyl phosphate} + 2\ ADP + P_i \qquad (14\text{-}4)$$

In this energy-consuming reaction, two moles of ATP are used per mole of carbamoyl phosphate made. The bicarbonate comes from carbon dioxide in a reaction catalyzed by an isozyme of carbonic anhydrase. There are actually two different isozymes of CPS, one in the mitochondrion and one in the cytosol; the cytosolic form is important in pyrimidine biosynthesis (see Chapter 15).

Importance of Transmembrane Carriers

Specific transmembrane carriers exist for ornithine (inward), citrulline (outward), ammonia (inward), and bicarbonate (inward). Because of the direction in which they work, defects in the transmembrane carriers for ornithine or citrulline could lead to hyperammonemia. Notice that nitrogen atoms from inside the mitochondria (the ammonium ions from oxidative deamination of glutamate) are combined with nitrogen atoms from amino acids in the cytosol. The latter are not derived from oxidative deamination, but instead are produced by transamination reactions with oxaloacetate, forming aspartate that enters the urea cycle.

Regulation of Urea Synthesis

Two general mechanisms provide for regulation of urea synthesis: induction of enzymes and allosteric activation of carbamoyl phosphate synthetase.

Enzyme Induction

Upon delivery of amino acids or ammonia to the liver, the synthesis of urea cycle enzymes is increased. This process leads to higher concentrations of the enzymes and hence greater throughput (urea synthesis). It is a relatively slow way to increase urea cycle throughput.

Allosteric Activation

N-*Acetylglutamate* acts as an allosteric activator of carbamoyl phosphate synthetase (**Figure 14-26**). This enzyme activation increases urea cycle throughput much more quickly than would induction of enzyme synthesis. *N*-Acetylglutamate is formed from the precursors acetyl-CoA and glutamate, by the enzyme *N*-acetylglutamate synthase (Figure 14-26). In turn, this enzyme is activated by arginine. Arginine is, of course, needed as an intermediate in the urea cycle, so its presence signals the availability of intermediates for urea synthesis; acetyl-CoA and glutamate serve as indicators of adequate supplies of cellular energy for the energy-demanding urea cycle.

Other Biochemical Uses of Ammonia

Ammonia is used biosynthetically, mainly in the form of the amino acids glutamine and glutamate. This is a sort of indirect use—for example, through glutamate in a transamination reaction—as the source of the α-amino groups in most of the common amino acids. Glutamine also serves as a nitrogen donor in many biosynthetic reactions; see, for example, the material in Chapter 15 on purine biosynthesis.

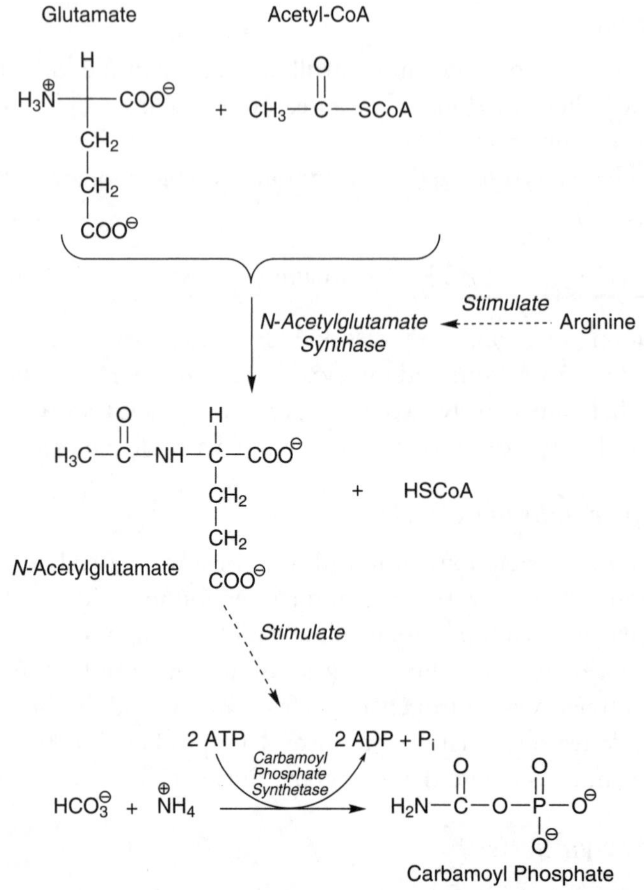

Figure 14-26 *N*-Acetylglutamate allosterically activates carbamoyl phosphate synthetase, allowing rapid response to an increase in ammonia levels. This allosteric activator is derived from glutamate and acetyl-CoA through the action of the enzyme *N*-acetylglutamate synthase. This latter enzyme is allosterically activated by arginine.

Clinical Applications

In this section we discuss several important diseases of amino acid metabolism, illustrating the consequences of interfering with regular amino acid metabolism, with utilization or regeneration of necessary cofactors, and with the delicate process of nitrogen excretion through the functioning of the urea cycle.

Phenylalanine Metabolism: Phenylketonuria and Catecholamines

Phenylketonuria

Figure 14-27 shows how Tyr is synthesized from Phe by the enzyme phenylalanine hydroxylase (also called phenylalanine 4-mono-oxygenase). An important catalytic metal ion, a Fe(II) ion, is found in the active site. The iron ion binds molecular oxygen, which is then converted to the hydroxy cation OH^+, a very powerful electrophile. In turn, it attacks the 4 position of the aromatic ring of a neighboring bound Phe molecule. The eventual product of the reaction is generation of an OH group at the 4 position on the ring—that is, the Phe has been converted to Tyr. The other oxygen atom of the O_2 is reduced to H_2O.

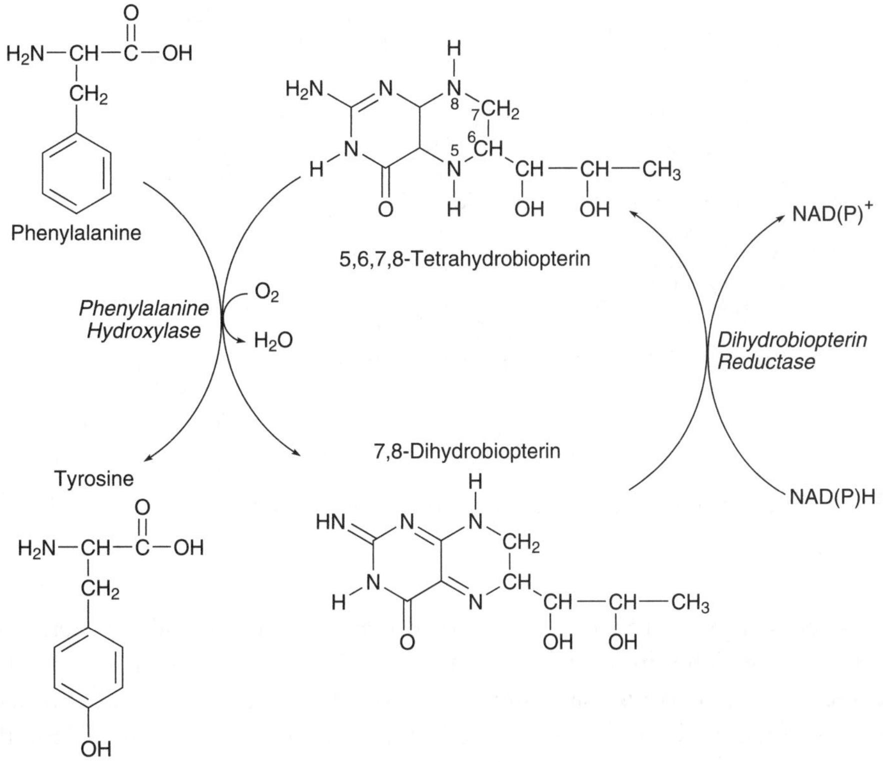

Figure 14-27 Conversion of Phe to Tyr is performed by a mono-oxygenase enzyme, phenylalanine hydroxylase, whose catalytic capacity depends on a reduced cofactor, tetrahydrobiopterin. Oxidized cofactor must be restored by a separate enzyme system, dihydrobiopterin reductase, using reduced nicotinamides as the source of reducing equivalents.

The proximal source of the electrons for this reduction is a molecule of tetrahydrobiopterin (a cofactor related to folate, as discussed later in this chapter); the tetrahydrobiopterin is oxidized to dihydrobiopterin in the process and must be regenerated. Regeneration is done by the enzyme dihydrobiopterin reductase, using NADH or NADPH as the source of electrons. Figure 14-27 summarizes this reaction cycle.

Phenylketonuria (PKU) is a classic example of an inborn error in metabolism—in this case, the metabolism of phenylalanine. Approximately 1 in 20,000 newborns have a defect in Phe metabolism. This disease is most commonly due to an autosomal recessive mutation in the gene for the enzyme that hydroxylates phenylalanine to form tyrosine (other, rarer forms are also known). PKU can lead to severe mental retardation and a short life span.

In classic phenylketonuria, the disease is caused by the absence or a deficiency of the enzyme phenylalanine hydroxylase. The absence of this activity blocks the (normal) conversion of Phe to Tyr, thereby resulting in the accumulation of Phe in all body fluids. Many side reactions then occur that normally would be at a very low level. For example, an appreciable transamination of Phe to form phenylpyruvate, a ketone, occurs—hence the name of the disease.

Figure 14-28 depicts the breakdown of phenylpyruvate to form phenylacetate and phenyllactate. The phenylacetate has a characteristic odor, and its aroma in the urine of newborns was an old-time diagnostic test for the disease.

The exact reasons why mental retardation occurs in patients with PKU are not well understood; perhaps the excess Phe competes with other amino acids for transport across the blood–brain barrier, or the phenylpyruvate acts to inhibit pyruvate transport into mitochondria.

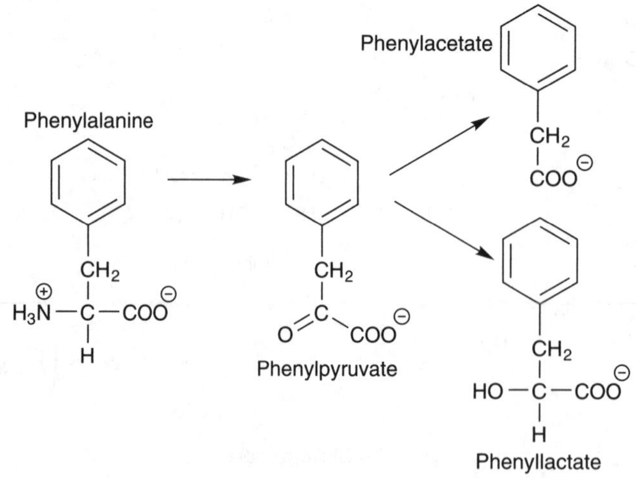

Phenylalanine → Phenylpyruvate → Phenylacetate; Phenyllactate

Figure 14-28 High levels of Phe, as in phenylketonuria, lead to unusual metabolic side reactions and their products.

Treatment for classic PKU involves a special (and fairly difficult to follow) diet, one that has very low Phe levels, which is instituted right after birth. Just enough Phe is provided for growth and replacement. Because Tyr is not being made from Phe, the patient will also need special dietary supplementation for tyrosine; in effect, tyrosine becomes "essential" for the PKU-affected patient.

Diagnosis of the disease is made through measurement of the blood levels of Phe in a newborn. Also, prenatal diagnosis is now possible, using genetic probes.

Catecholamines

Catecholamines are amines linked to catechol, *o*-dihydroxybenzene. Three principal catecholamines are derived from the metabolism of tyrosine: norepinephrine (noradrenaline), epinephrine (adrenaline), and dopamine. They function as neurotransmitters and as hormones, particularly in preparing the organism for stress. In this respect we have already seen how epinephrine affects metabolism, stimulating the breakdown of lipids and glycogen.

The catecholamines are derived from tyrosine (**Figure 14-29**). *S*-Adenosylmethionine (discussed in the next section) is the source of the methyl group added to norepinephrine in synthesizing epinephrine.

Adrenergic drugs act on the sympathetic nervous system through various mechanisms including direct binding to membrane-bound receptors (as we have seen in connection with lipid and carbohydrate metabolism). They are among the most commonly prescribed drugs, with different drugs being used to control blood pressure, glaucoma, asthma, and other disorders. An understanding of the pharmacology of these drugs requires an understanding of their storage, release, reuptake, and metabolism, and is beyond the scope of this text.

Folate and S-Adenosylmethionine

Folate

Dietary supplement studies performed in the 1930s found that certain types of megaloblastic anemia (characterized by large immature erythrocytes) could be cured by extracts from yeast or

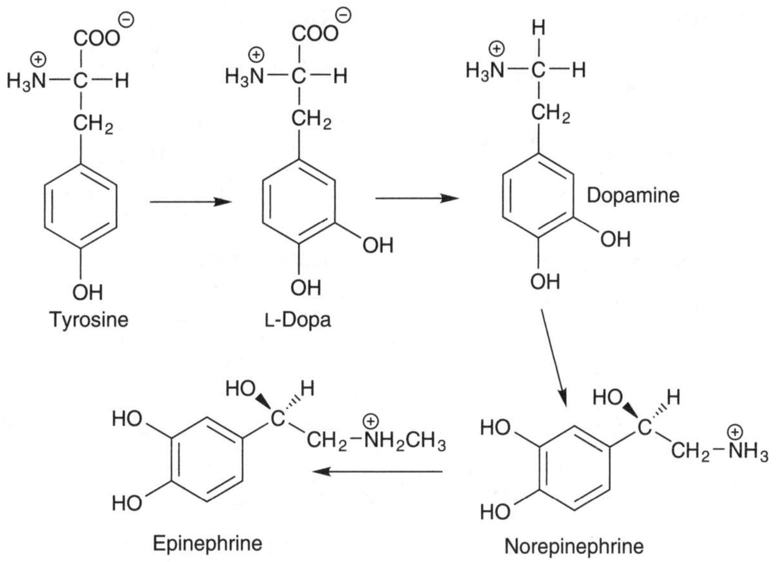

Figure 14-29 Conversion of Tyr to three important catecholamines—dopamine, norepinephrine, and epinephrine.

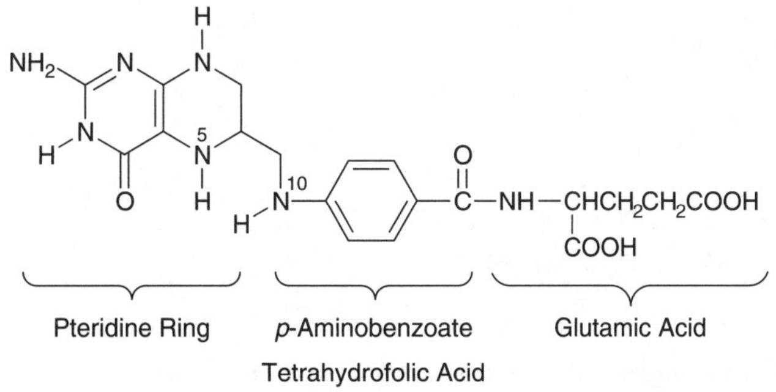

Figure 14-30 Structure of tetrahydrofolic acid (THF), showing its three building blocks of a pterin ring, *p*-aminobenzoic acid, and glutamic acid.

from liver cells. Later, the key component was identified as folic acid, or *folate*. This compound, or rather its reduced form *tetrahydrofolate*, is a cofactor in both anabolic and catabolic reactions, where it serves as a carrier of one-carbon units. Common abbreviations for tetrahydrofolate are *THF* and FH_4.

Tetrahydrofolate contains three distinct parts (**Figure 14-30**): a substituted pteridine ring; *p*-aminobenzoate (PABA); and glutamate. PABA is often found in sunscreen preparations; an inexpensive compound, it has a high extinction coefficient for UV rays. Pteridine rings appear in many biological pigments (e.g., in insect wings and eyes, and in the skin of certain amphibians).

When folate serves as a one-carbon carrier, this one-carbon group may be in various oxidation states, such as a simple methyl group, a formyl group, or a methenyl group. The group is bonded to the folate carrier at N-5 or N-10, or to both nitrogens simultaneously

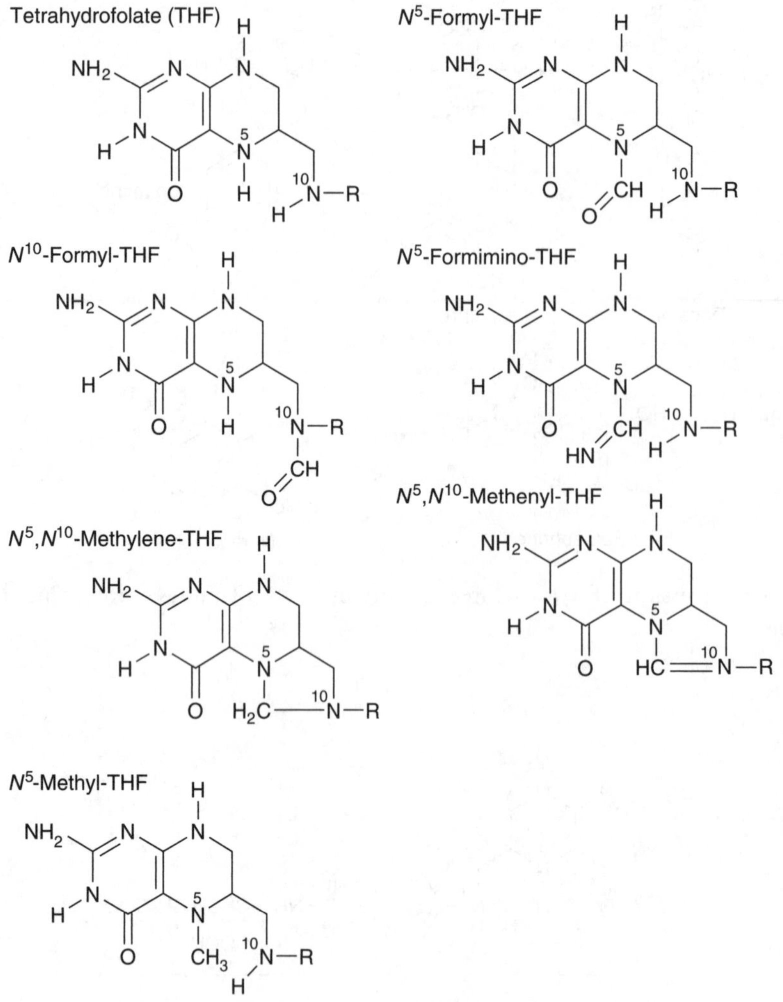

Tetrahydrofolate (THF)

N^5-Formyl-THF

N^{10}-Formyl-THF

N^5-Formimino-THF

N^5,N^{10}-Methenyl-THF

N^5,N^{10}-Methylene-THF

N^5-Methyl-THF

Figure 14-31 Common single-carbon–carrying variants of folate.

(depending on the oxidation state of the group). **Figure 14-31** illustrates most of the common possibilities.

THF accepts one-carbon groups in various catabolic reactions, as in the breakdown of Ser or His. Also, THF donates one-carbon groups in anabolic reactions; examples can be seen in nucleotide synthesis and in the formation of methionine from homocysteine (in a reaction assisted by coenzyme B_{12}).

As shown in **Figure 14-32**, THF is generated from folate in a two-stage reaction catalyzed by the enzyme dihydrofolate reductase (DHFR). Note the use of NADPH as the source of reducing power here. DHFR is a major target for antibacterial drug therapy. The mammalian and bacterial forms of this enzyme differ in sequence and shape, which allows them to be distinguished by antifolate drugs.

5-Methyl THF plays a key role in the biosynthesis of methionine, while simultaneously reducing levels of a toxic metabolite, homocysteine (**Figure 14-33**). In humans, higher than normal serum levels of homocysteine have been linked to an increased risk of developing cardiovascular disease.

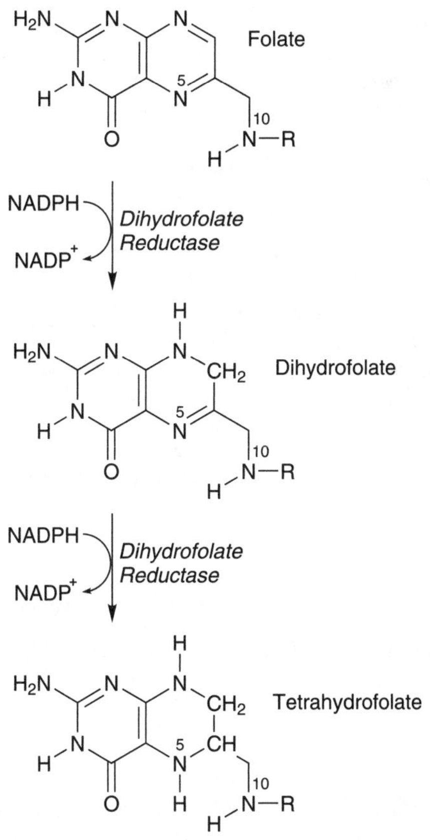

Figure 14-32 Two stages in the action of dihydrofolate reductase in reducing folate to tetrahydrofolate.

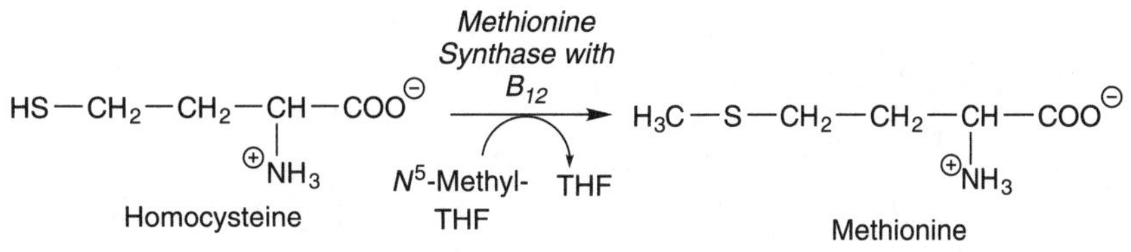

Figure 14-33 Use of N^5-methyl-tetrahydrofolate in converting homocysteine to Met.

Figure 14-34 summarizes the overall linkage of folate metabolism and cysteine regeneration. The methyl group is transferred from 5-Me THF to the homocysteine chain, in a reaction that depends on coenzyme B_{12}. This appears to be the only reaction by which 5-Me THF may lose its methyl group and be converted back to THF. If there is a deficiency in coenzyme B_{12}, then the 5-Me THF will tend to accumulate (the "methyl trap hypothesis"), at the expense of the pool of regular THF. Because THF is needed for other important folate-requiring reactions, this buildup can lead to pathology, particularly anemia. Treatment would involve supplementation with vitamin B_{12} or folate, or both.

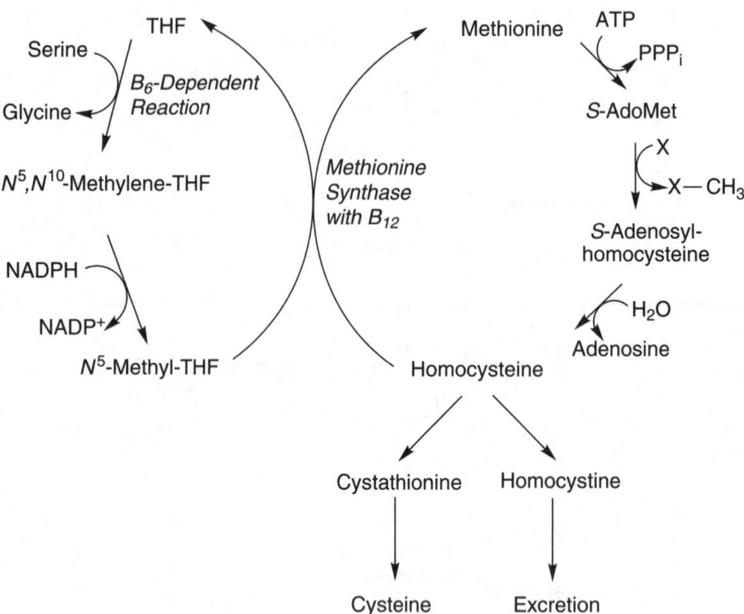

Figure 14-34 Interlocking pathways of folate and AdoMet metabolism. "X" represents one of any number of acceptors of methyl groups.

Folate Antagonists

Blockage of the regeneration ofTHF is one way to block the biosynthesis of nucleotides, a major biochemical activity in rapidly dividing cells. Agents (drugs) that do so are *folate antagonists*, which are important in anticancer therapy and in treating some microbial infections. Two important folate antagonists are trimethoprim and methotrexate (**Figure 14-35**). In Figure 14-35, note their similarities in chemical structure to folate; this is how they bind to the enzyme dihydrofolate

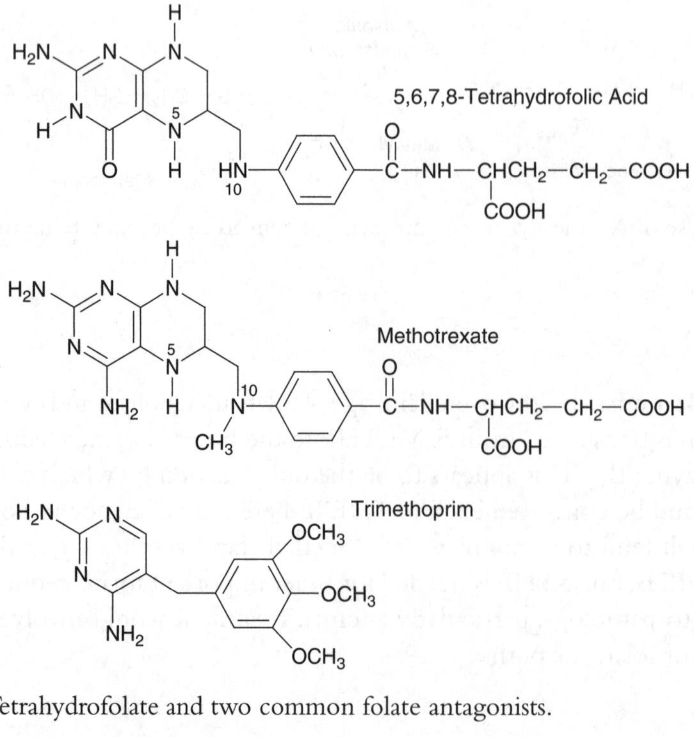

5,6,7,8-Tetrahydrofolic Acid

Methotrexate

Trimethoprim

Figure 14-35 Tetrahydrofolate and two common folate antagonists.

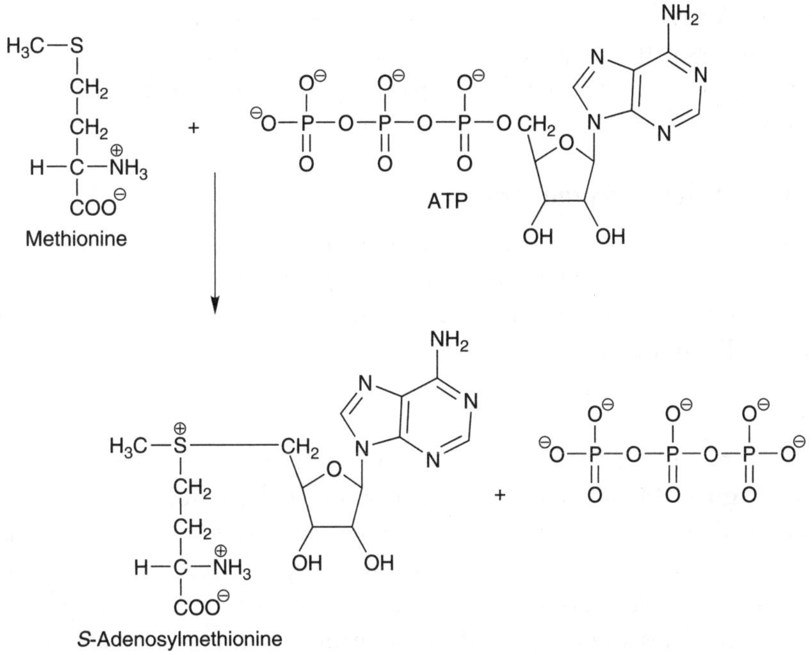

Figure 14-36 Biosynthesis of S-adenosylmethionine from Met and ATP.

reductase (which regenerates THF from folate). Trimethoprim has a higher affinity for the microbial enzyme versus the human enzyme, so it can be used at low concentrations to selectively inhibit the microbial enzyme without interfering with normal enzyme function in human cells.

S-Adenosylmethionine

Figure 14-36 shows the biosynthesis of *S-adenosylmethionine* (*S*-AdoMet or SAMe) from methionine and ATP. *S*-AdoMet is actually the major donor in vivo of methyl groups, participating in many more reactions than the path involving homocysteine and THF. The sulfur atom can donate electron density and accept a positive charge; this activates the attached methyl group, and makes it more reactive than methylated forms of THF.

Some important *S*-AdoMet–dependent reactions include synthesis of epinephrine from norepinephrine, synthesis of phosphatidylcholine from phosphatidylethanolamine, synthesis of creatine from guanidinoacetic acid, and methylation of bases in DNA or tRNA. Additionally, *S*-AdoMet can be decarboxylated and then serve as a donor of propylamine groups. This activity is important in the biosynthesis of polyamines such as spermidine and spermine (**Figure 14-37**),

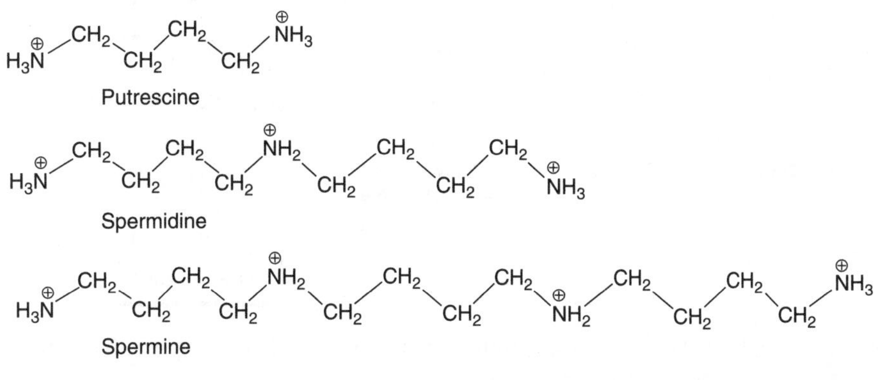

Figure 14-37 Common polyamines derived from *S*-adenosylmethionine.

which bind to DNA and help to pack it in more compact structures in the cell. Also, in plants, *S*-AdoMet is a precursor to the plant hormone ethylene. Release of this gaseous compound triggers ripening in fruit. Consequently, the pathway (and its regulation) from *S*-AdoMet to ethylene is of obvious importance to the agricultural industry.

Diseases of Amino Acid Metabolism

Many different disorders of amino acid metabolism have been identified. While PKU is the most common, two other disorders that have an appreciable frequency of occurrence are alcaptonuria (involving the metabolism of Tyr) and maple syrup urine disease (involving the breakdown of Val, Ile, and Leu).

Alcaptonuria

The breakdown and excretion of phenylalanine and tyrosine leads to an intermediate, homogentisate (**Figure 14-38**). Homogentisate is normally oxidized to maleylacetoacetate, which can be further broken down to fumarate and acetoacetate. In *Alcaptonuria*, the activity of homogentisate oxidase, the enzyme catalyzing the oxidation of homogentisate to maleylacetoacetate, is deficient. As a consequence of this enzyme deficiency, the intermediate homogentisate accumulates and is excreted in the urine. The homogentisate polymerizes upon standing to form a dark-colored substance, which can produce a startlingly ink-colored urine. The condition is relatively harmless.

Maple Syrup Urine Disease

The breakdown of Val, Ile, and Leu first involves transamination to the corresponding α-keto acids. The keto acids would then normally be oxidatively decarboxylated for further metabolism. In *maple syrup urine disease* (MSUD; also called branched-chain ketoaciduria), however, there is typically a deficiency in a specific dehydrogenase (branched-chain α-keto acid dehydrogenase, or BCDH) that blocks further metabolism of the α-keto acids (**Figure 14-39**). This defect leads to accumulation of the α-keto acids, which causes the characteristic odor associated with the disease. However, because the enzyme has several subunits (it is similar to the enzyme α-ketoglutarate dehydrogenase in the TCA cycle, and to the pyruvate dehydrogenase complex), several variants of the disease are possible, depending on which subunit is affected and the particular change in that subunit.

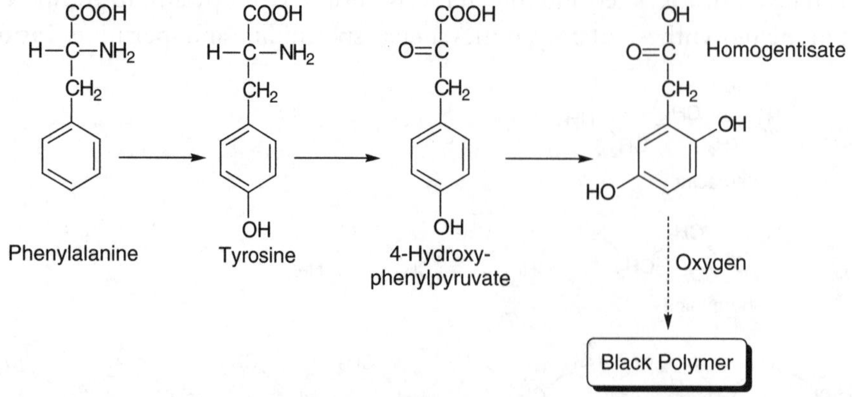

Figure 14-38 Alcaptonuria results in accumulation of homogentisate, which polymerizes in the presence of oxygen to form a black polymer.

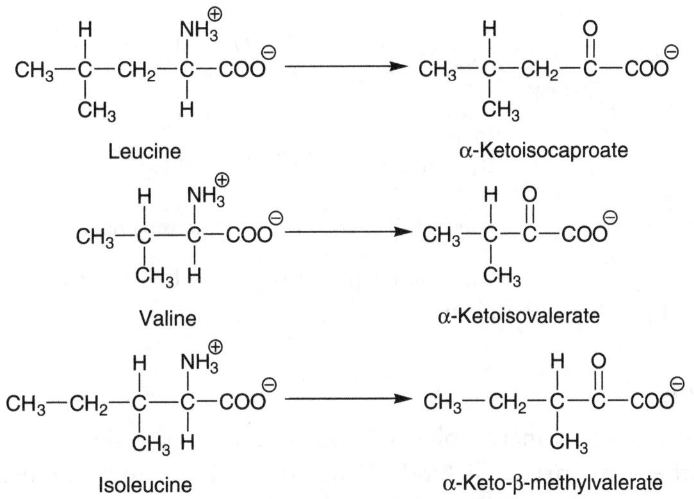

$$CH_3-CH(CH_3)-CH_2-C(H)(NH_3^{\oplus})-COO^{\ominus} \longrightarrow CH_3-CH(CH_3)-CH_2-C(=O)-COO^{\ominus}$$

Leucine → α-Ketoisocaproate

$$CH_3-CH(CH_3)-C(H)(NH_3^{\oplus})-COO^{\ominus} \longrightarrow CH_3-CH(CH_3)-C(=O)-COO^{\ominus}$$

Valine → α-Ketoisovalerate

$$CH_3-CH_2-CH(CH_3)-C(H)(NH_3^{\oplus})-COO^{\ominus} \longrightarrow CH_3-CH_2-CH(CH_3)-C(=O)-COO^{\ominus}$$

Isoleucine → α-Keto-β-methylvalerate

Figure 14-39 In maple syrup urine disease, breakdown of the branched-chain amino acids (Val, Leu, Ile) stops after transamination and formation of the corresponding α-keto acids. Breakdown of the α-keto acids is blocked by lack of activity of the dehydrogenase responsible for their further catabolism.

Early symptoms of MSUD include lethargy and loss of appetite. The newborn may also go into ketosis, which is followed by vomiting and seizures. Mental retardation is a common outcome if the newborn is not promptly treated; severe cases can result in coma and even death. Diagnosis requires a simple blood test for the serum levels of the three key amino acids and their corresponding α-keto acids.

Treatment consists of a diet that has much lower than normal levels of the three amino acids involved. Because Ile, Val, and Leu are all essential amino acids, this diet must be very carefully regulated to supply just the amount needed for growth and development, but not so much that the body starts to build up the toxic keto acid metabolites. Some variants of MSUD respond well to dietary supplementation with thiamine. These variants may be characterized by some defect in binding this cofactor to the BCDH enzyme, and higher levels of thiamine may help drive the binding equilibrium toward uptake of the cofactor; alternatively, thiamine binding may restore proper folding and functioning of a subunit in the enzyme.

Drug-Induced Vitamin Deficiencies

Pyridoxal phosphate is synthesized by the body from pyridoxine, vitamin B_6. Nutritional requirements for B_6 are rather low, and dietary deficiencies are rarely seen in humans. However, certain drugs may cause a deficiency, usually by reacting with the aldehyde group on the pyridoxal. Such a reaction reduces the amount of available PLP; in turn, a deficiency can arise, even though the diet is apparently adequate.

One pertinent example of such a drug-induced deficiency is that caused by the reaction with isoniazid. Isoniazid is used to treat tuberculosis, but it reacts with pyridoxal, forming a hydrazone (**Figure 14-40**). This hydrazone cannot then be phosphorylated by pyridoxal kinase, so PLP is not made. Treatment for tuberculosis typically continues for several months, if not longer, so there is a real possibility of a patient experiencing a deficiency in PLP as a result of the therapy for tuberculosis.

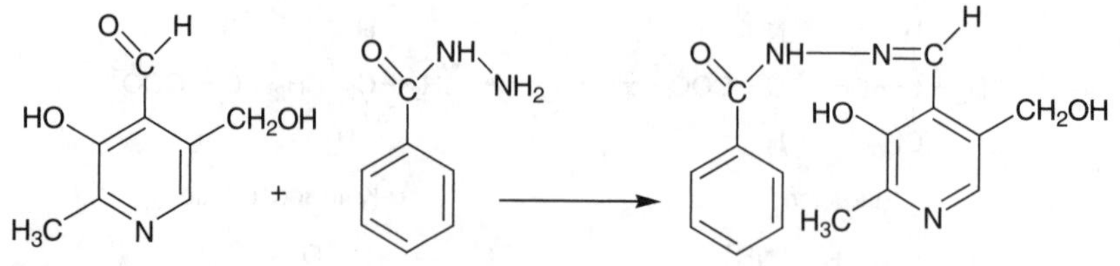

Figure 14-40 A drug-induced vitamin deficiency may arise when isoniazid reacts with pyridoxal, blocking formation of pyridoxal phosphate.

Hyperammonemia

An excess level of ammonia in the blood is characteristic of a defect in the urea cycle, at one point or another. Two principal kinds of hereditary hyperammonemia exist: a defect in carbamoyl phosphate synthetase (CPS) and a defect in ornithine transcarbamoylase (OTCase). The latter is the most frequent defect. Other defects in the cycle are possible, but are rare. Both CPS and OTCase are mitochondrial enzymes. CPS has a cytosolic counterpart that is important for pyrimidine biosynthesis, and that can take up some ammonia if the mitochondrial enzyme is defective.

If the defect is in mitochondrial CPS, then carbamoyl phosphate inside the mitochondria will not be made in adequate amounts to sustain the urea cycle. As a consequence, ammonia builds up and leaks out to the cytosol. Some of it may be accommodated there by the cytosolic CPS, which makes carbamoyl phosphate. This, is turn, can be used with aspartate to make orotate and uracil, which may then be excreted. In the cytosol, glutamate can also accept ammonia, forming glutamine in an ATP-dependent reaction; the glutamine can then be excreted.

If the defect is in OTCase, then carbamoyl phosphate is still made. As it builds up inside the matrix, some will leak out into the cytosol. Once in the cytosol, this product can be used to make orotate and uracil.

Basic therapy for these hereditary forms of hyperammonemia involves hemodialysis and transfusions as soon as the disease is diagnosed to avoid brain damage in the patient. A strict diet must also be followed—one that is limited in protein—to avoid generating ammonia.

In adults, another major cause of hyperammonemia is liver cirrhosis (from alcoholism, among other causes). Here there is a progressive loss of hepatocytes, and hence a loss of the ability to perform the urea cycle reactions and excrete ammonia nitrogen as urea.

QUESTIONS FOR DISCUSSION

1. Why would additional methionine be required in the diet, if the diet is deficient in cysteine?
2. Suppose that you are kidnapped by space aliens and put on a very restricted diet, such that you are fed only the amino acids isoleucine, lysine, leucine, phenylalanine, tryptophan, and tyrosine, plus all necessary vitamins. Within a couple of days you notice that your exhaled breath has a "chemical smell" like that in your organic chemistry lab.
   a. Explain the origin of the bad breath and relate it to the peculiar diet.
   b. Now the space aliens put you on a regular balanced diet ("lab chow for humans"), that is complete for carbohydrate, protein, lipids, minerals, and most vitamins, but lacks

vitamin B_{12}. They keep you on this diet for four months. Predict the consequences for your serum levels of methionine, homocysteine, and simple tetrahydrofolate, compared to your serum levels before this kidnapping. Which other biochemical perturbations might you experience from this diet?

3. Aspartame, the artificial sweetener, is a dipeptide that contains phenylalanine (as the methyl ester) and aspartate. Why would foods sweetened with aspartame pose a risk to individuals with phenylketonuria?
4. How might a defect in the enzyme dihydrobiopterin reductase lead to the symptoms of phenylketonuria?
5. The neurotransmitter serotonin is synthesized in the body from tryptophan. **Figure 14-41** sketches the biosynthetic pathway. Suppose this pathway were blocked by loss of activity of tryptophan hydroxylase. What would be the biochemical consequences?
6. In the bacterium *E. coli*, the enzyme glutamine synthetase catalyzes the synthesis of glutamine from glutamate. The amide nitrogen of glutamine serves as the source of the nitrogen atoms in a variety of products, including glutamate, tryptophan, glycine, alanine, carbamoyl phosphate, AMP, and CTP. The enzyme has 12 identical subunits and is subject to allosteric regulation (inhibition) by many of these small molecules, as shown in **Table 14-3**. Individually, these different inhibitors bind to distinct regulatory sites on the enzyme, and they produce only partial inhibition.
   a. Why is partial inhibition a reasonable metabolic strategy here?
   b. Explain how the combination of tryptophan plus carbamoyl phosphate is more effective than either inhibitor alone.
   c. Using the observed individual effect for each inhibitor, can you verify by a suitable calculation that a combination of all six inhibitors would produce 7–8% of the net activity remaining for the enzyme?
7. Pyridoxine oxidase acts on vitamin B_6 to convert pyridoxine into pyridoxal. Predict the biochemical consequences of a partial loss of activity by the pyridoxine oxidase enzyme.
8. "Chinese restaurant syndrome" is a collection of symptoms including headache, flushing, and sweating, noted after a meal with dishes heavily flavored with monosodium glutamate, such as have traditionally been common in many Chinese and Japanese restaurants. Monosodium glutamate is also found in many prepared or canned foods such as soup and snack foods.
   a. Suggest a physiological basis for the syndrome. *Hint:* Glutamate is a neurotransmitter.
   b. Proponents of dietary supplementation with vitamin B_6 have proposed that such supplementation would avoid or alleviate the symptoms that make up "Chinese

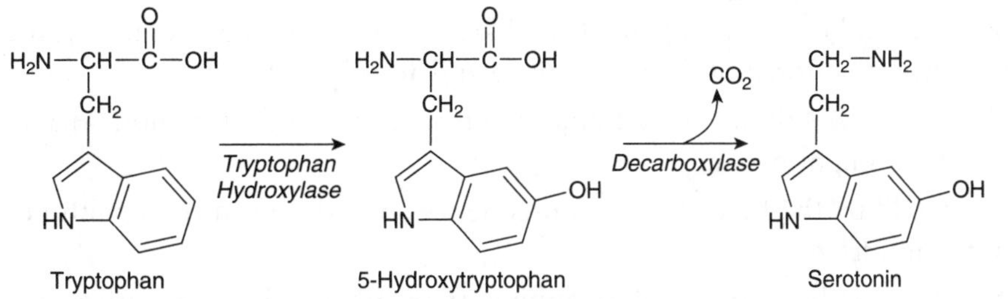

Figure 14-41 Biosynthesis of serotonin from tryptophan.

Inhibitor Added	Observed Net Remaining Enzymatic Activity (%)	Predicted Net Activity (%)
Tryptophan (Trp)	84	
Carbamoyl phosphate (CP)	86	
Glycine (Gly)	87	
Adenosine monophosphate (AMP)	59	
L-Alanine (Ala)	52	
Cytosine triphosphate (CTP)	37	
Trp + CP	72	72
Trp + CP + Gly	60	63
Trp + CP + Gly + AMP	41	37
Trp + CP + Gly + AMP + Ala	22	19
Trp + CP + Gly + AMP + Ala + CTP	8	7

Table 14-3 Inhibition of Bacterial Glutamine Synthetase

Source: C. A. Woolfolk and E. R. Stadtman. (1964). *Biochem. Biophys. Res. Commun.* 17:313–319.

restaurant syndrome." Suggest a biochemical basis for how vitamin B_6 supplementation would achieve this outcome.

9. What would be the biochemical consequences of a loss of sensitivity of glutamate dehydrogenase to the cell's energy charge?
10. A deficiency in either carbamoyl phosphate synthetase or ornithine transcarbamoylase leads to a block in the urea cycle, and causes accumulation of excess nitrogen as ammonia. In turn, this process leads to higher levels of glutamine in the body.
    a. Trace the path from high levels of ammonia to increased levels of glutamine.
    b. Excess glutamine can be absorbed by reaction with phenylacetyl-CoA; the product is phenylacetylglutamine, which is excreted via the kidney. In fact, patients suffering from either of these enzyme deficiencies are given phenylacetate instead of the CoA derivative. Why is this supplement used instead of adding phenylacetyl-CoA to their diet?
11. Suppose that a defect is present in the mitochondrial citrulline transporter. Trace the sequence of events leading to hyperammonemia.
12. Review why *N*-acetylglutamate is an apt choice as an allosteric activator of carbamoyl phosphate synthetase. Then predict the likely consequences of a defect in the activity of the synthase that forms it from glutamate and acetyl-CoA.
13. High serum levels of uracil are found in a patient with hyperammonemia. Explain how this buildup might occur.
14. What would be the biochemical consequences of a defect in the ornithine transporter in mitochondria?
15. Deficiency in the activity of ornithine transcarbamoylase or carbamoyl phosphate synthetase I can lead to hyperammonemia. How might dietary supplementation with L-citrulline help alleviate the hyperammonemia?

16. Two days after birth, a newborn infant suddenly becomes irritable, stops feeding, and starts vomiting. Lab tests indicate a disorder in the functioning of the urea cycle, leading to hyperammonemia. The infant is put on a protein-restricted diet (only carbohydrates and lipids) for 48 hours, but not longer.
    a. Why not use a longer period for the protein-free diet?
    b. During this period, the infant is fed intravenously a hypercaloric protein-free solution, and dosed with insulin. Why is the feeding hypercaloric, and why is the insulin given?
17. Suppose that a patient who is being treated for tuberculosis suffers a toxic overdose of isoniazid. How might administration of vitamin B_6 be helpful here?
18. The breakdown of methionine, valine, and isoleucine all lead to propionyl-CoA. How does the body metabolize propionyl-CoA to succinyl-CoA, and why is vitamin B_{12} important here?

REFERENCES

M. L. Batshaw, R. B. MacArthur, and M. Tuchman. (2001). "Alternative pathway therapy for urea cycle disorders: Twenty years later," *J. Pediatr.* 138:S46–S55.

D. A. Bender. (1985). *Amino Acid Metabolism* (2nd ed.), Wiley, New York.

P. Felig. (1975). "Amino acid metabolism in man," *Annu. Rev. Biochem.* 44:933–955.

D. A. Hood and R. L Terjung. (1990). "Amino acid metabolism during exercise and following endurance training," *Sports Med.* 9:23–35.

M. J. Jackson, A. L. Beaudet, and W. E. O'Brien. (1986). "Mammalian urea cycle enzymes," *Annu. Rev. Genet.* 20:431–464.

R. Matalon et al. (1989). "Hyperphenylalaninemia due to inherited deficiencies of tetera-hydrobiopterin," *Adv. Pediatr.* 36:67–90.

C. Phornphutkul et al. (2002). "Natural history of alkaptonuria," *N. Engl. J. Med.* 347:2111–2121.

T. J. Smith and C. A. Stanley. (2008). "Untangling the glutamate dehydrogenase allosteric nightmare," *Trends Biochem. Sci.* 33:557–564.

M. D. Toney. (2005). "Reaction specificity in pyridoxal phosphate enzymes," *Arch. Biochem. Biophys.* 433:279–287.

S. L. C. Woo. (1989). "Molecular basis and population genetics of phenylketonuria," *Biochemistry* 28:1–7.

C. A. Woolfolk and E. R. Stadtman. (1967). "Regulation of glutamine synthetase. III. Cumulative feedback inhibition of glutamine synthetase from *Escherichia coli*," *Arch. Biochem. Biophys.* 118:735–755.

CHAPTER 15

Nucleotide Metabolism

Learning Objectives

1. Define and use correctly the following terms: *salvage recovery, 5-phosphoribosyl-1-pyrophosphate (PRPP), nucleoside monophosphate kinase, nucleoside diphosphate kinase, ribonucleotide reductase, thymidylate synthase, 5-fluorouracil, gout, Lesch-Nyhan syndrome, hypoxanthine, inosine, hypoxanthine-guanine phosphoribosyl transferase (HGPRT), urate/uric acid*, and *xanthine oxidase*.
2. Describe the steps in the pathways leading to the de novo synthesis of pyrimidines and of purines. Explain why pyrimidine and purine bases are not regarded as "essential" components of the diet.
3. Explain why folate analogs may be powerful inhibitors of cell growth. Relate this activity to their uses as drugs.
4. Explain and describe the mechanism of action of 5-fluorouracil in the inhibition of thymidylate synthase.
5. Relate the breakdown of purines to two diseases—gout and Lesch-Nyhan syndrome. Describe the basis of action of various drugs used to treat gout.
6. Recognize the structures of PRPP, F-dUMP, 5-fluorouracil, carbamoyl phosphate, *N*-carbamoyl-L-aspartate, folic acid (folate), ribose, deoxyribose, uracil, adenine, thymine, guanine, cytosine, hypoxanthine, inosine monophosphate (IMP), and uric acid. Distinguish among the structures of the bases, nucleosides, and nucleotides.
7. Describe the action of ribonucleotide reductase, relating it to the cycling of thioredoxin and the use of NADPH by thioredoxin reductase.
8. Explain how sulfa drugs can inhibit bacterial growth, noting their target, and explain why the combination of trimethoprim with sulfamethoxazole is an especially effective antibacterial combination.

Introduction

Structures of nucleotides and their corresponding bases were introduced in Chapter 4. **Figure 15-1** and **Figure 15-2** are reminders of the structures of the major nucleic acid bases and nucleotides. Recall that nucleotides function in many important roles in the cell besides serving as building blocks for DNA or RNA: They are constituents of many important cofactors (e.g., coenzyme A,

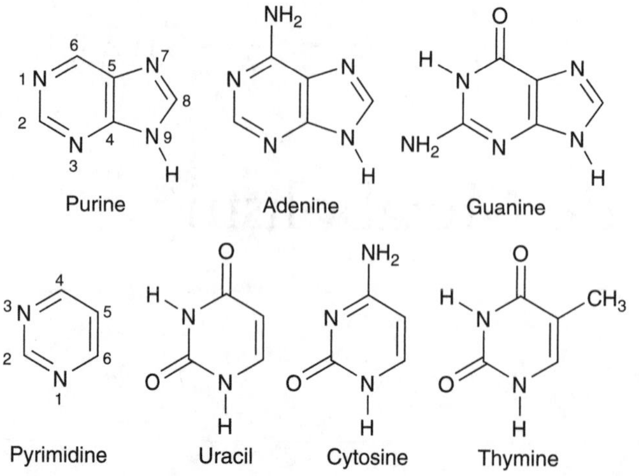

Purine Adenine Guanine

Pyrimidine Uracil Cytosine Thymine

Figure 15-1 Purine and pyrimidine ring numbering, and the five common nucleic acid bases.

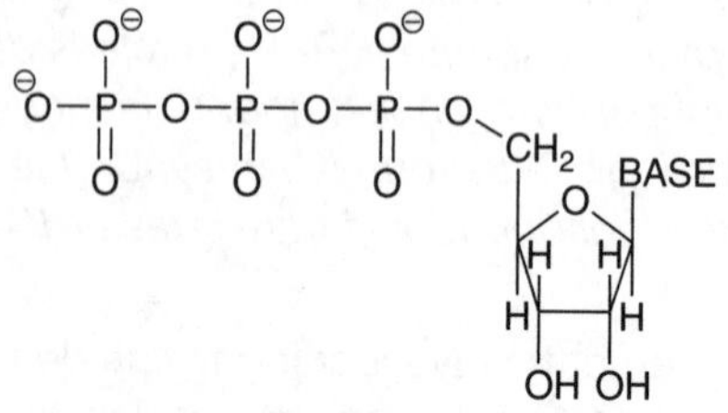

Figure 15-2 Nucleotides have three structural components: a base, a sugar, and a phosphate group (a monophosphate, diphosphate, or triphosphate). The sugar shown here is ribose.

the nicotinamide coenzymes); they help to activate sugars for metabolism; and ATP hydrolysis is the major source of free energy driving many cellular processes. Analogs of nucleotides might then be expected to be powerful drugs, affecting many diverse biochemical processes. Also, agents that affect nucleotide biosynthesis could have major consequences for the cell.

Catabolism of the nucleic acid bases occurs by two pathways:

- The purines can be catabolized to *uric acid* (*urate*) and excreted.
- Pyrimidines can be broken down to malonate and methylmalonate (both of which are soluble and can be excreted via the urine), along with ammonia and carbon dioxide.

The breakdown of pyrimidines usually proceeds without difficulty, but defects in the catabolism of purines can be clinically important, and they are associated with some significant human disease states.

Purine Biosynthesis

There are two major pathways for the construction of nucleotides. One pathway recovers DNA and RNA components from the diet and uses them to build up to nucleotides. The other pathway biosynthesizes the entire nucleotide from much simpler precursor molecules. Purine nucleotide biosynthesis starts with assembly of the purine ring, followed by attachment of the sugar–phosphate moieties. This pathway uses amino acids and products of carbohydrate metabolism and is regulated through feedback mechanisms using the end products of the pathway.

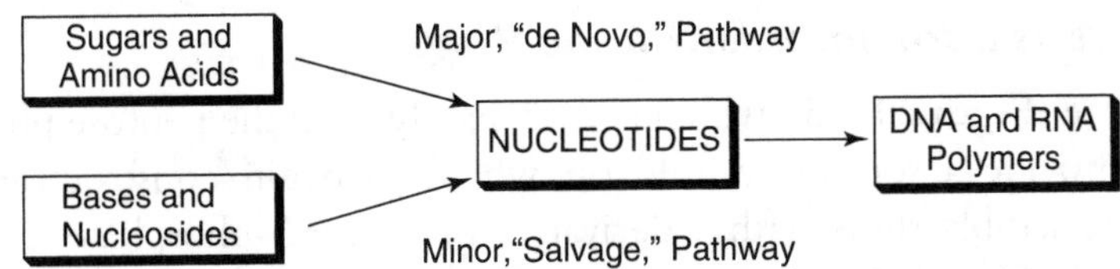

Figure 15-3 The two major pathways for biosynthesis of nucleotides: salvage and de novo synthesis.

Two Major Pathways for Biosynthesis of Nucleotides: De Novo and Salvage

The term *de novo* comes from Latin, meaning "from the new." Here it implies the synthesis of nucleotides from simpler and more basic building blocks. Purines have a different de novo biosynthetic pathway from pyrimidines. For both purines and pyrimidines, de novo biosynthesis takes place in the cytosol.

The term *salvage* or *salvage recovery* refers to the reuse of already synthesized compounds. Catabolism of nucleic acids from the diet or from DNA and RNA turnover within the cell yields free bases, which can then be reacted with an activated sugar–phosphate compound to give nucleotides. This process avoids the metabolic expense of synthesizing the ring structures, and represents a more efficient use of resources for the cell. **Figure 15-3** schematically compares de novo synthesis to salvage recovery.

The purine nucleotides AMP and GMP are derived from a precursor purine, *inosine monophosphate* (IMP). Note that the purine base in IMP is called *hypoxanthine*, not inosine. For the pyrimidine bases, uridine monophosphosphate (UMP) is synthesized first, then modified to give cytidine and thymidine nucleotides.

Although humans can absorb purine and pyrimidine bases from the diet, by far the greater part of cellular demand for nucleotides is satisfied by de novo synthesis. These bases are not considered to be "essential"; they are readily synthesized by normal healthy humans. Dietary sources that are especially rich in bases include liver and yeast extract.

Sources of Purine Skeleton Atoms

Figure 15-4 summarizes the contributions to the purine ring from several sources:

- Amino acids contribute both carbons and nitrogens to the ring: Glycine contributes at C-4, C-5, and N-7; aspartate at N-1; and glutamine at N-3 and N-9.
- Tetrahydrofolate contributes carbons (through activated derivatives, indicated by formic acid) at both C-2 and C-8.
- CO_2 contributes a carbon atom at C-6.

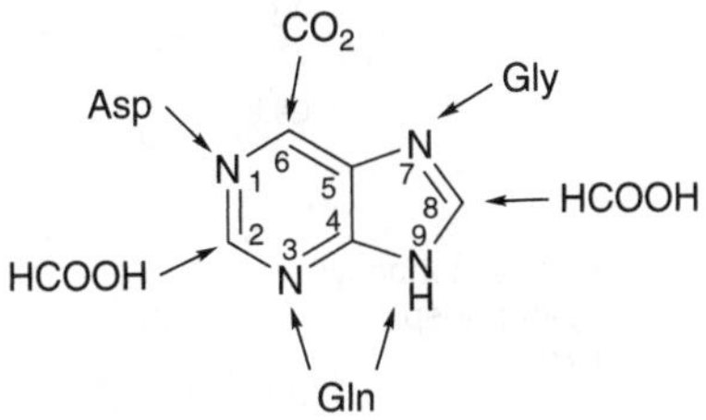

Figure 15-4 Sources of the atoms of the purine ring skeleton.

Ribose Phosphate as a Precursor for Purine Rings

Ribose 5-phosphate (**Figure 15-5**), which comes mainly from the pentose phosphate pathway, is used here to provide a sort of scaffold on which to begin construction of the purine ring. Purine ring assembly starts with a derivative of ribose 5-phosphate: *5-phosphoribosyl-1-pyrophosphate* (PRPP; **Figure 15-6**).

- PRPP is made from ATP and ribose 5-phosphate (**Figure 15-7**); the enzyme here is PRPP synthetase.
- The reaction mechanism involves the nucleophilic attack of the sugar C-1 hydroxyl group on the β-phosphorus of ATP; AMP is displaced and the pyrophosphate group is now attached to the sugar. Pyrophosphate is a good leaving group, so the sugar is now activated for the next reaction in the pathway.
- Because PRPP is used in several other pathways (e.g., in pyrimidine biosynthesis), this step cannot be regarded as the committed step for purine synthesis.

Synthesis of Inosine Monophosphate

The next set of steps converts PRPP into an amino sugar, attaches an amino acid, forms a five-membered ring, and finally makes the full purine ring in the form of *inosine monophosphate* (IMP).

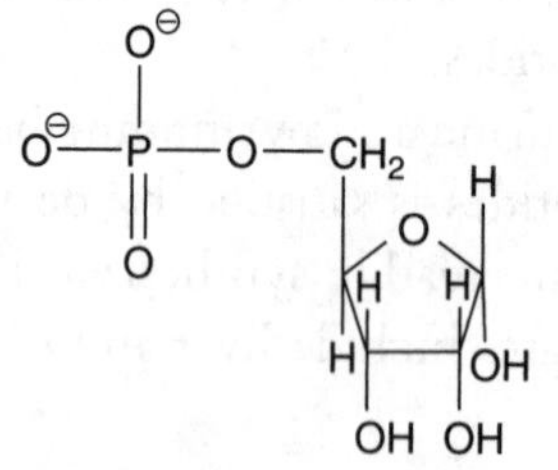

Ribose 5-Phosphate

Figure 15-5 Ribose 5-phosphate from the pentose phosphate pathway is a key starting material for purine biosynthesis.

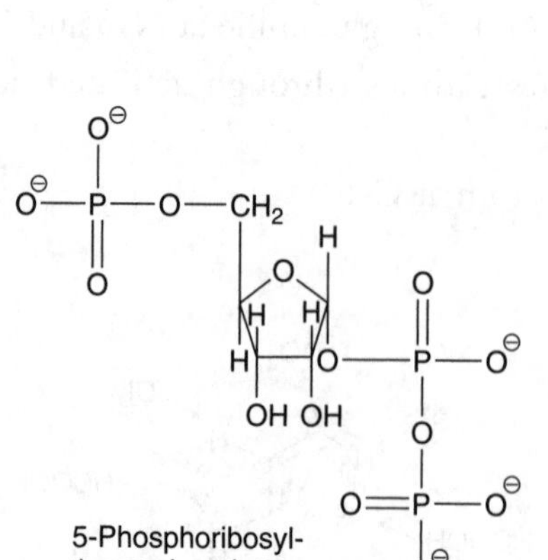

5-Phosphoribosyl-1-pyrophosphate (PRPP)

Figure 15-6 PRPP is an activated form of the ribose sugar.

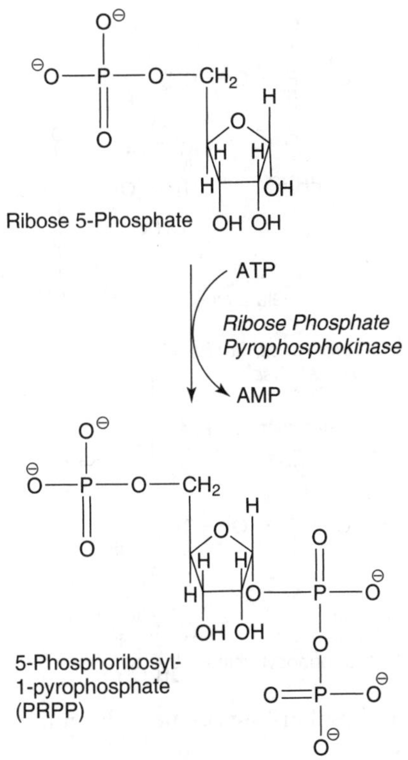

Figure 15-7 The pyrophosphate group of PRPP is derived from ATP.

The route to inosine monophosphate (from which AMP and GMP will be made) can be divided into the following stages.

PRPP and Gln React

- An amino group is transferred to the sugar, with release of PP_i.
- This is a major branch point in PRPP utilization; PRPP is also used in several other important biosyntheses, including those for pyrimidines, nicotinamides, histidine, and the conversion of guanine to GMP.
- The reaction here, catalyzed by amidophosphoribosyl transferase, can be regarded as the *committed step* in purine synthesis.
- The enzyme is regulated by purine nucleotides in a feedback inhibition system. Failure of regulation at this point can lead to severe disease.
- The amino group comes from glutamine (**Figure 15-8**).

Glycine Is Added to Phosphoribosylamine

- The product here is known as glycinamide ribonucleotide (GAR; **Figure 15-9**).
- The reaction uses ATP in helping to form the amide linkage of glycine to the sugar's nitrogen.
- The ribose phosphate is preserved—hence the designation of this compound as a "ribonucleotide."

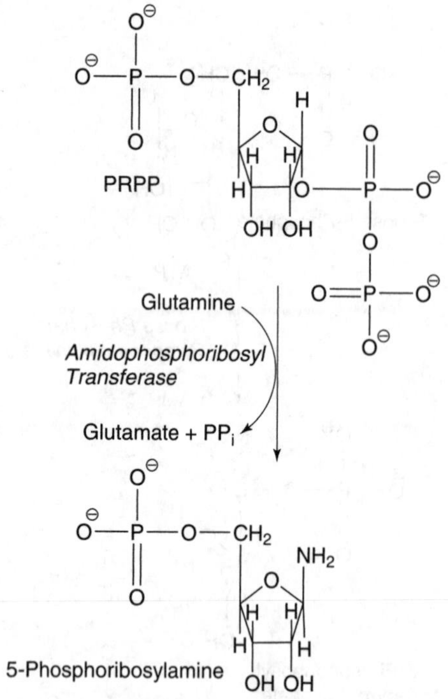

PRPP

Glutamine

Amidophosphoribosyl Transferase

Glutamate + PP_i

5-Phosphoribosylamine

Figure 15-8 The synthesis of 5-phosphoribosylamine is the committed step in purine biosynthesis.

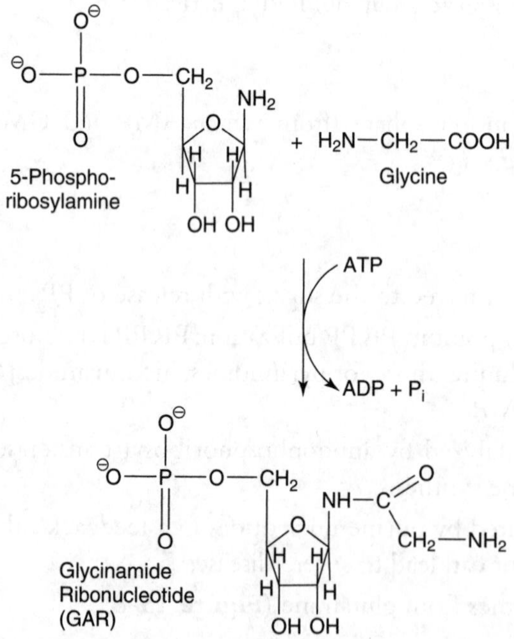

5-Phospho-ribosylamine

+ $H_2N—CH_2—COOH$

Glycine

ATP

ADP + P_i

Glycinamide Ribonucleotide (GAR)

Figure 15-9 Glycinamide ribonucleotide (GAR) is formed from 5-phosphoribosylamine through an amide linkage to glycine.

Formation of a Five-Membered Ring

In multiple reaction steps, we next have addition of a formyl moiety (from a folate derivative), another nitrogen from glutamine, and ring closure. A five-membered ring is formed, attached to the ribose phosphate (**Figure 15-10**).

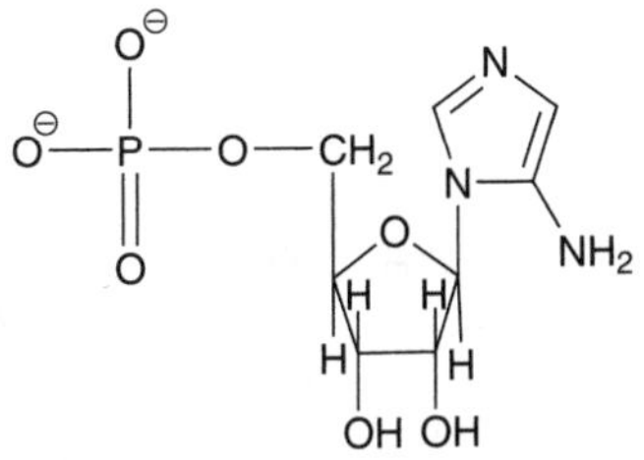

5-Aminoimidazole
Ribonucleotide
(AIR)

Figure 15-10 Multiple steps lead to the formation of a five-membered ring attached to the sugar–phosphate backbone: 5′-phosphoribosyl-5-aminoimidazole.

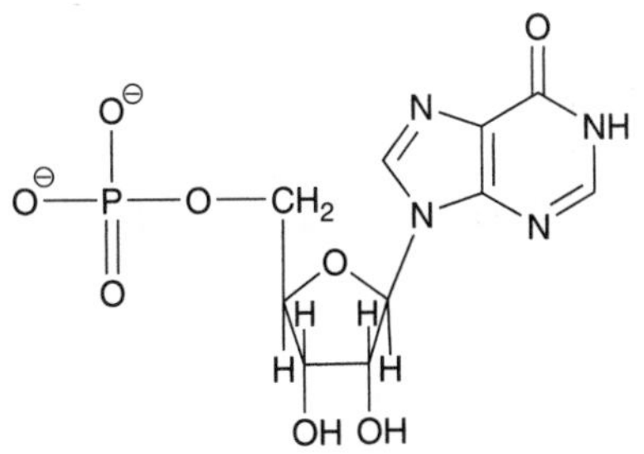

Inosine Monophosphate
(IMP)

Figure 15-11 In several more steps, a six-membered ring is added, giving inosine monophosphate (IMP).

Formation of a Six-Membered Ring

A six-membered ring is formed using CO_2, Asp, and formyl-THF (**Figure 15-11**). Folate (as THF) here donates the single carbon unit. The purine base that results is *hypoxanthine*, but the full nucleotide is called inosine monophosphate.

Synthesis of AMP and GMP

IMP is the precursor to both AMP and GMP; there is a branch point in the pathway here. **Figure 15-12** lays out the two branches:

- AMP is made by substituting $-NH_2$ for the carbonyl oxygen at C-6.
- GMP is made by oxidizing at C-2 and then substituting $-NH_2$ for the carbonyl oxygen.

Feedback Inhibition in Purine Synthesis

Figure 15-13 shows key points of regulation in the path from ribose 5-phosphate to the purine nucleotides. Recall that the committed step is the conversion of PRPP into phosphoribosylamine. This step is inhibited by IMP, AMP, and GMP, all of which are end products.

Other key steps where feedback is exerted are the branch point reactions at IMP, and at PRPP synthesis. Notice that "fine-tuning" of the rate of biosynthesis is allowed by feedback inhibition at checkpoints before and after the committing step.

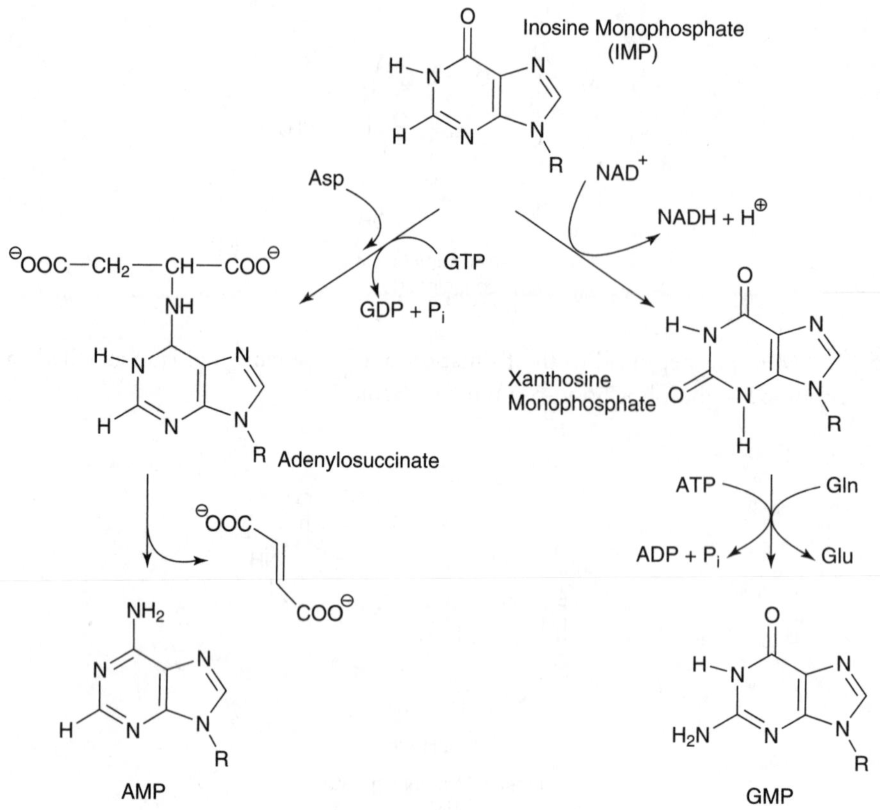

Figure 15-12 IMP is the precursor to both GMP and AMP.

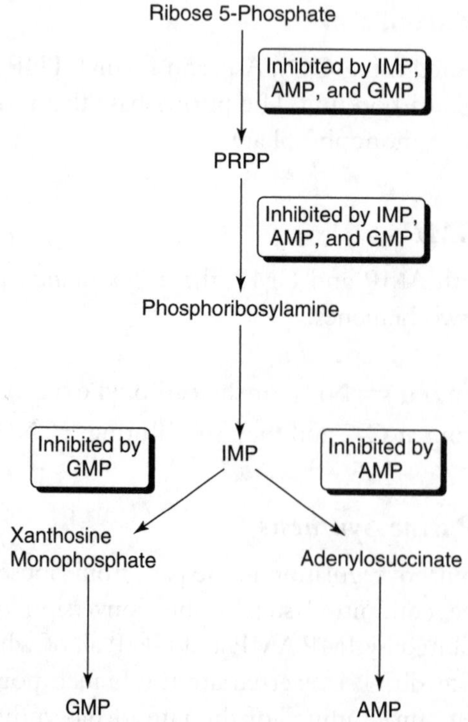

Figure 15-13 Purine biosynthesis is regulated by feedback inhibition at several points.

Pyrimidine Biosynthesis

Pyrimidine biosynthesis follows a pathway quite distinct from that for purines. Different precursors are used, and the sugar–phosphate moiety is attached before the actual pyrimidine ring is fully assembled.

Carbamoyl Phosphate

Recall that carbamoyl phosphate (**Figure 15-14**) is an intermediate in the urea cycle, where it is synthesized and used inside mitochondria. In eukaryotes, synthesis for nucleotides is compartmentalized in the cytosol, using carbamoyl phosphate, which is also made in the cytosol. This process involves a different carbamoyl phosphate synthetase from that in mitochondria; the cytosolic form is called carbamoyl phosphate synthetase II (CPS II), whereas the mitochondrial form is CPS I.

Glutamine is the nitrogen donor here, not free ammonia—another difference from the mitochondrial reaction. CPS II hydrolyzes glutamine specifically to release ammonia, which is then channeled through the enzyme to a site where it reacts with carboxyphosphate to form carbamoyl phosphate.

Committed Step

Carbamoyl phosphate reacts with aspartate to form *N*-carbamoylaspartate; this is the *committed step* in pyrimidine biosynthesis (**Figure 15-15**). The reaction is catalyzed by aspartate transcarbamoylase (ATCase). The bacterial form of this enzyme is a multisubunit enzyme with multiple binding sites for substrate and inhibitors, which uses allosterism for control. In eukaryotes, the enzymatic formation of carbamoyl phosphate, carbamoyl aspartate, and dihydro-orotate are catalyzed by one large trifunctional enzyme, located in the cytosol. Thus this biosynthesis pathway has greater efficiency because the intermediates do not have to leave the enzyme, only to then rediffuse back to reach the enzyme for further reaction.

Steps to UMP, UTP, and CTP

Biosynthesis of UMP precedes the biosynthesis of the cytidine and thymidine nucleotides. The pathway can be broken down into the following steps.

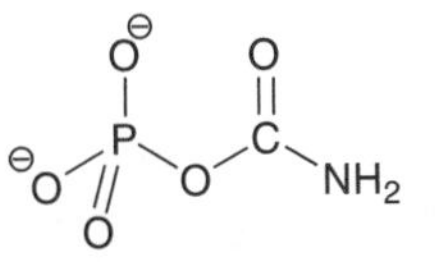

Carbamoyl Phosphate

Figure 15-14 Carbamoyl phosphate is the starting material for pyrimidine biosynthesis.

Carbamoyl Phosphate

Aspartate

Carbamoyl Aspartate

+ P_i

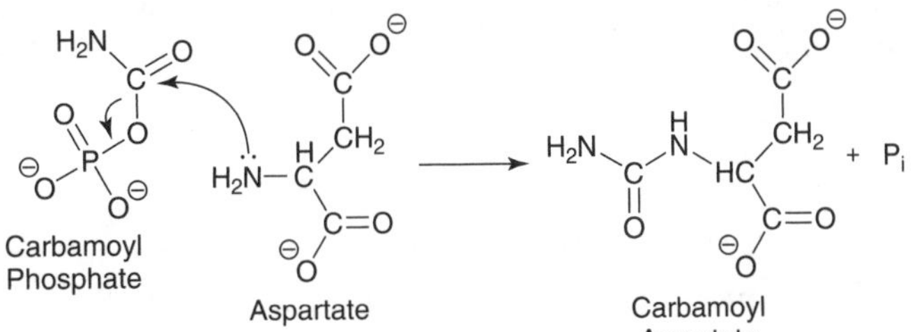

Figure 15-15 Carbamoyl aspartate is synthesized from carbamoyl phosphate in the committed step of pyrimidine biosynthesis, by the enzyme aspartate transcarbamoylase.

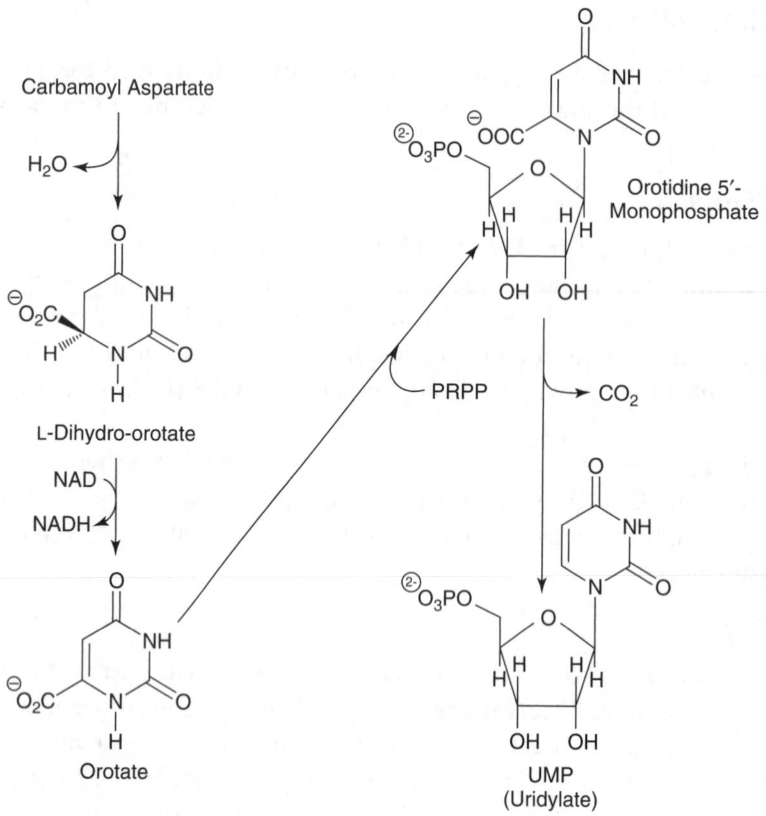

Figure 15-16 The pathway from carbamoyl aspartate to UMP.

Orotate Formation

First, ring closure of carbamoyl aspartate yields dihydro-orotate through a dehydration. Next dehydrogenation yields orotate (**Figure 15-16**).

UMP Formation

Now a ribose phosphate group is attached, to give orotidine 5′-monophosphate. PRPP supplies the ribose phosphate moiety here. (Note that PRPP is used in pyrimidine synthesis *after* the ring has already been formed; this is unlike the process involved in purine biosynthesis, where PRPP is used *before* ring formation.) The ring is then decarboxylated at C-6 to yield UMP. The UMP can, of course, be drawn off at this point for use in building RNA or in activating sugars for their metabolism.

UTP and CTP Formation

UMP is converted to the nucleotide triphosphate by donation of phosphate (twice) from ATP through kinase action. This conversion is followed by replacement of the carbonyl oxygen at C-4 by an amino group (derived from glutamine) to give CTP (**Figure 15-17**).

Figure 15-18 gives a general flowchart view of the route to UMP.

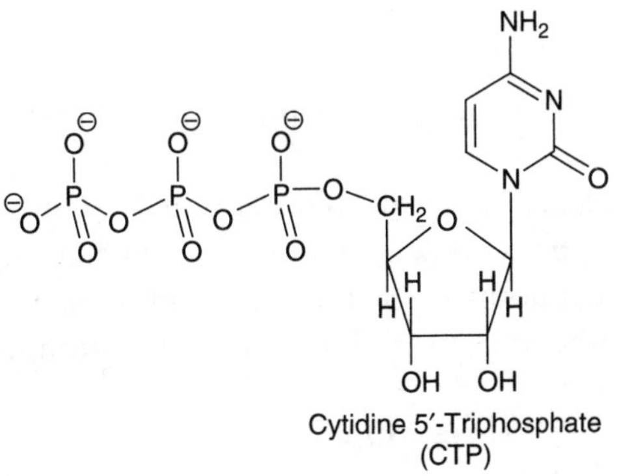

Cytidine 5′-Triphosphate
(CTP)

Figure 15-17 Cytidine 5′-triphosphate is derived from UTP.

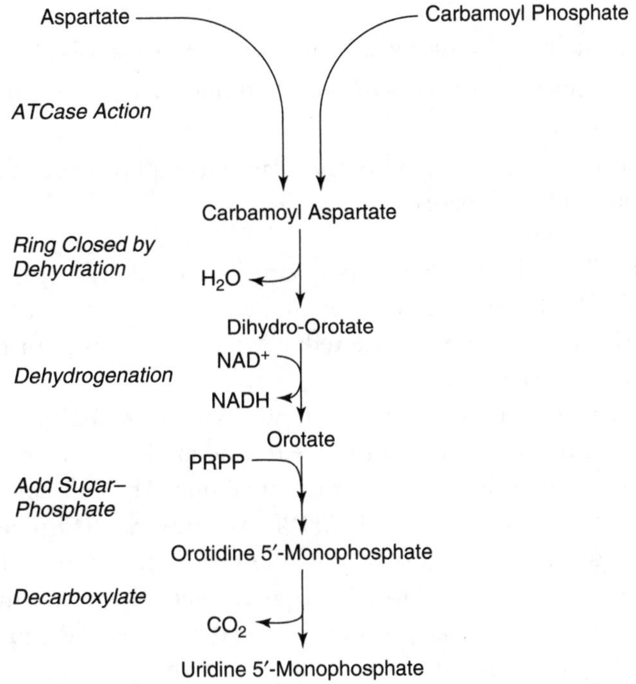

Figure 15-18 Overview of UMP biosynthesis.

Formation of NTPs and dNTPs

Nucleotides with More Phosphates

Nucleotide monophosphates (NMPs), whether the base is a purine or a pyrimidine, are readily converted to the corresponding nucleotide diphosphates (NDPs), and nucleotide triphosphates (NTPs) are converted through the action of various kinases.

NDPs Come from NMPs

$$\text{ATP} + \text{NMP} \rightarrow \text{ADP} + \text{NDP} \quad (15\text{-}1)$$

The reactions in which NDPs come from NMPs are catalyzed by *nucleoside monophosphate kinases*. Because the concentration of ATP is much greater than any other NTP, it makes sense to use it as the source of the phosphoryl group in forming the NDP.

NTPs Come from NDPs

$$\text{NTP}_{\text{donor}} + \text{NDP}_{\text{acceptor}} \rightarrow \text{NDP}_{\text{donor}} + \text{NTP}_{\text{acceptor}} \qquad (15\text{-}2)$$

The reactions in which NTPs come from NDPs are catalyzed by *nucleoside diphosphate kinase*, which has a very broad specificity: It will accept either purine or pyrimidine nucleotides. A wide variety of nucleotide triphosphates can donate a phosphate group, although usually the donor is ATP because it is present in much higher concentration than the others.

Deoxynucleotides and dTTP Formation

Ribonucleotide Reductase and Deoxyribose Formation

Deoxyribonucleotides are made from ribonucleotides.

- The conversion is catalyzed by *ribonucleotide reductase* (**Figure 15-19**).
- This enzyme acts specifically on ribonucleoside diphosphates, not the monophosphate or triphosphate nucleosides.
- The monophosphates can be easily phosphorylated to diphosphates through the action of nucleoside monophosphate kinases.

The reduction at the 2′-carbon requires two equivalents of hydrogen. These come from NADPH, although NADPH is not used directly in the reaction. Instead, the NADPH is used to regenerate the active form of ribonucleotide reductase, by the transfer of reducing equivalents through a chain of intermediates.

Ribonucleotide reductase uses a pair of thiols (which are oxidized to a disulfide) to perform the reduction of the sugar. The thiols are regenerated by similar thiols on the enzyme thioredoxin. The disulfides on thioredoxin, in turn, are reduced by another enzyme, thioredoxin reductase, which is a flavoenzyme that uses NADPH as a substrate (**Figure 15-20**).

Ribonucleotide reductase is regulated by allosteric interactions. Binding at specific regulatory sites can reduce or enhance overall enzymatic activity. For example, dATP serves to lower the activity, but ATP (with the ribose, not the deoxyribose sugar) stimulates it. The overall pattern of regulation by nucleotides is rather complex, with pyrimidine nucleotides affecting purine nucleotide reduction, for example.

Thymidylate Synthase and dTTP Formation

Formation of deoxythymidylate is essential for the synthesis of DNA and for cellular replication; deoxyuridylate cannot be substituted.

- The process starts with UMP, which is phosphorylated to UDP; this nucleotide still has the ribose sugar, however.

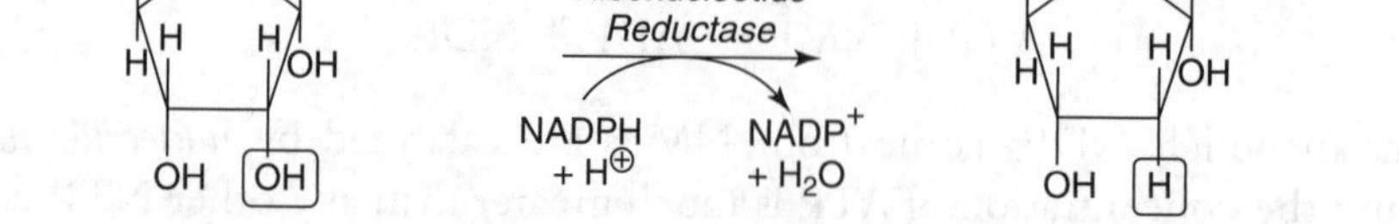

Figure 15-19 Ribonucleotide reductase converts ribonucleotide diphosphates to deoxyribonucleotide diphosphates.

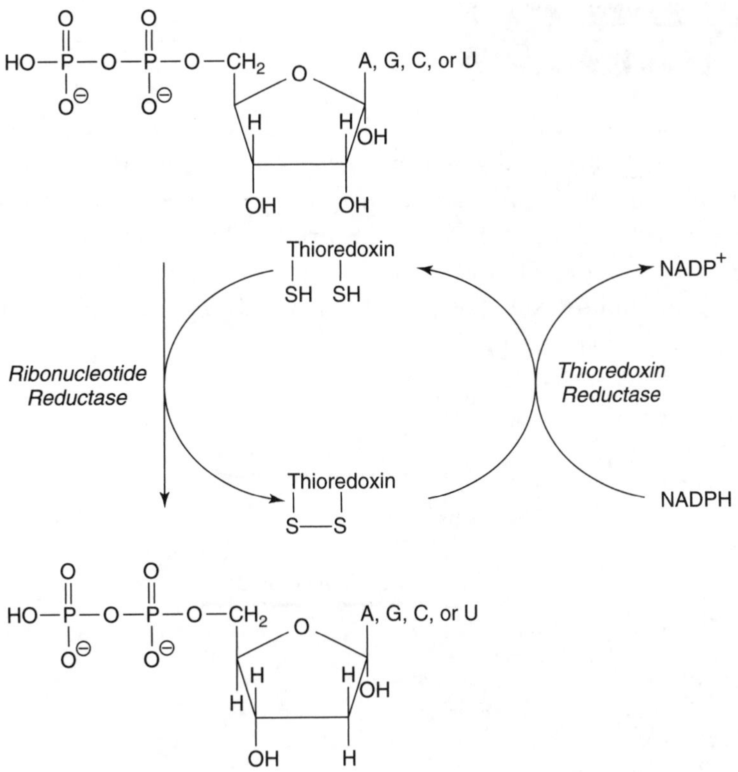

Figure 15-20 The reduction by ribonucleotide reductase is coupled to redox cycling of thioredoxin.

- Next, the ribose sugar on UDP is reduced to the deoxyribose sugar through the action of ribonucleotide reductase.
- The resulting dUDP can be readily dephosphorylated to dUMP through the action of kinases.
- The next step is to methylate dUMP, a reaction catalyzed by *thymidylate synthase*. The enzyme specifically acts on the *deoxy* form of uridylate. The methyl donor is a derivative of tetrahydrofolate, N^5, N^{10}-methylene-tetrahydrofolate.
- Finally, kinases add two more phosphates to convert to it to the triphosphate nucleotide dTTP, which is ready for biosynthesis of DNA (**Figure 15-21**).

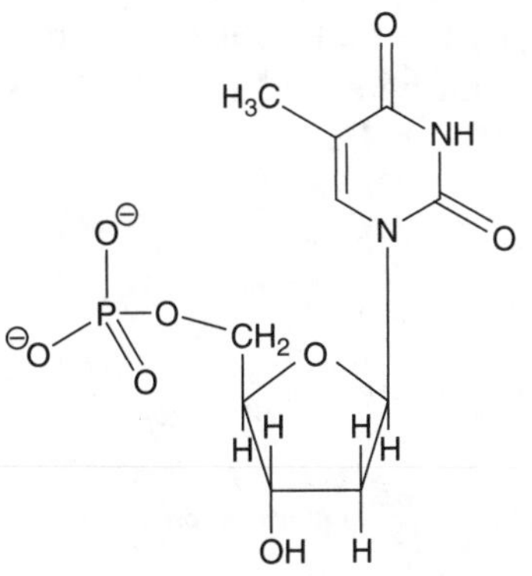

Figure 15-21 Deoxythymidylate is derived by methylation of deoxyuridylate, with N^5, N^{10}-methylene tetrahydrofolate acting as the donor.

Clinical Application

Cancer cells are especially vulnerable to a block of dTMP synthesis because the cancer cells generally are growing rapidly and thus need a lot of pyrimidine nucleotides. Two key enzymes are *thymidylate synthase* and *dihydrofolate reductase* (DHFR), both of which are the targets of several anticancer drugs (**Figure 15-22**). Additionally, the conversion of serine to glycine, as tetrahydrofolate goes to the N^5, N^{10}-methylene tetrahydrofolate, depends on pyridoxal phosphate. The path thus depends on three different vitamins and cofactors—folate, pyridoxine, and niacin.

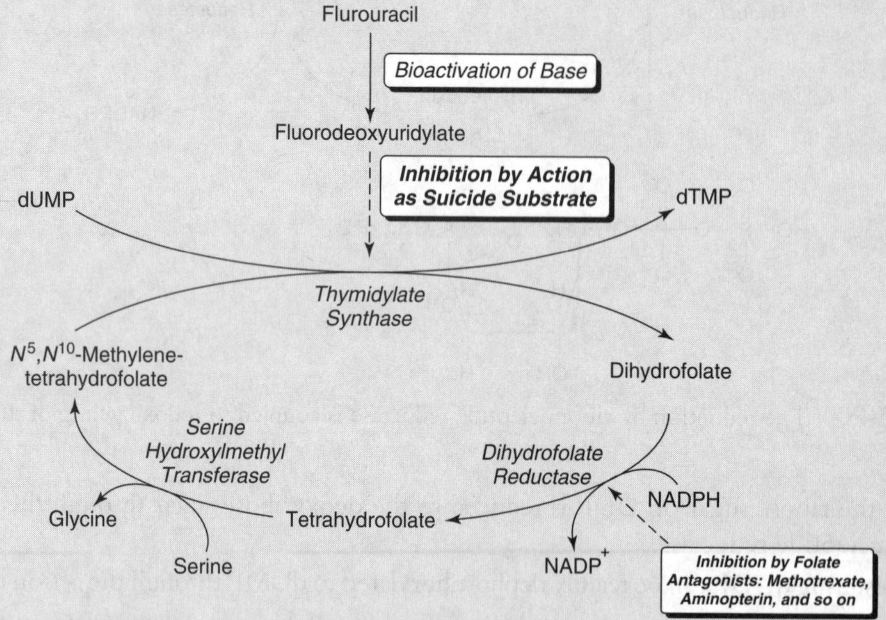

Figure 15-22 Inhibition of deoxythymidylate synthesis can be achieved by targeting two enzymes—thymidylate synthase and dihydrofolate reductase.

Thymidylate Synthase Inhibition

A main target, linked by metabolism to folate metabolism, is the enzyme thymidylate synthase. This enzyme is responsible for the methylation conversion of dUMP to dTMP, where N^5, N^{10}-methylene-tetrahydrofolate is the source of the methyl group. A medicinally important compound here is F-dUMP (**Figure 15-23**). This compound is

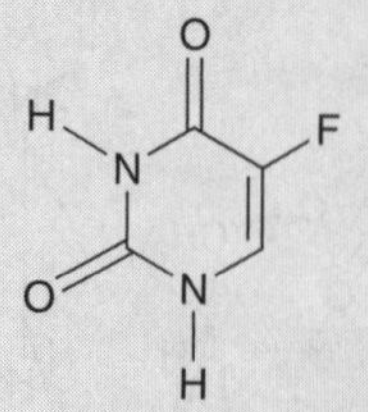

5-Fluorouracil (5-FU)

Figure 15-23 5-Fluorouracil is an analog of uracil. It is activated in the body to 5-fluorodeoxyuridylate (F-dUMP), a suicide substrate for thymidylate synthase.

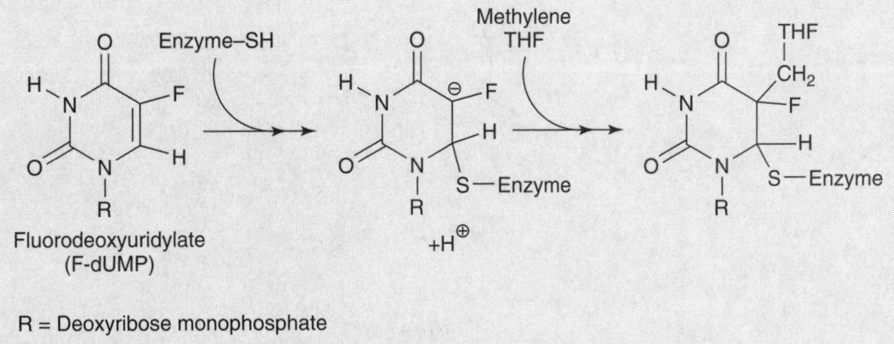

Fluorodeoxyuridylate (F-dUMP)

R = Deoxyribose monophosphate

Figure 15-24 F-dUMP becomes covalently bound to the active site of thymidylate synthase when the enzyme tries to use it as a substrate.

formed in the body from *5-fluorouracil* (given exogenously). F-dUMP acts to irreversibly inhibit the thymidylate synthase. Consequently, less dTMP is made, so less DNA is available for cellular replication, and the growth of the cancer is inhibited.

As a part of the reaction mechanism for transferring a methyl group to the uracil pyrimidine ring, the nucleotide is covalently bound to a sulfur atom on the enzyme through the C-6 position on the uracil ring, and the methylene–THF then covalently attaches to the C-5 atom on the ring. In the next step, a proton would normally be extracted from this C-5 atom. The fluorine replacement at this position makes this impossible, however: F^+ cannot be extracted. The fluoro-nucleotide remains covalently attached in the active site, irreversibly blocking the enzyme from further action (**Figure 15-24**). Because the substrate F-dUMP is consumed in its action as inhibitor, it is called a suicide substrate.

Dihydrofolate Reductase Inhibition

THF must be regenerated after use in biosynthesis, and DHFR is the enzyme responsible for its manufacture. A block here will affect both purine and pyrimidine biosynthesis, so DHFR is an especially important target. Aminopterin and methotrexate are reversible, competitive inhibitors of DHFR. These compounds are analogs of folate; they bind strongly (but noncovalently) to DHFR, thereby blocking the active site.

Selectively targeting cancer cells with inhibitors of folate metabolism (*antifolates*) is unfortunately not yet possible because both "normal" and cancerous cells use the same enzyme, DHFR. When antifolates are given to patients as cancer chemotherapy, great caution must be taken to avoid too much damage to "normal" cells.

Antifolates as Antibacterials

Antifolates are also useful antibacterial agents. Bacterial DHFR differs from mammalian DHFR in the amino acid sequence and in the structure around the active site. The bacterial enzyme can be selectively inhibited by trimethoprim (TMP), a competitive inhibitor. However, TMP will not bind nearly as strongly to the mammalian DHFR, so it is selective for killing bacteria.

Bacteria synthesize their own folate from *p*-aminobenzoic acid (PABA), pteridine, and glutamate. Aryl sulfonamides ("sulfa" drugs) are analogs of PABA and compete with the PABA in the bacterial enzyme dihydropteroate synthase (**Figure 15-25**);

(Continued)

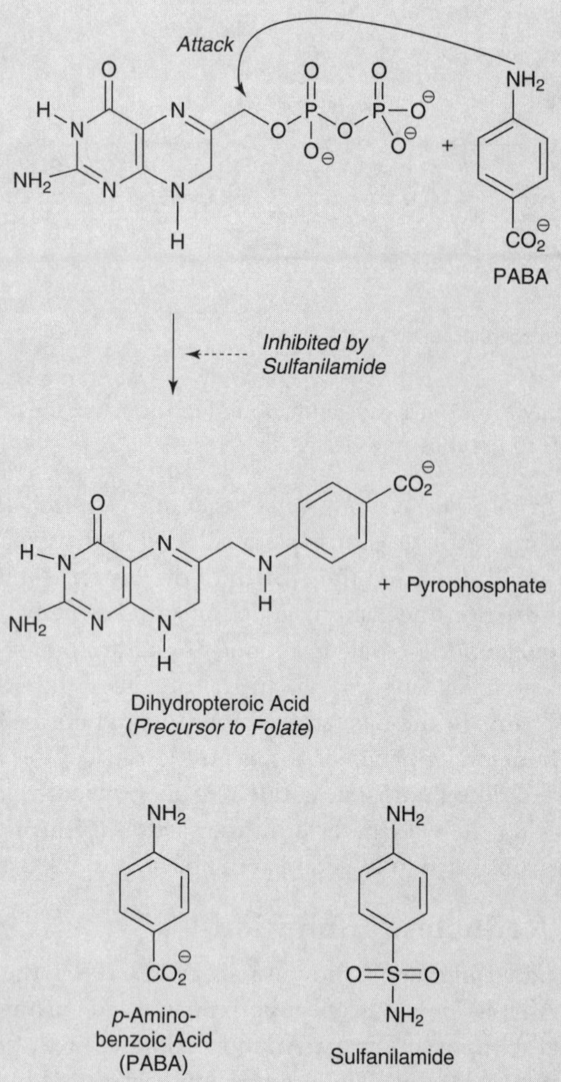

Attack

PABA

Inhibited by Sulfanilamide

+ Pyrophosphate

Dihydropteroic Acid
(*Precursor to Folate*)

p-Amino-benzoic Acid (PABA)

Sulfanilamide

Figure 15-25 Sulfa drugs such as sulfanilamide are analogs of *p*-aminobenzoic acid (PABA) and competitively inhibit the biosynthesis of folate, thereby producing an antibacterial action.

sulfonamides are competitive inhibitors of this enzyme. The bacteria are then unable to synthesize adequate amounts of folate, and their growth is inhibited (bacteriostatic action).

Co-trimoxazole is a combination of sulfamethoxazole with trimethoprim. With this combination, the sulfamethoxazole will inhibit folate formation, and trimethoprim will inhibit folate utilization (if any is made).

Purine and Pyrimidine Breakdown

A continuous turnover of nucleotides occurs within the cell. Some bases are recycled by salvage pathways, whereas others are degraded and the products are excreted. Breakdown of pyrimidine and purine rings involves removal (by oxidation) of exocyclic amino groups and oxidation of

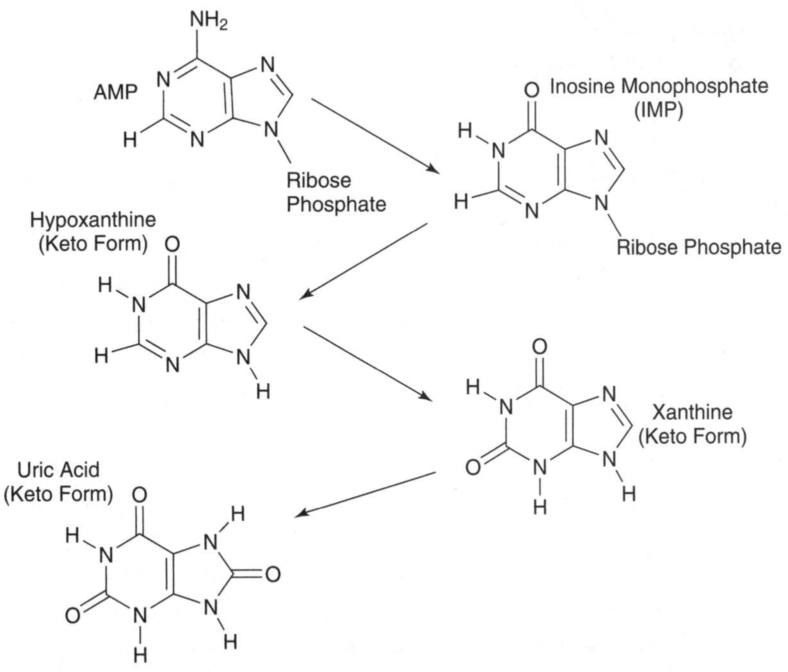

Figure 15-26 Uric acid is the excreted end product of purine catabolism in humans.

the ring structure. Pyrimidine catabolism leads eventually to simple ammonia and CO_2 as products. The catabolism of purines, however, is more complex. The compound *urate* (*uric acid*) is the final product of purine catabolism in humans (**Figure 15-26**); humans excrete urate in the urine. Other organisms break down urate further for excretion.

Urate is an antioxidant and an efficient scavenger of reactive oxygen species (e.g., hydroxyl radicals). Thus a high serum level of urate helps protect the body's tissues against these oxidative species. Unfortunately, urate is only moderately soluble, and urate levels in human serum are typically close to the solubility limit, which can lead to problems.

Gout

Because of its poor aqueous solubility and high serum concentration, sodium urate can precipitate in kidneys or in joints. When deposited in joints, inflammation of the joint results. The joints of the big toes are typical points of inflammation, but knees, fingers, and other joints can also be affected. This kind of joint inflammation is referred to as *gout*.

Excessive levels of urate in serum may be caused by inherited metabolic disorders of one type or another (e.g., compromised excretion of urate, over-synthesis of purines). They may also arise in certain types of cancer chemotherapy. In addition, urate buildup is associated with a diet that is rich in protein and nucleic acids and with alcohol consumption. Consumption of purines would obviously raise urate levels; a high-protein diet would likewise contribute to higher concentrations because certain amino acids go into the de novo synthesis of purines. Alcohol acts as a diuretic and tends to cause dehydration, leading to urate precipitation; the acidosis associated with over-indulgence further exacerbates this effect. Small wonder, then, that gout is historically associated with "high living."

Clinical Application

Allopurinol

Allopurinol (**Figure 15-27**), an analog of hypoxanthine, is used to treat gout. This compound is an irreversible inhibitor of *xanthine oxidase*; this inhibition then lowers urate production, reduces serum urate levels, and helps avoid further precipitation of urate (**Figure 15-28**). Notice that allopurinol can inhibit both the xanthine-to-urate reaction and the hypoxanthine-to-xanthine reaction because both are catalyzed by the same enzyme. Allopurinol does not, however, inhibit the guanine-to-xanthine reaction; it is catalyzed by a different enzyme.

Colchicine

Colchicine (**Figure 15-29**), a plant alkaloid, relieves the symptoms of gout not by directly interfering with the production of urate, but rather by retarding the inflammation associated with urate crystal deposition. It appears to inhibit the migration and phagocytic action of polymorphonuclear leukocytes, probably by binding to and depolymerizing tubulin (microtubules are needed for the cells to migrate and perform phagocytosis). Colchicine also inhibits the synthesis and release of leukotrienes, which tends to reduce inflammation as well.

Uricosuric Agents

Uricosuric agents (probenecid, sulfinpyrazone; see Figure 15-29) improve excretion of urate by exerting their action in the kidney. Urate is passed freely at the glomerulus in the kidney, but it is also reabsorbed, then reexcreted, in the proximal tubule by certain active transport proteins that are specific for weak acids like urate. Uricosuric drugs inhibit

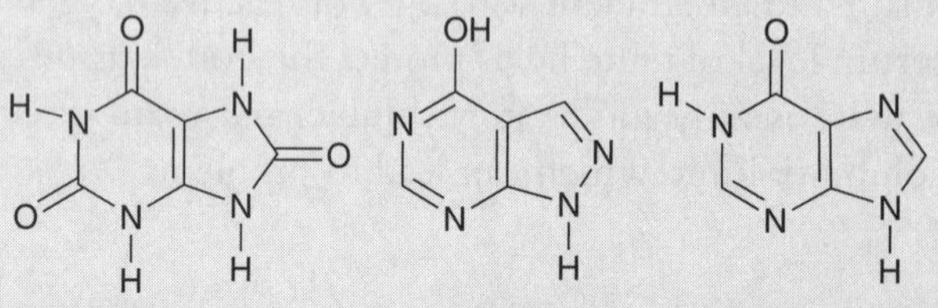

Uric acid (Keto Form) | Allopurinol | Hypoxanthine (Keto Form)

Figure 15-27 Allopurinol is an unreactive analog of hypoxanthine or uric acid. It inhibits the key catabolic enzyme xanthine oxidase.

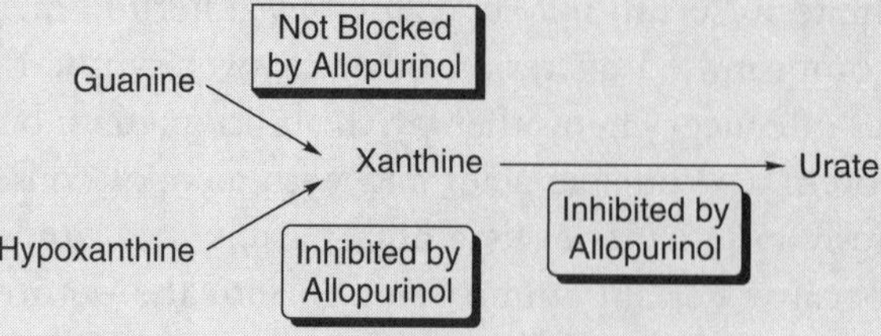

Figure 15-28 Allopurinol acts at two closely related steps in the degradation of purines to uric acid.

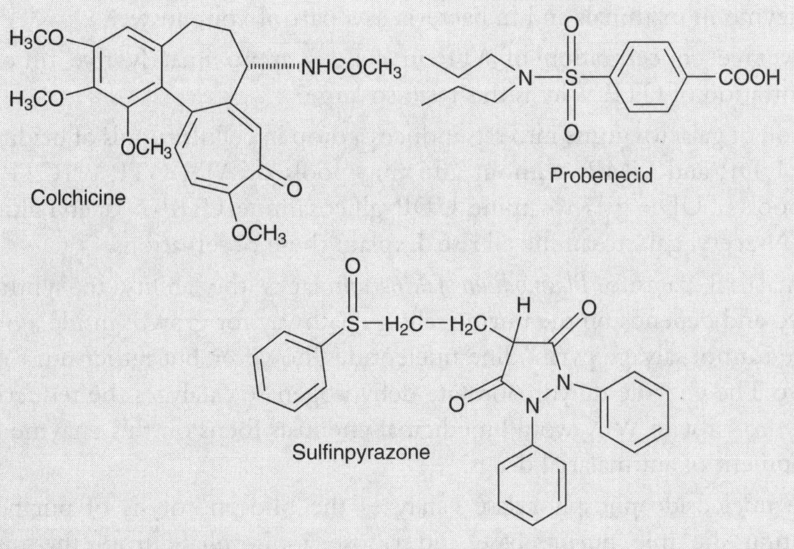

Colchicine

Probenecid

Sulfinpyrazone

Figure 15-29 Antigout agents. Colchicine reduces gout-associated inflammation, while probenecid and sulfinpyrazone help the excretion of uric acid.

these active transporters, such that the net result is to reduce the reabsorption of urate in the proximal tubules of the kidney, thereby promoting excretion of urate in the urine. With other weak acids, the *net* effect (the balance between release, reabsorption, and reexcretion) may be in the opposite direction. For example, probenecid *increases* the half-life of penicillin by *reducing* its excretion; probenecid is used clinically for this purpose. Unfortunately, probenecid also inhibits the renal excretion of several other drugs, which can lead to complications if a patient is taking one or more of these medications (e.g., methotrexate, rifampin, naproxen, sulfonamides in general, indomethacin).

Lesch-Nyhan Syndrome

Symptoms of *Lesch-Nyhan syndrome* include compulsive self-destructive behavior, mental deficiency, and spasticity. This disorder is caused by a sex-linked recessive gene that leads to loss of activity for the enzyme *hypoxanthine-guanine phosphoribosyl transferase* (HGPRT). Under normal circumstances, this enzyme attaches the phosphoribosyl group to the purine ring in the salvage pathway. Deficiency in activity here may lead to an increased level of PRPP, which then accelerates overall purine synthesis by the de novo pathway. As a consequence, the excess purines are degraded to urate. Gout is associated with this syndrome.

QUESTIONS FOR DISCUSSION

1. Why would loss of the activity of PRPP synthetase interfere with both histidine biosynthesis and purine biosynthesis?
2. In mammals, pyrimidine biosynthesis is regulated primarily through modulation of the activity of carbamoyl phosphate synthetase. How does this process contrast with

regulation of this pathway in bacteria? Review the differences in enzyme structure for this enzyme in mammals and in bacteria as a part of your answer.

3. The average concentration of ATP in cells is approximately five times the average concentration of GTP. Why is this ratio so large?
4. Injection of galactosamine into rats induces a drop in cellular pools of uridine nucleotides (UTP, UDP, and UMP) without affecting pools of ATP, GTP, or CTP. At the same time, pools of UDP-galactosamine, UDP-glucosamine, UDP-*N*-acetyl glucosamine, and UDP-*N*-acetyl galactosamine all rise. Explain these observations.
5. The malarial parasite *Plasmodium falciparum* lacks the ability to synthesize purines de novo and depends on the purine salvage pathway for growth inside a host's cells. The parasite cannot salvage pyrimidine nucleotides, however, but rather must make them all de novo. The enzyme dihydro-orotate dehydrogenase catalyzes the reduction of orotate to dihydro-orotate. Why would medicinal chemists focus on this enzyme as a target for development of antimalarial drugs?
6. Purine nucleoside phosphorylase catalyzes the phosphorolysis of purine nucleosides, generating the free purine base and ribose 1-phosphate from the nucleoside and inorganic phosphate.
   a. Write a balanced reaction for this phosphorolysis.
   b. 9-Deazainosine inhibits the enzyme with affinity in the micromolar range. Draw a structure for this compound, and suggest reasons why it is an inhibitor and not a substrate.
   c. Thermodynamics for the phosphorolysis reaction favors formation of the purine nucleoside and free phosphate, yet in vivo the enzyme-catalyzed reaction functions in the opposite direction to generate the free purine base and ribose 1-phosphate. Consider the metabolic fates of the cleavage products, and explain why the reaction functions in this direction in vivo.
   d. Deficiency in this enzyme results in very low concentrations of uric acid in plasma and urine. Explain why.
7. It is thought that in ancient Rome, as well as in Victorian England, there was significant chronic lead intoxication, due to the use of lead in food and drinking vessels (especially for wine, whose acidity would promote extraction of the lead from the vessel). Among its other toxic effects, lead is known to inhibit renal excretion of uric acid. Was lead responsible for the epidemics of gout that occurred during the Roman Empire and at the height of the British Empire? What other causes might there have been for such outbreaks?
8. 6-Azauridine is a clinically useful antimetabolite that is phosphorylated in vivo to 6-aza-UMP. Its administration produces drops in the concentrations of both uracil and cytosine nucleotides. Suggest a candidate for the molecular target for 6-azauridine, and explain why this compound inhibits synthesis of both cytosine nucleotides and uracil nucleotides.
9. The committed step in purine biosynthesis is the conversion of PRPP into phosphoribosylamine. The nucleotides IMP, AMP, and GMP are all inhibitors of the enzyme (glutamine-PRPP amidotransferase) catalyzing this step. Explain this pattern of inhibition in terms of cellular efficiency.
10. Cytidine deaminase removes the 4-NH_2 group of cytidine in a hydrolytic reaction. The enzyme is inhibited by 3,4-dihydrouridine and 3,4-dihydrozebularine (**Figure 15-30**).

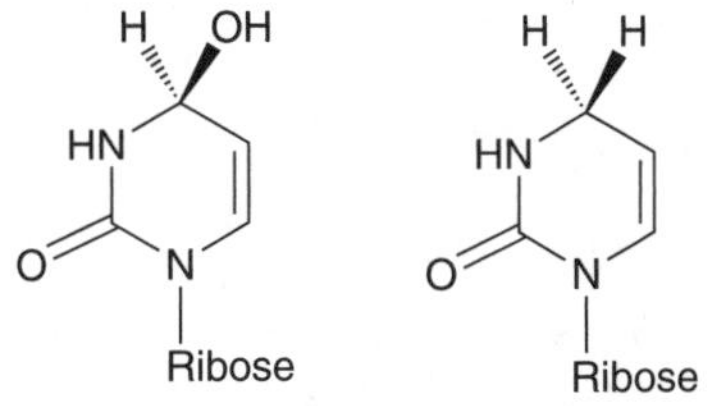

3,4-Dihydrouridine 3,4-Dihydrozebularine

Figure 15-30 Inhibitors of cytidine deaminase.

Propose a structure for the transition state in the deamination of cytidine, and explain the effectiveness of these two inhibitors.

11. Folate antagonists such as methotrexate (MTX) are used in anticancer therapy because cancer cells are often metabolically much more active than normal cells and, therefore, are more sensitive to any blockage in metabolism. In treating cancer patients, potentially toxic doses of this compound are given, and the level of MTX is closely monitored. As the MTX level approaches the toxic level in the blood, a bolus of leucovorin (N^5-formyltetrahydrofolic acid) is given to "rescue" the patient. Explain the potential toxicity of MTX, and explain how leucovorin prevents the lethal effects of MTX on normal cells.

REFERENCES

R. L. P. Adams et al. (1976). *Davidson's the Biochemistry of the Nucleic Acids*, Academic Press, New York.

C. W. Carreras and D. V. Santi. (1995). "The catalytic mechanism and structure of thymidylate synthase," *Annu. Rev. Biochem.* 64:721–762.

H. K. Choi et al. (2004). "Purine-rich foods, dairy and protein intake, and the risk of gout in men," *N. Engl. J. Med.* 350:1093–1103.

A. Holmgren. (1989). "Thioredoxin and glutaredoxin systems," *J. Biol. Chem.* 264:13953–13966.

R. J. Johnson and B. A. Ridout. (2004). "Uric acid and diet: Insights into the epidemic of cardiovascular disease," *N. Engl. J. Med.* 350:1071–1073.

M. E. Jones. (1980). "Pyrimidine nucleotide biosynthesis in animals: Genes, enzymes, and regulation of UMP biosynthesis," *Annu. Rev. Biochem.* 49:253–279.

P. Nordlund and P. Reichard. (2006). "Ribonucleotide reductases," *Annu. Rev. Biochem.* 75: 681–706.

W. B. Parker. (2009). "Enzymology of purine and pyrimidine antimetabolites used in the treatment of cancer," *Chem. Rev.* 109:2880–2893.

J. R. Schnell, H. J. Dyson, and P. E. Wright. (2004). "Structure, dynamics, and catalytic function of dihydrofolate reductase," *Annu. Rev. Biophys. Biomol. Struct.* 33:119–140.

CHAPTER 16

Synthesis of DNA, RNA, and Proteins

Learning Objectives

1. Define and use correctly the following terms: *Central Dogma, cell cycle, mitosis, template, DNA polymerase, semiconservative replication, replisome, primer, primase, helicase, topoisomerase, DNA ligase, ssDNA-binding protein, nuclease, DNA proofreading, exonuclease, chain catenation, leading strand, lagging strand, Okazaki fragment, replication fork, telomeres, telomerase, transcription, RNA polymerase, promoter, operator, operon, initiation, elongation, termination, transcription bubble, intron, exon, RNA splicing, spliceosome, alternative splicing, ribozyme, 5′-cap, poly(A) tail, translation, ribosome, codon, reading frame, anticodon, aminoacyl-tRNA, aminoacyl-tRNA synthetase, mutation, substitution, deletion, insertion, transition, transversion, nonsense mutation, silent mutation, mutagen, xeroderma pigmentosum,* and *reverse transcriptase*.
2. Describe the four stages of the cell cycle, relating each stage to protein and nucleic acid synthesis.
3. Explain why the DNA helix must be unwound for its faithful replication. Describe in general terms how the cell accomplishes this task.
4. Describe the structure of eukaryotic genes in terms of introns and exons.
5. Relate the sequence of telomeres to their structure and presumed biological function.
6. Review how DNA polymerase achieves high fidelity in DNA replication.
7. Describe the process of DNA replication, explain how it is semiconservative, and compare synthesis on leading and lagging strands.
8. Describe the process of transcription, including how RNA polymerase functions. Identify the roles of initiation and elongation factors. Describe the processing of a transcript to produce a mature mRNA.
9. Describe the process of translation, including how the ribosome functions. State the roles of tRNA and the tRNA synthetases in this process. Note the special role of fMet-tRNA^{fMet}.
10. Describe important structural features of the ribosome and of tRNA.
11. Describe what is meant by "degeneracy" in the genetic code, and give examples of it.

12. Describe how alternative splicing of a primary RNA transcript can produce different polypeptide chains from the same gene.
13. Compare the process of translation in eukaryotes to that in prokaryotes, noting similiarities and differences.
14. List the three basic types of mutation. Describe common causes of mutations in a gene. Relate these phenomena to errors made in DNA replication and to chemical damage to DNA.
15. List drugs that act to block action by DNA polymerase, by RNA polymerase, and by the ribosome.

Introduction

The Central Dogma

Although DNA is the central repository for genetic information in the cell, DNA itself does not directly regulate the synthesis of proteins (gene products). Instead, the information carried by DNA is copied into an intermediate form, RNA, which is then used as a template to direct the proper assembly of amino acids into the protein gene product. Nevertheless, DNA does act as a template for its own replication. These ideas are summarized in the Central Dogma of molecular biology, as shown in **Figure 16-1**. This chapter provides a brief introduction to the three processes shown in that figure—the replication of DNA, its transcription into the intermediate messenger RNA, and the translation of that message into a polypeptide chain. Additionally, the causes of genetic mutations are briefly covered. Because replication, transcription, and translation are all central life processes, any interruption of them is potentially life threatening. This relationship is the basis for the development of many antibiotic agents and anticancer agents, and this chapter provides a short introduction to the basis of action of the major classes of these agents.

Bacterial Cell Replication

In bacteria, DNA replication starts at a unique site on the chromosome, an origin of replication, which has a defined sequence of nucleotides. The bacterial replication machinery, involving a large set of proteins, recognizes the DNA sequence there and assembles at that point. The DNA is copied bidirectionally; that is, two DNA replication complexes are formed at the origin of replication, operating on different strands of the chromosome and moving away from each other (**Figure 16-2**).

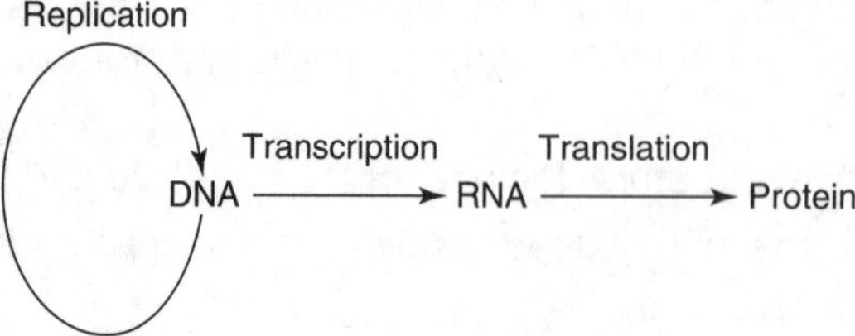

Figure 16-1 The Central Dogma of molecular biology: DNA is the primary genetic repository and directs its own replication; it is transcribed into RNA; messenger RNA is translated into a polypeptide gene product.

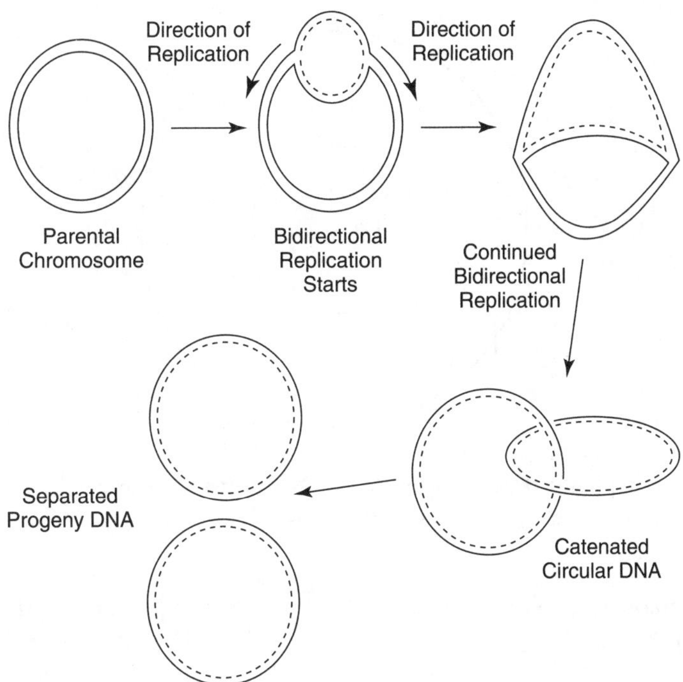

Figure 16-2 Bidirectional replication of DNA in a bacterial chromosome starts at an origin of replication and proceeds in two directions away from that origin. After both of the original DNA strands have been copied, the result is two interlocked (catenated) double-stranded DNA molecules, which are subsequently resolved into two separate daughter chromosomes.

After the bacterial chromosome has been replicated, the two new chromosomes begin to separate. A cell septum starts to form. The cell finally divides in two, with each half receiving one of the chromosome copies. Replication is complete.

In rapidly growing bacterial cells, DNA replication can be reinitiated before the previous round of chromosomal copying is complete. In this situation, cell division tends to lag behind DNA replication, and there is no necessary separation of distinct phases of polynucleotide and polypeptide biosynthesis, as there is for eukaryotic cells.

The Eukaryotic Cell Cycle

Eukaryotic cell replication is more complicated and subject to much more regulation than occurs in prokaryotic cells. In eukaryotes, cell replication follows a common pattern of four stages, called the *cell cycle* (**Figure 16-3**), with clearly defined phases of nucleic acid and protein biosynthesis.

- The cell cycle begins with the M phase. In this phase, the cell nucleus divides (*mitosis*) and extensive reorganization of the cell occurs, leading to division of the cell into two daughter cells, each with its own nucleus.
- Next comes the gap phase, denoted G_1, during which there is extensive synthesis of proteins and RNA, but not of DNA. Alternatively, mature and terminally differentiated cells may, after mitosis, pass to what is called the G_0 phase, with no further cell replication.
- After the G_1 phase, there is the S (synthesis) phase, during which cellular DNA is replicated; there is also substantial synthesis of RNA and protein in this phase.

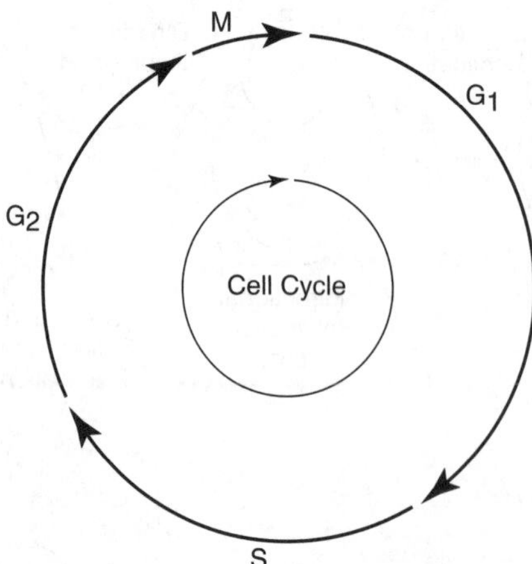

Figure 16-3 The four phases of the cell cycle. M = mitosis; G_1 = pre-DNA synthesis; S = DNA synthesis; G_2 = stage between DNA synthesis and mitosis.

- A second gap phase, G_2, follows, during which RNA and protein synthesis continues, but not DNA synthesis.

The cell is now prepared for another mitotic round of cellular division.

Cyclin-Dependent Kinases

A family of protein kinases controls the timing of the cell cycle. These kinases depend on association with a regulatory subunit, cyclin; hence they are called cyclin-dependent kinases (CDKs). They phosphorylate a large number of other proteins in the cell, thereby regulating their activity. Various CDKs are active at different times during the cell cycle, which is a key part of how the cell cycle phases are initiated or ended.

CDKs are themselves subject to regulation in several different ways.

- Association of the kinase subunit with the regulatory cyclin subunit is required to activate the kinase activity.
- Cyclin itself is subject to turnover and degradation in the cell, due to the timed activities of different proteases during the cell cycle.
- The rate of synthesis of both cyclin and the kinases is regulated. Binding of certain kinds of proteins (cytokines and growth factors) on the outside of the cell membrane can initiate signaling cascades that stimulate the synthesis of the CDKs as well as the transcription of genes for proteins involved in DNA synthesis.
- CDKs are regulated by cycles of phosphorylation and dephosphorylation at key residues. The phosphorylases and phosphatases that perform these actions are themselves responding to activity along cellular signaling pathways.
- Other proteins can specifically bind to and inhibit one or another of the CDKs. The activities of these inhibitory proteins may also depend on cell signaling pathway activities.

Key cellular targets acted on by CDKs include laminin and a subunit of the contractile protein myosin. Laminin is a protein that forms the filaments that help to maintain the structure of the cell nucleus. When phosphorylated by a CDK, the laminin filaments fall apart and the cell's nuclear envelope then breaks up. This action exposes the replicated DNA and allows the separation of sister chromatids as the cell begins to divide. During cell division, filaments of the contractile protein actin–myosin draw the cell contents toward two opposite ends of the parent cell; pairs of sister chromatids are separated in this way so that each daughter cell receives only one of the two copies of each chromosome. This contractile machinery must be shut down after finishing the segregation process. A CDK phosphorylates a subunit of myosin, causing myosin to dissociate from actin and halting the contraction exerted by actin–myosin. A later dephosphorylation by a phosphatase will reactivate myosin and permit actin–myosin filaments to reassemble; this step effectively recycles the filaments for a new cell division.

Clearly, this can be a very complicated business to unravel. Changes in activity among all these pathways and proteins may occur, depending on the stage of differentiation or development of the organism, its general state of health, and other factors.

Chromosomal Domains and DNA Replication

Eukaryotic cells, with their larger genomes, employ multiple sites along a given chromosome to start replication. In contrast, prokaryotes typically depend on a single origin of replication for their single chromosome. In eukaryotes, the genome can be divided into replication domains. A single domain may contain millions of base pairs, and each domain may contain one to perhaps several tens of origins of replication. Further, the replication of different domains may take place at different times; that is, some domains are consistently replicated early in S phase, whereas in others the DNA may be scheduled for duplication later in S phase. The timing here is connected, at least in some cases, to the activity of gene expression within the domain.

The origins for DNA replication for metazoans are not as well defined in terms of DNA sequence as they are for prokaryotes. The origins are not random, however, and their selection appears to depend on a number of factors, including the chromatin structure and histone acetylation, local supercoiling of the DNA, positioning of the DNA segment within the nucleus (eukaryotic chromosomes occupy distinct positions with the nucleus, and proximity to the nuclear periphery can affect both transcription and timing of replication), and transcription of nearby genes.

DNA Replication

For eukaryotic cells, DNA synthesis occurs during the S phase. In this phase, the cell must copy the entire genome and distribute copies to daughter cells. The key to faithful transmission of genes to progeny is the accurate replication of the genes—that is, of the cell's DNA. The DNA double helix, with its complementary strands, provides the necessary mechanism. The cell's general strategy is to use DNA as a *template* to direct the accurate synthesis of new DNA copies. Because DNA is double stranded, the cell needs to copy both strands; this activity is performed by *DNA polymerases*, along with accessory proteins. A special problem is the replication of DNA at the ends of chromosomes; special enzyme complexes must be used here.

Semiconservative DNA Replication

DNA replication is *semiconservative*. To ensure that the new strand contains the correct sequence of bases, the mechanism for DNA replication must unwind the original duplex to expose bases for pairing with incoming nucleotides in forming the new strands. The two strands in a parent DNA molecule are separated, and two new daughter strands are synthesized, one for each of the parent strands. The parent strand sequences are used to direct synthesis of the proper complementary sequence in the daughters; in other words, the parent strands are *template strands* in this process. The daughter duplexes thus contain one new strand and one old strand—this is what is meant by semiconservative replication. The top part of Figure 16-2 shows this process for a single bacterial chromosome, but the same general principles apply to the replication of eukaryotic chromosomes, albeit with replication proceeding from multiple points of origin on a single eukaryotic chromosome. In contrast, a "conservative" mechanism would give a daughter duplex, both of whose strands were wholly new.

Enzymes of DNA Replication

Cells not only replicate their genomic DNA, but also must repair copying errors and any damage to the DNA. The latter functions are performed by different species of DNA polymerase. These polymerases are typically large, multisubunit enzymes with a variety of enzymatic activities or functions, and they are assisted by a number of accessory proteins. **Table 16-1** compares the three principal enzymes from *E. coli* (other polymerases have been found in this bacterium, but these are the three main enzymes). Note the distinct biological roles for the three enzymes, and observe how they correlate with the catalytic properties of the respective enzymes. Eukaryotic cells likewise have a variety of DNA polymerases, which perform different functions in the cell. These eukaryotic polymerases are generally more complicated than their prokaryotic counterparts, having more subunits and accessory proteins.

For both prokaryotes and eukaryotes, DNA polymerases share a general structural plan but they differ in their details.

- The general structure is that of a right hand, with a "thumb," "palm," and "fingers."
- The thumb is involved in positioning the duplex DNA, and with translocation of the enzyme along the DNA.
- The fingers interact with the incoming dNTP and with the template DNA.
- The palm is where bond formation is catalyzed.

For DNA replication, the DNA polymerase is assisted by a number of accessory proteins that, together with the polymerase, form the *replisome*. These protein assistants include helicases, topoisomerases, single-stranded DNA binding proteins, primases, and ligases.

	Pol I	**Pol II**	**Pol III**
Main function	Erases primer and fills in gaps on lagging strand; DNA repair	DNA repair	Principal enzyme for DNA replication
Proofreading activity	Yes	Yes	Yes
$5' \rightarrow 3'$ Exonuclease activity	Yes	No	No
Polymerization rate (nucleotides/second)	16–20	40	250–1000
Processivity (nucleotides/enzyme dissociation)	3–200	1500	More than 500,000

Table 16-1 DNA Polymerases of *E. coli*

- *Helicases* are enzymes that unwind the DNA double helix into single-stranded regions. Because the helix is thermodynamically stable under conditions in vivo, unwinding calls for expenditure of free energy. Helicases use ATP hydrolysis as the source of this free energy.
- *Topoisomerases* act on the DNA to reduce the supercoiling stress caused by unwinding during replication.
- The exposed single-stranded DNA formed during replication is stabilized in that form by the binding of particular proteins with an affinity for single-stranded DNA, or *ssDNA-binding proteins*.
- *Primases* are enzymes that synthesize short RNA molecules (*primers*) that are complementary to the DNA sequence; these RNA primers form a short double-stranded region on which the DNA polymerase can start the polymerization process.
- *Ligases* are enzymes that repair broken covalent linkages ("nicks") on the phosphodiester backbone of DNA strands.

DNA polymerase acts on single-stranded DNA, but requires a short duplex region, containing a primer strand, to start polymerization. These primers are short oligonucleotides, approximately five nucleotides in length and complementary in sequence to the DNA. They have an exposed hydroxyl group at the 3′ end, onto which the polymerase will add a chain of nucleotides. In DNA replication, these primers are made of RNA, not DNA, and the enzyme that makes the RNA primer is called a primase. The RNA sequences are later digested by *nucleases* (enzymes that cleave the polynucleotide sugar–phosphate backbone), and are replaced by deoxynucleotides.

The polymerase complex acts processively: Once polymerization has started, the complex does not dissociate after each act of attaching a nucleotide. Instead, it stays attached to the template DNA and synthesizes a complementary new strand consisting of a few hundred nucleotides. Chain elongation by the complex is quite rapid. For example, a typical bacterial chromosome of 4×10^6 base pairs can be replicated in approximately 40 minutes. The rate of DNA synthesis in eukaryotic cells is much slower, however, perhaps by factor of 10 to 20.

DNA polymerases of course use deoxyribonucleotides to make new DNA.

- Addition is to the 3′-OH end of a growing strand (synthesis is thus said to be 5′-to-3′).
- The polymerase moves along the template strand in the 3′-to-5′ direction and "reads" it to determine the correct base to be added to the growing strand.
- The reaction on the growing strand is

$$(\text{DNA})_n + \text{dNTP} \rightarrow (\text{DNA})_{n+1} + \text{PP}_\text{i} \qquad (16\text{-}1)$$

The general mechanism for phosphoryl transfer is common to all nucleotide polymerases.

- The 3′-OH of the sugar on the primer strand is polarized and attacks the α-phosphoryl group of an incoming dNTP.
- DNA polymerases use two metal ions to help in catalysis. One of these enters with the incoming dNTP, bound to the triphosphate moiety; the other metal ion is held in the active site of enzyme, where it helps to polarize the 3′ hydroxyl group of the growing strand and promote its ionization for action as a nucleophile (**Figure 16-4**). The metal ions also may help to stabilize the structure and charge of the transition state, and they facilitate the departure of the pyrophosphate residue as it is displaced.

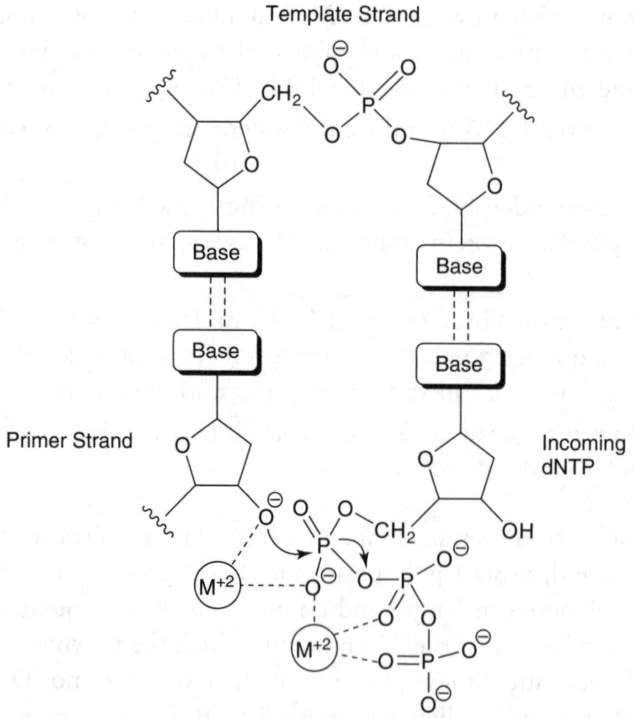

Figure 16-4 The nucleotide addition mechanism. Two metal ions are bound by the polymerase and are essential to catalysis.

- Hydrolysis of the pyrophosphate helps to drive the process, as do the hydrogen bonding of the newly incorporated nucleotide to its partner base on the template strand and the stacking of the new base pair at the end of the duplex.

The accuracy of the polymerase in incorporating the correct sequence of bases is high; DNA polymerases make approximately one mistake per 10^6 bases added. The sources of this fidelity include proper hydrogen bonding of complementary base pairs, and the proper geometric fit of the prospective new base pair in the active site of polymerase before the phosphodiester bond is formed. If the fit is wrong, then the dNTP is rejected and a new dNTP is inserted. It is possible, however, to "fool" the polymerase with base analogs that do not form hydrogen bonds but that do satisfy the geometric shape for a proper base pair; these analogs can be accepted by the polymerase and incorporated into the new DNA strand.

Further *proofreading* for errors in replication is performed by the *exonuclease* activity of the polymerase complex (an exonuclease hydrolyzes phosphodiester bonds at the end of a polynucleotide, and an *endonuclease* cleaves such bonds in the interior of a polynucleotide chain). If an incorrect nucleotide is incorporated, then before the next dNTP is added, the DNA polymerase complex reverses the reaction, cleaves the newly formed bond, releases the mismatched nucleotide, and reverts to its polymerization activity to synthesize more DNA. In addition, a separate enzyme system checks for errors after strand synthesis finished (the mismatch repair system). Altogether, this chain of error checks reduces the net error rate to approximately one in 10^9 bases.

Bacterial chromosomes are closed circular DNA duplexes. Bacterial chromosomal replication starts from a unique site on the bacterial chromosome and proceeds bidirectionally around the chromosome until the replication complexes meet at a termination site. After synthesis is

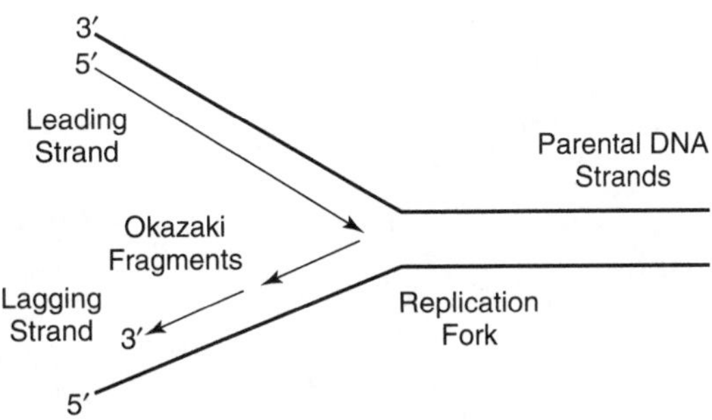

Figure 16-5 Schematic of a DNA replication fork, showing parental DNA strands (thick lines) and daughter strands (thin arrows). Arrowheads indicate the direction of synthesis for both leading and lagging strands. Synthesis is continuous on the leading strand, but discontinuous on the lagging strand, leading to so-called Okazaki fragments.

complete, the result is two circular chromosomes that are *catenated*, or joined like two chain links (Figure 16-2). The individual chains are covalently closed, so they cannot pass through one another. These catenated DNA circles are resolved by the action of a topoisomerase, and the two chromosomes are separated; later they will be partitioned into daughter cells during cell division. Eukaryotic chromosomes are much larger, and they have multiple sites where bidirectional DNA replication is initiated. Eukaryotic cells tightly coordinate DNA synthesis across these sites so that chromosomal replication occurs at a uniform time in the cell cycle.

At the point of DNA replication on a chromosome, the DNA structure resembles a fork with two tines (**Figure 16-5**), known as a *replication fork*.

- The replication complex synthesizes one of the two daughter strands in a continuous manner; this daughter strand is referred to as the *leading strand*.
- The other daughter strand (the *lagging strand*) is synthesized in a discontinuous manner, in runs of a few hundred to a few thousand nucleotides, called *Okazaki fragments*.
- Synthesis on both strands takes place in the 5′-to-3′ direction.
- The Okazaki fragments must later be joined covalently through the action of DNA ligase. This enzyme forms phosphodiester bonds at nicks in duplex DNA, between 3′-OH groups and 5′-phosphates. It uses ATP as the energy source for bond formation.

Telomeres

The ends of a linear eukaryotic chromosome pose a special problem for the cell in replicating the DNA (this is not a problem for prokaryotes, as their single chromosome is circular). An exposed chromosome end would be recognized as a break in a chromosome by cellular nucleases, and these enzymes would degrade the DNA. Alternatively, the cell might try to join the exposed ends of two chromosomes. In either case, genetic instability would result, possibly shortening the life of the cell. Furthermore, the regular DNA replication machinery of the cell will not function at the ends of DNA molecules. The solution to these problems is to create (and replicate) special DNA–protein complexes at the tips of chromosomes, to protect the chromosome.

Telomeres are the special DNA sequences and structures located at the ends of eukaryotic chromosomes. Their name derives from the Greek words *telos* (meaning "end") and *meros* (meaning "component"). Human telomeres have tandem repeats of a hexameric sequence, TTAGGG. One strand in the telomere is both longer than the other and richer in guanine

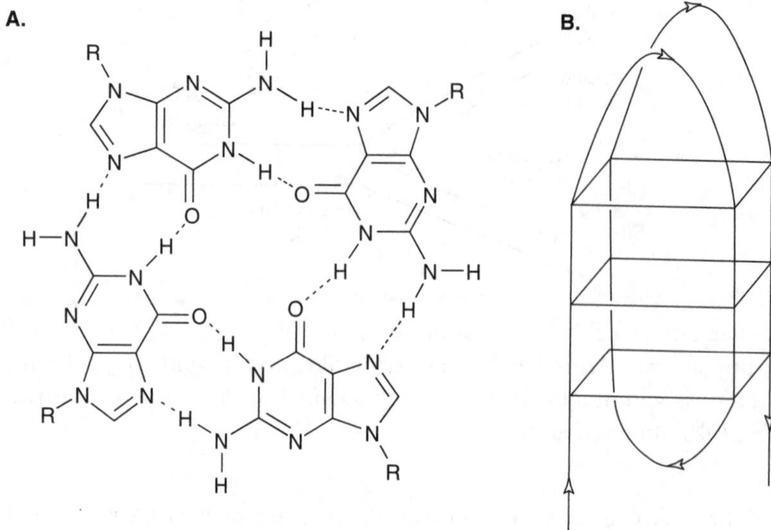

Figure 16-6 Telomere structure. **A.** Structure of a G-quadruplex, showing the pattern of hydrogen bonding. **B.** Possible strand folding, such as might be found in a telomere. Arrowheads indicate the direction of strand polarity; parallelograms indicate the three stacked G-quadruplexes contributing to this particular structure.

nucleotides. This strand loops back and pairs up with preceding DNA sequences in the same strand (**Figure 16-6**), forming stacked G-quadruplexes. G-quadruplexes are formed from four coplanar guanine bases, linked by hydrogen bonds. They can be stacked on top of one another, much as regular Watson–Crick base pairs are stacked.

The special structure of the telomere, with its stacked G-quadruplexes, makes it resistant to attack by nucleases in the cell. It also prevents end-joining of chromosomes. In these ways, telomeres protect the integrity of the chromosome.

Replication at telomeres is not performed by the usual replisome complex, but instead is carried out by a special enzyme, *telomerase*. This enzyme contains a template RNA strand that directs the synthesis of the telomere's hexameric repeated sequence. Telomerase can also add TTAGGG sequences to the ends of a chromosome where the telomere may have been eroded.

Transcription

What Is Transcription?

- *Transcription* is the process of synthesizing RNA molecules complementary to gene sequences on DNA.
- Transcription includes the synthesis of rRNA, tRNA, and mRNA.
- Transcription is carried out by RNA polymerases, with the aid of accessory proteins.

Transcription in Prokaryotes

In this section, we focus on the events leading to messenger RNA synthesis and set aside the synthesis of the various other molecules (e.g., tRNA, rRNA). In prokaryotes, a gene is transcribed directly into a messenger RNA, which can be read directly by a ribosome.

- Transcription starts at a DNA sequence called a *promoter* and proceeds in one direction along the duplex DNA ("downstream"); this direction, and hence which strand is copied

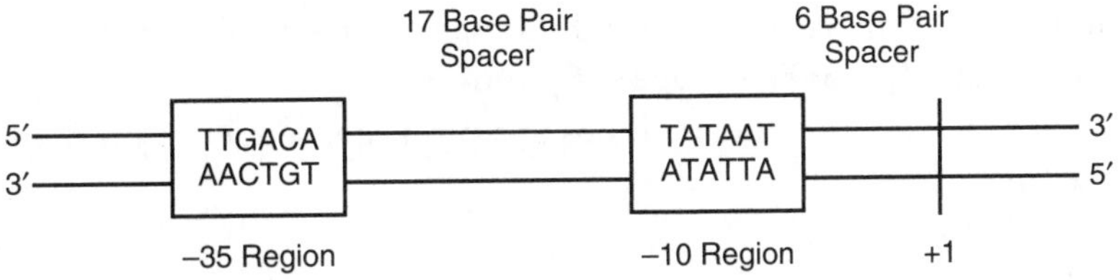

Figure 16-7 Consensus prokaryotic promoter structure, showing conserved sequences upstream (at −10 and −35) and nonconserved sequences separating these from each other and from the starting point of transcription (at +1).

into RNA, is specified by the sequence of the promoter. **Figure 16-7** shows the main sequence features of a typical bacterial promoter.

- A short distance downstream from the promoter, and perhaps overlapping in sequence with the promoter, will likely be a control site, an *operator*, where a regulatory protein (a repressor) can bind to DNA and inhibit the action of RNA polymerase.
- Additionally, DNA sequences may be found "upstream" of the promoter where other control proteins may bind to stimulate the action of RNA polymerase; these gene activation sites bind proteins called activators.
- Downstream from the promoter there may be only one gene or several genes (sequences coding for different polypeptides) that are separated by noncoding DNA sequences. When there is only one gene, the RNA polymerase forms a monocistronic transcript. When two or more such adjacent genes are present, the RNA polymerase will form a transcript of both the coding and noncoding sequences between them (a polycistronic transcript); the ribosomal machinery will read the transcript later to determine where to start polypeptide polymerization. The collection of activator binding site, promoter, operator, and downstream genes constitutes an *operon*.

Figure 16-8 summarizes these features of the DNA sequences in a typical bacterial operon.

RNA polymerase makes RNA chains by using DNA to specify the RNA base sequence. The general mechanism is like that for DNA polymerase—specifically, a nucleophilic attack by an activated hydroxyl group of a sugar (ribose), with displacement of pyrophosphate from a ribonucleotide triphosphate:

$$(\text{RNA})_n + \text{rNTP} \rightarrow (\text{RNA})_{n+1} + \text{PP}_\text{i} \tag{16-2}$$

The bacterial form of the polymerase is exemplified by that from *E. coli*. The enzyme has the subunit composition $\alpha_2\beta\beta'\omega(\sigma)$. The sigma ($\sigma$) subunit is responsible for recognizing and directing the polymerase to different promoter sequences on the DNA; it dissociates from the rest of the subunits after polymerization starts, so it is shown in parentheses to indicate its part-time

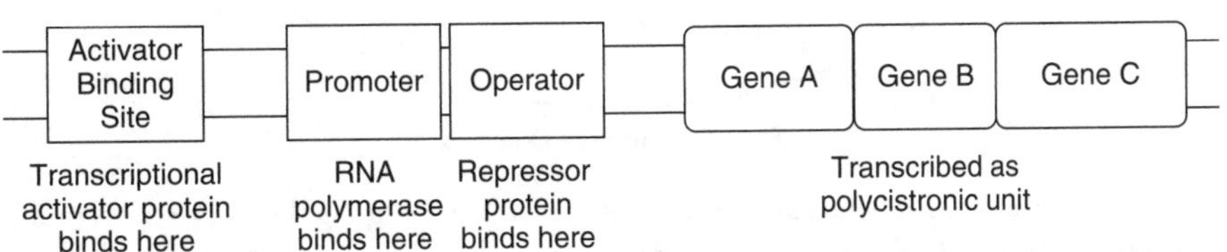

Figure 16-8 The structure of a bacterial operon, showing the locations of the promoter, the activator, and the start of the coding sequence for the gene product.

association with the rest of the enzyme. Several subtypes of the σ subunit exist, and the different types of σ have specificity for different types of promoters.

In the *initiation* phase, the polymerase binds at a promoter sequence on the DNA and starts RNA polymerization.

- First, the polymerase opens the double helix to form a transcription bubble. This action exposes the single-stranded DNA over a short region of about 17 base pairs (about 1.6 turns of the DNA helix).
- Inside this *transcription bubble*, the enzyme polymerizes a short RNA oligonucleotide of about eight bases, which pairs with an exposed single-stranded DNA to form a DNA–RNA hybrid duplex (**Figure 16-9**). This oligonucleotide itself does not code for any amino acids; coding sequences are located downstream from its position.
- No primer oligonucleotide is needed to initiate RNA synthesis.

After the transcription bubble is fully established, the *elongation* phase begins.

- The RNA polymerase ratchets down the template DNA strand, extending the complementary RNA chain. (Recall that the coding strand is the other DNA strand, which the RNA duplicates in sequence, except where U replaces T).
- The polymerase iteratively extends the transcription bubble, separating the downstream duplex DNA into exposed single strands, while the DNA duplex re-forms behind the bubble.
- The polymerase may occasionally pause, or halt polymerization, without dissociating from the DNA, but then resume polymerization. Pausing may be controlled partly by the folding of the extruded RNA into stem-loop structures of greater or lesser stability. If a very stable stem-loop structure is formed, the pausing may lead to a premature termination of polymerization, along with release of the polymerase and the (incomplete) transcript.
- RNA chain extension here is processive and relatively rapid (approximately 50 nucleotides per second), but it is more prone to errors than is DNA replication.

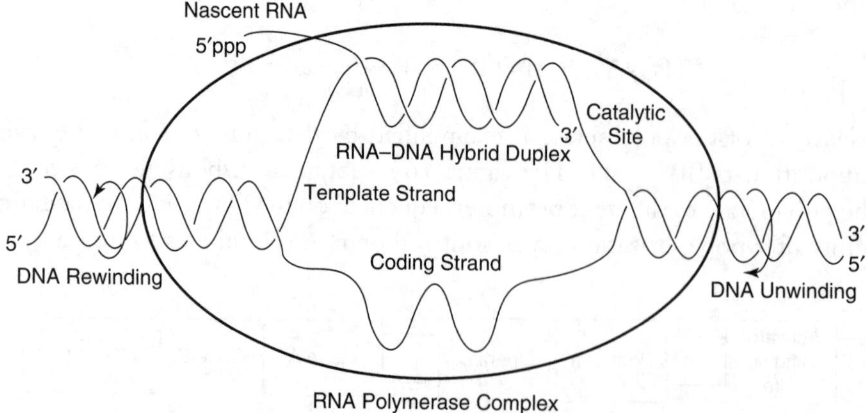

Figure 16-9 A schematic representation of a transcription bubble. As the RNA polymerase moves to the right, it unwinds the DNA; the DNA rewinds as it leaves the complex. A short RNA–DNA hybrid structure is formed as the RNA is polymerized at the catalytic site, and the nascent transcript is extruded from the complex.

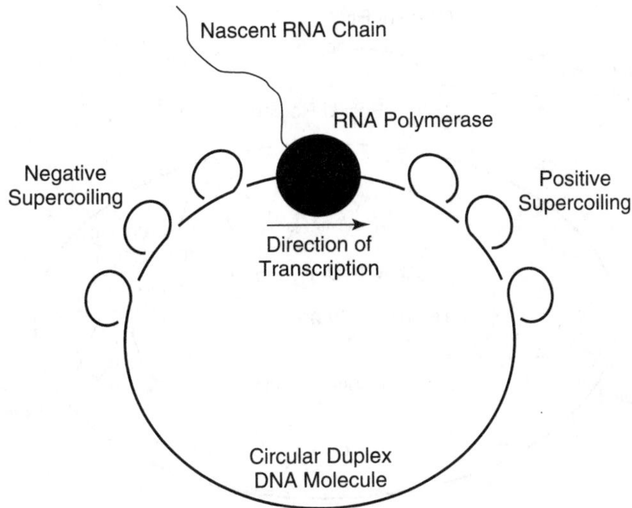

Figure 16-10 The unwinding and rewinding of DNA during transcription causes DNA supercoiling around the transcription bubble if the ends of the DNA are constrained. Here, that constraint is due to the closed circular DNA, but in the cell DNA-binding proteins may restrict DNA strand rotation and lead to DNA supercoiling.

The unwinding of the DNA helix during this process induces supercoiling in the DNA, with positive supercoiling appearing in front of the transcription complex, and negative supercoiling behind it (**Figure 16-10**). Topoisomerases promptly act to relieve the positive supercoiling stress, which, if allowed to accumulate, would inhibit the motion of the transcription complex.

RNA polymerase action terminates (*termination phase*) when certain sequences have been transcribed.

- In bacteria, the RNA transcript at such sites is typically a self-complementary palindrome with many possible G–C pairings, which folds into a hairpin; the RNA hairpin stem structure is characteristically followed by a run of four or more uridine residues (**Figure 16-11A**).
- The folding of the RNA transcript here is thought to disrupt the RNA–DNA pairing in the transcription bubble. It may also affect how the polymerase binds the RNA transcript.
- Depending on the details of the termination sequence, an accessory protein may help to bring the RNA polymerase to a halt (the ρ protein in bacteria; **Figure 16-11B**). This accessory protein uses ATP hydrolysis to destabilize the RNA–DNA hybrid duplex, causing the RNA polymerase to pause in the process of transcription.
- The polymerase and the RNA transcript then dissociate from the DNA, the transcript is released, and the RNA polymerase is free to begin another round of transcription.

Transcription in Eukaryotes

Eukaryotes contain three forms of RNA polymerase, denoted as RNA Pol I, Pol II, and Pol III. RNA Pol II is the enzyme mainly responsible for making mRNA; the other polymerases are responsible for synthesizing tRNA, rRNA, and a variety of smaller RNA species needed by the cell. Regardless, the basic RNA synthetic process is the same for prokaryotes and eukaryotes, and follows the same three stages: initiation, elongation, and termination. Note that these processes in eukaryotes take place in the cell nucleus; in prokaryotes, which lack a nucleus, transcription occurs in the cytosol. To keep our focus on mRNA synthesis leading to protein synthesis, we shall discuss only the behavior of RNA Pol II.

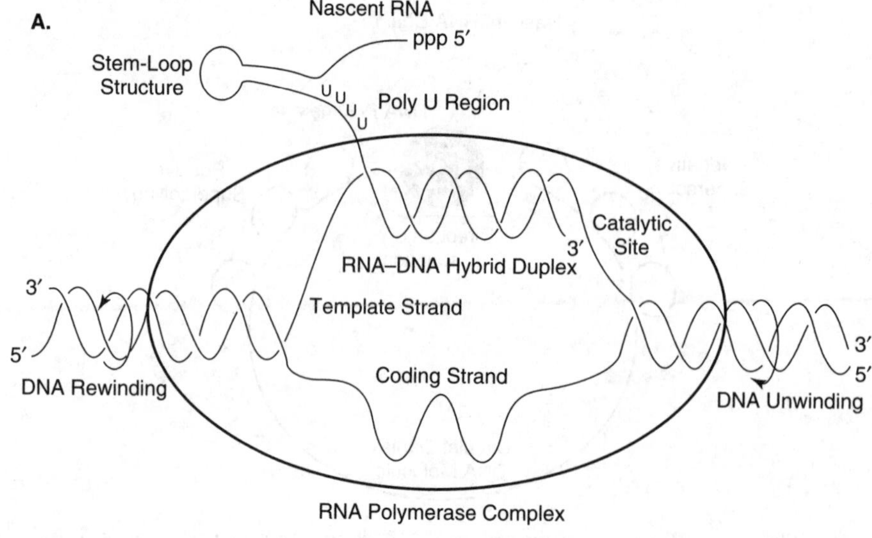

Figure 16-11 Transcription termination. **A.** Rho-independent termination occurs when the transcribed RNA folds into a stable stem-loop structure, followed by several uridyl residues that form less-stable hybrid base pairs with the DNA. **B.** Rho protein hydrolyzes ATP and destabilizes the RNA–DNA hybrid duplex during transcription, leading to termination.

As with prokaryotes, eukaryotic genes have promoters for the binding of the RNA polymerase. For RNA Pol II, these promoters have two common features, a so-called TATA box and an initiator (Inr) sequence (**Figure 16-12**). Unlike prokaryotic RNA polymerases, eukaryotic RNA polymerases typically do not have high affinity for the promoter sequence, although they do have a general nonspecific binding affinity for DNA. This nonspecific affinity is augmented by interaction of the polymerase with proteins that themselves do have relatively high site specificity in DNA binding. These auxiliary proteins bind to specific sites upstream and downstream of the promoter, and they help to hold the polymerase in proper position for the start of transcription. In this way, they help to stimulate or enhance transcription. The enhancer binding sites, however, may be separated from the promoter by quite long stretches of DNA.

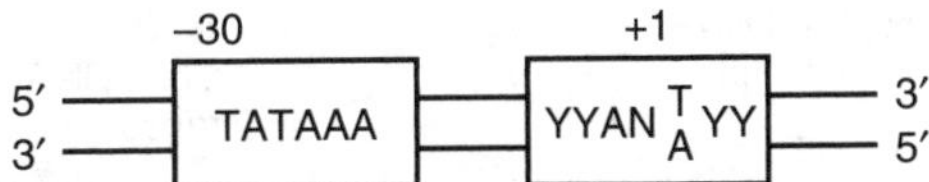

Figure 16-12 Features of a typical eukaryotic promoter sequence for RNA Pol II, showing the conserved TATA box at −30 relative to the starting point for RNA synthesis, and the initiator (Inr) sequence centered at +1, the starting point for RNA synthesis. Only the sequence of the "top" strand is shown, reading 5′ to 3′; here Y symbolizes a pyrimidine base (T or C), and N symbolizes any base (G, A, T, or C). This base is followed in sequence by either a T or an A.

Accessory proteins called transcription factors help Pol II to form an active transcription complex with DNA (e.g., helping to open the DNA helix so that it can be read). Another set of proteins, called elongation factors, suppress pausing by the polymerase and help coordinate post-transcriptional processing of the RNA. Additionally, a separate multisubunit assembly, known as the mediator complex, associates with RNA Pol II to convey regulatory information from activators and repressor proteins.

Complicating matters is the bundling of eukaryotic DNA into nucleosomes and the packing of nucleosomes into higher-order chromatin structures. The DNA must be unbundled to allow action by RNA polymerase. Covalent modification of the histone proteins in nucleosomes is an important factor in this unbundling, and hence plays a major role in regulating expression of a gene. For example, acetylation of histones at lysine residues tends to reduce the protein's affinity for DNA, making it easier to displace the nucleosome from a promoter or active gene sequence, thereby allowing for more frequent transcription of that gene. Eukaryotes have a complex system of enzymes for histone modification and remodeling of chromatin to enhance or reduce gene expression.

Transcript Processing

Unlike prokaryotic transcripts, eukaryotic transcripts can be extensively processed before they meet the ribosome.

- After transcription has terminated but before the transcript leaves the nucleus, the transcript receives special nucleotide sequences at the 3′ and 5′ ends.
- The 5′ end receives a *cap* of 7-methylguanine, attached through an unusual 5′-5′ triphosphate linkage (see Figure 4-17), and the last two ribose residues in the transcript may be methylated at the 2′-hydroxyl group.
- The 3′ end often carries a run of a few hundred adenylate residues, called a *poly(A) tail.*

These modifications protect the RNA transcript against attack by endogenous nucleases that might otherwise degrade the transcript. (Some bacterial mRNAs also have poly(A) tails, but these are not protective; instead, they mark the mRNA for rapid degradation.) The cap also helps to orient the transcript appropriately for ribosome binding, which facilitates translation of the mRNA.

Another difference from prokaryotes is that eukaryotes commonly have "split genes," where regions coding for protein sequences are interrupted by noncoding, intervening segments of DNA (see Figure 4-1). In prokaryotes, such intervening, noncoding sequences are very rare. The regions coding for protein are called *exons*, while the noncoding, intervening sequences are called *introns*. Not all eukaryotic genes have introns, but many do. Interestingly, the amount of DNA in the introns can greatly exceed the amount actually used for coding. The role of such introns in the control of gene expression is under active study.

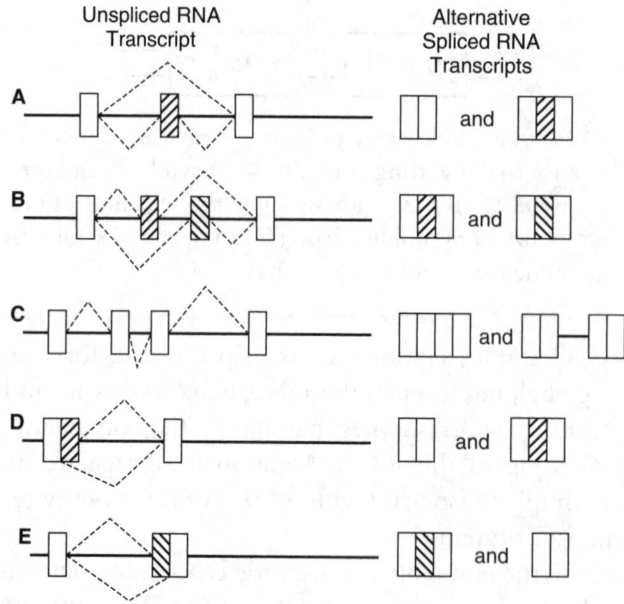

Figure 16-13 Examples of alternative mRNA splicing. The heavy line represents the primary RNA transcript; the dashed lines indicate introns that are removed by splicing. Open boxes represent exons that are expressed constitutively; shaded boxes represent alternative exons that may or may not be expressed. **A.** An alternative exon that may or may not be included in the mRNA. **B.** Mutually exclusive alternative exons. **C.** Retention of an intron in the mRNA. **D** and **E.** Alternative 5′ and 3′ splice sites generate different mRNA species.

To form a mature mRNA, the introns must be removed and the exons joined to give a continuous coding sequence for the ribosome to translate. The process of removing the introns is called *RNA splicing*. Some introns are self-splicing, meaning that they can cleave and re-form phosphodiester linkages without help from any protein. Most introns are not capable of self-splicing, however; for them, splicing is performed by a complex assembly of proteins and RNA, known as the *spliceosome*. The RNA molecules in this complex are small nuclear RNAs (snRNAs) of a few hundred nucleotides, which associate with polypeptide chains to form small nuclear ribonucleoproteins (snRNPs; pronounced "snurps").

Given a transcript containing multiple introns, it is possible that splicing at alternative sites could generate quite different final mature mRNAs; that is, *alternative splicing* of the transcript is possible. Multiple alternative splicing patterns could be possible on the same original RNA transcript, and **Figure 16-13** illustrates a few of the simpler possible scenarios. The resulting processed mRNAs would then specify polypeptides of different lengths and amino acid sequences. In this way, a single gene could lead to quite different gene products. Such processes in higher organisms play a major role in diversifying the proteins produced from a genome of a few tens of thousands of genes.

Translation

Translation is the overall process of synthesizing a polypeptide chain in a sequence specified by mRNA. It is carried out by the *ribosome*, and uses activated amino acids as the substrate for polymerization.

Codon Triplets Specify Amino Acids

The translation process reads the mRNA as blocks of three sequential nucleotides (a *codon*), which specifies a particular one of the 20 possible amino acids. Codons along the mRNA do not overlap. There are three possible *reading frames* for an RNA transcript because reading could start at any base; the correct reading frame is specified by an initiation codon, generally AUG.

There are 64 possible codons, resulting from the $4^3 = 64$ possible triplet combinations of the four "letters" of DNA (G, A, T, and C). Not all triplets are used to specify an amino acid; some are used as signals to indicate the starting point and the ending point of the polypeptide chain ("start" and "stop" codons). **Table 16-2** is a standard representation of the genetic code. Notice that many amino acids are specified by more than one codon; an example is leucine, which is specified by six different codons. For this reason, the genetic code is sometimes referred to as "degenerate." However, it is important that no codon specifies more than one amino acid. Thus there is no ambiguity about which amino acid is indicated at a particular codon in the mRNA.

The genetic code is nearly universal among living organisms. Some variations on the basic set of codons have been found in mitochondria and in some microorganisms, involving changes in which codon specifies which amino acid.

UUU	Phe	UCU	Ser	UAU	Tyr	UGU	Cys
UUC	Phe	UCC	Ser	UAC	Tyr	UGC	Cys
UUA	Leu	UCA	Ser	UAA	Stop	UGA	Stop
UUG	Leu	UCG	Ser	UAG	Stop	UGG	Trp
CUU	Leu	CCU	Pro	CAU	His	CGU	Arg
CUC	Leu	CCC	Pro	CAC	His	CGC	Arg
CUA	Leu	CCA	Pro	CAA	Gln	CGA	Arg
CUG	Leu	CCG	Pro	CAG	Gln	CGG	Arg
AUU	Ile	ACU	Thr	AAU	Asn	AGU	Ser
AUC	Ile	ACC	Thr	AAC	Asn	AGC	Ser
AUA	Ile	ACA	Thr	AAA	Lys	AGA	Arg
AUG	Met	ACG	Thr	AAG	Lys	AGG	Arg
GUU	Val	GCU	Ala	GAU	Asp	GGU	Gly
GUC	Val	GCC	Ala	GAC	Asp	GGC	Gly
GUA	Val	GCA	Ala	GAA	Glu	GGA	Gly
GUG	Val	GCG	Ala	GAG	Glu	GGG	Gly

Table 16-2 The Standard Genetic Code

AUG specifies the initial methionine residue that begins a polypeptide chain ("start") as well as any internal methionine residues. UAA, UGA, and UAG specify the end of a polypeptide chain ("stop").

tRNA Carries Activated Amino Acids for Polymerization into Polypeptide Chains

Formation of peptide bonds between amino acids is not a thermodynamically spontaneous reaction, and involves an appreciable activation energy. Therefore, amino acids must be activated in the cell before they can be polymerized into peptide chains. The activation has two steps, which are catalyzed by enzymes called *aminoacyl-tRNA synthetases.*

- The first step is formation of a mixed anhydride link between the carboxylate group of the amino acid and the phosphate group of AMP, giving an aminoacyl adenylate (**Figure 16-14A**) plus pyrophosphate.
- The second step, which occurs without dissociation of the aminoacyl adenylate from the enzyme, reacts this intermediate with the 3′-end of a tRNA molecule to form an *aminoacyl-tRNA*, a charged tRNA (**Figure 16-14B**). The charged tRNA serves as the substrate for polymerization by the ribosome into a polypeptide chain.
- The reactions can be summarized as follows:

$$\begin{aligned}\text{Aminoacid} + \text{ATP} &\rightarrow \text{Aminoacyl-AMP} + \text{PP}_i \\ \text{Aminoacyl-AMP} + \text{tRNA} &\rightarrow \text{Aminoacyl-tRNA} + \text{AMP}\end{aligned} \tag{16-3}$$

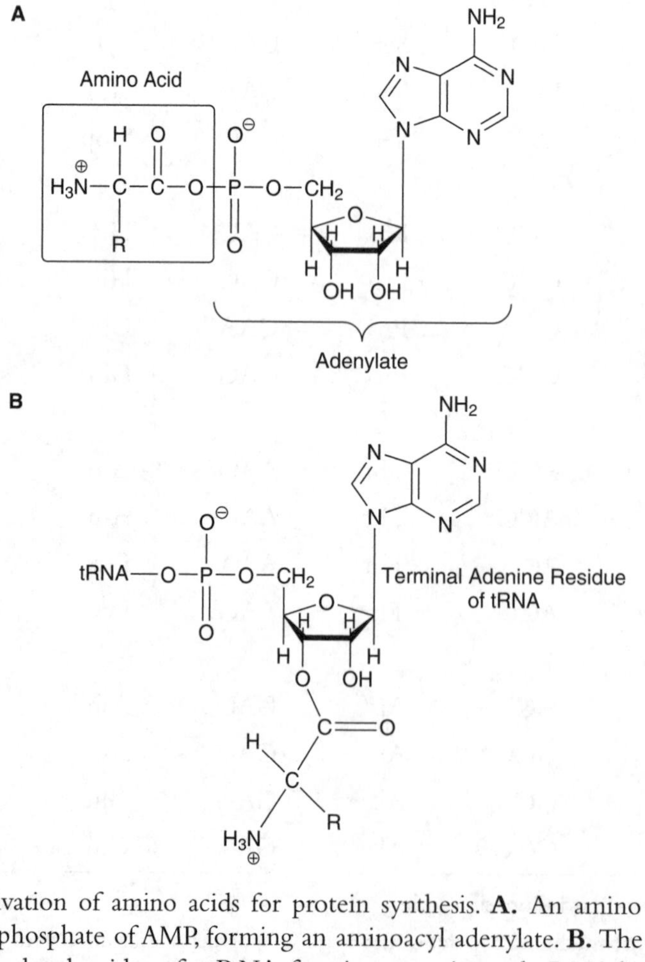

A

Amino Acid

Adenylate

B

Terminal Adenine Residue of tRNA

Figure 16-14 Activation of amino acids for protein synthesis. **A.** An amino acid is activated by attachment to the 5′ phosphate of AMP, forming an aminoacyl adenylate. **B.** The amino acid is transferred to the terminal adenyl residue of a tRNA, forming an aminoacyl–tRNA linkage.

- The aminoacyl link to the tRNA is at the CCA (3′) end of the tRNA and joins the amino acid's carboxyl group to a hydroxyl group of the terminal ribose.
- The net $\Delta G'^{\circ}$ for forming the aminoacyl-tRNA is close to zero, but the hydrolysis of pyrophosphate helps drive the reaction toward the product side.

Each of the 20 common amino acids is associated with one or more species of aminoacyl-tRNA synthetase, located in the cytosol, that perform this activation. The enzymes are quite specific in their amino acid preferences, coupling the correct amino acid to the correct tRNA with error rates of less than 1 in 10,000. This specificity, of course, greatly helps in maintaining the fidelity of the end product, the polypeptide chain, to the original DNA gene sequence coding for that chain.

To indicate the tRNA specific for a particular amino acid, a convention is used in which the three-letter abbreviation for proper amino acid is appended as a superscript. Thus the tRNA whose codon specifies valine would be named as tRNA^{Val}, while the tRNA for methionine would be named tRNA^{Met}. Furthermore, the charged tRNA species is named by placing the proper three-letter amino acid abbreviation in front; thus Val-tRNA^{Val} is a tRNA whose codon specifies valine, and which is charged with a valine residue at its 3′ end.

Ribosome Structure

The ribosome is a massive complex of proteins with RNA. In fact, approximately two-thirds of the mass of an intact ribosome is attributable to RNA; this is the origin of "ribo" in the term "ribosome."

- Ribosomal proteins are located mainly on the exterior surface of the ribosome, while RNA occupies the interior.
- Ribosomal RNA is folded into domains, with each domain containing a few hundred nucleotides. Domains are composed of A-type helices, many terminating in hairpin turns, and with bulges or loops of unequal numbers of bases that introduce bends into the helix.
- In addition to the usual Watson–Crick base pairings, there are many other base-to-base interactions, base–phosphate and base–sugar interactions, and interactions with ribosomal proteins, metal ions, and polyamines.
- Additionally, many of the nucleotides are modified. **Figure 16-15** shows the structures of some of the more common modified bases found in tRNA and rRNA.

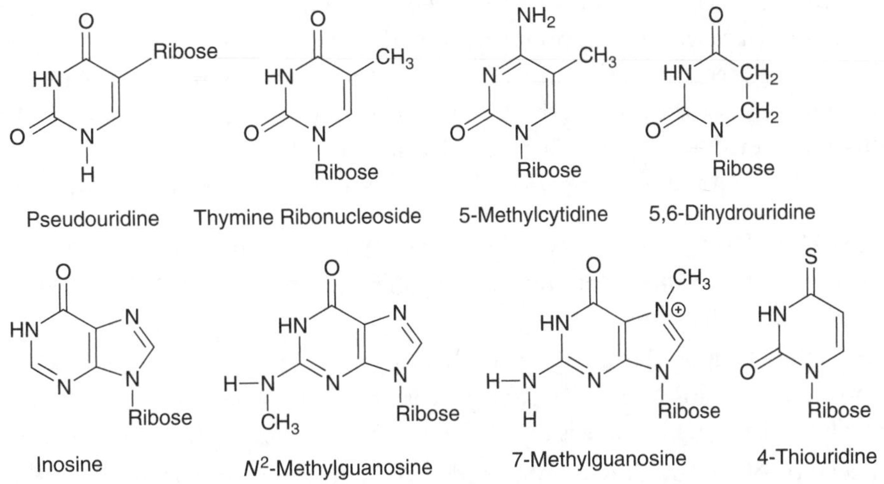

Pseudouridine | Thymine Ribonucleoside | 5-Methylcytidine | 5,6-Dihydrouridine

Inosine | N^2-Methylguanosine | 7-Methylguanosine | 4-Thiouridine

Figure 16-15 Structures of some of the most common modified bases found in tRNA and mRNA.

Macromolecular complexes such as the ribosome are often characterized by their sedimentation behavior during centrifugation.

- A quantity called the sedimentation coefficient measures this behavior and provides a rough measure of molecular weight. The sedimentation coefficient has units called Svedbergs (abbreviated S), after the scientist who developed the measurement method.
- The bacterial ribosome has a molecular weight of about 2.7×10^6 and a sedimentation coefficient of about 70S.
- The eukaryotic ribosome is larger, with a molecular weight of about 4.2×10^6 and a sedimentation coefficient of 80S.
- For both bacterial and eukaryotic ribosomes, two major ribosomal subunits are present, each with multiple polypeptide chains and distinct rRNA chains. In bacteria, the larger subunit has a sedimentation coefficient of 50S, and the smaller subunit a coefficient of 30S; it is common to use the shorthand notation of "50S subunit" or "30S subunit" to distinguish these assemblies. The corresponding eukaryotic subunits have sedimentation coefficients of 60S and 40S.
- In bacteria, the 50S subunit contains a 23S RNA and a 5S RNA, and the 30S subunit contains a 16S RNA. In eukaryotes, the large subunit contains three RNAs (28S, 5S, and 5.8S), and the small subunit contains a single 18S RNA.

Stages in Polypeptide Synthesis

In prokaryotes protein synthesis occurs in the cytosol, whereas in eukaryotes it takes place mainly on the outer face of the membranes of the endoplasmic reticulum. Protein synthesis occurs in three stages: initiation, elongation, and termination. For simplicity, we will concentrate on the process occurring in bacteria; the translation process in eukaryotes is much the same except for the initiation phase.

Polypeptide chain initiation starts with the binding of the mRNA to the smaller ribosomal subunit. The mRNA associates with the subunit's 16S rRNA using a purine-rich sequence upstream of the AUG start codon on the mRNA; it matches and pairs up with a complementary sequence on the 16S rRNA. This upstream sequence is referred to as a Shine–Dalgarno sequence, after the two scientists who discovered it.

There are three sites for binding tRNA on the bacterial ribosome: the A (aminoacyl) site, the P (peptidyl) site, and the E (exit) site. The A and P sites are formed from residues contributed by both the small and large ribosomal subunits, while the E site is primarily formed from residues on the large subunit. Because of the initial pairing of the mRNA with the 16S rRNA, the start codon of the mRNA is positioned at the P site. Recall that the anticodon loop of tRNA has an exposed single-stranded loop containing a nucleotide triplet that can pair with a codon triplet on the mRNA. Thus an initial charged tRNA binds the start codon on the mRNA.

- In bacteria, the start codon is usually AUG, specifying the amino acid methionine.
- In prokaryotes, the position of the initiation codon on the mRNA is indicated by an upstream Shine–Dalgarno sequence.
- In bacteria, the initiating tRNA is a specially charged tRNA carrying *N*-formylated methionine, known as fMet-tRNA^{fMet}. It pairs up with the initiating codon and is bound in the P site. (The formylated methionine is usually later removed from the finished polypeptide chain.)
- This special tRNA is the only one to bind initially to the P site; tRNAs that follow it will bind first to the A site.

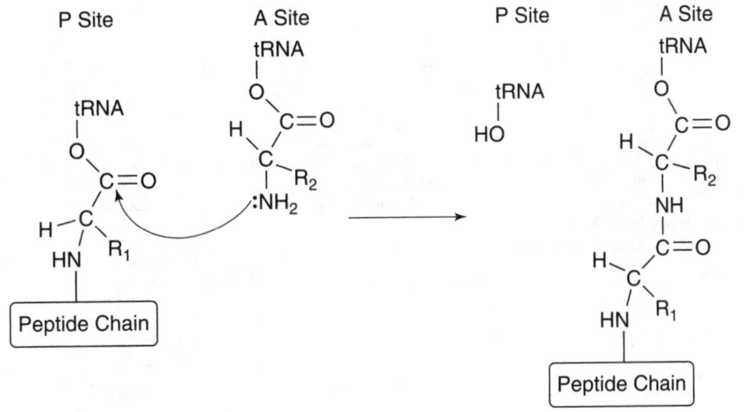

Figure 16-16 The mechanism of peptide bond formation, as performed by the ribosome.

Next, the large ribosomal subunit associates with the small subunit. This process, which is aided by proteins called initiation factors, requires GTP hydrolysis.

The elongation phase now commences with the uptake of a charged tRNA, at the A site. The anticodon of this charged tRNA matches the next codon on the mRNA. The amino acids are joined by attack of the amino group of amino acid held at the A site on the acylated tRNA in the P site. **Figure 16-16** shows the mechanism involved.

At this point in the synthesis process, the ribosme must remove the discharged tRNA, take up a freshly charged tRNA, and move down the messenger to the next codon.

- The discharged tRNA moves to the exit site. The growing polypeptide chain is now attached to the just-arrived tRNA.
- The mRNA ratchets along by one codon, and the acyl-tRNA shifts into the P site.
- Another charged tRNA enters the A site, and the reaction joining the amino acids is repeated.
- This cycle is repeated multiple times, with the ribosome reading successive codons on mRNA and extending the peptide chain by one amino acid unit at a time.

The peptide chain grows in the amino-to-carboxyl direction, and the ribosome reads the mRNA in 5′-to-3′ direction. The growing peptide chain is extruded from the ribosome through a "tunnel" in the large subunit.

This elongation process is assisted by proteins called elongation factors, which bind and deliver the charged tRNA molecules to the ribosome. Hydrolysis of GTP occurs as these charged tRNAs are transferred to the ribosome. Also, GTP hydrolysis occurs with translocation of the mRNA and the tRNAs across sites in the ribosome.

Figure 16-17 illustrates the process of starting a peptide chain, with a bacterial ribosome that is ready to start polymerization. In the figure, the ribosome has already bound the mRNA and has the fMet-tRNA^{fMet} at the P site. Another charged tRNA is taken up in the A site, and a peptide bond is formed. The tRNA and mRNA molecules shift their positions on the ribosome, leading to release of the discharged tRNA and the uptake of the next charged tRNA.

The process continues until finally a termination codon on the mRNA is reached; no amino acids are incorporated beyond this stopping point. Three codons are used for termination (UAA, UGA, and UAG), and there are no tRNAs with anticodons for these three. Instead, the proteins RF1 and RF2 (release factors 1 and 2) recognize these codons, bind there, and

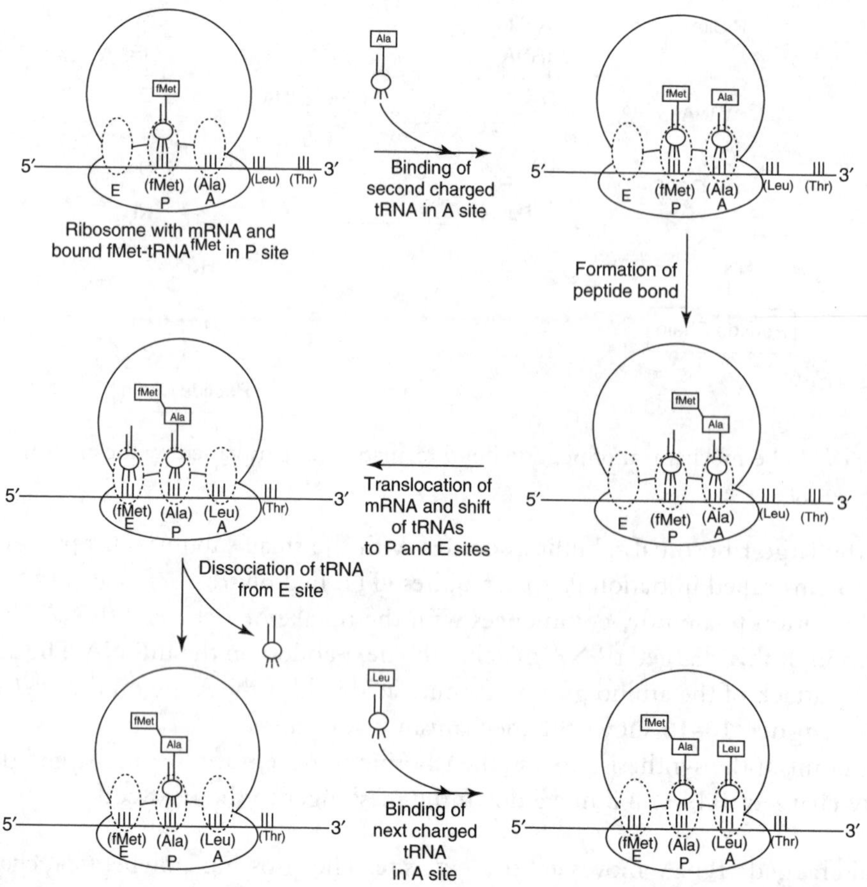

Figure 16-17 Movement of mRNA and tRNA molecules across the A, P, and E sites on the ribosome.

promote hydrolysis of the peptidyl-tRNA link, leading to release of the peptide chain. They are assisted in this task by another protein, RF3. The ribosome now dissociates into its small and large subunits, and the mRNA and tRNA molecules dissociate, assisted by yet more protein factors. At this point, the subunits can reassemble into a new functional ribosomal complex.

Processing of the new polypeptide chain then follows. This step may entail proper folding of the chain and covalent modification by chain cleavage or attachment of sugars, or phosphoryl, acetyl, or other groups. **Figure 16-18** summarizes the entire process for a bacterial ribosome; the process is rather more complicated for eukaryotic cells, as discussed in the next subsection.

The mRNA may demonstrate considerable secondary and tertiary folding structure. Such regions in the untranslated regions at the 5′ and 3′ ends of the molecule can, in turn, play a role in regulating the process of protein synthesis. If these regions remain structured, a substantial loss in efficiency of translation of the message may occur due to difficulties in having proteins recognize the appropriate sequences in single-stranded RNA versus paired and folded RNA; in addition, the energetic cost of unfolding such (presumably) stable structures can exact a toll on efficiency.

Lastly, a single mRNA may simultaneously undergo translation by several ribosomes. The assembly of multiple ribosomes on a single mRNA is referred to as a polysome. Polysomes are found in both prokaryotes and eukaryotes. Such usage of a single messenger molecule by several ribosomes at the same time will, of course, increase the overall rate of translation.

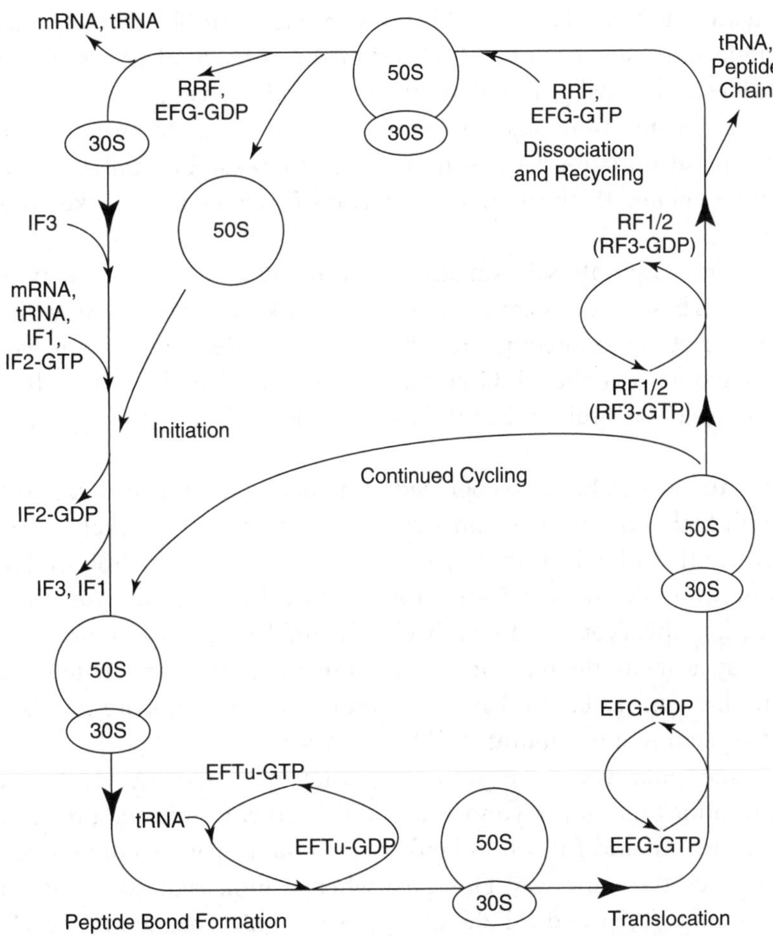

Figure 16-18 Ribosomal cycling through the stages of initiation, peptide bond formation, translocation of the ribosome along the mRNA, and finally dissociation and re-association of the 30S and 50S subunits.

Comparing Prokaryotic and Eukaryotic Translation

While both prokaryotic and eukaryotic ribosomes are assembled from two large subunits, the size and composition of the respective subunits, and hence of the ribosomes, are different. The eukaryotic subunits and assembled ribosome are larger; the eukaryotic 80S ribosome is assembled from 40S and 60S subunits, and the bacterial 70S ribosome is made up of 30S and 50S subunits. These subunits also differ in the associated ribosomal RNAs, both in numbers and in their sizes, as discussed earlier.

The start codon for both prokaryotes and eukaryotes is typically AUG (specifying methionine); much less frequently used are GUG and UUG (specifying valine and leucine, respectively). Prokaryotes have a special sequence (the Shine–Dalgarno sequence) on the mRNA that specifies the position of the initiating codon, and a prokaryotic mRNA may contain one or several such points of initiation of protein synthesis. For chain initiation, eukaryotes use the AUG codon nearest the 5′ end of the mRNA.

Bacteria start protein synthesis with incorporation of a formylated methionine residue (fMet), carried by a special tRNA. In protein synthesis at the endoplasmic reticulum in eukaryotes, the formylated amino acid is not required, but the first amino acid incorporated into a nascent polypeptide chain will still be methionine, which is carried by a special initiating tRNA. This initiating tRNA ($tRNA_i$) differs from a related tRNA that also carries a charged methionine residue and reads the same AUG codon; this latter tRNA is used for incorporating methionine residues at internal points along the polypeptide chain.

Eukaryotes have many more auxiliary proteins to help initiate protein synthesis than do prokaryotes. At least 14 initiation factors are involved in eukaryotic initiation, some of which are multisubunit assemblies. In contrast, the bacterium *E. coli* seems to make do with just three initiation factors.

The mature eukaryotic mRNA contains a 5′ cap and a 3′ poly(A) tail, which are added in the cell's nucleus. These features are not present on prokaryotic mRNAs, which are released, ready for use by a ribosome, directly after their synthesis. Because the eukaryotic ribosome will start protein synthesis at the AUG codon nearest the 5′ end of the mRNA, it is quite important that the cell mark this end of the message distinctively—the cap structure provides such a marker.

The cap structure is specifically recognized by a eukaryotic initiation factor (eIF-4E). This protein binds with high affinity there and serves as an orientation marker for another protein (eIF-4A) to unwind the folded structures, at the expense of ATP hydrolysis. The poly(A) tail region is also bound by the same eIF-4E protein, aided by other accessory proteins. Thus a mRNA molecule in a eukaryote is effectively circular, unlike the linear message in a prokaryote. This difference may facilitate the recycling of ribosomes that have terminated translation: On a circular template they can readily find another start codon and reinitiate translation, instead of dissociating and separating into subunits and free mRNA.

Prokaryotes and eukaryotes are similar in their requirements and mechanisms for polypeptide elongation and for termination of the polymerization. Prokaryotes use two elongation factors, EF-Tu and EF-Ts, and eukaryotic counterparts to these two proteins exist that function in much the same way. However, whereas prokaryotes use two protein factors to terminate translation (RF1 and RF2), eukaryotes use only one, denoted eRF1 (eukaryotic release factor 1).

Eukaryotic cells need to direct proteins to a variety of cellular locations, while in a bacterium the choices are basically twofold: the cytosol or the cell membrane. Eukaryotes use signaling sequences on the nascent peptide chains as they are synthesized at the endoplasmic reticulum for this purpose, to help direct their processing. Proteins that are to be released to the cytosol can, of course, be synthesized by a free cytosolic ribosome and released directly into the cytosol. Proteins that must be embedded in a membrane, or that must be passed through the cell membrane to an extracellular site, will contain a special sequence to help direct this process.

For this latter set of proteins, the ribosome starts translation, but halts this process temporarily as it moves to dock with the endoplasmic reticulum (ER). There protein synthesis resumes, but the polypeptide chain is extruded into the lumen of the ER. This temporary halt and redirection of synthesis involves attachment of a signal-recognition particle (SRP) to a particular kind of amino acid sequence on the nascent polypeptide chain. This amino acid sequence consists of 9 to 12 amino acids whose side chains are characteristically hydrophobic, but that occasionally have some positively charged side chains (e.g., lysine residues). The SRP acts as an escort, guiding the ribosome to the ER ("guiding" is perhaps an overstatement—the process apparently relies on random diffusion). When bound to the ribosome, the SRP also blocks the action of an elongation factor, which is why protein synthesis is temporarily interrupted.

At the ER, the SRP guides the ribosome to a particular receptor, an integral membrane protein that helps the ribosome to associate with another set of integral membrane proteins.

This latter set of proteins forms a channel through the ER membrane, and the nascent polypeptide chain from the ribosome is directed into the channel. Protein synthesis then resumes, with the protein chain now appearing in the ER lumen, where it folds and undergoes appropriate modifications. Transport vesicles then bud off the ER and carry the proteins to the Golgi apparatus for further processing, or to other compartments in the cell, or to the plasma membrane for release to the cell's exterior.

Mutations

Different Types of Mutations

A mutation is an inheritable change or variation in a gene—that is, a change in the DNA nucleotide sequence of a gene. Three basic types of mutations are distinguished: substitution, deletion, and insertion (**Figure 16-19**).

- A *substitution* occurs when one base (or base pair) in a gene is replaced by another.
- A *deletion* is a loss of one or more base pairs in a gene.
- An *insertion* arises when there is introduction of one or more base pairs into the sequence of a gene.

Insertions and deletions may be introduced by the replication complex when a short run of bases around the replication fork forms a single-stranded loop and the bases are left unpaired, on either the template or the growing strand. If the template strand forms the loop, the result is a deletion mutation; if the growing strand forms the loop, the result is an insertion mutation. This type of mutation tends to occur in regions of the DNA containing runs of identical bases, where the looping strand can rejoin the duplex with normal base pairing. Large deletions or insertions, or rearrangements of gene sequences, are usually the result of genetic recombination systems acting aberrantly.

Mutation by substitution is the most common type of mutation, and there are two types of these mutations (**Figure 16-20**). A *transition* occurs when a purine is replaced by another purine (or a pyridine by the other pyridine). A *transversion* occurs when a purine is replaced by a pyrimidine, or vice versa. For example, deamination of cytosine yields the base uracil, which will pair with adenine and so be "read" as thymine; this would be a transition mutation. As

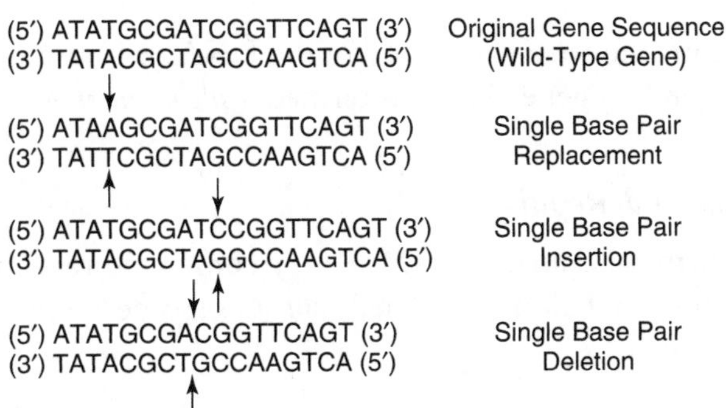

Figure 16-19 The three types of DNA mutation, shown as single base pair changes: substitution, insertion, and deletion.

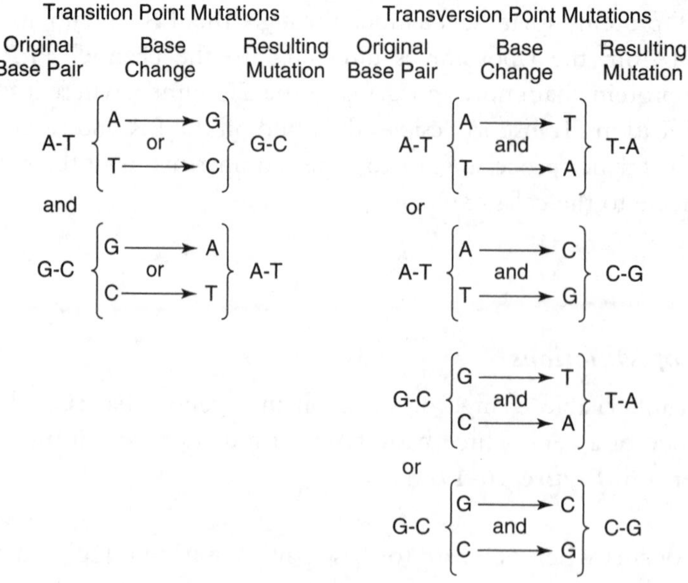

Figure 16-20 Transition and transversion mutations.

another example, deamination of adenine yields hypoxanthine, which pairs with guanine and so is "read" as a cytosine; this would be a transversion mutation.

- Base replacements sometimes have no effect on the protein synthesized, due to the degeneracy of the genetic code. In this case, the replacement of a base may simply give an alternative codon specifying the same amino acid.
- An alteration to a codon may sometimes lead to an entirely different amino acid being specified, which might well change the properties of the resulting polypeptide (e.g., change the folding pattern of the protein, alter an enzyme's affinity for substrate or inhibitors, block the addition of a prosthetic group).
- A mutation may yield a stop codon and a truncated transcript; these are termed *nonsense mutations*. Such a change could obviously have a drastic effect on the properties of the resulting polypeptide.
- Mutations in control sequences, such as promoters or operators, may interfere with the overall level of expression of a gene. Mutations around the boundaries between introns and exons can affect how the transcript is spliced and, therefore, change the type of protein synthesized.
- If the mutation lies in a nonessential region of the DNA or if it results in no change in the expression or function of a gene, then it is termed a *silent mutation*.

Mutagens, Mutations, and Repair

Chemical and photochemical damage to DNA is a constant threat to the integrity of the genome. Agents that cause mutations are called *mutagens*. Some typical types of spontaneous damage are highlighted here:

- Oxidation of guanine, yielding 8-oxoguanine, which mispairs with adenine, leading to a transversion mutation (**Figure 16-21**)

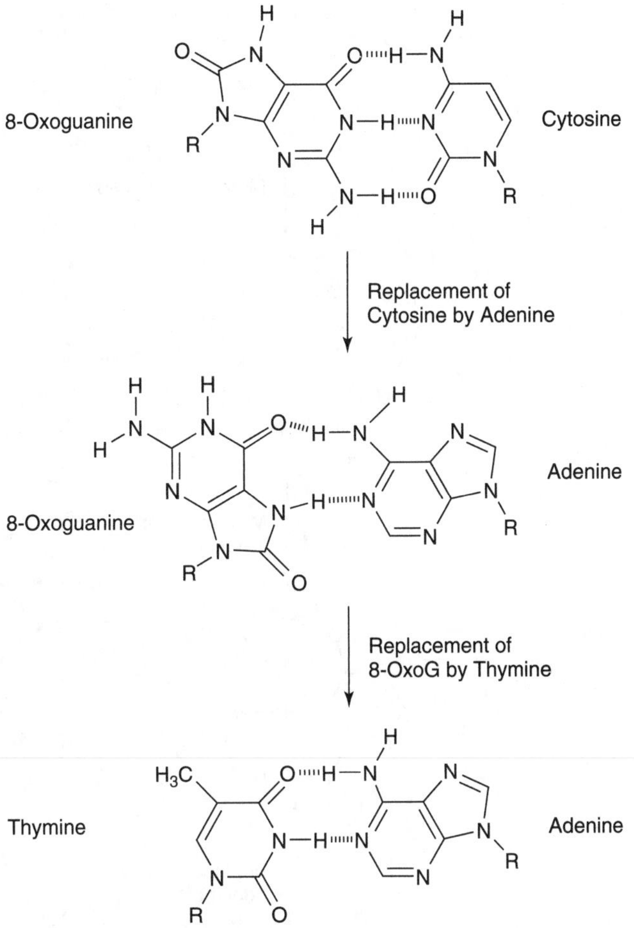

8-Oxoguanine — Cytosine

Replacement of Cytosine by Adenine

8-Oxoguanine — Adenine

Replacement of 8-OxoG by Thymine

Thymine — Adenine

Figure 16-21 Oxidation of a guanine residue, forming 8-oxoguanine, can lead to a transversion mutation, where a G-C base pair is replaced by a T-A pair.

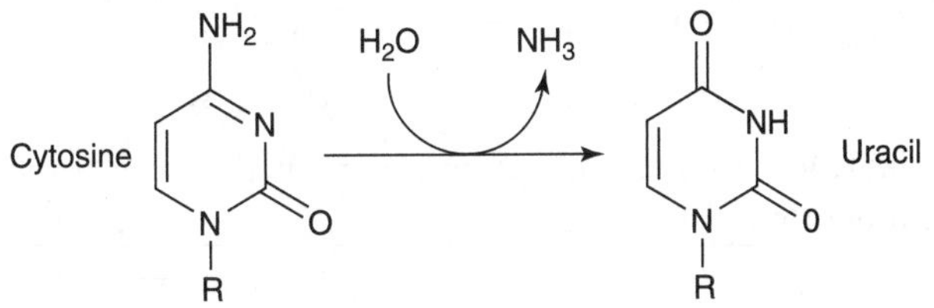

Cytosine $\xrightarrow{H_2O \quad NH_3}$ Uracil

Figure 16-22 Deamination of cytosine leads to uracil, which can pair with adenine and cause a transition mutation.

- Deamination of cytosine, adenine, or guanine (by, for example, nitrous acid or HNO_2, or as generated from nitrosamines), leading to mutations (**Figure 16-22**)
- Attack by alkylating agents on the bases, leading to incorrect base pairs (e.g., formation of O-6-methylguanine, which mispairs with thymine, leading to a G-C to A-T transition mutation; see **Figure 16-23**)
- Dimerization of adjacent pyrimidine residues by ultraviolet rays, forming a cyclobutane ring that cross-links the bases and that blocks replication and transcription (**Figure 16-24**)

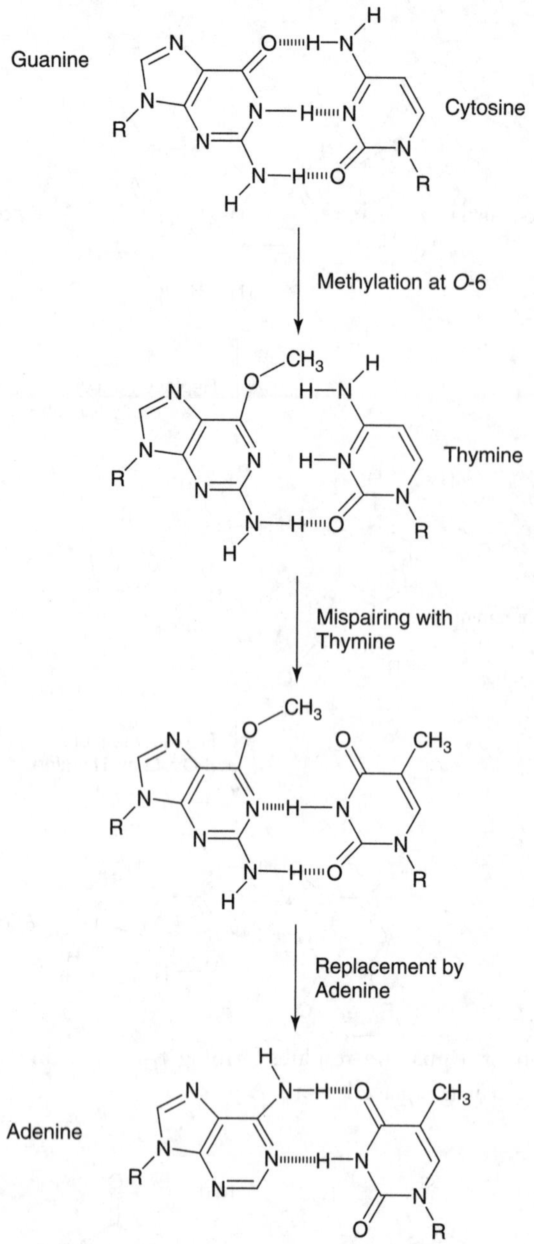

Figure 16-23 DNA alkylation can cause mutations. Here, methylation at the O-6 of guanine causes a G-C to A-T transition mutation.

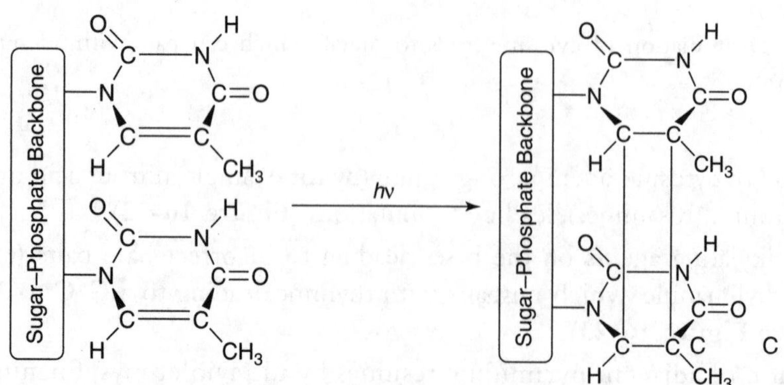

Figure 16-24 Ultraviolet radiation can cross-link two thymine residues on the same strand, thereby blocking replication or gene expression.

Additionally, cleavage of the *N*-glycosyl linkage may lead to release of the base even as the backbone remains intact (a so-called apurinic/apyrimidinic [AP] site). In addition, single- or double-strand breaks may be caused by ionizing radiation such as X-rays or the emissions from radioactive elements.

The cell has several systems to carefully repair damaged DNA: mismatch repair, base-excision repair, nucleotide-excision repair, and direct repair.

- Direct repair systems act on modified bases, such the pyrimidine photodimers produced by ultraviolet light, to restore the original base structures while the bases are still attached to the DNA strand. Other direct repair systems can remove methyl groups from methylated bases such as *O*-6-methylguanine (carried out by the *O*-6-methylguanine-DNA methyl-transferase), or 1-methyladenine and 3-methylcytosine (repair performed here by the AlkB protein).
- The excision repair systems remove damaged bases or nucleotides and replace them with new bases or nucleotides. The replacement may actually extend over several residues or even tens of residues to either side of the original DNA lesion.

Mismatch repair is rather special, in that there is no obvious chemical lesion on the bases or the backbone, so it is not clear which strand has incorporated the incorrect base. The question is resolved by enzymatic systems that detect the state of methylation of the strands. Shortly after a strand is replicated, methyl transferase enzymes act on selected bases to attach methyl groups, and the methylation does not appreciably affect proper base pairing. The parent strand has already been methylated during the previous cell cycle, but the daughter strand, being newly synthesized, is not yet methylated. The repair system senses the unmethylated state of the daughter strand and acts on it—not on the (correctly synthesized) parent strand—to replace the mismatched base (actually, a wide swath of hundreds or thousands of nucleotides are repolymerized by the enzyme system).

In *E. coli*, the main methylation system (the Dam methylase) acts on GATC sequences to methylate the adenine residue at the N-6 position. GATC sequences occur sufficiently frequently that, when methylated, they provide a reliable marker for the parent strand.

In mammalian systems, the DNA methylation is specific to cytosine bases in CpG dinucleotide sequences (**Figure 16-25**). This dinucleotide sequence tends to cluster in short

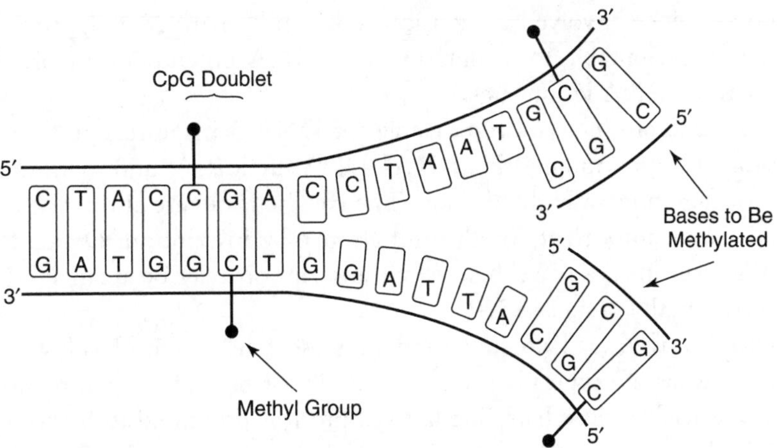

Figure 16-25 DNA methylation at CpG doublets helps to identify strands in mismatch repair.

stretches of DNA, 400 to 500 base pairs in length, that are called CpG islands. These islands are frequently found in the promoter regions of genes. In normal cells, the islands tend not to be methylated. Those in cancer cells are often hypermethylated, however, and it is thought that this hypermethylation is connected with the aberrant gene silencing often found in tumor cells.

Additional repair systems deal with the extensive DNA damage that arises from ionizing radiation or heavy oxidative attacks, causing double-strand breaks or covalent cross-links that join two strands. These repair systems attempt to synthesize DNA past the damaged region, but the polymerase activities here are much more prone to errors than is the regular replicative complex. There is a trade-off here: While the repair may introduce errors, the lack of repair would likely lead to cell death. To deal with this issue, evolution has opted for toleration of a certain low level of mistakes.

Defective DNA Repair Can Lead to Cancer or Other Diseases

DNA repair is obviously of high importance, and mutations in genes responsible for the repair systems would present a serious challenge to the cell or organism. Indeed, certain types of cancer are closely connected to defects in one or another of these repair systems. For example, defects in mismatch repair have been associated with a certain type of colon cancer (hereditary nonpolyposis colon cancer), and defects in recombinational repair (which can involve large insertions or deletions) have been associated with certain types of breast cancer. One of the best-characterized repair defects results in the disease xeroderma pigmentosum.

Clinical Application

Xeroderma pigmentosum (XP) is a genetic disorder caused by a defect in the excision repair system for ultraviolet damage to DNA. Skin cancer is a common consequence in this disease, and there is evidence for an increased incidence of internal tumors as well. Neurological abnormalities are also associated with XP, perhaps due to the relatively high rate of oxidative metabolism in nerve tissue leading to oxidative DNA damage.

The disease is genetically complex. Seven genetic groups are distinguished by the loss of function of one or another member of the excision repair system (there are seven different gene products involved in excision repair in humans). An eighth variant form of the disease is attributable to a mutation in a DNA polymerase involved in DNA synthesis across the DNA lesion sites.

Three XP gene products are responsible for DNA damage recognition, two more are responsible for unwinding the DNA (DNA helicases), and two nucleases are responsible for digesting away the damage. The two helicases are also involved in a basal transcription factor, important for the initiation of transcription. Depending on the particular mutation in these two helicases, transcription may be unaffected but repair would be deficient; this results in XP.

If transcription is instead affected, then a disease called trichothiodystrophy results. Patients with this disease typically show growth abnormalities, mental retardation, and, most characteristically, brittle hair. The last symptom is presumed to be connected to a transcriptional deficiency in the synthesis of sulfur-rich proteins found in hair.

Antimicrobial Agents

The fundamental life processes of DNA replication, gene transcription, and polypeptide synthesis are common to all life forms. Any interference with these processes will have severe consequences for the viability of a cell or organism; thus drugs that introduce such interference are extremely powerful agents. The discovery and application in medicine of drugs that will selectively act on pathogenic microorganisms has been one of the triumphs of modern medical science. The selectivity of these antibiotics is ultimately due to differences in target structure between mammals and the pathogenic microorganisms (or, in some cases, to the existence of a unique but essential protein target present in the pathogen but not in mammals). This section provides a brief survey of antibiotic action on the three fundamental life processes.

DNA Polymerase Inhibitors

Certain viruses encode their own DNA polymerase for replication (for example, herpes viruses), and inhibition of this polymerase will interrupt the viral life cycle and block the viral infection. Acyclovir is a representative example of the class of inhibitors developed for such a purpose.

- Acyclovir is an analog of guanosine, but the carbohydrate ring here is now acyclic (**Figure 16-26**).
- To be active, acyclovir must be phosphorylated inside the host cell. The compound is monophosphorylated by a viral thymidine kinase, then converted to the triphosphate by host cell enzymes. The phosphorylated form then competes with dGTP for incorporation into DNA; the compound is selective for the viral DNA polymerase.
- Acyclovir lacks a 3′-OH group, so if it is incorporated, the DNA chain cannot be extended beyond this residue. This constraint causes premature chain termination during DNA replication, thereby blocking viral replication.

Reverse Transcriptase Inhibitors

Retroviruses, such as the human immunodeficiency virus (HIV), are a class of viruses whose viral particles carry RNA, not DNA. In a retrovirus, the viral particle generally carries one or more copies of an RNA-dependent DNA polymerase, or *reverse transcriptase.*

- The enzyme, which is essential to the life cycle of the retrovirus, first synthesizes a DNA strand complementary to the viral RNA, forming a DNA–RNA hybrid duplex.

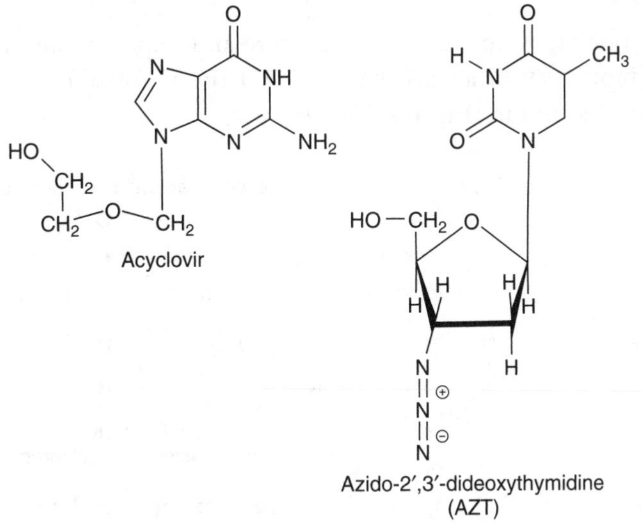

Acyclovir

Azido-2′,3′-dideoxythymidine (AZT)

Figure 16-26 Inhibitors of DNA polymerase: acyclovir and AZT.

- The reverse transcriptase then degrades the RNA strand and synthesizes a new DNA strand to replace it in the duplex.
- Frequently, the viral duplex DNA may be inserted into the host genome. The inserted duplex DNA can then be transcribed by the host cell's RNA polymerase, leading to the expression of viral gene products, and eventually the formation of new viral particles that incorporate viral genomic RNA transcribed from the duplex DNA.

Azidothymidine (AZT; Figure 16-26) is an analog of thymidine and an effective inhibitor of HIV replication. AZT is taken up by the cell and converted to AZT triphosphate, which is a substrate for HIV reverse transcriptase. It is also a substrate for normal human DNA polymerases, albeit with a much lower affinity. Like acyclovir, AZT lacks 3′-OH. Thus, if it is incorporated at the end of a growing strand of DNA, there is no way to extend the DNA chain past it. This will block DNA synthesis and inhibit viral replication.

Topoisomerase Inhibitors

Quinolones are a class of compounds that inhibit DNA topoisomerases. The cell is then unable to relieve the superhelical stress generated by replication and transcription, which eventually leads to cell death. Human topoisomerases differ from the bacterial enzymes and are not as susceptible to inhibition by quinolones, so with proper dosing, a bacterial infection can be fought off.

Nalidixic acid was the first quinolone to be marketed. The fluoroquinolones were discovered later and proved to be highly potent antibiotics, active against a wide variety of microorganisms. Ciprofloxacin and norfloxacin are representative members of this class of drugs (**Figure 16-27**).

RNA Polymerase Inhibitors

Rifampin and rifapentine (**Figure 16-28**) are antibiotics based on rifamycin, which is a natural product derived from *Streptomyces mediterranei*. Rifampin and rifapentine inhibit DNA-dependent RNA synthesis in bacteria by binding to the β-subunit of the bacterial RNA polymerase. Interestingly, rifampin inhibits elongation of RNA transcripts but does not seem to block the initiation of RNA synthesis. These drugs are active against a variety of microorganisms and are especially valuable in the treatment of tuberculosis.

Ribosome Inhibitors

Bacterial and eukaryotic ribosomes differ in structure and sequence, and these differences can be targeted for antibiotic action against bacteria. A large number of agents are known that inhibit bacterial ribosome action (**Figure 16-29**).

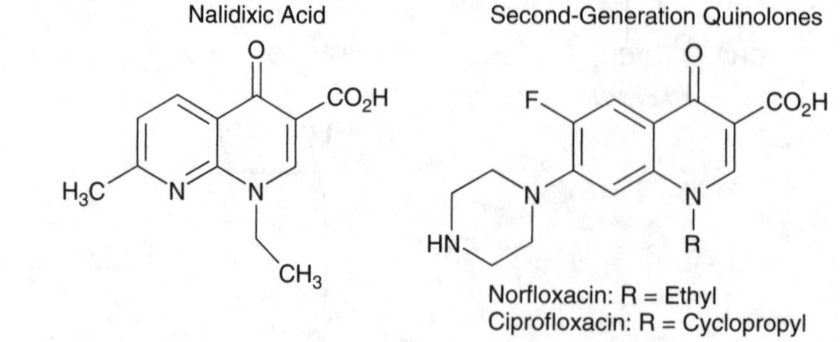

Nalidixic Acid

O
CO_2H
H_3C N N
CH_3

Second-Generation Quinolones

O
F
CO_2H
HN N N
R

Norfloxacin: R = Ethyl
Ciprofloxacin: R = Cyclopropyl

Figure 16-27 Inhibitors of DNA topoisomerases: nalidixic acid, and two quinolone antibiotics developed from it.

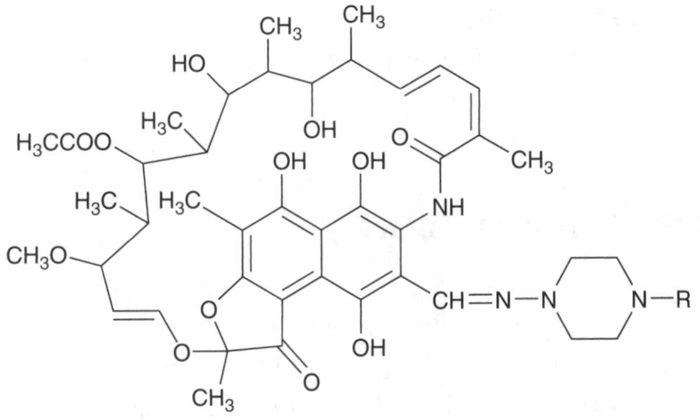

Rifampin: R = CH_3
Rifapentine: R = Cyclopentyl

Figure 16-28 Inhibitors of RNA polymerase: rifampin and rifapentine.

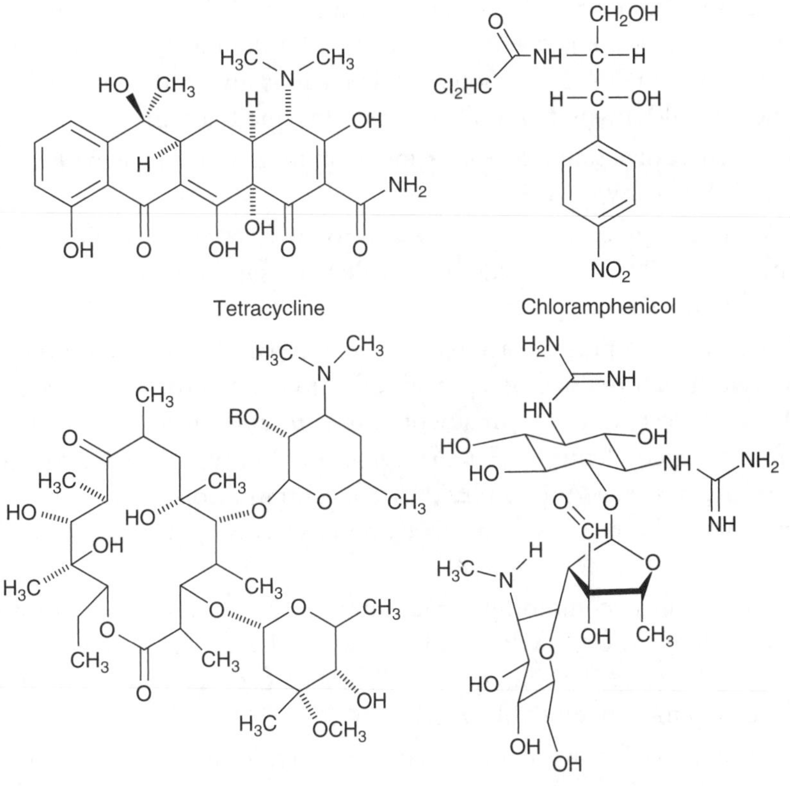

Tetracycline

Chloramphenicol

Erythromycin A

Streptomycin

Figure 16-29 Inhibitors of ribosomal action. These drugs act on the ribosome to inhibit translation: tetracycline, chloramphenicol, erythromycin A, and streptomycin.

For example, tetracycline interferes with the decoding of mRNA by blocking tRNA from binding in the A site. Chloramphenicol interferes with peptide bond formation by blocking the A site. Aminoglycoside antibiotics like streptomycin can interfere with chain translocation; they can also interfere with the way in which the ribosome proofreads the mRNA, which may lead to errors in amino acid incorporation in the polypeptide, which in turn can lead to nonfunctional ("nonsense") proteins that are toxic to the cell. Macrolide antibiotics such as erythromycin A act by binding in the region around the exit tunnel on the large ribosomal subunit. This binding arrests the motion of the nascent peptide chain through the tunnel and consequently blocks peptide elongation.

QUESTIONS FOR DISCUSSION

1. Hemoglobin C is an abnormal hemoglobin in which the glutamic acid in the sixth position of the β-chain is replaced by lysine. The original DNA gene sequence for the wild-type β-chain has (5′)GAG (3′) as the codon specifying glutamic acid in the sixth position. Which triplet codon sequence would you suggest for the gene coding for the mutant β-chain in which the glutamate is replaced by lysine? Which kind of mutation is this?
2. Purine nucleoside phosphorylase deficiency can arise when a certain CGA codon (at position 234 in the polypeptide chain) is changed to CCA. Which amino acid is coded for by CGA? In the mutant enzyme specified by the CCA codon, which amino acid replaces it? Position 234 in the polypeptide chain is involved in a very tight turn of the chain. How would the mutation likely affect enzyme folding?
3. Would two successive single base-pair insertion mutations in a gene be likely to correct each other? Why or why not?
4. Compare the energy cost to a chicken cell for synthesizing a molecule of the enzyme lysozyme (with 129 amino acids) versus that for synthesizing the protein ovalbumin (with 385 amino acids).
5. Diphtheria toxin is a protein secreted by the bacterium *Corynebacterium diphtheriae*. The toxic protein has an unusual mechanism of action: The protein is cleaved after it binds to a cell surface receptor, and a fragment of the protein enters the cell. This fragment acts as an enzyme to covalently attach an ADP-ribosyl group from NAD^+ onto a specific residue of the host cell's protein, EF2. A concentration of 10^{-8} M in the cytoplasm is sufficient to kill the cell. Explain this extreme sensitivity of the cell to the diphtheria toxin.
6. Certain strains of the common gut bacterium *E. coli* can produce a toxin called colicin E3, which inhibits the growth of other bacteria by enzymatically cleaving their 16S ribosomal RNA. Trace the consequences for the target bacterium upon its encountering and taking up a molecule of colicin E3.
7. The DNA and RNA polymerases of viruses are typically more prone to making errors in polymerization than are regular cellular polymerases. Why would viruses be more tolerant of errors than are cells?
8. Suppose that you find a mutation in *E. coli* in which transcription now frequently starts at promoter sites that are ignored by the wild-type bacterium. Which subunit of the polymerase is most likely to have the mutation, and why?
9. How might a C-to-T transition mutation at a CpG site affect mismatch repair?
10. The N-7 position of guanine or adenine in DNA is much more susceptible to alkylation than are the N-1 or N-3 nitrogens. Why?

REFERENCES

S. J. Benkovic, A. M. Valentine, and F. Salinas. (2001). "Replisome-mediated DNA replication," *Annu. Rev. Biochem.* 70:181–208.

D. L. Black. (2003). "Mechanisms of alternative pre-messenger RNA splicing," *Annu. Rev. Biochem.* 72:291–336.

F. Brueckner, J. Ortiz, and P. Cramer. (2009). "A movie of the RNA polymerase nucleotide addition cycle," *Curr. Opin. Struct. Biol.* 19:294–299.

A. L. Gnatt, P. Cramer. J. Fu, D. A. Bushnell, and R. D. Kornberg. (2001). "Structural basis of transcription: An RNA polymerase II elongation complex at 3.3 Å resolution," *Science* 292:1876–1882.

A. Kornberg and T. A. Baker. (1992). *DNA Replication*, 2nd ed., W. H. Freeman, New York.

A. Korostelev, S. Trakhanov, M. Laurberg, and H. F. Noller. (2006). "Crystal structure of a 70S ribosome–tRNA complex reveals functional interactions and rearrangements," *Cell* 125:1065–1077.

H. Masai, S. Matsumotom, Z. You, N. Yoshizawa-Sugata, and M. Oda. (2010). "Eukaryotic chromosome DNA replication: Where, when, and how?", *Annu. Rev. Biochem.* 79:89–130.

W. C. Merrick. (2010). "Eukaryotic protein synthesis: Still a mystery," *J. Biol. Chem.* 285:21197–21201.

K. Nierhaus and D. N. Wilson. (2004). *Protein Synthesis and Ribosome Structure*, Wiley-VCH, New York.

H. F. Noller. (2005). "RNA structure: Reading the ribosome," *Science* 309:1508–1514.

T. A. Steitz. (1999). "DNA polymerases: Structural diversity and common mechanisms," *J. Biol. Chem.* 274:17395–17398.

J. D. Watson, T. A. Baker, S. P. Bell, A. Gann, M. Levine, and R. Losick. (2004). *Molecular Biology of the Gene,* 5th ed., W. H. Freeman, New York.

A. Yonath. (2005). "Antibiotics targeting ribosomes: Resistance, selectivity, synergism and cellular regulation," *Annu. Rev. Biochem.* 74:649–679.

Glossary

A

Acetal: Product of the reaction of a hemiacetal and an alcohol in the presence of acid, with the general formula (R)CH(OR′)(OR″).

Acetyl-CoA carboxylase: Enzyme that carboxylates the acetyl group of acetyl-CoA to yield malonyl-CoA; the reaction is coupled to the hydrolysis of ATP to ADP and inorganic phosphate.

Acid dissociation constant (K_a): Equilibrium constant for dissociation of an acid to its conjugate base, with release of a proton.

Acidosis: The physiological condition of a blood pH of 7.35 or lower.

Active site: Region on an enzyme where substrate binds and catalysis occurs.

Active transport: Transport of a substance, mediated by a carrier, that uses ATP and that can move substances against a concentration gradient.

Acyl carrier protein (ACP): Protein carrying a phosphopantetheine group, which is responsible for linkage to acyl groups during fatty acid synthesis.

Adenine: 6-Aminopurine.

Adenosine 5′-triphosphate (ATP): A ribonucleoside 5′-triphosphate; the major carrier of free energy in the cell, serving as a phosphate group donor.

***S*-Adenosylmethionine (AdoMet; SAMe):** Cofactor used in methyl-transfer reactions by enzymes.

Aerobic: Requiring the presence of oxygen.

Alcaptonuria: Disorder in amino acid metabolism caused by the absence of the enzyme homogentisate oxidase.

Aldimine: Aliphatic nitrogen compound having the characteristic structure RCH=NH.

Aldolase: Enzyme that interconverts fructose 1,6-bisphosphate and the triose phosphates, glyceraldehyde 3-phosphate and dihydroxyacetone phosphate.

Aldose: A simple sugar whose carbonyl group is an aldehyde.

Allosteric effector: A ligand that, upon binding, causes a conformational change in its receptor molecule.

Allosteric protein: A protein that undergoes appreciable changes in conformation, typically in response to its binding of a ligand.

α-Helix: A common helical secondary structure of polypeptides, stabilized by a characteristic pattern of intrachain hydrogen bonding.

α-Ketoglutarate dehydrogenase: Enzyme in the TCA cycle that oxidatively decarboxylates α-ketoglutarate to succinyl-CoA while reducing NAD^+ to NADH.

α-Oxidation: Minor pathway for oxidation of fatty acids, involving attack at the α-carbon adjacent to the carboxyl group.

Amino acid: Carboxylic acid with an α-amino group, used in protein biosynthesis.

Aminoacyl-tRNA: A molecule of tRNA attached via an ester linkage to an aminoacyl moiety.

Aminoacyl-tRNA synthetase: Enzyme catalyzing the ester linkage of a tRNA to an aminoacyl group, using ATP to drive the reaction.

Amphiphile: A molecule with distinct, separate polar and nonpolar regions.

Anabolism: The collection of primary biosynthetic metabolic reactions.

Anaerobic: Occurring in the absence of oxygen.

Anaplerosis: Replenishment of metabolic intermediates of the citric acid cycle through enzyme reactions.

Anemia: A physiological condition in which the blood contains fewer red blood cells (or equivalently, less hemoglobin) than normal.

Anomer: One of a pair of sugar stereoisomers, which differ only in the configuration about their carbonyl carbon.

Anticodon: The three contiguous ribonucleotides in a tRNA molecule that bind to the cognate codon in a mRNA.

Antiport: Concurrent transport of two solutes across a membrane in opposite directions.

AP site: A site in a polynucleotide chain lacking a purine or pyrimidine base.

Apoprotein: The polypeptide part of a protein, without any cofactors.

Ascorbic acid: Vitamin C; an antioxidant that is important in the prevention of the disease of scurvy.

Aspartate transcarbamoylase (ATCase): Enzyme catalyzing the condensation of aspartate and carbamoyl phosphate to form *N*-carbamoylaspartate.

ATP synthase: Membrane-bound multisubunit enzyme mainly responsible in the cell for ATP synthesis from ADP and inorganic phosphate, in the process of oxidative phosphorylation.

B

Base pair: Two nucleotides joined by hydrogen bonding between the bases.

Beri-beri: Vitamin deficiency disease caused by inadequate intake of thiamine.

β-Oxidation: Degradation of fatty acids, with attack at the second (β) carbon.

β-Sheet: A common secondary structure in proteins involving two or more polypeptide chain segments hydrogen-bonded to one another, forming a roughly planar array.

β-Turn: A type of protein secondary structure characterized by a sharp turn in the polypeptide chain involving four amino acids.

Bile acid: Amphiphilic derivatives of cholesterol, secreted by the gallbladder to help solubilize dietary lipids.

Bilirubin: Red pigment derived from the breakdown of heme groups.

Binding change model: Proposed mechanism for the action of ATP synthase, involving concerted conformational changes, rotational motions, catalysis, and substrate binding and release.

Binding site: Region on a macromolecule where a ligand binds.

Biopterin: Enzyme cofactor used in redox reactions.

Biotin: Enzyme cofactor used in carboxylation reactions.

Brown adipose tissue (BAT): Collections of specialized fat cells whose mitochondria contain the uncoupling protein thermogenin, and which generate heat for the body.

C

Calorie: The amount of energy needed to raise the temperature of one gram of water from 14.5°C to 15.5°C.

Carbamoyl phosphate synthetase: Enzyme that synthesizes carbamoyl phosphate from ammonia and bicarbonate, using two ATP molecules per reaction.

Carbohydrate: A polyhydroxy aldehyde, polyhydroxy ketone, or other substance that yields these compounds upon hydrolysis.

Carbonic anhydrase: Enzyme that interconverts CO_2 and carbonic acid (or bicarbonate).

Carnitine: Molecule to which fatty acids are conjugated for transport across the inner mitochondrial membrane.

Carnitine palmitoyl transferase (CPT1 and CPT2): Enzyme catalyzing the extramitochondrial *O*-acylation of carnitine using an acyl-CoA (by CPT-1) and the subsequent intramitochondrial deacylation of carnitine and transfer of the acyl group to CoA (by CPT-2).

Catabolism: The collection of metabolic reactions that degrade foodstuffs to extract energy.

Catalysis: Acceleration of a reaction; an increase in the rate of reaction, produced by a catalyst.

Catalyst: Substance that accelerates a chemical reaction rate but is itself unchanged at the end of the reaction.

Catecholamine: A member of a class of compounds with hormonal action, which are based on amine derivatives of *o*-dihydroxy benzene (catechol).

Catenation: Noncovalent linking of two or more circular, covalently closed molecules, as in the formation of the links of a chain.

ccc DNA: Covalently closed circular DNA; a circular duplex DNA in which the individual strands are completely covalently bonded, without any breaks in their backbone linkages.

Cell cycle: The coordinated replication of DNA and cellular constituents, occurring in defined stages and leading to cell division in eukaryotes.

Central Dogma: The principle that information in the cell passes from DNA to RNA and then to protein.

Centromere: Site on a chromosome serving as the attachment point for a spindle in meiosis or mitosis.

Cerebroside: Sphingolipid carrying a single sugar residue.

Chemiosmotic model: Model of energy extraction and storage in cells, in which redox reactions are used to generate a transmembrane gradient in voltage and ion concentration, which is then used to drive the synthesis of ATP.

Cholesterol: The main sterol found in higher animals.

Chromatin: A complex of DNA, histones, and other proteins, made up of repeating nucleosomal units.

Chromosome: DNA molecule carrying multiple genes.

Chylomicron: Lipoprotein complex containing principally triglycerides, which is largely responsible for dietary fat transport.

Chymotrypsin: Serine protease that specifically cleaves peptides next to residues with aromatic or large nonpolar side chains.

Cistron: DNA base sequence that specifies one polypeptide.

Citrate synthase: Enzyme in the TCA cycle that synthesizes citrate from acetyl-CoA and oxaloacetate.

Citric acid cycle: Set of reactions that form a cycle whose first step involves formation of citrate and that degrades acetyl-CoA to CO_2, with extraction of energy.

Closed system: In thermodynamics, a system that can exchange energy, but not matter, with its surroundings.

Cobalamin: Cofactor derived from vitamin B_{12} used in rearrangements of substrate carbon skeletons.

Codon: The three contiguous bases in a molecule of mRNA that specify a particular amino acid in a polypeptide chain.

Coenzyme: Organic molecule serving as a cofactor for an enzyme.

Coenzyme A: Cofactor with pantothenic acid group that serves as an acyl group carrier.

Coenzyme Q (ubiquinone): Quinone derivative with long hydrophobic tail that serves as an electron carrier between respiratory complexes.

Cofactor: Non-proteinaceous part of an enzyme; includes both metal ions and small organic molecules.

Collagen triple helix: A three-stranded polypeptide helix with a right-handed twist, composed of three polypeptide strands, each containing a glycine residue at every third position.

Combination chemotherapy: The simultaneous use of two or more drugs, each with a distinct mechanism of action, and each at a level expected to be effective on its own.

Committed step: The first unique step in a metabolic pathway involving a large, favorable, free-energy change.

Compartmentalization: In eukaryotic cells, the separation of competing metabolic pathways into different organelles.

Competitive inhibition: Type of reversible enzyme inhibition that can be overcome by increasing the concentrations of substrate.

Concerted model (MWC model): Model of cooperative enzyme action for multisubunit enzymes that requires simultaneous conformational switching of all of the subunits.

Cooperativity: In binding thermodynamics, the influence of a bound ligand on the uptake of a second ligand; positive cooperativity results in greater affinity for the second ligand, while negative cooperativity results in lower affinity for the second ligand.

Cori cycle: The flow of lactate from muscle to liver, coupled to the flow of glucose from liver to muscle.

Corticosteroid: Steroid synthesized in the adrenal cortex.

Coupled reactions: Two chemical reactions sharing one or more chemical species or intermediates.

Cristae: Infoldings of the inner membrane of the mitochondrion.

Crossover Theorem: Model of the effects of inhibiting a biochemical pathway, where inhibition at one step of the pathway causes an increase in the concentration of precursor substrates and a decrease in the concentration of subsequent products.

Cruciform: In the form of a cross or the letter X; in nucleic acids, a secondary structure having this form.

Cyclic AMP (cAMP): Adenosine 3′,5′-phosphate; a second messenger in several signal transduction pathways.

Cyclin-dependent kinase (CDK): Protein kinase that is activated by the binding of a cyclin protein.

Cyclo-oxygenase (COX): Prostaglandin H_2 synthase.

Cytochrome: Protein carrying a heme group; electron carriers in redox reactions in the cell.

Cytoplasm: The fluid portion of cell bounded by the plasma membrane, excluding the nucleus but including other organelles.

Cytosine: 4-Amino-2-pyrimidinone.

Cytosol: The fluid portion of a cell bounded by the plasma membrane, exclusive of the nucleus or other organelles.

D

Deletion mutation: Mutation resulting from the removal of one or more nucleotides in a DNA sequence in a chromosome.

Denaturation: Unfolding of a protein or nucleic acid, resulting in loss of higher-order structure and activity.

De novo synthesis: Synthesis of a biochemical from simpler precursors.

Deoxyribonucleoside: Nucleic acid base covalently joined to deoxyribose.

Deoxyribonucleotide: Nucleic acid base joined covalently to deoxyribose phosphate.

Diabetes mellitus: Metabolic disease resulting in reduced catabolism of carbohydrates and increased catabolism of lipids and amino acids, often accompanied by high circulating levels of glucose.

Diastereomer: One of a set of stereoisomers that are not mirror images of one another.

Dihydrofolate reductase (DHFR): Enzyme responsible for the reduction of dihydrofolate to tetrahydrofolate.

Disaccharide: Carbohydrate consisting of two covalently joined simple sugars.

Dissociation constant (K_d): Equilibrium constant for the breakup of a complex, as in a protein releasing a ligand.

Disulfide bond: Sulfur-to-sulfur covalent bond; in proteins, it is typically formed by oxidation of the thiols of two adjacent cysteine residues.

DNA: Deoxyribonucleic acid.

DNA polymerase: Enzyme that catalyzes the polymerization of deoxynucleotides.

Domain: Distinct, compact, folded region of a protein.

Double-reciprocal (Lineweaver-Burk) plot: Graphical format used in enzyme kinetics; a plot of the reciprocal of the initial reaction velocity as a function of the reciprocal of the initial substrate concentration.

E

Eicosanoid: A class of fatty acids containing 20 carbon atoms; the class includes prostaglandins, leukotrienes, and thromboxanes.

Electrochemical potential: In thermodynamics, the sum of the chemical potential for a species and a term representing the contribution of an electrostatic potential.

Electromotive force (emf): In thermodynamics, the maximum potential developed when an electrochemical cell is operated reversibly; it is related to the free energy change ΔG by $\Delta G = -nF\Delta E$, where n is the number of moles of electrons exchanged in the balanced cell reaction and F is the Faraday constant.

Electron transport chain: A series of mitochondrial membrane proteins responsible for redox reactions leading to the generation of a transmembrane electrochemical potential that is used to drive ATP synthesis.

Electrophile: A generalized electron acceptor; a Lewis acid that is kinetically efficient.

Enantiomer: One of a pair of mirror-image isomers.

Endocytosis: Uptake of extracellular material in a vesicle that is formed by folding and pinching off part of the plasma membrane.

Endonuclease: An enzyme that cleaves a polynucleotide at an internal point.

Endoplasmic reticulum: Subcellular organelle containing a highly folded set of membranes, where much protein synthesis and modification take place.

Energy: Generally, the capacity to perform work; in thermodynamics, the internal energy E is a conserved quantity that depends on the internal state of the thermodynamic system (e.g., temperature, pressure, composition).

Energy charge: A measure of the degree to which the collection of adenylate nucleotides possess phosphoanhydride bonds; also known as the adenylate charge.

Enthalpy: In thermodynamics, the sum of the internal energy and the product of pressure and volume: $H = E + PV$.

Entropy: A thermodynamical measure of disorder.

Enzyme: A protein or RNA molecule that catalyzes a specific chemical reaction.

Epimer: One of a pair of diasteromers, differing only in configuration at one asymmetric center.

Equilibrium constant: For a given chemical reaction, the ratio of the concentrations of products to the concentrations of products, with the individual concentration terms being raised to their respective stoichiometric coefficients for the reaction.

Essential amino acids: The set of amino acids, needed for protein synthesis, that cannot be synthesized by humans but that must be obtained through the diet.

Essential fatty acids: The set of fatty acids, containing multiple double carbon–carbon bonds, that cannot be synthesized by humans but that must be obtained through the diet.

Eukaryote: Organism whose cells contain a membrane-bound nucleus and membrane-bound internal organelles.

Exon: Segment of a eukaryotic gene that encodes a portion of an expressed protein chain.

Exonuclease: An enzyme that cleaves a polynucleotide at one or both ends of the chain.

F

$FADH_2$: Flavin adenine dinucleotide; coenzyme used in redox reactions.

Faraday constant: The amount of charge, in coulombs, per mole of electrons; numerically equal to 96,485 coulombs per mole of electrons.

Fatty acid: A class of carboxylic acids with long, typically linear, alkyl chains with two or more carbon atoms in the chain.

Fatty acid synthase: Enzyme principally responsible for biosynthesis of fatty acids from acetyl-CoA and malonyl-CoA.

Feedback inhibition: Use of the result or product of a process to reduce its own production; negative feedback.

Fermentation: Anaerobic catabolism of nutrients, generating energy.

Fibrous protein: Insoluble protein, generally used for mechanical, structural, or protective coating roles.

First law of thermodynamics: Energy is conserved.

Flavin nucleotide: Cofactor containing riboflavin.

Flavoprotein: Protein containing a flavin nucleotide.

Fluid mosaic model: Model of biological membranes as lipid bilayers with embedded, mobile proteins.

$FMNH_2$: Flavin mononucleotide; coenzyme used in redox reactions.

Folate (folic acid): Cofactor used in single-carbon transfer reactions, with multiple redox states; consists of a pteridine ring linked to *p*-aminobenzoic acid, and a chain of one or more glutamate residues; reduced states include dihydrofolate and tetrahydrofolate.

Folate antagonist: Compound that blocks the action of folate.

Free energy: In thermodynamics, the energy of a system that is available to do work; the Gibbs free energy G is defined as $G = H - TS$.

Furanose: A sugar with a five-membered ring, based on the resemblance of the ring structure to that of furan.

G

Galactosemia: An unnaturally high level of galactose in the circulation, due to a defect in its metabolism.

Ganglioside: Sphingolipid with attached oligosaccharide chain.

Gene: Segment of chromosomal DNA that encodes a polypeptide chain or RNA molecule.

General acid–base catalysis: Catalysis involving proton transfer mediated by a species other than water.

Genetic code: The set of triplet codons specifying amino acids to be incorporated into a polypeptide, plus the three codons specifying the terminus of such a sequence of amino acids.

Genome: The complete set of genes, control sequences, and other genetic information for a cell, an organism, or a virus.

Genotype: The genetic composition of an individual cell or organism.

Globoside: Class of sphingolipids, carrying two or more sugar residues.

Glucogenic/glycogenic: Leading to the synthesis of glucose (or glycogen), as applied to the catabolism of amino acids.

Gluconeogenesis: The biochemical anabolic pathway leading from simple precursors, such as pyruvate or oxaloacetate, to glucose or related carbohydrates.

Glucose 6-phosphate dehydrogenase: Enzyme in the pentose phosphate pathway that oxidizes glucose 6-phosphate to 6-phosphoglucono-1,5-lactone while reducing NADP to NADPH.

Glucuronide: Metabolite to which a residue of glucuronic acid has been attached.

GLUT: Family of glucose transporter proteins; membrane-embedded proteins that transfer glucose across lipid bilayers.

Glutamate dehydrogenase: Enzyme that catalyzes the oxidative deamination of glutamate to yield ammonia and α-ketoglutarate, while reducing NAD^+ to NADH.

Glutathione: Tripeptide containing a thiol group, serving as an antioxidant.

Glutathione reductase: Enzyme that converts oxidized glutathione to its reduced state, using NADPH as a source of reducing power.

Glycan: Polysaccharide.

Glycerol-phosphate shuttle: Multistep pathway for the transfer of reducing equivalents across the inner mitochondrial membrane.

Glycogen: Branched polymer of glucose; major storage form of glucose in animals.

Glycogenolysis: Process of breaking down glycogen into its constituent glucose units.

Glycogen phosphorylase: Enzyme that breaks down glycogen, releasing glucose 1-phosphate.

Glycogen storage disease: One of several genetic defects in enzymes responsible for glycogen metabolism.

Glycogen synthase: Enzyme that synthesizes glycogen from UDP-glucose.

Glycolipid: Lipid carrying a carbohydrate group.

Glycolysis: Main catabolic pathway for glucose, which yields pyruvate and ATP.

Glycoprotein: Protein carrying one or more carbohydrate groups.

Glycosaminoglycan: Polysaccharide consisting of repeating disaccharide units, one of which is an amino sugar and the other of which is a uronic acid.

Glycoside: A sugar acetal; the product of the reaction of an aldose with an alcohol or amine.

Glycosidic linkage/bond: In a sugar acetal, the bond between the sugar and the alcohol (an *O*-glycosidic bond) or between the sugar and an amine (an *N*-glycosidic bond).

Glycosylation: Covalent attachment of a carbohydrate group to a protein, sphingolipid, etc.

Golgi apparatus/complex: Eukaryotic organelle that is responsible for post-translational processing of proteins and their sorting to lysosomes, the plasma membrane, or secretory vesicles.

Gout: A disease of the joints caused by high serum levels of uric acid (urate).

Guanine: 2-Amino-6-hydroxypurine.

H

Hairpin: Element of nucleic acid secondary structure, in which a single strand of polynucleotide containing a palindromic sequence folds back on itself to form an antiparallel double-stranded structure by pairing the complementary bases in the palindromic sequence.

Half-reaction: The electrochemical reaction associated with one or the other of the two electrodes in an electrochemical cell.

Helicase: Enzyme that catalyzes the unwinding of a DNA double helix.

Helix-coil transition: For polypeptides or polynucleotides, the process of converting the helical secondary structure to a disorganized, random, coil-like structure.

Heme: Prosthetic group formed from porphyrin, with a central atom of iron.

Hemiacetal: Product of the reaction of an aldehyde with an alcohol, with the general formula (R)CH(OH)(OR′); it is both an ether and an alcohol.

Hemiketal: Product of the reaction of a ketone with an alcohol, with the general formula (R)(R′)C(OH)(OR″); it is both an ether and an alcohol.

Hemoglobin: Oxygen transport protein found in red blood cells.

Hemolytic anemia: Anemia due to the breakdown of red blood cells.

Heparan sulfate: Variably sulfated proteoglycan whose polysaccharide chains consist of heparin.

Heparin: Linear variably sulfated polysaccharide; a glycosaminoglycan consisting of alternating units of *N*-acetylglucosamine and either glucuronic acid or iduronic acid.

Hexokinase: Enzyme catalyzing the phosphorylation of a hexose, using ATP.

Hexose: Simple sugar with six carbons.

High-density lipoprotein (HDL): A major type of lipoprotein, largely responsible for cholesterol ester transport to the liver from peripheral tissues (reverse cholesterol transport).

Histone: Member of a family of basic proteins that associate strongly with DNA in chromosomes.

Holoenzyme: Enzyme containing all subunits and cofactors necessary for its full activity.

Hormone: A substance synthesized in and released by an endocrine gland, which acts in small amounts as a messenger to regulate specifically the function of one or more tissues.

Hydrolase: Enzyme that catalyzes a hydrolysis reaction, with transfer of a functional group to water.

Hydrophilic: Easily dissolved in water.

Hydrophobic: Resisting dissolution in water.

Hydrophobic effect: Tendency for nonpolar substances to segregate themselves away from contact with water.

Hydroxymethylglutaryl CoA reductase (HMG-CoA reductase): Enzyme catalyzing a key step in cholesterol biosynthesis—namely, the conversion of hydroxymethylglutaryl CoA to mevalonic acid.

Hyperammonemia: Higher than normal levels of ammonia in the blood.

Hyperglycemia: Higher than normal levels of glucose in the blood.

Hypoglycemia: Lower than normal levels of glucose in the blood.

Hypoxanthine: 6-Hydroxypurine.

Hypoxanthine-guanine phosphoribosyltransferase (HGPRT): Enzyme involved in the purine salvage pathway; a lack of this enzyme leads to Lesch-Nyhan syndrome.

Hypoxia: Lower than normal levels of oxygen in tissues or blood.

I

Induced-fit model: Model of enzyme action in which uptake of substrate causes conformational changes in the enzyme (and possibly in the substrate) for more efficient catalysis; applied more generally to adaptive conformational changes occurring in ligand–macromolecule associations.

Initiation: In the action of polymerizing enzymes, the chemical events leading to the first covalent bond linking two monomers; the beginning phase of polymerization.

Inosine: Purine nucleotide in which the base is hypoxanthine.

Inositide: A phospholipid containing inositol.

Inositol: A hexahydroxycyclohexane.

Insertion mutation: Mutation caused by introduction of one or more new nucleotides into a chromosome.

Integral membrane protein: Protein strongly associated with a lipid bilayer membrane through extensive hydrophobic interactions.

Intron: An intervening sequence in a gene; a region that is not expressed in the mature mRNA.

Inverted repeat: Short sequence of DNA repeated in an inverted orientation.

Iron–sulfur complex: Prosthetic group containing both iron and sulfur atoms.

Irreversible inhibition: Inhibition of an enzyme by covalent attachment of an inhibitor, such that the inhibition cannot be overcome.

Irreversible process: In thermodynamics, a change in state involving nonequilibrium or out-of-balance processes.

Isocitrate dehydrogenase: Enzyme in the TCA cycle that converts isocitrate to α-ketoglutarate.

Isoenzyme (isozyme): Member of a set of enzymes that catalyze the same reaction but differ in amino acid sequence or some other property.

Isomer: Member of a set of compounds having the same molecular formula but differing in structure.

Isomerase: Enzyme that catalyzes a rearrangement of chemical groups in a molecule (an isomerization).

Isoprene: 2-Methyl-1,3-butadiene.

Isoprenoid: Natural product derived from two or more isoprene units.

J

Joule: S.I. unit of energy.

K

K_a: Acid dissociation constant.

K_d: Dissociation constant.

Katal: S.I. unit of enzyme activity; one katal is sufficient to convert one mole of substrate to product in one second under standard conditions.

Kelvin: S.I. unit of temperature.

Keratin: Fibrous protein with characteristic coiled-coil structure used in hair, horn, and some other bodily structures.

Ketimine: Aliphatic nitrogen compound having the characteristic structure $R_2C{=}NH$.

Keto–enol tautomerization: Isomerization of a compound from a ketone form to an enol form.

Ketogenic amino acids: Amino acids whose catabolism leads to acetoacetyl-CoA.

Ketone body: One of the three compounds—acetone, β-hydroxybutyrate, and acetoacetate—that serve as fuel substitutes for the body when glucose supplies are low.

Ketose: Monosaccharide whose carbonyl carbon is a ketone.

Ketosis: Physiological condition in which circulating levels of ketone bodies are above normal.

Kinase: Enzyme that uses ATP to phosphorylate substances.

Krebs cycle: Citric acid cycle.

L

Lactate dehydrogenase: Enzyme catalyzing the reduction of pyruvate to lactate, and vice versa.

Lagging strand: DNA strand that is synthesized in the opposite direction of movement of the replication complex.

Leading strand: DNA strand that is synthesized in the direction of movement of the replication complex.

Lectin: Protein that specifically binds a particular carbohydrate chain with high affinity, promoting intercellular adhesion and communication.

Lecithin: Phosphatidyl choline; membrane phospholipid composed of glycerol esterified with two fatty acids chains and a phosphate group that bears a choline moiety.

Lesch-Nyhan syndrome: A rare inheritable disorder that is due to a lack of activity of the enzyme hypoxanthine-guanine phosphoribosyltransferase.

Leukotriene: Member of a family of molecules obtained from arachidonic acid, which serve as signaling agents.

Ligand: In a macromolecular binding equilibrium, the small molecule that attaches specifically to the larger partner.

Ligase: Enzyme that catalyzes a condensation reaction between two substrate molecules, with concomitant hydrolysis of ATP.

Lipase: Enzyme that hydrolyzes triglycerides to release fatty acids.

Lipid: Small nonpolar biochemical that is related to fatty acids, sterols, or isoprenoids.

Lipid bilayer: Two lipid sheets joined so that the nonpolar groups are oriented to the interior and the polar groups are exposed externally to solvent.

Lipid raft: Region of a biomembrane that is physically distinguishable by its rigidity and lesser fluidity and that contains a higher level of cholesterol, sphingolipids, and certain types of proteins.

Lipoic acid (lipoate, lipoamide): Prosthetic group that transfers acyl groups and hydrogen atoms.

Lipolysis: The set of reactions leading to the breakdown of triglycerides into the constituent fatty acids.

Lipoprotein: Assembly of lipids and certain proteins for lipid transport in the circulation.

Lock-and-key model: Model for enzyme action in which the substrate and the enzyme active site fit together like a hypothetical key in a lock, without any conformational changes in either component.

Low-density lipoprotein (LDL): A major type of lipoprotein that is largely responsible cholesterol transport in the blood.

Lyase: Enzyme that either catalyzes removal of a group to form a double bond or adds a group to a double bond.

Lysosome: Eukaryotic organelle that serves to degrade and recycle damaged cellular components as well as exogenous material.

Lysosomal storage disease: Defect in one of several different enzymes, leading to accumulation of lipids in lysosomes.

M

Malate–aspartate shuttle: Multistep pathway for the transfer of reducing equivalents across the inner mitochondrial membrane.

Maple syrup urine disease (MSUD): Defect in the metabolism of branched-chain amino acids, a symptom of which is the characteristic odor of the urine.

Maximal velocity (V_{max}): The highest rate of an enzyme-catalyzed reaction, occurring when the enzyme is saturated with substrate.

Membrane potential: Electrical potential (voltage) difference across a lipid bilayer membrane.

Messenger RNA (mRNA): Class of RNA molecules responsible for conveying genetic information on polypeptide sequences from DNA to the ribosome.

Metabolism: The complete collection of all enzyme-catalyzed reactions in the cell, including both catabolic and anabolic reactions. Primary or intermediary metabolism is the subset of metabolic reactions dealing with the extraction of energy from foodstuffs, the synthesis of the main cellular constituents, and the disposal of wastes from these processes.

Metalloprotein: Protein containing a metal ion cofactor.

Metazoan: Multicellular eukaryote.

Micelle: Globular or tubular assembly of amphipathic molecules, whose nonpolar moieties are oriented to the interior of the assembly and whose polar moieties are exposed to water.

Michaelis constant (K_M): The concentration of substrate that produces half of the maximal velocity in an enzyme-catalyzed reaction.

Michaelis–Menten model: Two-step model of enzyme action, with reversible association of enzyme and substrate followed by irreversible conversion to product.

Mitochondrial matrix: Inner compartment of a mitochondrion, inside the inner membrane.

Mitochondrion: Organelle responsible for ATP production, containing the enzymes for oxidative phosphorylation, the citric acid cycle, and fatty acid oxidation.

Mitosis: In eukaryotes, the process of cellular replication and division.

Mixed inhibition: A type of reversible enzyme inhibition in which the inhibitor may bind to either the free enzyme or the enzyme–substrate complex, to cause loss of enzyme activity.

Monosaccharide: A single simple sugar.

Motif: Combination of two or more elements of protein secondary structure into a recognizable superstructure.

Mutagen: Chemical that causes genetic mutations.

Mutase: Any of a class of enzymes that catalyze transposition of chemical groups.

Mutation: Change in chromosomal nucleotide sequence that can be inherited.

N

NADH: Nicotinamide adenine dinucleotide; cofactor used in redox reactions.

NADPH: Nicotinamide adenine dinucleotide phosphate; cofactor used in redox reactions.

Native conformation: The properly folded and active conformation of a protein or nucleic acid.

Niacin: Vitamin precursor to the nicotinamide cofactors.

Nitrogen fixation: Process in which atmospheric nitrogen gas (N_2) is reduced, mainly to ammonia, and made available for biological use.

Noncompetitive inhibition: Special case of mixed inhibition of an enzyme, in which the inhibitor binds with the same affinity to either the free enzyme or the enzyme–substrate complex.

Non-heme iron: Iron cofactor in a protein, not in the form of a heme group.

Nonsense mutation: Change in gene nucleotide sequence that causes premature truncation or termination of a polypeptide chain.

NSAID: Nonsteroidal anti-inflammatory drug.

Nuclease: Enzyme that hydrolyzes nucleic acids.

Nucleophile: A generalized electron donor; a Lewis base that is kinetically efficient.

Nucleoside: A nucleic base joined covalently to a pentose.

Nucleoside diphosphate kinase: Enzyme catalyzing the transfer of a terminal phosphate group from a nucleoside triphosphate to a nucleoside diphosphate.

Nucleoside monophosphate kinase: Enzyme catalyzing the transfer of a terminal phosphate group from ATP to a nucleoside monophosphate.

Nucleotide: A nucleic acid base joined covalently to a pentose phosphate.

Nucleosome: A protein–DNA complex, part of chromatin, consisting of a histone octamer core wrapped around by double-stranded DNA of approximately 140 base pairs.

Nucleus: In eukaryotes, the membrane-bound organelle that contains the chromosomal DNA.

O

Okazaki fragment: One of the small segments of DNA on the lagging strand that are synthesized discontinuously by the replication complex.

Oligomer: Short sequence of covalently joined monomer units.

ω-Oxidation: Minor route of oxidation of fatty acids in which the terminal ω-carbon is first oxidized instead of the carbon adjacent to the carboxyl group.

Open system: In thermodynamics, a system that can exchange both energy and matter with its surroundings.

Operator: Sequence or region of DNA to which a repressor protein binds, generally in close proximity to a promoter region.

Operon: Cluster of (bacterial) genes under the control of a single regulatory region of DNA.

Order of reaction: The sum of the exponents of the concentration terms in a chemical rate law.

Ornithine transcarbamoylase: Enzyme of the urea cycle that makes citrulline from carbamoyl phosphate and ornithine.

Oxidase: Enzyme that catalyzes an oxidation reaction, using molecular oxygen as the electron acceptor, without incorporating oxygen into the product.

Oxidation: Loss of electrons by an atom or molecule.

Oxidation–reduction reaction: Reaction in which electrons are passed between reactants.

Oxidative phosphorylation: The coupling of electron transfer reactions through respiratory complexes, with the phosphorylation of ADP to ATP.

Oxidoreductase: Enzyme catalyzing an oxidation–reduction reaction.

Oxygenase: Enzyme that catalyzes an oxidation reaction and that incorporates oxygen atoms into the reaction product, forming a hydroxyl or carboxyl group.

P

P/O ratio: In connection with oxidative phosphorylation, the number of moles of ATP formed per mole of atomic oxygen ($\frac{1}{2}$ mole of O_2) consumed.

Palindrome: Duplex DNA segment that has two-fold rotational symmetry in its base sequence.

Pantothenic acid: A vitamin that is a precursor to coenzyme A and to some prosthetic groups in enzymes, consisting of D-pantoic acid and β-alanine.

Pathway: Ordered set of biochemical transformation reactions, leading from precursors to products.

Pellagra: Disease due to dietary deficiency in niacin.

Pentose: Sugar with five carbon atoms.

Pentose phosphate pathway: Minor oxidative pathway for glucose, producing NADPH, ribose 5-phosphate, and other carbohydrates.

Peptide: Compound of two or more amino acids joined by peptide bonds.

Peptide bond: Amide bond between the α-amino group of one amino acid and the α-carboxyl group of a second amino acid.

Peptidoglycan: Cross-linked linear heteropolysaccharide chains, in which the cross links are short peptide chains; the principal component of bacterial cell walls.

Peripheral membrane protein: Protein bound loosely to the surface of a biomembrane.

Pernicious anemia: Anemia due to a deficiency in vitamin B_{12}.

pH: Measure of the concentration of hydrogen ions in aqueous solution; the negative logarithm of the hydrogen ion concentration.

Phenotype: The set of observable characteristics of a cell or organism.

Phenylketonuria (PKU): Metabolic disease due to a deficiency in the processing of phenylalanine to tyrosine.

Phosphatase: Enzyme that hydrolyzes phosphate esters or anhydrides.

Phosphatidate: A lipid, diacylglycerol 3-phosphate.

Phosphoanhydride: Anhydride formed by the condensation of two phosphoryl groups.

Phosphodiester linkage: Phosphate group esterified to two alcohol groups.

Phosphoester: Organic compound analogous to an ester, in which a phosphate group is bonded to an acyl group.

Phosphofructokinase (PFK): Glycolytic enzyme responsible for conversion of fructose 6-phosphate to fructose 1,6-bisphosphate.

Phosphoglyceride: Phospholipid containing glycerol (not sphingosine) as the backbone to which the fatty acid and phosphate–alcohol groups are attached.

Phospholipid: Member of a major class of membrane lipids, which consist of one or more fatty acid chains, a glycerol or sphingosine moiety, a phosphate group, and an alcohol attached to the phosphate.

Phosphorolysis: Cleavage of a compound with phosphate as the attacking agent.

Phosphorylase: Enzyme that catalyzes phosphorolysis.

Phosphorylation: Attachment of a phosphate group to a biomolecule.

Pleated sheet: Characteristic planar secondary structure of proteins, in which neighboring strands lie side-by-side and are connected by interstrand hydrogen bonds.

Plectonemic supercoiling: A type of supercoiling in which the coiled strands are wound around each other like a twisted thread.

Poly(A) tail: Polymer of adenosine nucleotide residues attached to the $3'$ end of an mRNA.

Polymer: A long sequence of covalently joined monomer units.

Polynucleotide: Polymer of nucleotides.

Polypeptide: Polymer of amino acids.

Polysaccharide: Polymer of sugar units.

Porphyrin: Ring of four substituted pyrrole residues, often found with a central metal ion.

Pressure: Force exerted per unit area. The S.I. unit of pressure is the pascal (symbol Pa), but other units (e.g., the atmosphere, where 1 atm = 101,325 Pa) are in common use.

Primary structure: The structure of covalent linkages of monomer units forming the backbone of a polymer, together with any cross links between monomers.

Primer: Short oligomer to which an enzyme adds more monomer units.

Primase: Enzyme responsible for forming RNA oligomers to be used as primers by DNA polymerase.

Processivity: With respect to polymerizing or depolymerizing enzymes, the property of continued enzymatic action on a substrate polymer without dissociation.

Prokaryote: An organism lacking a membrane-bound nucleus.

Promoter: DNA sequence recognized and bound by RNA polymerase prior to initiation of RNA synthesis.

Proofreading: Enzymatic removal of incorrectly incorporated monomer units during biosynthesis of polymers such as DNA, RNA, and proteins.

Prostaglandin: Member of a class of lipids that are derived from unsaturated fatty acids (principally arachidonic acid) and that serve as hormone-like messenger molecules.

Prosthetic group: A metal ion or small organic molecule (other than an amino acid) bound covalently to a protein, needed for activity of the protein.

Protease: Enzyme that cleaves peptide linkages in a protein substrate.

Proteasome: Large multisubunit assembly responsible for the breakdown and turnover of damaged or unneeded proteins in the cell.

Protein: Heteropolymer of amino acids, linked by peptide bonds.

Proteoglycan: Polypeptide carrying one or more polysaccharide chains in which the polysaccharide component dominates the physico-chemical properties of the molecule.

Proton gradient: Difference in proton concentration across a biomembrane.

Proton pump: Transmembrane protein that transfers protons across the membrane against a gradient in free energy.

Purine: Heterocyclic aromatic compound containing both a pyrimidine ring and an imidazole ring.

Pyranose: A sugar containing a six-membered ring, based on the resemblance of the ring structure to that of pyran.

Pyridoxal phosphate (PLP): Coenzyme containing pyridoxal (vitamin B_6), used in amino group transfer reactions.

Pyrimidine: 1,3-Diazine.

Pyruvate carboxylase: Enzyme that carboxylates pyruvate to yield oxaloacetate.

Pyruvate dehydrogenase complex: Multisubunit enzyme, with multiple cofactors, that generates acetyl-CoA from pyruvate while reducing NAD^+ to NADH.

Pyruvate kinase: Glycolytic enzyme responsible for conversion of phospho*enol*pyruvate to pyruvate, and phosphorylation of ADP to ATP.

Q

Quadruplex: Four-stranded nucleic acid secondary structure.

Quaternary structure: The three-dimensional structure of a multisubunit macromolecular assembly; it may consist solely of protein but may also contain nucleic acids.

R

Rate constant: Constant of proportionality between the time rate of change of the concentration of a reactant (the velocity or rate of reaction) and the concentration(s) of the reactant(s).

Rate law: Algebraic expression connecting the velocity of a chemical reaction and the concentration(s) of reactant(s) and product(s).

Rate-limiting step: The slowest step in a chain of reactions or metabolic pathway.

Reaction intermediate: Chemical species in a reaction pathway with appreciable stability and lifetime.

Reaction rate: The time rate of change of concentration of a reactant in a chemical reaction.

Reading frame: Contiguous nonoverlapping groups of three nucleotides or codons in a polynucleotide, used to specify a polypeptide sequence.

Redox reaction: Reduction–oxidation reaction; a reaction in which electrons are passed between reactants.

Reducing agent: Electron donor in a redox reaction.

Reducing sugar: Carbohydrate with a free anomeric carbon that is susceptible to oxidation by Fehling's, Benedict's, or Tollens' reagent.

Reduction: Gain of electrons by an atom or molecule.

Relaxed DNA: Unstrained DNA; for covalently closed circular DNA, the form without any supercoiling.

Relaxed state (R state): In an allosteric enzyme, the conformation with greater ligand affinity or enzymatic activity.

Renaturation: Refolding of a protein or nucleic acid to regain its original secondary (and higher) structure and activity.

Replication fork: Y-shaped DNA structure, found at the point where DNA is undergoing replication.

Replisome: Large assembly of enzymatic and accessory proteins that carries out DNA replication in the cell.

Repressor protein: DNA-binding protein that regulates gene expression by binding to the operator sequence and blocking transcription.

Residue: In a polymer, the fundamental repeating chemical unit (e.g., an amino acid in a polypeptide).

Respiration: Metabolic process that consumes oxygen, oxidizes organic or inorganic substrates, and generates ATP.

Respiratory chain: Ordered set of electron-carrying proteins and associated small molecules, responsible for transferring electrons from substrates to molecular oxygen during respiration.

Respiratory complex: Multisubunit member of the set of electron-carrying proteins involved in respiration.

Reverse transcriptase: DNA polymerase that uses RNA as the template.

Reversible inhibition: Type of enzyme inhibition in which the inhibiting molecule may dissociate from the enzyme, thereby allowing restoration of enzymatic activity.

Reversible process: In thermodynamics, an idealized change of system properties that proceeds through a series of equilibrium states that are only infinitesimally different.

Riboflavin: Vitamin B_2; cofactor containing an isoalloxazine ring attached to ribitol.

Ribonuclease: Enzyme that cleaves RNA.

Ribonucleoside: Nucleic acid base joined to ribose.

Ribonucleotide: Nucleic acid base joined to a phosphorylated ribose.

Ribonucleotide reductase: Enzyme that converts ribonucleotide diphosphates to deoxyribonucleotide diphosphates, with concomitant oxidation of NADPH to $NADP^+$.

Ribosomal RNA (rRNA): Class of RNA molecules that are essential components of the ribosome.

Ribosome: Large multisubunit assembly of RNA and protein chains, responsible for synthesizing polypeptides in sequences directed by mRNA.

Ribozyme: Species of RNA capable of catalytic action.

RNA: Ribonucleic acid.

RNA polymerase: Enzyme that polymerizes ribonucleotides.

RNA splicing: Processing of an RNA transcript to remove intervening sequences and covalently link exons.

S

Salvage pathway: Biosynthetic pathway that uses or recycles intermediates from the corresponding degradative pathway.

Saturated fatty acid: Fatty acid with only single carbon–carbon bonds.

Schiff base linkage: Chemical bond formed by reaction of a primary amine with the carbonyl carbon of an aldehyde or ketone, giving an aldimine or ketimine, respectively.

Secondary structure: A regular three-dimensional pattern of folding in a biopolymer.

Second law of thermodynamics: In a reversible thermodynamic process, the change in entropy for the universe is zero; for an irreversible process, the change in entropy of the universe is positive.

Second messenger: An intracellular molecule, serving as a messenger or intermediary in a signal transduction pathway; examples include cAMP, cGMP, calcium ions, diacyl glycerol, and inositol 1,4,5-trisphosphate.

Sedimentation coefficient: Measure of the rate of sedimentation of a species in a centrifuge.

Sequential model of cooperative enzyme action (KNF model): Model of cooperative enzyme action for multisubunit enzymes that allows individual subunits to change conformation one at a time.

Serine protease: Proteolytic enzyme with a serine residue in its active site that plays a key catalytic role.

Shine-Dalgarno sequence: Sequence in bacterial mRNA for recognition and binding by the ribosome.

Signal transduction: Process by which a chemical signal, external to a cell, causes an internal physiological or metabolic change in the cell.

Signaling cascade: Series of enzymatic amplifications of an external chemical signal into metabolic changes in a cell.

Silent mutation: Inheritable genetic change without a change in phenotype.

Solenoidal supercoiling: A type of supercoiling in which the coiled strands are wound up to form a tube with a central channel.

Specific acid–base catalysis: Catalysis involving proton transfer mediated by solvent water molecules.

Sphingolipid: Type of lipid formed from sphingosine, a fatty acid, and a fatty alcohol.

Spliceosome: Enzyme assembly responsible for removing intervening sequences from immature messenger RNA molecules.

Standard free energy change ($\Delta G°$): In thermodynamics, the change in Gibbs free energy for a reaction occurring under standard state conditions.

Standard reduction potential: The electromotive force (voltage) for a reduction half-cell reaction in an electrochemical cell, with the cell set up under standard conditions.

Standard state: For reactions in aqueous solution, conditions consisting of a pressure of one atmosphere and a temperature of 298 K, with unit activity of all reactants; typically the molarity concentration scale is used in biochemistry.

Statin: Member of a class of drugs that competitively inhibit the enzyme hydroxymethylglutaryl-CoA reductase and that resemble mevalonate; used therapeutically to reduce serum levels of cholesterol.

Stereoisomer: An isomer differing from its fellows only in the way its atoms are arranged or oriented in three dimensions.

Steroid: Lipid with a characteristic planar structure of four fused rings (the steroid nucleus).

Sterol: An alcohol built from the steroid nucleus.

Substitution mutation: Mutation in which one base is replaced by another.

Substrate: The particular compound acted upon by an enzyme.

Suicide substrate: Compound that is normally stable but that, when acted upon by an enzyme, will react with residues in the enzyme's active site to irreversibly inactivate the enzyme.

Sulfatide: A type of sphingolipid; a sulfate ester of a cerebroside.

Sulfhydryl buffer: Agent that serves to maintain the reduced state of sulfhydryl groups.

Supercoiling: Twisting of a coiled molecule upon itself.

Surroundings: In thermodynamics, the part of the universe that is not the system; the part of the universe that is outside the system.

Svedberg (S): Unit for sedimentation coefficients, defined as 1×10^{-13} second.

Symport: Concurrent transport of two solutes across a membrane in the same direction.

Synthase: Enzyme that catalyzes a condensation reaction without the use of ATP.

Synthetase: Enzyme that catalyzes a condensation reaction with the use of ATP.

System: In thermodynamics, a part of the universe separated from the rest of the universe by boundaries.

T

T_m: Midpoint temperature of an order–disorder transition in a biopolymeric system.

Taut state (T state): In an allosteric enzyme, the conformation with lesser ligand affinity or enzymatic activity.

Tautomerism: Ability of a compound to react as if it had more than one structure, due to the existence of relatively stable but interconvertible isomers.

Telomerase: Enzyme responsible for replication of the telomere structures at the ends of eukaryotic chromosomes.

Telomere: An unusual DNA structure, rich in guanine residues and having a characteristic four-stranded structure, that is found at the ends of linear eukaryotic chromosomes.

Temperature: Measure of the degree of hotness or coldness of a system; the S.I. unit of temperature is the Kelvin (K).

Template strand: Nucleic acid strand used to guide the selection of the correct base sequence in the synthesis of a second nucleic acid strand by a polymerase.

Termination: The final phase of a polymerization process.

Terpene: Organic compound whose carbon skeleton is synthesized from isoprene units.

Tertiary structure: Three-dimensional folded structure of a polymer.

Tetrose: Carbohydrate with four carbon atoms.

Thermal energy: Heat.

Thiamine pyrophosphate (TPP): Coenzyme used in activated aldehyde transfers, derived from vitamin B_1.

Thioester: Organic compound analogous to an ester, in which a thiol group is bonded to an acyl group.

Third law of thermodynamics: The entropy of a perfect crystalline substance is zero at the absolute zero of temperature.

Thymidylate synthase: Enzyme that methylates deoxyuridylate to form deoxythymidylate.

Thymine: 5-Methyl-2,4(*1H,3H*)-pyrimidinedione; 5-methyluracil.

Topoisomer: One of a set of forms of the same species of covalently closed, circular DNA molecule that differ only in the number of times the strands are wound about each other.

Topoisomerase: Enzyme that can change the degree of supercoiling in a covalently closed circular DNA molecule.

Transamination: Transfer of an amino group from an α-amino acid to an α-keto acid.

Transaminase: Enzyme catalyzing a transamination reaction.

Transcription: Synthesis of RNA using a DNA template.

Transcription bubble: Region on a double-stranded DNA molecule where the strands are parted by an RNA polymerase complex as it performs transcription.

Transfer RNA (tRNA): Class of RNA molecules that carry amino acids to the ribosome for polymerization into polypeptide chains.

Transferase: Enzyme that moves a chemical group.

Transition mutation: Substitution of an A · T base pair for a G · C base pair, or vice versa.

Transition state: In a chemical reaction, a distorted state of the reactants, having a higher energy than the equilibrium state, and corresponding to the highest point of energy along the reaction path; an activated complex of reactants.

Transketolase: Enzyme with a cofactor of thiamine pyrophosphate that catalyzes transketolization reactions among intermediates in sugar metabolism.

Translation: Synthesis of protein as directed by an mRNA template.

Transporter: Membrane-bound protein that spans the membrane and serves to carry specific compounds, ions, and other substances across the membrane.

Transversion mutation: Substitution of a (purine) · (pyrimidine) base pair for a (pyrimidine) · (purine) base pair, or vice versa.

Tricarboxylic acid cycle (TCA cycle): The citric acid cycle.

Triglyceride: Glycerol esterified with three fatty acids.

Triose: Carbohydrate with three carbon atoms.

Triose phosphate isomerase: Glycolytic enzyme that interconverts dihydroxyacetone phosphate and glyceraldehyde-3-phosphate.

Turnover number (k_{cat}): The number times per second that an enzyme converts substrate to product, under conditions of maximal velocity.

U

Ubiquinone: Coenzyme Q; lipid-soluble benzoquinone used in mitochondrial electron transport.

Ubiquitin: Small protein used to mark intracellular proteins for degradation.

Uncompetitive inhibition: Type of reversible enzyme inhibition that cannot be overcome by increasing substrate concentration, typically involving the formation of a ternary complex of enzyme, substrate, and inhibitor, but not a complex of inhibitor and free enzyme.

Uncoupling agent: Molecule that decouples electron transport through respiratory complexers from the phosphorylation of ADP to ATP.

Unsaturated fatty acid: Fatty acid with one or more double bonds.

Uracil: 2,4-Pyrimidinedione.

Urea cycle: Cyclic metabolic pathway that accepts nitrogens in the form of amino groups and discharges them as urea.

Uric acid (urate): 2,6,8-Trihydroxypurine, or 7,9-dihydro-1*H*-purine-2,6,8(3*H*)-trione.

Uronic acid: Aldose whose end carbon forms carboxylic acid.

V

V_{max}: Highest reaction rate for an enzyme-catalyzed reaction, occurring when the enzyme is saturated with substrate.

Vesicle: A closed lipid bilayer containing an aqueous interior.

Vitamin: Organic compound that is a precursor to a coenzyme.

W

Watson–Crick pairing: Pattern of hydrogen bonding that matches adenine with thymine, and guanine with cytosine, in the double-stranded form of DNA.

Wernicke-Korsakoff syndrome: Moderate thiamine deficiency, leading to memory loss, partial paralysis, and other symptoms.

X

Xanthine: 2,6-Dihydroxypurine.

Xeroderma pigmentosum: Human skin disease caused by a genetic defect in DNA repair.

X-ray crystallography: Analysis of X-ray diffraction patterns by crystalline substances; used to determine atomic structures of compounds.

Z

Zwitterion: Dipolar ion whose opposite charges are spatially separated.

Zymogen: Inactive precursor to an enzyme.

Index

Note: Page numbers followed by *d* indicate discussion questions; those followed by *f* indicate figures; those followed by *t* indicate tables.